NEW REMEDIES:

THEIR

PATHOGENETIC EFFECTS

AND

THERAPEUTICAL APPLICATION

IN

HOMŒOPATHIC PRACTICE.

BY

EDWIN M. HALE, M. D.,

Late Lecturer on Materia Medica and Therapeutics in Hahnemann Medical College;
Author of "Monograph on Gelseminum;" "Abortion and its Homœopathic Treatment;"
Corresponding Secretary of the Western Institute of Homœopathy, etc.

DETROIT, MICHIGAN:

E. A. LODGE, HOMŒOPATHIC PHARMACY, 266 JEFFERSON AVENUE.

HENRY TURNER & Co., 77 Fleet street, E. C., London. HENRY TURNER & Co., Manchester, England.
WM. RADDE, 550 Pearl street. J. T. S. SMITH & SONS, 484 Broadway. C. T HURLBURT, 437 Broome st., N. Y.
F. E. BŒRICKE, 635 Arch street. A. J. TAFEL, Ninth street, below Arch street, Philadelphia.
OTIS CLAPP, Boston. H. C. G. LUYTIES, St. Louis. JOHN B. HALL, Cleveland.
C. S. HALSEY, Chicago. SMITH & WORTHINGTON, Cincinnati.
J. G. BACKOFEN & SON, Pittsburgh. E. B. SPRAGUE, Owego, N. Y.

Detroit:
ADVERTISER AND TRIBUNE STEAM PRINTING ESTABLISHMENT.

TO THE

HOMŒOPATHIC PHYSICIANS

OF

AMERICA

THIS VOLUME IS RESPECTFULLY DEDICATED

BY

THE AUTHOR.

PREFACE.

The object in the preparation of this work has been to furnish the physicians and students of the homœopathic school of medicine, with full and accurate information relative to a class of remedies, mostly indigenous, but few of which have had any place in the published Homœopathic Materia Medica. Some of the provings have been incorporated into the Symptomen Codex (*Phytolacca, Podophyllum and Sanguinaria*), others have been published in the various journals of our School (*Rumex, Cimicifuga, Cornus c., etc.*), but the great majority have never been proven until now, and the only mention of them has been in occasional clinical or empirical suggestions. To the first and second classes I have added many pathogenetic symptoms gleaned from various sources, re-provings, poisonings, etc., and added also all the clinical observations that could be collected from reliable sources. The latter class may be divided into two others; namely; those which have been proven, and those of which we have only empirical data upon which to base clinical use, and suggestive or theoretical deductions.

As we gather experience in the use of these remedies, and institute accurate provings, the necessity for these suggestions and theoretical deductions will be done away. Each physician should consider himself bound to collect all the symptoms which are really pathogenetic, and note down all reliable curative experience belonging to these medicines, and faithfully report the same to our journals.

The causes which led me to investigate the properties and virtues of the remedies mentioned in the following pages, will be patent to every progressive mind. After using for many years those invaluable remedies found in our standard Materia Medica, most of which were handed down to us by Hahnemann and his colleagues, I found that although their curative scope was very wide, it did not apparently include many symptoms and diseases. I was led to investigate the field of indigenous remedies for these reasons: (1) the suggestion of

Teste,* that plants are adapted to cure the diseases which infest the same localities: and (2) the many cures which had come under my observation, made by these remedies in the hands of eclectic and domestic practitioners (some of the cases will be mentioned in the body of this work). These reasons, together with a natural ambition to enlarge the sphere of homœopathic Materia Medica, induced me to throw away all prejudice, and devote my energies to the task of introducing, by *provings* and clinical experience, the indigenous medicines which so largely abound in the United States. A few others had started before me, and Cimicifuga, Cornus, Podophyllum, and Sanguinaria had been proven, and their pathogeneses published. But from some cause they have not attracted the attention which they deserve. After several years spent in the investigation and study of the new remedies, publishing from time to time items from my experience with them, I was induced to attempt the work of collecting all that had been published concerning the indigenous plants of this country, and to add to such all the knowledge, clinical and theoretical, which could be gleaned from my colleagues, together with my own.

To this I have taken the liberty of adding the testimony and empirical experience of physicians of the allopathic and eclectic schools, relative to the medicines under consideration. If any object to this method, I would refer them to the writings of Hahnemann and his colleagues,—Dudgeon, Madden and Drysdale, of England; Teste and Roth, of France; and Joslin, Marcy, Hempel, and others of this country. I contend that the experience of others, besides members of the Homœopathic school, is often useful in building our pathogeneses, and adding to reliable clinical knowledge.

I shall not be held responsible for the opinions of any writer quoted in the following pages. Let each be judged upon his own merits. I do not claim that this work is in any way *complete*. Indeed, I shall be satisfied if it is only pronounced by the profession as eminently *suggestive*. Many of the provings are very imperfect, and some of the Clinical remarks, open to criticism. Let the wheat be separated from the chaff by the inexorable test of honest trial.

---

* "Introduction of Materia Medica."

INTRODUCTION.

He who undertakes to write a Materia Medica which shall come up to the high standard necessary to meet the scientific requirements of the Homœopathic School of Medicine, has before him a really herculean task. The work even of expunging *worthless symptoms*, will compare with the cleansing of the Augean Stables.

The Allopathic Materia Medica, is not susceptible of much improvement, so long as that school adheres to the dogmas which form the basis of that system of practice; the Homœopathic, on the contrary, is capable of immense improvement.

I have found that the task of writing a monograph on any one drug, as Gelseminum, was really a laborious undertaking; and the work of collecting, compiling and arranging the material for the elucidation of *several* drugs, is, of course, proportionately greater.

That the profession may see how high an appreciation I have for a scientific Materia Medica, and how much this work has fallen short of my ideal, both in the matter, and the manner of its composition, I will insert an extract from my introductory to a course of lectures, delivered to the class of Hahnemann Medical College, in the winter of 1863 and '64:

"Since the time of Hahnemann, nearly all our works on Materia Medica, have been moulded upon the same plan, notwithstanding the progress of all the sciences which properly pertain to medicine; and while a knowledge of chemistry, pathology, and physiology is deemed essential to every homœopathic physician.

"The great desideratum of our school at this time is a purely scientific Materia Medica. Hahnemann laid the foundation upon the imperishable rock of natural truth. Let us build upon it a magnificent temple, which time nor change can ruin, but will ever increase its grand proportions and massive solidity.

" *Gentlemen:*—Would you have my individual conception of an '*Ideal Materia Medica*' With a few preliminary remarks on the action of medicines, I will give it you. All drugs, and by this I mean all substances which can by any possibility be used as remedial agents, have three modes of action upon the animal economy.

" FIRST—*Mechanically.*—This action is only by virtue of their physical conformation. This includes bulk, and the shape of the particles which compose the medicine.

" SECOND—*Chemically.*—The chemical action of nearly all medicines, when given in appreciable doses, is fully admitted by every authority; thus, we have acids, and alkalies, and numerous compounds, which, by their chemical union with the solids and fluids, effect changes in the constituents of the body.

" THIRD—*Dynamically.*—This method of action may be entirely independent of the two former. But a medicine may have at the same time a mechanical, chemical, and a dynamic action; or if properly administered, it may have only the latter action. It was a knowledge of this dynamic action that Hahnemann strove to attain. This he attempted to do by stripping his remedial agents of all material forms, or chemical power, and so diluting them as to leave nothing but the 'spirit' of the drug wherewith to oppose disease.

" Now, it is an indisputable fact, which I shall point out to you more fully in my course of lectures, that our Materia Medica abounds with symptoms due to the mechanical and chemical effects of drugs, and these are so mixed up with the symptoms having a dynamic origin, that they mislead us when we are engaged in the selection of a remedy. Upon almost every page of our Materia Medica, is to be found, too many of the *natural* sensations to which every person is liable.

" In view of these facts, I would have a rational revision of our Materia Medica, expunging all but undoubted dynamic symptoms; and I would have these symptoms arranged in natural groups, in strict accordance with their rise and progress.

"In order to elucidate more clearly my views in relation to drug proving, we will suppose that a society is formed, by a number of patient, conscientious, and self-sacrificing men, whose object is to make a perfect and complete proving of a drug or number of drugs.

We will suppose that the drug selected be *Phosphorus*—that most excellent of all polychrests, The first desideratum would be to ascertain the exact physiological and pathological condition of each person who intends to experiment upon his own person. We should ascertain if every organ performs its functions properly; whether any organic disease be present, and if so, what is its character. We should inquire into the nature of all the secretions and excretions, aiding our investigations by the use of the microscope, and those delicate tests which science has applied to such uses. If the prover is in perfect health, the fact should be noted; if not, his condition and symptoms should be carefully recorded.

"The drug selected should then be taken by each one, in similar quantities, and at the same time. The quantity of the drug should be just enough to induce symptoms and pathological changes in the organism, by its dynamic influence, and not by any chemical action. It would be next to impossible to administer Phosphorus in sufficient quantities to set up any mechanical action; but with such drugs as Mercury, Stannum or Podophyllum, such effects might readily be obtained.

"The chemical action of Phosphorus upon the surfaces with which it comes in contact, would be the most important to be guarded against. It is doubtful if inflammation of the stomach could be produced by minute quantities of this drug; but we know that material doses will cause gastritis, by its actual combustion while in contact with the mucous coats of the stomach. Such chemical symptoms would be worthless to us, when obtained. Only the specific, dynamic affects of a medicine are of value in a strictly therapeutic point of view.

"Immediately after the ingestion of the drug, the first symptoms should be watched for and carefully noted; then all the unmistakable drug-symptoms which arise, should be recorded in the natural order in which they appear. The objective and subjective symptoms should be considered of equal importance. It matters not how minutely the subjective symptoms, the aches, pains, and sensations be recorded, but we insist that all the objective phenomena, should have an equally conspicuous place. Hahnemann himself once insisted upon this very proposition, for in speaking of *Belladonna* particularly, he says:—'We want to know what organs it deranges functionally, what it modifies in other ways, what nerves it principally benumbs or excites, what alterations it effects in the circulation and in the digestive operations, how it affects the mind, how the disposition, what influence it exerts over secretions, what modifications the muscular fibre receives from it, how long its action lasts, and by what means it is rendered powerless.'

"Now, the investigation of the properties of a medicine in this way would leave nothing to be desired. Could Hahnemann have availed himself of the labors of a Brown, a Sequard, a Lehmann, or Rokitansky, what a complete Materia Medica he could have written. But this requirement was far beyond what his times afforded, and he did the best that was possible under the circumstances.

"Dr. Dudgeon asks: 'Ought we not to strive to attain the theoretical standard proposed by Hahnemann? And how is this to be obtained?' I answer, by a more scientific character to our Materia Medica; by treating our pathogenetic provings in a thoroughly physiological manner; by bringing to bear on the action of medicines, the aids and appliances of the microscope, chemical analysis, and the ascertained principles (*not* the theoretical surmises) of modern physiology. This is now being done by some members of our school; and if we were all animated by the same noble zeal, we should soon rescue the school from the reproach of its unscientific character, which is so continually urged against it by adherents of so-called rational medicine.

"When we shall have recorded all the subjective and

objective symptoms in the manner above stated, we shall have what we will term a true *physiological* proving. But we must consider that it would endanger the life of any individual, to carry our experiments so far as to get all the objective phenomena desirable. What shall we do to perfect our pathogeneses? I answer, by subjecting to the slow action of drugs, some of the lowest animals, after the manner of some of the greatest physiologists of the age. Already have Curie in France, and some members of our profession in this country, begun the laudable work. Such experiments I would term *pathological provings*. By such investigations we could learn the ultimate effects of drugs; what structural changes they cause in the tissues, and what extreme organico-pathological conditions they can induce. The experiments of the physiologists of the allopathic school were crude and unsatisfactory. They destroyed life with huge mechanical or chemical doses of drugs, and the results are of little value to our school. Our aim should be, not only to cause death, but to cause *disease*, of longer or shorter duration, and then by a careful scientific analysis of the artificial malady, classify it, and determine its character, in order that we may use it as a guide in the selection of a remedy wherewith to combat a similar, and ascertained disease, existing in the human body.

"Do not deem these views utopian in their character! Much more than is here advised will yet be attained, and some of you will live to see the day when just such provings shall be made. Aye, more! Some of you may live to look upon the realization of a dream which has haunted me for years—an *Inconographic Materia Medica*. Let me illustrate. Going back to our first proposition of a proving of Phosphorus, we will suppose all the subjective and objective symptoms recorded in strictly scientific language, but in addition to this written pathogenesis we have correct drawings of all the pathological changes; of all the organic alterations in various organs and tissues, upon which the drug exerted its poisonous influence. Let us call to our aid the photographer and the painter, and invest the delineations of morbid specimens, with all the wonderful similitude which those arts are capable of creating.

"With such an illustrated Materia Medica would not the Art of Healing be so far perfected as to leave little to be desired, and so enhance our skill in the management of disease as to rob it of half its terrors?

"We will now suppose such a Materia Medica attainable, we will also suppose the existence of works on Diagnosis and Pathology, similarly illustrated, or, that all are combined in one complete work, in beautiful and massive volumes. What then would be the status of the practice of medicine?

We will imagine the young physician just returned from his visit to a child, ill with malignant scarlatina. He turns to his library and finds written down the subjective symptoms of similar cases; and he also finds a written description of the objective symptoms, the latter illustrated with colored plates, the whole giving a striking portrait of the case he has just visited.

"He now turns to his Iconographic Materia Medica, and finds, it may be, in the pathogenesis of Belladonna or Apis, all the subjective symptoms of the case; and more satisfactory still, he finds that the objective symptoms correspond, and the conditions of the skin, the throat and the mucous surfaces, are in every way similar to the case under investigation.

"What, I ask, would be the result of this method of study? What the consequence of this correspondence between the malady, the illustrated pathology and pathogenesis of a drug in the materia medica?

"Would it not be the selection of a remedy whose action would be eminently specific to the totality of the symptoms, and therefore *curative?* Would it not elevate medicine to the position of one of the *exact* sciences? Would it not strip disease of half its terror, and much of its fatality?"

* * * * *

In the British Journal of Homœopathy, number 87, will be found a Review of Coe's "Concentrated Medicines," in which the writer, Dr. Stokes, seems to have the idea that the book belonged to the literature of the homœopathic school, at least one easily gets such an impression from some remarks the writer makes, relative to certain opinions and assertions put forth by Dr. Coe. I cannot account for the stupidity which could entertain such an idea. Dr. Coe is a sort of mongrel, half allopath, half eclectic, and quite an enthusiast in regard to indigenous remedies. When Keith & Co. established their manufactory of concentrated medicines in New York city, Dr. Coe was selected by them as a proper man to set forth the merits of indigenous remedies in general, and their preparations in particular. Consequently, Dr. Coe's work abounds in extravagant assertions and unreliable opinions. I consider Keith's medicines generally unfit for use in homœopathy. Their concentrated powders do not come up to the required standard of chemical purity. Tinctures are to be preferred. In the provings, more symptoms were elicited from tinctures than from the resinoids of the same plant. The tinctures should be carefully prepared from the fresh plants. Tinctures of the allopathic pharmaceutists, made from old dried herbs, etc., are, for homœopathic uses, always unreliable and unsatisfactory.

NOTE.—It will be noticed that after the few first pages of this work, the word "female" is not used, but the term "woman" is substituted. This was not done without considerable deliberation, and from the best of motives. This alteration was suggested to me by the talented authoress, Mrs. Sarah J. Hale. While on a visit to Philadelphia, in June, 1864, I visited my gifted relative, and in the course of a conversation, I happened to use the term "female" as applied to *woman.* Mrs. Hale called my attention to the impropriety of this mode of expression. Is it not a little strange, that men of education, scholars, divines, and others, should have overlooked this matter so long? Yet, writers and speakers have used the term "female" instead of "woman," for the last several centuries, and the thought of its impropriety never occurred to them; or if it did, they failed to mention it. To Mrs. Hale, is due the honor of arresting the improper use of "female," as a synonym for "woman." In the "Lady's Book," for July, 1856, will be found her able and incontrovertible arguments against the practice. I will state a few, enough to convince any person of their importance: 1st.—"The word "female" is only used twelve times in the Bible, and in contra-distinction to man, as male, while the word "woman" is used over thirteen hundred times, and in each case as designating the human feminine. Any one will immediately recognize the impropriety of using the term "female," if he substitutes it, in any of the latter instances, thus: "*Man* that is born of a *female,* &c." A *female* what—Dog, Horse, or Sheep? How absurdly it sounds! This brings us to the 2nd.—"The term "female," does not imply anything pertaining to a *woman,*—it cannot be construed to mean a *lady,*—it does not even imply anything *feminine,* for feminine means—literally—pertaining to woman. The word *female,* then, should never be used except in contra-distinction to man *as a male.* Its appropriate place is to designate the *sex of an animal.* To use this term in any other way, is to degrade woman. "The poets are the best expounders of language, because they must use the most appropriate words in their truest sense, which is their noblest signification, in order to exalt, beautify, and perfect their themes of song." If we take a few examples, changing the style in regard to woman, to the vulgar word of "female," the following will be the result:

"For none of *female* born shall harm Macbeth."—*Shakspeare.*

"O! *female* in our bowers of ease."—*Milton.*

The intense absurdity is at once apparent.

LIST OF MEDICINES TREATED OF IN THIS WORK.

DIRECTIONS TO PHARMACEUTISTS.

ALL the medicines treated of in this book can be prepared in TINCTURE, and this form is generally preferable.

Æsculus Glabra, Æsculus Hippocastanum, and Arum Triphyllum, are also frequently required in form of TRITURATION. Triturations are also made of the Resinoids *Aletrin, Asclepedin, Baptisin, Caulophyllin, Cornin, Cypripedin, Dioscorein, Eupatorin, Eupurpurin, Gelseminin, Hydrastin, Irisin, Phytolaccin, Sanguinarin, Senecionin, Trillin, and Xanthoxylin.*

Some have prepared tinctures of the *resinoids,* such as Aletrin, Baptisin, Caulophyllin, etc., etc., but these are very unreliable preparations. They will never produce all the symptoms upon the healthy, that the tinctures made directly from the fresh plants will develop, and are consequently not as potent for the cure of disease. The tinctures should be prepared from fresh plants, gathered during their time of flowering, soon after the dew has dried off and when they are free from dust. They should be collected where indigenous, and should not be made from cultivated plants.

We make use of—

ROOTS. Aletris, Apocynum a., Apocynum c., Arum t., Asclepias s., Asclepias t., Caulophyllum, Cimicifuga, Collinsonia, Cypripedium, Dioscorea, Erigeron can., Eryngium, Euphorbia c., Eupatorium aromat., Eupatorium purp., Gelseminum, Gossipium, Helonias, Hydrastis c., Iris v., Leptandria, Nuphar l., Phytolacca, Podophyllum, Rumex c., Sanguinaria, Silphium, Trillium p., Veratrum viride.

WHOLE PLANTS. Baptisia, Chimaphila u., Eupatorium perf., Polygonum hyd., Sarracenia, Scutellaria l., Senecio g., Sticta p.

NUTS. Æsculus glabra, Æsculus hyppocastanum.

BARKS. Cornus c., Cornus f., Hamamelis v., Xanthoxylum f.

ÆSCULUS GLABRA (OHIOENSIS).

(*Buckeye.*)

THIS tree is so well known, that it does not need description. It grows on the banks of streams, in rich alluvial soils. The *fruit* contains its most active poisonous principles, although the leaves, bark, and roots possess active toxical powers.

It is often eaten by domestic animals; cattle, in particular, are apt to partake freely of the fruit. In my boyhood, I have seen a great many cows fall victims to their careless imprudence in diet. Even when a student of medicine, I have witnessed deaths in cattle from its effects; and it is a matter of sincere regret, now, that I did not make a careful *post mortem* examination of the animals. The general symptoms exhibited in cases of poisoning in animals may be summed up as follows:

1. Distention of the stomach and abdomen; staggering; reeling; apparent loss of sight; constipation.
2. Falling; paralysis of the hinder extremities; "Palsy; wry neck; convulsions; fixed eyes, and death."

There have been cases of poisoning in men and children, who ate of this fruit, but I have not been able to obtain any account of the symptoms exhibited. Two of my pupils once attempted to prove the Buckeye, but did not continue the experiments, on account of the apparent gravity of the few symptoms which manifested themselves.

It caused—

1. Vertigo, severe, with reeling like drunken men; vertigo with *nausea;* vertigo with dimness of sight; fullness and heaviness of the head; confusion of ideas; a confused stupor; "thickness" of speech; loathing of food; nausea; cramp in the stomach; sensation of fullness of the stomach.
2. Great weakness; trembling of the lower limbs; a strong tendency to contractions of the legs; constipation.

It seems to stand in relation both to Opium and Nux vomica,—possessing some of the narcotic properties of the former, and the cerebro-spinal affinities of the latter. It may be called a *cerebro-spinal irritant.*

The fruit is used to *stupefy* fish, by the Indians—a decoction of the nut is thrown into the water.

3

Dr. McDowell, who tested the properties of the *rind* of the fruit, says, "*Ten* grains of it are equivalent to three grains of Opium."

The following theoretical and clinical remarks are all that we have to offer in relation to this medicine :

1. It should prove curative in some forms of vertigo, congestion or gastric cephalalgia, dyspepsia, nausea, vomiting and constipation.

2. In some severe brain affections the symptom "wry neck" in animals is quite suggestive. Wry neck is not always a rheumatic affection. It may arise from irritation at the base of the brain, or in the cervical region of the cord. It is a symptom of *tubercular* meningitis, apoplexy, meningitis, and many other brain diseases. When this symptom occurs, during these affections, the Æsculus glabra will be indicated.

It will probably prove useful in paralysis of the lower extremities, when Nux vomica fails to cure.

It has been used in the treatment of some typhoid symptoms.

But its principal use up to this time has been in hemorrhoidal affections. It is a popular belief with many of the country people in Ohio, that the fruit of the Buckeye, carried in the pocket, or worn as an amulet, will act as a prophylactic and curative remedy against the piles.

Dr. Hill (Surgery, p. 371,) says, "A number of cures have been reported to us, effected by the use of the Buckeye, taken in repeated small doses."

Dr. J. S. Douglas considers it quite specific in some severe hemorrhoidal diseases.

I have prescribed it in constipation and piles, and in some instances got good effects from its use; in other cases it did not seem to cause any curative action. I gave the 1-10th and 1-100th dilution.

ÆSCULUS HIPPOCASTANUM.*

(*Horse-Chestnut.*)

BY H. M. PAINE, M. D.

History.—The horse-chestnut is a highly ornamental tree, and is greatly admired for its majestic proportions, and for the beauty of its flowers and foliage. It grows rapidly, and often attains the height of forty or fifty feet. It is a native of middle Asia, but flourishes well in the temperate climates of both hemispheres. Its genus comprises about twelve known species, the genus *æsculus*, however,

* Although the Æsculus hippocastanum is not indigenous to this country, yet, as it has been naturalized, and proven by American physicians, I have thought best to include it in this work. It is a near analogue of the Æsculus glabra, and will doubtless prove a valuable remedy.

is incomparably the finest, and is the only one found in the Northern States, and this even is not indigenous in New England.

It was introduced into Europe nearly three centuries ago by Baron Ungnad, ambassador of the Ottoman Porte, who, in the year 1576, sent the seeds of the common horse-chestnut to Clausius, at Vienna. It is now extensively cultivated as an ornamental tree in Europe as well as in this country.

The name æsculus was originally applied to a species of oak, also to a tree which bore esculent fruit, and probably is derived from esca—"food." It was transferred to this genus by Linnæus to the exclusion of the earlier and more appropriate name of "hippocastanum" (*horse-chestnut*), on account of the resemblance of the large seeds to chestnuts, and because the Turks often grind them into a coarse flour, which is mixed with other food, and given to horses which are broken-winded.

In the Southern and Western States there are several species, which bear the name of buckeye, from a resemblance of the seeds to the eye of that animal.

Botanical Description.—In the language of flowers this tree symbolizes luxury.

The beauty of the horse-chestnut consists chiefly in its inflorescence—surpassing that of almost all our native trees; the huge clusters of gay blossoms, which every spring are distributed with such luxuriance and profusion over the surface of the foliage, and at the extremity of the branches, give the whole tree the aspect of some monster flower, than of an ordinary tree of the largest size. Early in June this beautiful tree puts forth large pyramidal racemes or thyrses of flowers, of pink and white, mottled with red and yellow—finely contrasting with the dark green of its foliage, which has great grandeur and richness in its depth of hue and massiveness of outline.

Order.—Hippocastanacæ (sapindaceæ, *Gray*,) ; *genus*, æsculus; *species*, hippocastanum. *Leaves* opposite, digitate, of seven obovate-cunate, acute, toothed leaflets, serrate and straight-veined. *Flowers* showy, in large terminal thyrsoid racemes or panicles; pedicels articulated. *Calyx* campanulate of five united sepals. *Corolla* spreading white, spotted with purple and yellow, and composed of four or five petals, which are irregular, unguiculate, and nearly hypogynous. *Stamens* usually seven, unequal, inserted on the hypogynous disc. *Ovary* large, round, echinate when young, dehiscent, loculicidal, three cornered, three celled, crowned with a single filiform, conical style, containing two ovules in each cell, only one of all of which, sometimes two or even three matures. These seeds are very large, shining, roundish, coriaceous, mahogany-colored, with a broad, round, pale hilum, without albumen.

The Æsculus Ohioensis (*Ohio buck-eye*) differs from the æsculus hippocastanum in having *five* leaflets—stamens red, curved, much longer than the corolla, which consists of *four* upright yellow petals. Fruit prickly when young, but *smooth* at maturity, about half the size of the hippocastanum. This tree is small in size, and exhales an unpleasant odor, particularly while in flower.

Medicinal Properties.—The timber is not valuable. The large farinaceous seeds contain a considerable amount of nourishment, which is rendered unavailable, because of the intensely bitter and narcotic principle with which they are charged. Common horse-chestnuts, nevertheless, with some precautions, are largely and advantageously used in Switzerland for fattening sheep. They are also eaten eagerly by deer, horses and oxen. Starch prepared from them, is superior to that of wheat, and excels as an article of diet, that of the potato. Paste prepared from them is preferable to any other, not only because possessing great tenacity, but also from the fact, that no moths or vermin will attack anything cemented with it. They have been recommended as a substitute for coffee. They contain sparingly a saponaceous principle.

The young leaves are aromatic, and have been used instead of hops in brewing beer.

The roots contain a mucilaginous and saponaceous matter, which is thought to be poisonous. Active and poisonous properties prevail in the root, seeds, bark and foliage.

The bark has little odor, but an astringent and bitter, though not disagreeable taste. It contains, among other ingredients, bitter extractive and tannin, and imparts its virtues to boiling water. Its active constituent is supposed to be tannin, hence it has been employed in tanning. It is recommended as a tonic, astringent, narcotic, and antiseptic; in fevers as a febrifuge, for gangrene, and as an errhine. A strong decoction is recommended as a lotion to gangrenous ulcers.

It has attracted much attention in Europe, as a substitute for Cinchona, although it certainly cannot be considered comparable to Peruvian Bark in its power over intermittents. It is at present seldom used, and never in this country. The bark of the branches from three to five years old is considered the best. It should be collected in spring.

The powdered kernel snuffed up the nostrils produces sneezing, and has been used with advantage as a sternutatory in complaints of the head and eyes. In Europe the oil at present is a fashionable remedy for gout and rheumatism. Maceration in an alkaline solution removes the bitter principle. Æsculine is the name given to the extractive matter.

Hahnemann thus speaks of it: "We can, from the morbid effects which the bark is able to produce, form a just estimate of its medicinal powers, and determine whether it is suitable for pure intermittent fever, or some of its varieties. The sole phenomenon we know belonging to it is, that it produces a constrictive feeling in the chest. It will accordingly be found useful in (periodical) spasmodic asthma."

Digest of Symptoms.—The following digest of the symptoms have been arranged from provings made by Dr. Woodward Warren, and by Dr. O. A. Buchmann, upon himself and six other persons—four females and three males, all in middle life:

In each instance the mother tincture or crude drug was employed, in doses of from five drops to twenty grains.

Dr. Buchmann introduces the provings in the following words: "Horse-chestnuts have been occasionally used as a popular remedy, and the favorable results heard from their use in glandular swellings of horses, in chronic catarrhs of the respiratory passages and of the intestinal canal, determined me to undertake a careful proving of them on the healthy, in order to ascertain if their vaunted curative powers were on the homœopathic principle."*

Symptoms.—Compiled from eighteen provings, by eight persons. The figures represent the number of times the preceding symptom was mentioned by the provers.

General Symptoms.—Feeling of extreme illness. Great weakness. Totters when walking (2). Weariness (3). Fatigued feeling, as from a long walk. Sensation as if she would faint. General feeling of malaise.

Duration of action, from two to six hours.

Sleep.—Inclination to sleep. Yawning and stupefying sleepiness. Constant yawning (2). Falls asleep when sitting. Sleep for a quarter of an hour. Slept well.

Fever.—Chilliness and goose-skin. Attack of rigor, lasting ten minutes. Cannot get warm. Rigor for half an hour. Rigors. General perspiration. Heat in the whole body.

Sensorium.—On waking cannot recognize what she sees; knows not where she is; nor whence come the objects about her (2). Inward cheerfulness and placidity of temper.

Head.—Feeling as if a board were on the head. Aching in the forehead. Feeling as during a cold in the head. Sensation as if intoxicated. Confusion of the head (2). Giddiness. Vertigo, with sensation of balancing in the head. Formication in the front of the temple. Heaviness in the head. Heat in the head and eyes. Headache over the left eye (2). Headache over the right eye. Dull pains in the head, here and there, chiefly in the right temple and occiput, followed by dull stitches in the forehead and left temple. Dull pressure in the forehead. Throbbing in the right frontal eminence. Fine stitches in the left temple. Dull pain in the left temple. Sharp pressing pain in the right temple. Dull stupefying pain in the head. Dull pain in the occiput (3). Bruised feeling in the occiput. Heat in the integuments of the occiput (3). Heat extending from the occiput to the ears (2).

Eyes.—Burning in the internal canthi. Burning and stinging deep in the left orbit, as if the pain surrounded the eye-ball. Weight and heat in the eyes. Coldness in the left eye. Jerking in the right eye. Quivering of the lids. Lachrymation (2). Flickering before the eyes (2). Can see well at a distance; can read without spectacles, which she could not do before.

Ears.—Burning of the ears. Heat in the occiput, extending to the ears.

Nose.—Severe fluent coryza (8). Burning in the nostril. Raw

* See *British Journal of Homœopathy*, Vol. XVIII., pages 88—194.

feeling throughout the whole nasal cavity. The nasal mucus becomes watery. Thin mucus from the nose, causing a frequent use of the pocket-handkerchief. Dry feeling and sensation of heat in the nose, especially its point, as when a severe coryza is about to come on. Disposition to sneeze. Feeling as after having taken a pinch of snuff. Formication in the nose (3). Sensitiveness of the nasal mucous membrane to the respired air (3). The respired air causes a feeling of coldness in the nose (2). Drawing in the right nostril, as in violent coryza. Twisting sensation in the front part of the nose. Shooting pain in the head.

Face—Looks ill. Pale miserable appearance (2). Flying heat and redness of the left side of the face (2). Burning in the left cheek.

Mouth—The taste was something like that of aloes. Bitter taste (3). Coppery taste, acting as an astringent in the mouth and œsophagus; at first bitter, then sweet. Sweetish taste (6), as after taking Dulcamara—like liquorice. Burning in the mouth (3). Biting and stinging at the tip of the tongue. Increased flow of saliva (9), producing an inclination to swallow.

Throat.—Contractive pain in the throat (2). Sort of constricted scraped sensation, causing a disposition to hawk. Irritation in the throat and œsophagus. All the throat was excoriated and constricted. Dryness and contraction of the throat. Dryness in the throat. Burning in the throat (12), like fire, when swallowing; at one time slight, then severe; with raw feeling. Constant shooting and raw pain in the throat. Scraping sensation in the throat. The mucus in the throat becomes thinner. Hawking of thick (2), afterwards watery mucus. Frequent call to expectorate mucus, which becomes watery. The mucus in the throat excites a cough. Tickling in the throat (2), causing a cough. Inclination to swallow. Formication in the fauces. Dull pressing and pricking in the fauces. Biting and stinging pain in the fauces. Stinging and burning in the soft palate and posterior nares. Increased pain in the throat, after eating a grape.

Stomach.—Nausea (15). Retching (2). Inclination to vomit. Violent vomiting. Burning in the stomach (4). Heart-burn for half an hour. Water-brash. Eructations of wind (16); of mucus; of thick mucus; of viscid mucus (3); empty eructations. Flying heat before the eructation. Fullness of the stomach (3). Periodical tightness in the scrobiculus cordis, with labored breathing. Twisting in the scrobicults cordis. Aching and rumbling in the stomach. Cutting stomach-ache. The aching in the stomach extends. Comfortable feeling in the stomach. Hunger.

Abdomen.—Constricted feeling in the bowels. Cramp-like constriction in the bowels, followed by stool (the fourth time). Griping in the bowels (2). Cramps in the bowels. Motions, preceded by pain in the bowels. Pinching below the navel. Fine pricking pains around the umbilicus. Pain from the bowels to the small of the back. Burning in the bowels. Pressing downwards in the abdomen. Rumbling in the bowels, half an hour, without pain. Distention of the abdomen. Pain in the hypochondria, through to the back, especially on inspiration. Tearing pain in the *right* side, above the hip, deeply seated. Colic, with pinching pains in the *right* hypochondrium. Stitches in the *right* hypochondrium. Stitches in the *left* side. Fine stitching in the *left* hypochondrium. Cutting in the *left* inguinal region. Rumbling in the hypogastrium.

Stools.—Eructations of wind, with desire to go to stool. Three moderate fœcal evacuations half an hour after taking the drug. Four loose evacuations within a quarter of an hour. In two hours several thin evacuations. In two hours after taking the drug, two moderate evacuations. Constant urging to stool, after two hours. Pressure in the rectum, with desire to go to stool. Ineffectual efforts to stool. Difficult scanty stool. Difficult hard stool, followed by burning and constriction in the rectum. Constriction in the rectum (2). Itching in the anus (2); with raw feeling. Stool of a mixed character. Two liquid motions, preceded by griping. Motions preceded by pinching in the bowels. Frequent expulsion of flatus (2.) The usual stool did not take place (2).

Urine.—Shoots in the orifice of the urethra. Call to urinate. On two occasions, at short intervals, urging to urinate.

Genital Organs.—Leucorrhœa. Burning in the mammæ.

Larynx.—Hoarse voice; speaking brings on a cough. Short cough, increased by swallowing and breathing deeply. The mucus in the throat excites a cough (2). Tickling in the larynx, causing a cough with mucus expectoration. Cough from irritation. Dry cough. Repeated cough. Dryness in the larynx. Frequent call to expectorate mucus, which becomes watery. Pressure in the throat-pit, as if something had stuck there which required to be expelled.

Lungs.—Hot feeling in the chest, with cold rising up (2). Burning and heat in the chest. Raw feeling in the throat and chest (2). Warm feeling in the chest. Shooting pain in the sternum. Pains in the sternum, as if a piece were torn out of the chest. Sudden stitches throughout the chest. Pains in the right scapula, and in the left side of the chest, increased on inspiration. Rheumatic pain in the right scapula. On the right side of the chest a sensation as if the lung painfully moved up and down at each respiration (2). Increase of the pain on drawing a deep inspiration. Pain in the chest, alternating with pain in the abdomen. Stitches leave the left side of the chest and go to the right. Twitching from the chest to the left shoulder. Tightness in the chest (6). Labored breathing (2). Palpitation of the heart (4); severe, periodic, frequent, with great anguish.

Upper Extremities.—The arm and hand of the left side become strikingly warmer, and feel as if they were heavier and swollen. Heat in the shoulders. Burning in the palms of the hands and soles of the feet. Constant jerking in the right arm. Paralysis of the right arm—cannot raise it.

Back.—Pains in the small of the back, and lame feeling. Pain extending from the abdomen to the small of the back (2). Weariness in the small of the back. Tearing pain in the back. Lameness and sensation at if strained in the right lumbar region, extending to the gluteal muscles. Heat in the back of the neck and shoulders. Weariness in the back of the neck. Lameness in the back of the neck (2).

SUMMARY.

General Symptoms.—Weariness, faintness.

Sleep.—Sleepiness.

Fever.—Rigors; chills.

Head.—Confused, dull, aching pain, as if from a cold.

Eyes.—Burning heat, as if from a cold.

Nose.—*Severe fluent coryza.*

Mouth.—*Increased flow of saliva.*

Throat.—*Burning; raw; stinging; dryness.*

Stomach.—*Eructations; nausea.*

Stools.—*Diarrhœa; burning, constriction, pressure, tenesmus, and itching in the rectum,* indicate the utility of this drug in *hœmorrhoids.*

Larynx.—*Laryngitis?*

Lungs.—*Bronchitis? Asthma? Palpitation?*

Back.—*Pains and lameness in the small of the back.*

These symptoms indicate a wide range of influence. They exhibit decided action upon the mucous surface of the air-passages, upon the stomach, bowels, and rectum.

The chills and rigors, stupifying sleep, confusion and dullness of the head, congestion of the liver and spleen, palpitation and impeded respiration, indicate an accumulation of blood in the central parts of the organism.

The burning in the eyes, fluent coryza, water in the mouth, burning in the throat, nausea and eructations, the evident bronchitis, and hemorrhoidal disturbance, indicate congestion of the capillary vessels, chiefly, we believe, *venous* congestion.

Dr. Buchmann thus concludes his article: "I trust these provings may induce others to institute more provings, and to test the therapeutic action of this drug. I may merely add, that I have succeeded in curing radically a *chronic cough* with emaciation—which had long been treated without effect—by daily administration of as much powdered chestnut as would lie on the point of a knife; and that I have heard from persons on whom I could rely, of the rapid cure of a *chronic diarrhœa*, in which many remedies have been used in vain, by a single dose of powdered horse-chestnut."

Let these abundant evidences of its usefulness become an incentive to renewed diligence in developing and perfecting the pathogenesis of this important remedy.

It is usually prepared by grating the nut, after removing the shell. When dry it can easily be reduced to a fine powder. Triturations are made as of any other homœopathic remedy. [It is also prepared in the form of tincture.—Ed.]

PROVINGS.

PROVING BY C. W. BOYCE, M. D., OF AUBURN, N. Y.

Read before the Oneida County Hom. Med. Society.

August 24. Took ten grains of the first decimal trituration at 9 A. M. Nausea immediately. Constant desire to swallow, with feeling of dryness and stiffness of the throat when swallowing.

August 28. At 11 A. M., took ten grains of the same preparation. Nausea immediately. Constant nausea. Feeling of dryness and roughness of the throat, as if from taking cold.

At 5 P. M., took ten grains more. Nausea. For two following days, constant tendency to diarrhœa. Almost constant inclination to stool, but without any, or very slight evacuations.

September 12. At 9 A. M., took ten grains of the same preparation. Nausea immediately. Sick feeling in the stomach all day, with increase of appetite.

At 4 P. M., took ten grains more. Nausea. Salivation. Metallic taste in the mouth. Sensation and dryness of the rectum.

At 8 P. M., took ten grains more. Nausea. The thought of the medicine is unbearable. Dryness of the throat. Dryness and itching in the rectum, with feeling of stiffness of the skin and adjacent cellular tissue, continuing for several days.

September 24. At 3 P. M., took ten grains. Nausea immediately. Diarrhœa for twenty-four hours following.

September 26. At 4 P. M., took ten grains. Nausea immediately. Increase of saliva. The taste of the drug remained in the mouth several hours. Diarrhœa of ingesta. For several days following there was a sensation as if the mucous membrane of the rectum was thickened, obstructing the passage of fæces. Dryness of the passage for several days, followed by a secretion of moisture. Soreness of the rectum, with a feeling as if something would pass off all the time I induced several other persons to make a few trials, but with no result except *increased salivation.*

October 3. At 3 P. M., took ten grains of the first decimal trituration. Nausea immediately, and continuing all the afternoon. Dryness of the throat. Dryness of the rectum.

October 4. At 1 P. M., took ten grains. Nausea. Increase of saliva. Dryness of the larynx, with tickling, scraping feeling of the laryngo-pharyngeal mucous membrane. Sensation of swelling of the nasal mucous membrane, as if from taking cold. Sneezing.

October 5. At 9 A. M., took ten grains. Sensation of dryness and stiffness of the glottis, and all the pharyngo-laryngeal mucous membrane. Slight nausea.

At 2 P. M., took ten grains. Increase of the dry feeling in the throat, followed by secretion of mucous, quite like the second stage of catarrh. Dry uncomfortable feeling in the rectum, which feels as if it were filled with small sticks.

October 6. At 2 P. M., took ten grains. Painful dryness of the throat, lasting six hours. Feeling of prostration of the whole system. Great repugnance to the drug.

October 7. At 10 A. M., took ten grains. Nausea. Increase of the saliva. At 4 P. M., took ten grains. Nausea. Desire for a passage from the bowels without result. Desire to remain at stool a long time, with straining. Excessive dryness of the rectum, with feeling of heat. At 9 P. M., took ten grains. Nausea immediately, with ineffectual attempts to evacuate the bowels. Feeling in the rectum as though folds of the mucous membrane obstructed the passage, and as if, were the effort continued, the rectum would protrude.

October 10. There has been during the past three days soreness in the rectum, with increased secretion of mucus. Frequent inclination for and ineffectual efforts at stool. At 3 P. M., took ten grains. Nausea as soon as the drug was taken. At 8 P. M., took ten grains. Nausea.

October 11. Early in the morning a feeling of emptiness and gnawing in the stomach. At 10 A. M., took ten grains. Nausea. Dryness of the throat after eating. After eating the stomach feels full, as if the walls were greatly thickened. Considerable pain in the stomach for four or five hours after eating, which continues until after taking food again. Dyspepsia. Quite severe pain in the right side of the head above the temple. Metallic taste in the mouth. Increase of secretion from the submaxillary glands. Good appetite. Dryness and soreness of the rectum. At 3 P. M., took ten grains. Soreness of the tip of the tongue, like that produced by ulcers. Thinking of the drug always produces nausea. The dryness of the rectum is followed by increased secretion of mucus.

PROVING BY W. WARREN, M. D., OF DEERFIELD, N. Y.

Read before the Oneida County Homœopathic Medical Society.

Dr. WOODWARD WARREN, aged thirty-six, nervo-bilious temperament, subject to bilious and gastric derangements.

May 22. Took two grains of first decimal trituration at 4 P. M. In half an hour felt a dull, pressing and pricking in the fauces, with a sensation of fullness in the epigastrium, with empty eructations, followed immediately by burning in the stomach and bowels. At 4.45, dull pains in the head, here and there, but principally in the right temple and occiput, followed by dull stitches in the forehead and temple. At 5.30, colic, with pinching pains in the right hypochrondrium ; empty eructations. At 6.30, fine, pricking pains around the umbilicus.

May 29. Took two grains of second decimal trituration at 2 P. M. At 2.25, felt a dull pressure in the forehead, with a slight feeling of nausea in the stomach, followed immediately by stitches in the right hypochondrium. At 2.45, bruised feeling in the occiput, with feeling of lameness in the back of the neck. At 3.30, pressure in the rectum with inclination to stool, with empty eructations. At 4.45, ineffectual efforts to stool. At 8.25, feeling of constriction in the rectum.

May 30. At 6 A. M., difficult scanty stool. At 8 A. M., took three grains of first decimal trituration. In ten minutes coppery taste in the mouth, with increased flow of saliva. At 8.30, dull pain in the occiput, extending to the ears; fine stitches in the left temple, with slight feeling of nausea in the stomach. At 9 o'clock, feeling of lameness and weariness in the back of the neck, and small of the back. At 10 A. M., empty eructations.

May 31. Took two grains of second trituration at 8.30 A. M. At 9, copious soft stool, followed by burning, and a feeling of swelling and constriction in the rectum. At 9.15, empty eructations. At 9.30, slight burning and nausea in the stomach, with increased flow of saliva; fine stitching in the left hypochondrium. At 9.45, confused feeling in the head; giddiness. At 10, dull pain in the occiput, with flushes of heat in the integuments of the occiput, back of the neck, and shoulders. At 11.25, burning in the ears.

June 7. Took five grains of second decimal trituration at 12 A. M. At 12.30, coppery taste, with increased flow of saliva, and a dull, pressing pain in the left hypochondrium. At 12.45, dull pain in the left temple; giddiness and confused feeling in the head; sharp, biting, and stinging pain in the fauces and tip of the tongue. At 1 P. M., rumbling in the hypogastrium, with cutting pains around the umbilicus; burning and stinging deep in the left orbit, as if the pain surrounded the ball of the eye, with a feeling of coldness in the eye. At 1.15, heat in the integuments of the occiput, extending to the ears. At 1.30, cutting in the left inguinal region; slight nausea with empty eructations. At 2.30, general feeling of malaise, with dull, stupefying feeling in the head. At 4 P. M., dull pain in the occiput, and lame feeling in the small of the back.

June 8. At 7 A.M., difficult, hard stool, followed by burning and feeling of constriction in the rectum. At 9 A.M., took three grains of second trituration. At 9.45, stinging and burning in the soft palate and posterior nares; bitter taste, and increased flow of saliva. At 10, vertigo, with sensation of balancing in the head; throbbing in the right frontal eminence. At 10.15, empty eructations, with burning in the stomach, and fine, pricking pains around the umbilicus. At 10.20, sharp, pressing pain in the right temple. At 2 P.M., lameness, and sensation as if strained in the right lumbar region, extending to the gluteal muscle.

PROVING BY H. M. PAINE, M. D., OF CLINTON, N. Y.

Read before the Oneida County Homœopathic Medical Society.

September 28. In usual health. Took ten drops of the pure alcoholic tincture at 10 P. M.

September 29. Took ten drops at 10 P. M.

September 30. Took thirty drops at 10 P. M.

October 1. Headache, general, through the whole head. A sensation of fullness in all the upper part of the head. Vertigo, very annoying all the afternoon. General malaise.

October 2. Experienced a repetition of similar symptoms again to-day. Disappeared after 4 o'clock, P. M. Took forty drops at 9 P. M. Observed a few minutes after a quick, severe, griping pain in the epigastric region. It continued about half an hour.

October 3. Feel miserably, cross, disinclination to perform any labor. Headache in the upper part of the head. The pain is uniform and constant. The sensation is that of fullness and pressure rather than acute pain. Vertigo, quite troublesome. The above symptoms continued till toward evening, and then disappeared. At 10 P. M., took forty drops. Experienced a severe griping pain in the epigastrium a few minutes after taking the drug. It continued until I fell asleep—about half an hour. It extended from the stomach to the umbilical region, and appeared to be produced by flatus, as there was at the same time quite a perceptible sensation of motion in the bowels.

October 4. Few abnormal sensations to-day. No headache. Slight vertigo. Took forty drops at 9 P. M.

October 6. Sore throat, quite troublesome in the forenoon; none in the afternoon. For the first time since commencing the proving had rather a difficult stool. Took forty drops at 9 P. M.

October 7. Slight soreness in the pharynx during the day. Rather a difficult stool about noon, followed for an hour by a slight soreness, aching and fullness in the rectum, indicating piles. Took fifty drops at 9 P. M.

The taste of the drug is at first intensely bitter, and is peculiarly unpleasant and nauseous. The bitter taste is soon displaced by a pleasant, sweetish flavor, very similar to that of ordinary liquorice root. This sweet taste remains about an hour.

Immediately on taking the drug there is a sensation of scraping, irritation, or burning, extending from the mouth to the stomach. It usually passes off in an hour or two. It remains longer in the stomach than in the throat.

Another very unpleasant sensation experienced immediately on taking the drug is nausea. It is transient, recurring at short intervals, and usually disappears in about half an hour.

Clinical Notes I. P.—Have been subject for several years to occasional attacks of hæmorrhoids, attended with little hæmorrhage, although considerable pain, aching, swelling, and rigid hardness of the rectum. The paroxysms usually accompany constipation. The pain commences about an hour after an evacuation, and continues from two to six hours.

About ten grains of the crude nut, finely pulverized, were placed in a half-ounce vial of alcohol and water, in equal parts. Of this ten or twelve drops were taken nearly every evening for about five weeks—commencing August 11, 1860.

The piles were uniformly relieved after three or four doses. Observed on two or three occasions, that when the remedy was discontinued for a few days, the symptoms soon returned. It is now four months since all symptoms of the disease disappeared. No other effects were discovered.

II. R.——Had been suffering severely from hæmorrhoids for ten or twelve days, with a constipated state of the bowels, and severe pain in the tumors—making it very unpleasant to stand on my feet or walk. Also more or less nausea, loss of appetite, furred tongue, a sensation of fullness about the navel, flatulent pains in the bowels, and very dark stools. About two weeks previous to the attack of hæmorrhoids, had a severe attack of bilious colic, which was relieved by Colocynth, Chamomilla, and Mercurius sol.

On the morning of June 13, 1860, took 200 pellets of the sixth centesimal attenuation of Æsculus. The only symptom referable to the drug was irritation of the throat and œsophagus—a sort of constricted, scraped sensation, causing a disposition to hawk. This occurred about an hour after taking the drug, and continued for several hours.

Continued the remedy for several mornings in succession. The piles are entirely relieved; the bowels act regularly; the appetite fair; nausea and flatulence gone; and, in short, enjoy my usual standard of health.

Dr. L. B. Wells, of Utica, has employed this remedy in all cases of hæmorrhoids occurring in his practice during the past two years, and generally with very good results.

Dr. Wm. M. Cuthbert, in N. A. Journal for February, 1864, says: "I proved the drug to a limited extent on my own person, not being subject to piles, using the first potency. The effects produced being *a painful weakness of the loins, with dull, aching pain, accompanied by severe tumors around the anus.* These symptoms becoming so severe as to interfere with professional duties, I was reluctantly compelled to end the proving, and one dose of Nux vomica antidoted in a few hours all the painful symptoms, since which I have experienced none of them."

Cases referred to by Dr. Cuthbert:

1. Man; aged 37; mechanic. One dose of third potency not only entirely relieved the piles, but also enabled him to lay off a truss which he had worn for years for an inguinal hernia.

2. Mrs. M. Piles (protruding at times) of ten years' standing, cured with three doses. It is now three years since, and she has never had any symptoms of it in that time.

3. Mr. B. External piles. Promptly cured with one dose; Nux vomica never having any effect.

4. Mr. L. Blind bleeding piles of twenty years' standing, cured with three doses, one every two weeks.

A cerate has been prepared from the Æsculus, which has been found a very efficacious and convenient external application to pile tumors.

PROVING BY W. H. BURT, M. D.

The following thorough proving by Dr. Burt, of Lyons, Iowa, I present to the profession without any clinical remarks. It speaks for itself. The Æsculus h. seems likely to prove a valuable remedy.—(*Hale*):

March 14th, 1864. At 10 A. M., took 10 grs. of the first dec. trituration of the dried nut; 11 A. M., neuralgic pain in the region of causality (right) darts towards the left, with a constrictive feeling of the skin of the forehead, followed by flying pains in the epigastric region (lower right lobe of the liver); constrictive feeling of the fauces; 12 M., neuralgic pain in the region of the heart lasted one minute, with frequent pains in the epigastric region. Dull, aching pain in the small of the back, very much aggravated by walking; 1 P. M., there has been very frequent neuralgic pains in the region of the apex of the heart and stomach, with a severe, dull, aching pain in the lumbar region; 4 P. M., constant, dull, aching pain in the small of the back, aggravated by motion—took 20 grs.; 5 P. M., slight frontal headache, acrid constrictive feeling in the fauces—there has been frequent sharp pains in the region of the apex of the heart and stomach, constant, quite severe, aching pain from the pit of the stomach to the right lobe of the liver, slight back-ache, knees ache severely; 10 P. M., there has been frequent flying pains in the forehead and temples, feeling as if something had lodged in the fauces that produces a constant inclination to swallow, good deal of distress in the stomach, and flying pains in the bowels, very severe and constant backache, knees ache severely—took 20 grs., no stool.

15th. Called up three times through the night, back ached very hard all night, and is still aching; 7 A. M., took 20 grs.; 12 M., dull frontal headache, fauces feeling very dry and constricted, burning distress in the stomach, frequent eructations of air, very tired and languid, back aches severely; 9 P. M., there has been frequent pains in the umbilical and hypogastric regions all day, but they were not very severe, dull backache; no stool.

16th. Up most of the night with the sick; very hard and dry stool at 7 A. M., followed by colicky pain in the umbilicus, and severe cutting pains in the anus. Took 10 grs. at 9 A. M. 10:30—For the last hour there has been constant burning distress in the epigastric and umbilical regions, with a very severe aching pain in the lumbar region, very painful when trying to walk; occasional neuralgic pains in the forehead and apex of the heart; dry feeling of the fauces with frequent inclination to swallow. 11 A. M., dull frontal headache; severe constrictive feeling of the fauces, with frequent inclination to swallow; constant burning distress, with a constrictive feeling of the lower part of the chest; frequent pains in apex of the heart; constant dull, aching distress in the umbilical region, with a very severe headache; walking is very painful. 12—Pulse 68, soft and weak; dull frontal headache, with fluent coryza; constant burning distress in the stomach; dull, aching pain in the lumbar region; took 40 grs. 3 P. M., slight frontal headache, with great tightness of the skin of the forehead. At 1 P. M. there was great constriction of the fauces, with great irritation of the epiglottis that produced a dry hacking cough; does not trouble me now; there has been constant burning distress in the stomach and bowels, with a severe fluttering sensation in the pit of the stomach, lasting five minutes at a time; came on five different times; empty eructations; frequent dull aching pains in the right hypochondriac region; dull pains in the umbilicus, sometimes they are very sharp; constant dull backache; weariness in the small of the back; tearing pains in the small of the back and hips when walking; weariness with faintness at the pit of the stomach. 5 P. M., dull headache; frequent neuralgic pains in the fauces, with frequent inclination to swallow; constant burning distress in the stomach; severe aching pain in the lumbar region. 9 P. M.—Frequent twitching of the muscles under the left eye; stomach and bowels distress me very much.

17th. Was up all night with my wife who has a violent attack of diphtheria, compelled to stop my proving; feeling very much prostrated; back aching violently; walking is almost impossible; great desire for stool. At 5 A. M., a very hard and dry knotty stool, voided with great difficulty; violent backache all day; almost impossible to get up after sitting down.

18th. Slight backache all day; no stool.

19th. Hard stool, followed by a prolapsed feeling of the anus.

20th. No stool.

21st. Natural stool.

22d. Feeling well; took 20 grs. of the pure pulverized nut at 10:30 A. M. 11 A. M.—Severe smarting of the eyes; tongue feeling as if it had been scalded, with great constriction of the fauces; constant dull pain in the region of the navel. 11:45 A. M.—Severe neuralgic pain in the region of the heart; it is so painful that it arrests the breathing; lasted 10 minutes; dull aching pain in the right hypochondriac region; back commencing to ache severely. 12 M.—Dull frontal headache, with a constricted feeling of the skin of the forehead; great dryness of the fauces, with frequent inclination to swallow; dull burning distress in the stomach; severe neuralgic pain in the right inguinal region; constant backache, affecting the sacrum and hips, very much aggravated by walking and stooping forward; pulse 70. 3 P. M.—Slight frontal headache; great dryness of the fauces; constant and severe burning in the stomach, with a very severe backache in the lumbar region. 6 P. M.—There has been frequent flying pains in the forehead and temples all day; fauces feeling constricted, with frequent dull pains on each side of the tonsils; they look very dark and congested; frequent eructations; constant burning distress in the stomach; frequent and long, lasting, dull pains in the right hypochondriac region; dull backache. 9 P. M.—Great distress in the umbilical and hypogastric regions, and a very urgent desire for stool, with rumbling in the bowels; a very large and hard stool, voided with great difficulty, followed by severe pains in the anus, with a feeling as if a portion of the anus was protruded, accompanied with dull pains in the umbilical and hypogastric regions; this feeling lasted all night and until late in the morning, with a very severe backache in the lower part of the lumbar and sacral regions.

23d. Slept soundly; feeling quite well, excepting a feeling as if a portion of the anus was prolapsed, with a dull backache; flat slimy taste in the mouth. 9 A. M., took 30 grs. 11 A. M.—Frequent flying pains through the temples; profuse secretion of mucus in the nostrils, with coryza. The acridity in the mouth and fauces is very slight; constant and severe burning distress in the stomach, with an inclination to vomit; constant dull, aching pain in the right hypochondriac region, and region of the gall bladder; burning, aching distress in the umbilicus; constant dull pain across the hips and sacrum; sharp pains in the region of the apex of the heart.

3 P. M.—Feeling very depressed and low spirited; constant dull, burning, aching pain in the epigastric and umbilical regions; the greatest pain is in the pyloric portion of the stomach; at 4:30 P. M. took 30 grains. 6 P. M.—Great congestion of the tonsils and soft palate; frequent sharp, neuralgic pains in the region of the heart, with a great burning in the same region; constant and very severe burning in the stomach and bowels; very hard to endure the burning distress; feeling faint and weak; very severe backache, worse by motion. 9 P. M.—Frequent flying pains in the temples; constant dull, burning pain in the pyloric portion of the stomach; constant dull pains in the right hypochondriac region, aggravated by walking; dull pains in the umbilicus; very urgent desire for stool. 7 P. M.—Very hard, dry stool, followed by pain in the anus; frequent stitches in the region of the heart; dull, aching pain in the sacrum.

24th. Slept well, but awoke three times and found I had a dull, burning pain in the stomach; sweet, flat, slimy taste in the mouth; tongue very much coated yellow; fauces congested; constant dull pain in the cardiac portion of the stomach; very severe pain in the small of the back and hips when getting up, not much after moving a minute or so; pulse 76. 10 A. M.—Severe burning distress in the stomach (superior cardiac portion). Took 30 grs. 12 M.; pulse 72; constant burning, aching distress in the epigastric region, with constant dull, aching pains in the right hypochondriac region; constant dull backache; frequent pains in the region of the apex of the heart and between the shoulders. 2 P. M.—Great desire for stool; stool, first part black and hard, the last part about the natural consistence, but almost white as milk, showing that the secretion of bile is almost completely suspended; the stool was followed by severe tearing pains in the anus; constant burning distress in the epigastric region; the small of my back aches so severely that it is almost impossible to stoop down, or to get up when sitting down. 4 P. M., took 40 grs. 6 P. M.—Severe congestion of the tonsils and soft palate, with a constant aching distress in them; constant aching, burning distress in the epigastrium; constant dull, aching distress in the right lower lobe of the liver; the backache is very severe when moving. 9 P. M.—Constant aching distress in the tonsils and fauces, with frequent inclination to swallow; the burning, aching distress in the epigastrium is almost unendurable, it makes me feel very faint and weak; constant dull, aching distress in the right lobe of the liver; great pain in the back and hips when trying to move; legs aching severely, feeling so weak that I must lie down all the time.

25th. Slept soundly; feeling so weak, and my back pains me so much when trying to move, that it is with great difficulty that I can get up; moving produces violent pains in the sacrum and hips; very severe frontal headache; flat, bitter taste in the mouth; tongue coated yellowish white; tonsils and soft palate very much congested, but no enlargement; constant pain in the cardiac portion of the stomach; dull, aching distress in the right liver; urine very high colored; good deal of dull, aching pain between the shoulders. 12 M., have had a very hard frontal headache all day; back and legs have ached so severely that I was compelled to lie down all the forenoon; feeling very feverish, hands hot and dry; pulse 66, soft and weak; disposition to stretch and yawn all the time; feeling as if I had the ague; great deal of distress in the epigastrium and liver. 3 P. M.—Feeling very weary and low-spirited. Took 30 grs. 6 P. M.—Constant distress in the stomach, with frequent pains through the bowels; back pains severely when moving. 9 P. M.—Great desire for stool; stool about natural consistence, followed by a prolapsed feeling of the anus.

26th. Slept soundly; back pains me when first moving, otherwise feeling well. 10 A. M.—Slight pain in the epigastrium; took 60 grs. 11 A. M.—For the last half hour there has been a constant dull, aching, burning pain in the region of the heart; pulse 66, soft and regular; constant aching distress in the tonsils; frequent inclination to swallow; constant pain in the stomach and right lower lobe of the liver; very severe pain in the lumbo-sacral region when stooping; dull, aching distress in the dorsal region; feeling very faint and weak. 5 P. M.—Dull pain in the tonsils, with frequent inclination to swallow; the tonsils are congested of a very dark color; constant dull and very severe aching pain just below the pit of the stomach, which produces a very weak, faint feeling; it is very hard to endure the distress; constant dull, aching distress in the right lobe of the liver, and between the shoulders along the dorsal region; dull pain when moving in the lumbar in the lumbar-sacral region; frequent rumbling in the bowels. 9. P. M.—Stool about natural consistence, but very white, showing a great deficiency of bile; constant dull pain in the liver and back.

27th. Slept well; feeling quite well excepting good deal of pain in the lumbar-sacral region when moving. 7 P. M.—For the last two hours there has been constant very severe pain about and just below the pyloric extremity of the stomach; severe pain in the sacrum and hips when moving; a very dry stool at 9 P. M., voided with difficulty; dull pains in the right lobe of the liver and dorsal region.

28th. Back is feeling very stiff when moving; dull pains in the small of the back and sacral region; constant dull, aching pain in the right hypochondriac region, with frequent pains in the stomach all day, with constant desire for stool; had two soft stools, without giving relief to the desire for stool; feeling very sad.

29th. Slept well; constant dull, aching pain in the right lobe of the liver all day, with frequent pains in the stomach and bowels, and constant desire to stool; stool at noon very black and soft, without relieving the desire for stool.

April 1st. There is still a good deal of pain in the lumbar region, with soft, mushy stool.

I believe if I had used nothing but the first trituration it would have produced large hæmorrhoidal tumors, the large doses that I took kept the bowels too loose. Not one of our remedies produce so many and so strongly marked symptoms of hæmorrhoids as the æsculus. I would also call the attention of our physicians to the *powerful effect* æsculus has on the liver. I intended to experiment on animals with the æsculus, but could not get the time to do it, but hope I will soon. It is a remedy that will well repay us for all our trouble. W. H. BURT, M. D.

ALETRIS FARINOSA.

(*Unicorn Root, Stone Grass.*)

This plant is the *true* Unicorn, as distinguished from the *false*, Helonias dioica. From all accounts it possesses many properties in common with the latter. The root is the officinal part, and is with difficulty distinguished from the Helonias.

Aletrin, or Aletridin, the active principle, is an Oleo-Resin, and is said to possess the medicinal virtues of the plant.

GENERAL EFFECTS.—No proving of this plant has yet appeared, and the clinical experience of our school, is very meagre. The eclectic school however, speak highly of its value.

"In the recent state, and in large doses it is considerably narcotic, with emetic and cathartic properties. When dried these properties are destroyed, and it becomes a bitter tonic." (*King.*)

"The aletris is tonic, stomachic, narcotic, discutient, emetic, cathartic and expectorant. In large doses it is said to produce nausea, vomiting, purging, dizziness and other unpleasant effects, which would seem to indicate that it is possessed of *acro-narcotic* properties." (*J. and S. Mat. Med.*) "It is believed, that no American plant exceeds the Aletris, in intense and permanent bitterness. In this respect it is not inferior to aloes or quassia. It seems to be a pure bitter, having also some emetic and cathartic properties. As a tonic stomachic, it is not surpassed by any of our indigenous plants, and for this purpose it is extensively employed as a popular remedy and in regular practice. It has long been held in high repute among the Indians. There is some reason to believe, that it possesses narcotic properties. Rafinesque, who seems to have experimented a good deal with it, says, that "only small doses must be used, because large ones produce nausea, dizziness and narcotic effects, and that the powdered root should not be given in larger doses than twelve grains. Its uses are the same as gentian and quassia. In some parts of the country it is used by botanics as a remedy for dropsy, dysentery and colic. We regard it as an alterative tonic, very similar to hydrastin."—(*Prof. Lee.*) It is highly probable that a thorough proving of this medicine would develop its value, and make it almost an equal with Helonias, or perhaps China, although it does not appear to possess the antiperiodic properties of the latter drug. It has, however, some reputation in Intermittents, and one of the common names of the plant is "ague root."

Special Effects.—**Sensorium, Head, etc.**—Vertigo; dizziness, *with* vomiting; purging; sleepiness; and even stupefaction.

Clinical Remarks.—Theoretically, I would suggest that it may be useful in certain *congestions* of the head, when the above symptoms are present. In certain cases of *Meningitis*, in children and adults, the disease is ushered in by a similar train of symptoms. A high dilution of the tincture of the *fresh* root might in such cases prove curative. It is highly recommended by Dr. King ("Diseases of Females") in *hysteria*.

Gastric Symptoms—Vomiting; purging; excessive nausea, with giddiness, etc.

Clinical Remarks.—Small doses are said to promote the appetite and assist digestion. It is used in cases of flatulent colic. It is highly recommended in cases of dyspepsia, with much general debility. All drugs which derange the digestive organs are, of course, homœopathic to some form of dyspepsia, or gastric disorder. Until we have a proving of Aletris, the indications for the use of this remedy cannot be given. It may, however, be used empirically as a *dernier resort* when other remedies fail. A case treated by me, may throw some light on its probable sphere of action. A lady in the fourth month of pregnancy became very much debilitated; had nausea, but no vomiting; disgust for all food; the least food caused distress in the stomach; very constipated; frequent attacks of fainting, with vertigo; sleepy all the time; emaciated. I used Pulsatilla, China, Iron, Sepia, Nux vomica, Ignatia, and many other remedies with no apparent result. Discouraged at the result of my treatment, she declared her intention to procure some "bitters." She "knew some *bitter* tonic would help her." I happened to have a drachm of *Aletridin* in the office. This I dissolved in four ounces of sherry wine, and ordered a teaspoonful three times a day. In a week she came into my office exclaiming, "Your bitters have cured me." The improvement was really great, and no other medicine was used. A constant *pressure* and pain in the uterine region was also removed by the medicine. In a similar case I have since used the *first* dilution with apparent good results.

Female Generative Organs.—Colic in the hypogastrium. Pressure in the region of the uterus. Labor-like pains at the time of the menses. Weight in the uterine region. Premature and profuse menses. Abortion. Leucorrhœa.

Clinical Remarks.—The *Aletris*, is by general consent of Eclectic physicians, considered to possess specific relations as a curative remedy, on certain diseases of the Uterus. I quote some of the testimony: "The root exerts a tonic or stimulating influence upon the reproductive organs of the female. In amenorrhœa, dysmenorrhœa, and engorged condition of the uterus, it will be found of especial benefit, removing the difficulties by restoring the uterus to its normal condition. It will also be found advantageous in those instances when there is an habitual tendency to *abort*, not depending upon syphilitic taint, or other causes independent of the reproductive organs. I have found it useful in *prolapsus uteri*, and am inclined to believe that it exerts a peculiar influence upon the uterine ligaments, having cured several severe cases of uterine prolapsus by this agent alone, without the aid of any mechanical means."—(*King's* Obstetrics, page 638.) "The Aletris is recommended in diseases peculiar to females, as an article of great value. In cases of frequent abortions, or when a disposition to abort exists, and uterine derangements in general."—(*J. & S. Mat. Med.*) If the aletris possesses the power of preventing recurring abortions, it is certainly worthy our investigation. A fragmentary proving even may establish the basis upon which this recommendation is based. Several physicians have verbally given me their testimony in favor of its power of preventing abortion, even after pains and hæmorrhage had set in. I have been assured that it has been used in domestic practice, to produce abortion in the early months. It is evidently homœopathic to *abortion* when accompanied by the symptoms named above, as arising from over doses of the fresh root; also in cases which seem to depend upon a want of tone in the uterine tissues and general system.

APOCYNUM ANDROSEMIFOLIUM.

(*Dog-bane, Milk Weed, Bitter Root.*)

This in an indigenous, perennial, herbaceous plant, from three to six feet in height, and abounding in a milky juice which exudes when any part of the plant is wounded. The stem is smooth and simple below, branched above, usually red on the side exposed to the sun, and covered with a tough fibrous bark. It grows in all parts of the United States, from Carolina to Canada; is found along fences, in wet places, the skirts of woods, and flowers in June and July. The leaves are opposite, petiolate, ovate, acute, entire, smooth on both edges and two or three inches long. The flowers are white, tinged with red and grow in loose nodding, terminal or axillary cymes. The peduncles are furnished with very small acute bractes. The tube of the corrolla is larger than the calyx, and its border spreading. The fruit consists of a pair of long, linear, acute follicles, containing numerous imbricated seeds, attached to a central receptacle and each furnished with a long seed-down. The root is the part employed, and is large, and like other parts of the plant, contains a milky juice. Its taste is unpleasant and extremely bitter.

Great care should be taken not to confound this plant with the apocynum cannabinum, which it closely resembles; for the medicinal effects of the two are very different, and the use of the one for the other might hazard the lives of our patients.

The allopathic and eclectic schools have used it in a crude empirical manner, as an *emetic*, alterative, tonic, aperient, diuretic, detergent, deobstruent, diaphoretic and anthelmintic, &c., much as they use other drugs, especially those of whose virtues they know the least.

What little we do know of its real sphere of action, and its pathogenetic effects, have been ascertained by Dr. J. H. Henry, a Southern homœopathist, who proved it upon himself and two ladies, in pretty large doses, ranging from 50 to 1,800 drops of the mother tincture, of the fresh root. (The tincture must have been a very weak preparation.) All the provers were well when they commenced taking the medicine, with the exception that one of the ladies had suffered from leucorrhœa, and Dr. H. himself had suffered from hæmorrhoids.

May 14th.—Each person took 50 drops fasting in the morning. Two of them felt *cramps in the bottoms of the feet*; the third had *violent heat* of the bottoms of the feet, with profuse *sweating* of the whole body.

May 15th.—Each took 100 drops. All felt *cramps* and *burning* in the bottoms of the feet, most severely in the *right* foot, with severe *pain in the joint of the left big toe*, and heat in the right leg and knee. One of the ladies and Dr. H. complained of great fulness and pain in the head, of an indescribable character. The next morning the three persons complained of *constipation* of the bowels.

May 16th.—All took 150 drops, and experienced about the same symptoms as on the 15th. Dr. H.'s feet *tingling pains in his toes*, sharp pains in the middle; *trembling* of the body in two provers; most delightful taste in the mouth of each. Everything smelled like honey to Dr. H. *All* complained of pains in different parts of the body, and Dr. H. of much pain in the *knee and right shoulder*. The ladies complained of *pain of all the teeth* of the lower jaw, left side.

May 17th.—Each took 200 drops. Neither, except Dr. H. felt cramps in the bottom of the feet. All experienced symptoms like those felt on the 16th; pains and stiffness in the back of the head and neck; dull heavy pain when breathing seeming to go from above downward.

May 18th.—Each took 250 drops. Dr. H. and one of the ladies sufferred from painful bilious diarrhœa.

May 19th.—Each took 300 drops, and experienced heaviness of the body, with a great desire to sleep; flying pains in different parts of the system; pain in the head and back of the neck, swollen sensations of the face and body, violent *itching* of body and face.

May 20th.—Each took 350 drops, and experienced all of the above symptoms, with profuse flow of clear urine; pulsating pain in back of the head, and between the right hand and elbow, constipation of two persons; diarrhœa of the third, with much pain and rumbling, only two evacuations, but copious and affording much relief.

May 21st.—Each took 400 drops and experienced much pain all over the head; stiffness of the neck; pain on turning of the left side; itching and burning of the face, much lassitude, frequent passing of clear urine.

May 22d.—Each took 450 drops, and felt all the previous symptoms, together with great sneezing, twitching of the face, most violent *pains in all the joints*, great itching and irritation in left nostril.

May 23d.—Each took 500 drops. Violent pain in the left zygomatic process, chilliness, lassitude, heat of head and neck, inability to sleep at night, violent dreams, sleep not refreshing, pain in the left groin of a shooting character.

May 24th.—Each took 550 drops. Ladies suffered from *profuse menstruation*, lasting eight days, with violent pressing pain; other symptoms as before.

May 26th.—Each took 650 drops. Some efforts to vomit; pain increased in back of neck, and extending to front; pains severe above each wrist. One prover had four bilious evacuations, another ten, and another, constipation.

May 27th.—Each took 1,800 drops. All sick; vomiting, purging, great prostration and trembling of the body.

This was truly heroic proving, bringing out boldly the characteristic symptoms of the drug.

General Symptoms. — *Nerves of Sensation.* — Although the remedy produces a great many pains, and pain implies that the nervous system is involved, still it would seem that these were not simple nervous pains or neuralgias, but rather simulated rheumatic or dyscratic pains. It may prove useful in rheumatic-neuralgias.

Nerves of Motion.—It produces cramps in the soles of the feet, pains and stiffness in back and neck, sneezing, twitching of the face, etc., yet it seems to act far more specifically upon the fibrous tissues and nerves of sensation, than upon those of motion.

Fever and Inflammation.—It causes violent heat in the bottoms of the feet, with a profuse sweating all over; heat and pain in the toes, legs, and knees. Swollen sensation of the face and body, with violent itching of those parts; pulsatory pain in head and back of neck, and between the right hand and elbow; chiliness, heat of head and neck, so that one cannot sleep at night.

Clinical Remarks.—According to Dr. Henry, it has been much used in the South, in bilious diseases and fevers; in the marsh fever of the rice plantations, in yellow fever, in colds and inflammation of the bowels and lungs, in dysentery and diarrhœa, of all these it seems most homœopathic to *bilious fever*, when attended with bilious diarrhœa, in rheumatic catarrhs, dysenteries and fevers.

On the Fibrous Tissues.—This seems to be the great field of its action. It has produced cramps in the feet, probably in the muscles and tendons; great pain in the joint of the big toe; heat in the right leg and knee; tingling pains in the toes, pains in different parts of the body, but especially in the knee and right shoulder; pains and stiffness in back of head and neck; dull heavy pain in the chest while breathing; flying pains all over the system; most violent pain in all the joints, etc.

Clinical Remarks.—All the above prominent symptoms were

brought on by tangible doses of the drug. They seem to have been specific, for all the provers felt them.

In Rheumatism and Rheumatic Gout.—It is perhaps the most homœopathic remedy that we are yet acquainted with; it may be most suitable in bilious subjects, or when there is a prominent bilious disorder in connection with the rheumatism. It seems to be absorbed into the system and to penetrate into the innermost portions of the body, similarly to the rheumatic poison, and even to produce those critical evacuations from the bowels, skin, liver and kidneys, which terminate an attack of rheumatism; and according to the law of "Similia," it ought to be specific for that protean disease.

Mucous Membranes.—We have no decided proof that it acts specifically upon this tissue, although it produces sneezing and itching of nostrils, still it would seem homœopathic to catarrhal affections of a rheumatic character.

Skin.—It causes profuse sweating when taken in large doses; also swollen sensation of the face and body, and itching all over, and burning itching of face, etc.

Clinical Remarks.—It may prove useful in those disagreeable perspirations which attend or follow rheumatic fever; and is certainly indicated in prurigo, especialy when attended with derangement of the liver.

Head.—Great fullness and pain in the head; pains and stiffness in back of head and neck, pain in head and back of neck. Pulsatory pain in back of the head, and between the right hand and elbow. Pain all over the head with stiffness of the neck. Heat of head and neck, and chilliness, lassitude, sleeplessness and troublesome dreams. Great pain in all of *left* side of head with pain above each wrist.

Clinical Remarks.—It is homœopathic to bilious, rheumatic, and congestive headaches, especially when attended with rheumatic pains in other parts, preceeded by constipation, followed by diarrhœa attended with swelling and itching of the face, and terminating with profuse flow of urine, or perspiration. It is also indicated in rheumatic or neuralgic hemicrania.

Eyes and Ears.—No symptoms involving these organs have yet been evolved, but judging from its general effects, it ought to prove useful in rheumatic affections of those organs.

Nose.—With the pains all over, had severe *sneezing* with great itching and irritation in nostril. Everything smelled like honey.

Clinical Remarks.—With the country people this plant in decoction, is considered a specific for worms and verminous fever, and in one case I saw good effects from it after Cina and Santonine had failed. Its moderate use expelled large quantities of ascarides. The above symptoms of the nose, are such as often indicate the presence of worms,

Face and Teeth.—Swollen sensation of the face and body; violent *itching* of body and face; itching and *burning* of face, *twitching* of the face. Pain in *all the teeth of the lower jaw, left side.*

Clinical Remarks.—The *sensation* of swelling of the face and body is also caused by *aconite*, and is probably a purely nervous sensation. The itching etc., is like that caused by Opium and Morphia, is probably of a nervous character, *not* like that caused by *Rhus*, which indicates an impending eruption. The twitching of the face and pain in the teeth, point it out as a remedy in those rheumatic neuralgias of a similar character.

Gastric Symptoms.—Most *delightful* taste in the mouth of each. Nausea and efforts to vomit. Vomiting, purging and great prostration. Nausea with constipation, bilious vomiting.

CLINICAL REMARKS.—So uniform is its emetic effects in large doses, that it was named by the Botanics, American Ipecac. It generally caused profuse vomiting of bile. When we have *bilious* vomiting with or without diarrhœa; but with pains in the limbs, cramps in the feet, etc., then the Apoc. Andros. will prove a specific remedy. In cases of gastric irritability and debility from habitual biliousness, it will improve the tone of the stomach.

Stomach and Bowels.—Flying pains in the stomach, fullness and pain in right side, (region of the liver,) with feeling as if something would pass the bowels, with slight nausea. *Constipation* (from small doses 50 drops.) Bilious and painful diarrhœa. Diarrhœa attended with pain and rumbling, but only two large evacuations, giving much relief; 650 drops caused four bilious evacuations in one prover, two in another, and constipation in a third; constipation and diarrhœa every alternate day. The largest dose caused sickness vomiting, purging, prostration, etc.

CLINICAL REMARKS.—It is indicated in bilious diarrhœa with pain in the bowels and region of the liver; in constipation like that caused by jaundice when the bile does not find its way into the bowels, but is retained in the blood and tissues. It is indicated in bilious headaches; also in bilious fever, when there is much heat and pain in the head, great tendency to drowsiness, or restlessness with troublesome dreams, and either bilious diarrhœa or constipation, with pains in the limbs.

Urinary Organs.—Profuse flow of clear urine. Frequent passing of clear urine.

CLINICAL REMARKS.—Previous to a bilious attack some persons have profuse flow of clear, limpid urine, with chilliness, headache, etc. This remedy would seem homœopathic to such symptoms. It has been used successfully in dropsy from diseased liver.

Genital Organs.—Profuse menstruation lasting eight days, and attended with violent pressing down pain. One of the ladies was troubled with leucorrhœa before taking the medicine. She was cured, and has not since had a return.

Prof. Lee says, "The Choctaw Indians use it extensively for the cure of venereal affections, for which they regard it as specific. They chew the fresh root, swallowing only the juice. There is no doubt of its efficacy in secondary and tertiary syphilis."

Back and Extremities.—It caused severe pains in different parts of the body, back of the head, arms, legs, feet, shoulder, and *violent pains in all the joints*. (See "General Symptoms," and "Fibrous Tissues.")

CLINICAL REMARKS.—No remedy seems more indicated by its

pathogenesis, for muscular and articular rheumatism, than this. It seems the analogue of Bryonia, Cimicifuga, Aconite, Phytolacca and Colchicum.

APOCYNUM CANNABINUM.

(*Indian Hemp.*)

This should not be confounded with the A. Androsemifolium, which it resembles only in appearance. The medicinal properties of the two are widely different.

It is a perennial plant, stems herbaceous, erect, branching, of a brown color, and two or three feet in height; the leaves are opposite, ovate, oblong, acute at both ends, and somewhat downy beneath; the cymes are pedunculate, many flowered and pubescent; the corolla is small and greenish, with a tube not longer than the calyx, and with an erect border, the internal parts of the flowers are pinkish or purple. The pod, or follicle is from three to five inches long, and resembles the pods of the asclepias syriaca, or common silk-weed, but are much smaller.

The stalk and root abounds in a milky juice which concretes into a substance closely resembling caoutchouc. It is the juice which contains the active principles.

The *root*, which is the officinal part, is horizontal, five or six feet in length, about one-third of an inch thick, dividing near the end into branches, which terminate abruptly, of a yellowish brown color when young, but dark chestnut when old, of a strong odor, and a nauseous, somewhat acrid, and a permanently bitter taste.

It grows in damp places, by marshes and running streams, and is indigenous to nearly every part of the United States.

The tincture should be dark red and intensely bitter. It is said by old authorities to be emetic and cathartic, sometimes diuretic, and like other emetic substances, promotes diaphoresis and expectoration.

When it does cause nausea, it is persistent and intense; it then diminishes the frequency of the pulse, and appears to induce drowsiness independently of the exhaustion consequent upon vomiting.

These crude notions however, convey but a faint idea of the qualities of this plant. No thorough and systematic proving of this plant has been made. A fragmentary but suggestive proving was once made by Dr. Peters. My own observations of its effects, enable me to record many of its pathogenetic symptoms.

Dr. Peters took half wine-glass full doses of Hunt's decoction, three times a day—morning, noon and night. For the first few days he noticed no perceptible effect, except an increased inclination towards constipation. (This decoction must have been very

6

weak, for a table spoonful of a decoction such as I have made, would have acted on him as a powerful cathartic.) He noticed a decided *scantiness* of *urine:* occasionally there was some flatulence, and slightly uneasy sensation in the bowels. About the fourth day, decided distention of the abdomen began to occur. Especially after a moderate dinner, all the sense of fullness seemed about the stomach, liver and spleen, while the lower bowels did not seem more flatulent than usual.

The sense of oppression about the epigastrium and chest was so great, that there was often the greatest difficulty in getting breath enough to speak with any comfort, and this happened after lighter meals than ordinary. He was confident that his urine diminished to one-third its usual quantity, but there was no pain or uneasiness about the kidneys or bladder, on the contrary these organs felt remarkably comfortable; they seemed simply torpid; the little water that was passed, flowed as easily as if it were oil, and there seemed to be but little expulsive power about the bladder. The urine was generally of a light golden sherry-yellow color, not depositing any sediment on exposure to cold. "This *torpid action* of the kidneys was rather peculiar as the weather was severely cold, and I was much exposed to it, and in my ordinary state, my kidneys act frequently and rather freely. It is right to add that during the experiment I was growing very stout, and had just recovered from fever and ague, which may account for the oppression of the chest and flatulence." (*Peters.*) This may be, but his own experiments afterwards brought on similar symptoms, even when the drug was taken in minute doses. The symptoms observed by him and others, will be found under their appropriate heads.

General Symptoms.—Weakness, lassitude. "I took for 6 days, 5 drops, three times daily, of the 3d dilution. No unusual sensations were observed until the fifth morning of the proving, when on waking we felt a sinking at the stomach, dryness of the mouth, thirst, nausea, irresistible disposition to sigh, short and unsatisfactory respiration, short and dry cough, scanty expectoration of white mucus. These symptoms continued during the day, and on retiring, we had in addition unusual heat of the skin, general restlessness and desire to sleep without the ability to do so. During the entire day, urine was natural in quantity, and gave the same color to test papers as in health. The night of the fifth was one of great restlessness and little sleep. On the morning of the sixth day we awoke at about five o'clock, unrefreshed by our sleep, and with the same symptoms as on the fifth day, with the exception of a diminution of the quantity of urine. During this day we were unable to detect any alteration in the composition of the urine, either by test paper or with acids. The symptoms of the seventh day and night were a continuation of the sixth, on the eighth day the stomach and chest symptoms had diminished, but the urinary secretion had increased in quantity and much lighter in color than in health. On the evening of the eighth day we experienced an unusual heaviness of the head, with dull aching pains in the small of the back and limbs. There was no tenderness of the region of the kidneys on pressure, but a slight soreness of the parts when bringing the muscles into action, indicating the muscles as the seat of the pains. From the ninth day the symptoms continued very gradually to decline until the thirteenth day, after which no further abnormal phenomena were observed. (*Marcy.*)

Clinical Remarks.—The above fragmentary proving, is a very suggestive one. The groups of symptoms resemble those of non-inflammatory dropsy, having a rheumatic or congestive origin. We often meet such symptoms in practice, where it is difficult to give a satisfactory diagnosis. Before we can know the real action of apocynum, we shall have to make pathological provings of the drug.

In cases of general debility, from a watery condition of the blood and poor digestion, if at the same time there is scanty urine, apocynum will restore the strength and tone of the system.

Skin.—Unusual heat of the skin. Cold skin—with nausea, vomiting, etc. Copious sweating.

Clinical Remarks.—In nearly all the dropsies, the skin is dry and harsh. When from natural processes or from the action of medicines the skin becomes moist and soft, we may be pretty sure that improvement will soon follow. Whenever I have been successful in the use of apocynum, the skin became moist before the urinary secretion became more abundant. It has been found useful in some inveterate eruptions, as psoriasis.

Sleep.—*Desire to sleep* without the ability to do so. Great restlessness with little sleep at night. On retiring unusual heat of skin; waking unrefreshed about 5 A. M. induces a tendency to sleep. Sleepiness with heaviness of the head.

Clinical Remarks.—In nearly all dropsies, especially post-scarlatinal, the patient is feverish at night, and very restless. This often occurs before the dropsical effusion is noticed. In this stage the apocynum will prevent the malady from being established.

Fever.—Unusual heat of the skin with general restlessness and desire to sleep with inability to do so—at night. Pulse very slow, with nausea.

Clinical Remarks.—Dr. Trent claims for the *apoc.* anti-periodic virtues, but he gave it combined with oil of black pepper. Such observations as made by the allopathic school are perfectly worthless, yet upon such flimsy foundations does their vaunted materia medica depend! It is probably not useful for the *ague* properly, but *is* of value in the dropsical sequelæ which so often follow that disease. It is homœopathic to the thoracic oppression, the bloating of the stomach and bowels after eating; the œdema and even night sweats; in all of which I have used it with advantage in the 2nd and 3d dilutions.

In *catarrhal* fever with nightly exacerbation, short dry cough with scanty expectoration of white mucus, and oppression of the chest, it will be found curative.

Head.—Heaviness in the head. Heavy stupid headache with drowsiness.

Clinical Remarks.—It is undoubtedly slightly narcotic in its effects. The drowsiness which it causes is very similar to that which occurs in all dropsical affections which have reached a high degree of intensity. In such cases sleepiness is an unfavorable symptom, and should warn us to be on our guard against coma and apoplexy. In such conditions we have in this medicine a prompt and reliable remedy. Several times in the course of my practice have I rescued my patients by giving promptly the *apocynum.* If the dilutions failed of effect, as they sometimes will in cases marked by such torpidity, I have not hesitated to resort to the decoction, for I have ever considered the life of my patients to be of more importance than a blind adherence to established forms. We should recollect moreover that the *tincture* is not always the best preparation. With many valuable plants the decoction is the best method of administration, because hot water alone, is capable of extracting all their medicinal virtues.

In a case of supposed *hydrocephalus* in a child of Prof. Renwick, of New York, aged 16 months, after all other remedies had been given up and the case regarded as hopeless, the use of a decoction of Indian hemp was followed by perfect recovery. "The sutures of the head were opened; the forehead projecting considerably; the sight of one eye totally lost; the other slightly sensible; the child lying in a stupor, with constant involuntary motion of one leg and arm. The urinary secretion had ceased for more than twenty-four hours. A tea of apocynum was prepared by dropping pieces of the root into a coffee cup until nearly full, covering with water, and steeping for half an hour: of this a teaspoonful was given every hour. In the course of a few hours free action of the kidneys was restored; the sight of both eyes were perfect; stupor and insensibility passed away. The child steadily convalesced, though the hemp was given for a fortnight, gradually diminishing the dose, until but half a teaspoonful was given in 24 hours." This was undoubtedly a case of hydrocephalus, and the *apocynum* as undoubtedly cured it. The lower dilutions may have done as well, perhaps as the higher; but in such a case, of a generally fatal disease, what conscientious physician would hesitate to use other preparations? The dose given was not more than 10 or 15 drops of a 1st decimal dilution would contain, and no pathogenetic symptoms were caused. One cannot but be struck with the similarity between the symptoms cured, and those for which Hartman so confidently recommends Helleborus. In fact, the two medicines are very nearly allied. Some undoubted cures of hydrocephalus have been made with Helleborus, but we have given it faithfully and in various potencies in that disease; and yet the little patients died. What physician has not lost patients with that dreaded malady in spite of Belladonna, Hellebore, Sulphur and Zinc? How gladly we would have resorted to any remedy, in any form, if we thought it would restore health? Let a fair trial, then, be given to the Apocynum.

Eyes.—"I was once waked up early in the morning with severe irritation of the left eye, as if several sharp grains of sand were in it, attended with much heat, irritation and redness, often lasting several hours. This disappeared as suddenly as it came on, not leaving a trace behind; although the symptoms were severe enough to make me believe I had an attack of catarrhal rheumatic ophthalmia, which would last at least three or four days."—*Peters.*

Clinical Remarks.—The above symptoms would indicate its usefulness in some forms of ophthalmia.

In the case of hydrocephalus, it restored sight to one eye. It may prove very useful in many diseases of the eye and disorders of vision due to effused fluids in the eye or brain.

Ears.—In hydrocephalus there is often more or less deafness, for which condition this remedy will prove curative.

Nose.—"A very peculiar catarrhal attack was experienced, viz: without any other sign of having taken cold, I would wake up in the morning with the nostrils and throat filled with thick and well cemented, yellow mucous, as if I had had a severe catarrh for at least seven or ten days, and which had skipped its first stage and commenced in the second."—*Peters.*

Clinical Remarks.—The action of *apocynum* on the mucous surfaces is not yet fully understood. I have cured one case of obstinate nasal catarrh with the 1st dil. It seems to cause catarrhal states similar in nature to those induced by Pulsatilla, Sumbul, Copaiva and Paris quadrifolia.

Mouth.—Dryness of the mouth, with nausea, thirst, &c. (See general symptoms.) Dryness of the tongue.

Throat.—Throat filled with thick, well concreted yellow mucus in the morning. Unpleasant degree of heat in throat.

Clinical Remarks.—Some persons are much troubled with hawking of yellow mucus from the throat and fauces every morning. In such cases the apocynum will probably give relief.

Stomach.—Distention of the stomach after meals. Sense of great oppression about the epigastrium, with great difficulty of getting breath, after lighter meals than ordinary, Occasionally a sense of *sinking* was experienced at the pit of the stomach, with general but transient debility. *Sinking* at the stomach (this is a prominent symptom of the drug). Intense nausea, but cannot vomit. Severe vomiting (from very large doses). Violent vomiting, with prostration *and* drowsiness. Increases the appetite and digestion (curative).

Clinical Remarks.—It causes symptoms of the stomach similar to those which are nearly always presented in cases of impending or existing dropsy. It should be tried in that troublesome symptom—"Sinking at the stomach"—which occurs in women at the climacteric period. In diabetes this symptom is nearly always present, and may be relieved by this drug. It seems quite homœopathic to the vomiting which occurs in the first stage of hydrocephalus, for "violent vomiting with drowsiness" is quite pathonomonic of that disease. Dr. Freligh cured with it an "irritable stomach so bad that the patient could not retain even a draught of water," which occurred as a complication of dropsy.

Abdomen.—Decided distention of the abdomen, especially after a moderate dinner. The upper bowels seemed distended—the lower not at all. Occasional flatulence, with slightly uneasy sensations in the bowels.

Clinical Remarks.—Of the great value of *apocynum* in *ascites* we have an immense amount of proof from the allopathic, eclectic, and homœopathic physicians. All unite in pronouncing it a generally useful remedy, a veritable "vegetable trocar," as Dr. Rush called it.

The mass of evidence in its favor would fill many pages, and we will only record a few of the most prominent cases.

The first accounts of its great value in ascites were from the reports of Dr. Griscomb, in the Amer. Jour. of Medical Sciences, Vol. XII. Afterwards, Prof. Merrill, Dr. Knapp, Dr. Valentine Mott, and Prof. Lee, and many others bore testimony to its great usefulness.

Prof. Merrill related to his class a case of ascites in a boy of 12 years old, which was promptly relieved by this remedy, after every other treatment had failed, and the disease had progressed so far that a time had been fixed for the operation of tapping. The extract was given, first in doses of one grain, afterwards increased to ten grains, three times a day. The effects were, moderate catharsis of a bilious and feculentc haracter, free diuresis, without being profuse, and copious perspiration. Great relief and relaxation was obtained in the first 24 hours, and in five days there was no hydrophic condition remaining." (Other cases of ascites will be found under the head of "General Dropsy.")

To Dr. John F. Gray, of New York, is due the the credit of fairly introducing this remedy in the treatment of dropsical affections. He could, if he would, make known hundreds of cases successfully treated by the Apocynum. But with advancing years he has an invincible dislike to making his great and varied experience public. Happily, other homœopathic physicians have reported cases of anasarca, &c., of great value to the profession.

Dr. Jas. T. Alley, in the N. A. Journal, reports a case of ascites, supposed to be caused by cirrhosis or hobnail liver. In this instance it was used in conjunction with apis and nitro-muriatic acid. He bears testimony to its value in cases of dropsy "when there is no organic derangement to impede its action." Even when there *is*, he thinks it may aid other and more specific remedies. In "abdominal drosy from hob-nail liver, I believe it to be a sure, though not rapid remedy." He gave quite large doses, "as much," he says, "as could be perfectly well borne without disturbance to the digestive organs.

In Hull's Jahr is reported a case of ascites caused by Quinine, cured by Apocynum.

Dr. Freligh (N. A. Jour., Vol. IV., p. 519,) reports several cases of ascites cured with this drug:—

"Mrs. C., aged 49, and Miss M., aged 23. The former was referable to a cessation of the menses, and the latter arose from congestion of the liver and portal system.

"Within six months I treated an aged lady, who had been under treatment for the best part of eight months by one of the professors of our city, who pronounced the case 'incurable organic disease of the heart,' cured with apocynum."

I once cured a notable case of ascites with this remedy. The patient was a lady, aged 45. Her climacteric period had passed without much disturbance. She caught a severe cold in the month of March; had some fever and pain in the bowels, and was treated by an eclectic physician for "inflammation of the bowels." When I first saw her she was much emaciated, very weak, no appetite, red tongue and sore throat, abdomen slightly distended, and the seat of a great deal of heavy, "bruised" pain. The urine was scanty, high colored; bowels costive. The treatment was commenced with Arsenicum 30th. No improvement following in a week, the 3rd, and finally the 1st trituration was given, but the ascites rapidly increased. For six weeks various remedies were tried, among which were Kali carb., Helleborus, China, Colchicum, Cantharis, Cannabis, and Kal. iod, but no benefit accrued from any thing. The effusion had now increased to an enormous extent. She was obliged to sit erect in a chair *all* the time. Lying down brought on fits of suffocative dyspnœa. Her body and extremities were exceedingly emaciated. No œdema of the feet. Urine nearly suppressed; only one or two ounces a day. Bowels very constipated, moving only every four or five days. At this time, an experienced allopathic physician was called in, who advised blue pill, gamboge, and a resort to tapping. This treatment was not tried. I then gave Apocynum 1st, for two days; no effect; then 10 drops of the tincture every two hours for two days. She got worse. Then I made a decoction of the dry root, half ounce to one pint of water. Of this she took a tablespoonful every four hours, but no effect was noticed. I proposed tapping to save her life, but she decidedly refused to submit to the operation. I then procured some of the fresh root (in the month of July), and made a decoction (one ounce to one pint of water). She took a tablespoonful of this every two hours. In 12 hours the urine became more profuse, the bowels moved freely, the skin became moist, no nausea or pain was produced. In a week she could lie down and sleep all night. Under the use of similar doses, four times a day, she ultimately recovered, and in two months was considered as healthy and strong as ever.

Bowels.—From small doses; loose feculent bilious stools, with slight uneasiness in the abdomen. Loose, but not very copious bilious stools. Sensation as if diarrhœa would occur. From very large doses; copious watery discharges with severe griping pains, nausea and vomiting, slow pulse, cool skin and copious perspiration.

Clinical Remarks—In moderate doses it does not seem to irritate the bowels much. The best Allopathic authorities do not deem it necessary to produce its hydrogogue effects, in the treatment of dropsy; Prof. Lee says it need not be given, even to nausea, all its best cures have been made without giving it to the extent of causing watery evacuations. It has even cured dropsy, while the bowels remained obstinately costive and the stools light colored. Dr. Payne, of Albany, states that it has been used successfully for diarrhœas and intestinal *hæmorrhages*, and suggests it in cholera morbus, and cholera-infantum. Its analogues are Elaterium, Helleborus niger, Euphorbia cor, Colocynth and Arsenicum, yet it has a specific effect upon the kidneys which these have not.

Kidneys and Urine.—Dull aching pain in the region of the kidneys, with increased secretion of straw-colored urine. No tenderness in the region of the kidneys on pressure, nor was the composition of the urine changed any. (Marcy's proving with 3d dil). Decided *scantiness of urine.* Urine diminished to one-third the usual quantity, but no pain or uneasiness about the kidneys or bladder. The little water that passed flowed as easily as if it were oil, and there seemed to be but little expulsive power about the bladder. The urine was generally of a light golden sherry-yellow color, not depositing any sediment on exposure to cold. Very peculiar *torpid action of the kidneys.* (*Peter's* proving with crude doses.) Very profuse, light colored urine. Several quarts, and even gallons of urine were passed every day. It causes copious diuresis when given in dropsy.

Clinical Remarks.—In all the provings, so far, it has caused no particular pain in the urinary organs, but a decided *scantiness* of urine. Probably the experiments were not thorough enough. My experience is, that it is the most reliable *diuretic* in use. No drug may be more confidently relied on to produce profuse urination, when given in disease.

Dr. Freligh says, "I have found it equally efficient in urinary difficulties, particularly dysuria, strangury and anury, and it appeared quite immaterial, judging from its effects, whether the symptoms depended upon common catarrh of the bladder, diseases of the prostrate, or upon a morbid irritation of the bladder, and whether from gravel, or from a want of tone in the parts concerned in its evacuation. I have never known it to fail even in cases of retention depending upon paralysis, having used it successfully, in a case of paralysis of the inferior extremities, caused by injury to the spine. Every remedy had been tried in vain, and the catheter afforded the only relief, which had been used once and sometimes twice a day for a fortnight. The first dose had the desired effect, I have treated many other interesting cases of urinary difficulty successfully with the apocynum. The doses administered in the case referred to, were from two to five drops of the tincture, (never more than seven) in a tumbler two-thirds full of pure cold water, a desert spoonful given, for the dropsical affections, every four hours; in urinary difficulties every hour until relief was afforded.

Dr. Freligh reports several cures of dropsy effected with the Apocynum:

"Mr. L. aged 64, who had been under medical treatment for several months, and gradually grew worse, until his symptoms were of the most alarming character, and threatened immediate suffocation. I found him laboring under the most agonizing difficulty of breathing, being supported in the sitting position in bed, by two or three persons alternately. His stomach was in such an irritable condition that he could not retain even a draught of cold water, countenance expressive of anguish, abdomen distended, urine entirely suppressed and very extensive œdema. This case was denominated organic disease of the heart, by his physician. In a fortnight from the time I recommended the treatment, he rode out with ease and comfort, and now appears perfectly well. If the diagnosis of the other physician was correct, the apocynum will not only cure dropsy depending upon organic disease of the heart, in a less time than would appear credible, but also the primary or original disease, pronounced incurable."

"Mr. G. aged 62, ascites, and anasarca, and œdema of the inferior extremities, succeeding typhus. His abdomen very much distended and painful, pulse small and irregular, skin dry and husky, urine high-colored, diminished in quantity, voided with difficulty, breathing very laborious."

"Master P. aged 8, post-scarlatinal dropsy, face much swollen, also neck, chest and extremities. When I was called they thought him dying; he was gasping for breath and could not utter a syllable although perfectly conscious and would answer by signs. "Dr. F. adds that during the last seven or eight years he has used the apocynum with the most decided success in almost every form of dropsy. He has succeeded with it in hydrothorax, ascites and general anasarca, when Arsenicum, Apis, Hellebore, Digitalis and Kali iod, with vapor baths, &c., have failed.

Dr. Peters has reported several interesting cases:—

Case 1. A gentleman aged 70, over six feet high and splendidly proportioned, became dropsical. The urine became scanty, bowels constipated, feet, legs and abdomen grew slowly larger, and gradually great difficulty in breathing from the slighest exertion or on lying down ensued. From the thickness of the abdominal walls, and the great quantity of fat in the omentum, fluctuation in the abdomen was long masked, but finally became very distinct. The thickness of the walls of the chest also rendered the physical signs of hydrothorax indistinct for a long time, but they finally became very manifest. The action of the heart became very feeble, but was always distinct, the pulse often vanished down to a mere thread, was often almost imperceptible for several beats, frequently so compressible that slight pressure would obliterate for the time, and altogether so strangely irregular, weak and intermitting, that the sudden death of the patient was expected as a matter of course. These symptoms progressed steadily in spite of the use of Arsenicum, Hellebore, Scilla, Digitalis, China, &c.. He was finally put upon the use of Hunt's decoction of apocynum. At the suggestion of Dr. Gray, commencing with tea-spoonful doses every two or three hours. In less than 48 hours the patient was comparatively comfortable, was able to lie down and sleep with pleasure, whereas previously he had looked forward to the approaching night with the utmost dread and horror; the urine increased moderately and steadily, and in a few weeks, the patient who had been ill for upwards of four months, was not only well, but felt better than he had for years. The bowels remained sluggish under the use of the Hemp. This improved state of things lasted for more than a year then a relapse was speedily cured by Hemp; a third attack was cured by Apis; a fourth by Digitalis, Squills and Mercurius; and a fifth by Iodide of Potash. During the larger portion of this time the patient had contracted a most invincible dislike to Apocynum; but in a sixth attack, all the other remedies failing, he was persuaded to resume the Hemp, after his condition was almost hopeless, and distressing in the extreme, from excessive oppression and difficulty of breathing, &c., hydrothorax and œdema of the lungs, inability to walk or step without being thrown into the most violent suffocating attacks, and in short from the numerous and complicated symptoms of general anasarca, ascites, hydrothorax, hydro-pericardium, &c. After using the apocynum three or four days, in doses of one-third of a wine-glass full three times a day, the urine increased from less than a pint in 25 hours, to fully three quarts, with a progressing diminution of all the symptoms. This case has since died without any return of the dropsy."

Case 2. "A man aged 32, had sufferred with anasarca, ascites and commencing hydrothorax for many weeks, under active Allopathic treatment by means of Cream of Tartar and Digitalis, Eleterium, &c. When I first saw him, his largest pantaloons had to be cut open and tied with strings, to accommodate his elephantine limbs; he was utterly unable to lie down or sleep; urine especially scanty and bowels costive. The apocynum was commenced in table-spoonful doses, gradually increased to a wine-glass full every four hours, by night and day; this was continued for upwards of ten days without any unpleasant symptoms, the urine slowly commenced to increase, and finally became enormous in amount. In less than a month he was entirely well; was soon able to go to sea, and remains well until this day, upwards of two years after.

Case 3. A gentlemen aged 67, had gradually been growing dropsical for eleven months; he had first been treated homœopathically in the country, by an exceedingly able, but excessively high dilutionist; he then fell into the hands of two of the most distinguished Allopathic profession of this city; then he was again treated with high dilutions for several weeks by one of our oldest and best-known homœopathists, finally he came into my hands and was immediately put under the use of Apocynum. One desert spoonful per dose, every four hours; his urine which had been excessively scanty for months and finally had decreased to a small half pint, in twenty-four hours, thick yellow and turbid, as if yellow clay had been dissolved in it, increased to upwards of two quarts in one night; two large chamber pots full were passed in one day. In less than 48 hours after commencing the apocynum the urine also became clear and of a light straw-yellow color; all the signs of ascites, anasarca, hydrothorax, and œdema of the lungs disappeared in less than ten days, after using about one pint of Hunt's preparation of Apocynum, (about one-half oz. of mother tincture).

Case 4. A gentleman, aged about 50, was attacked with inflammatory rheumatism, and treated by an eminent old school physician for about eight weeks, when he became discouraged from the severity of his sufferings and placed himself under our care. He had taken the usual routine medicines of the other school, Colchicum, Mercury, Iodide of Potash, Opium, etc., etc., and when he came into my hands, was reduced by the combined influence of the disease, and the drug to the following condition:

Severe rheumatic pains in the back, shoulders, elbows and wrist joints, dull pains and great stiffness, and immobility in the lower extremities, œdematous condition of both legs, effusion of water in the chest and abdomen, excessive dyspnœa with constant sense of suffocation, acute pains in the cardiac region at every respiration, pulse rapid, feeble and very irregular, almost entire suppression of urine, dry and hot skin, thirst, dull headache, excessive anxiety and constant dread of suffocation, inability to assume the recumbent position, dryness of the tongue and mouth, inability to sleep from constant feeling of suffocation, short dry and painful cough. For this group of symptoms we prescribed the first dil. of Bryonia every hour. After a few hours the rheumatic and cardiac pains were ameliorated, and the oppression of the chest and difficult breathing were somewhat better. At the expiration of ten hours we prescribed Aconite 1st, in alternation with Bryonia every hour. During the night, some ten hours after the first dose of aconite, the patient had profuse perspiration for several hours, followed by an amendment of the entire condition. These two remedies were continued for two days longer, but caused no further improvement. The first dilution of apis, was next ordered in drop doses, every two hours. This was continued for three days without any notable improvement.

The patient was now ordered to take a teaspoonful of Hunt's apocynum every two hours. In a few hours the urinary secretion was much increased and it continued for several days, until the dropsical effusions, and the œdematous condition of the limbs, had entirely disappeared. While under the use of apocynum occasional scarifications were made upon the legs and feet, giving exit to much serum. As the dropsical effusions diminished, nearly all of the symptoms, first enumerated, gradually disappeared, until finally the patient complained of debility, and occasional paroxysms of palpitation of the heart, the remains of the rheumatism. After a few weeks the patient returned to his home in the West, remained in a comfortable condition for several months, was again attacked with dropsy and after an illness of about two months, died. (*Marcy.*)

"Apocynum is utterly useless in Bright's disease, except to remove the dropsy. I ought to add that albuminaria was present in none of the above cases. It is also comparatively useless when inflammation is present." (*Peters.*)

"I have seen it very effectual in ascites in the hand of Dr. Okie of Providence, and have seen it remove the dropsical accumulations in Bright's disease, but never knew it to cure the disease."

(*Watson.*)

Dr. Wm. P. Fowler says he prolonged the lives of three dropsical patients, in which the disease was hepatic cirrhosis, (proved by post mortem) for several years, by the use of apocynum.

In *Dropsy after Scarlatina* the apocynum has not been as

thoroughly tested as it should be. Before I became acquainted with its value, I relied almost entirely upon Apis, Colchicum and Digitalis, and with very good success. But now and then a case would occur, marked by bloody urine, very scanty, with general œdema, which would utterly resist the action of these remedies. My first case treated with apocynum, was a little girl, aged about 2 years, who had been given up to die by the allopathic attendants, who had given squills, calomel, cream of tartar, etc. No urine had been voided for 24 hours, and all that had passed for several days previously was thick and black (from blood). I commenced with apocynum, 10 drops of the tincture in half a tumbler of water, a spoonful every hour. She was cured in a week, of the dropsy. The urine became *profuse* in 48 hours. Since this case, I have treated twenty or thirty, and with uniform success. I never got much effect from the 3d. dil. Sometimes the tincture, even in drop doses failed to act, but a resort to a weak decoction of the fresh root always had prompt effects, (one-half oz. of fresh root to one pint hot water, steep an hour or two.) In several cases marked by excessive debility, and typhoid symptoms, I gave 10 drops of a tincture prepared with *spirits nitre dulc.* instead of alcohol. It acted beautifully. I am inclined to think this mode of preparation a good one.

Prof. Lee, who claims to have had large experience with this drug, says: "It is more certain as a diuretic, if the skin is kept cool, and cool drinks used. As the chief causes of dropsies are certain pre-existing lesions of certain organs, as the heart, liver, and kidneys, we, of course can only expect our remedies to act as palliative, unless these organic lesions can be removed. In cases of idiopathic dropsy, when the exciting causes are external or physical agents, as cold, conjoined with moisture, malaria, suppression of eruptions, or accustomed discharges, excessive depletions, etc., etc., we may expect curative effects from apocynum, aided by other remedies adapted to the pathological state."

In chronic and asthenic forms of dropsy, connected with a watery, non-albuminous state of the blood, and general weakness of the system, the apocynum is most efficacious, in small and frequently repeated doses. In cases dependent on mere debility and mal-nutrition, this remedy aided by suitable diet, will often effect a permanent cure. In advanced stages of albuminuria when there is considerable effusion, great relief may often be obtained from its use.

Case 1. "General dropsy in a man of 68, of plethoric habits, brought on by exposure to cold. Small doses of the decoction were given, and in a short time all the dropsical symptoms disappeared."

Case 2. A lady of 58, of a full and plethoric habit, subject to congestion of the brain, and paralytic seizures of a hemiplegic nature, in which repeated bleedings had been practiced with apparent good effect, but followed by serous effusion into the pleural, pericardial, and peritoneal cavities, and cellular tissues generally, the effusion was successfully removed by small doses of the decoction."

Case 3. A gentleman of 66, a gentleman of spare habit and accustomed to luxurious living, began to be affected with cough, shortness of breath and symptoms of aqueous deposit in the pleural cavity followed by œdema of the extremities. The apocynum was found to exercise complete control over the disease for many years. He finally died of dropsy.

Dr. Griscomb reports many cases of the same character, in which the apocynum was successful. In idiopathic dropsies it generally effected a cure, while in dropsies depending on disease of the liver, heart or kidneys, its effects were mainly palliative, prolonging life for years. Probably, had it been aided by proper remedies, homœopathic to the pathological conditions present, permanent cures might have been effected.

From the foregoing, the physician should get a pretty plain idea of the sphere of action of this valuable drug, in the treatment of dropsical affections. As the result of my individual experience, I would lay down the following rules for its administration.

1) *In cases of acute idiopathic dropsies, use the dilutions beginning with the highest and descending more or less rapidly, according to the progress of the disease.*

2) *In chronic or atonic dropsies,* (*secondary*) *use the tincture, or if necessary the decoction, in one or two dram doses.*

Sexual Organs.—The few experiments which have been made with the hemp, have not developed any pathogenetic symptoms of the male sexual organs. None of the provers were females, and its action on the uterus, is only known by some curative effects noticed by *D. H. Marsden, M. D.*, who gives the following cases:

He says—"For about ten years, I have been in the habit of using the apocynum in arresting menorrhagia as well as some other forms of uterine hæmorrhage."

Case 1. "A lady was laboring under alarming uterine hæmorrhage. It was her regular catamenial period, the flow had been moderate for a day or two, and then suddenly set in with so much violence that she soon became too weak to be out of bed. She was about 25 years of age, the mother of three children; in her last labor she had hæmorrhage previous to delivery. When I arrived at the bed side she was almost pulseless and disposed to faint, whenever she attempted to raise her head from the pillow. There was great irritability of the stomach, and vomiting. The hæmorrhage which ceased at intervals, always resumed when the vital powers rallied, and the heart resumed in some degree its wonted action. The blood was usually expelled in large clots, but sometimes was fluid. I prescribed one after the other, all the remedies laid down in the books, but with no good results. Several days had now elapsed, and I now resolved to try the Apocynum cann. I prepared some extempore tincture from the fresh root. Hastening to the bedside, I found the hæmorrhage still going on undiminished. I prescribed one drop of my tincture (of uncertain strength) every hour. Almost immediately after commencing the medicine the flow became less profuse, and regularly and rapidly declined, without a single recurrence of its violence."

Case 2. The patient was a house-keeper, about 40 years of age, accustomed to hard service, and but little careful of her health. She was the mother of one child, born about 15 years before. She had been suffering from the most exhausting menorrhagia for about six weeks, and had been taking medicine from an allopathic physician, but without benefit. I found her greatly debilitated, pulse feeble and quick, palpitations very troublesome whenever she attempted to move about the house, stomach excessively irritable. She had been obliged to leave off her occupations, and passed her time for the most part in bed, or seated on a chair by the bedside. The discharge was fluid, and still undiminished. I left apocynum to be taken in drop doses at an interval of two hours (same tincture as used in first case.) The next day she had severe vomitings. Her stomach was too irritable to bear the dose I had prescribed, and which was probably unnecessarily large. The discharge seemed, however, to be diminished. After givivg some medicines to allay the irritability of the stomach, I again gave the hemp, a few drops in a teaspoonful of water. I believe I decreased the strength more than once, before the remedy could be borne without creating nausea. The flow, however, still continued to diminish, and in about a week from the time of my first visit was reported to have nearly ceased. It was, of course, some time before the patient regained her strength. Upon inquiry made some months afterwards, I was informed that at one or two periods immediately subsequent, the flow was somewhat above the normal amount, but soon subsided spontaneously, and that then she was as regular as is usual at her time of life.

Dr. Marsden says he could furnish many other cases in his own practice equally striking, but will only give the following, reported to him by his friend and former pupil, Dr. W. H. Cook :—

"Mrs. N., aged 38 years, was taken ill in June, 1863, with uterine hæmorrhage, and was attended by an Allopathic physician until about the middle of December following. During this period she experienced the most frightful floodings, as she termed them, and for more than three months of the time the flow was continuous, requiring her to keep her bed for weeks together. After having hæmorrhage for several weeks, she expelled a mass of membrane, (as she has since informed me,) which I supposed to be the deciduous lining of the uterus. But, even after this the hæmorrhage continued, and in exhausting quantities—so much so, that there was not a blood-vessel perceptible upon the surface of the body, and the emaciation was extreme. She had only had a cessation of a couple of weeks together, and but two or three times since the commencement in June. The flow was excessive at the time of my first visit. I saw her at 12 M., and after inquiring into the case, I left her four grs. of the 1st dec. trit. of apoc. can. (bark of the root) to be dissolved in 2 oz. of water, a teaspoonful to be taken every hour until the hæmorrhage should cease, or I should see her again. By 12 o'clock, midnight, the hæmorrhage had almost entirely ceased, and she left off the medicine. I then gave her other remedies to assist in recruiting her almost exhausted system, under the use of which she improved rapidly. In about two weeks the hæmorrhage set in again, when I left her the same prescription, and in less than 24 hours all was right. Since that time there has been no return, except at her catamenial periods, and then not excessive. I am now, (April, 1864,) treating her, with a prospect of success, for an ulcerated os tincæ. I also gave the same prescription as the foregoing to another lady who had suffered with uterine hæmorrhage about three-fourths of the time for several months. Some three months have since passed, and she now reports herself entirely rid of the trouble and regular. When I first employed the Apocynum, as above stated, I had seen no proving of that drug. In my own practice, however, I have seen enough of its pathogenesis to satisfy me that it is homœopathic to uterine hæmorrhage. On two different occasions, when I gave it to a lady past the turn of life, in doses of ten drops of the tincture three or four times a day, for ascites, it had not the slightest perceptible influence on that affection, but was followed in both instances, after a few days, by the return of the catamenial flow, very much in the natural manner. I also remember the case of a young girl, in whom the catamenia had ceased without any apparent cause. She still retained her health and usual appearance. After taking the medicine in pretty large doses for a few days, she was reported all "right." By the way, I would suggest that in cases where amenorrhœa depends not upon deranged health, but upon some strong revulsion diverting the female circulation into other channels, this remedy might be legitimately used, with the hope that by its primary effects it would restore the accustomed discharge, and break up the abnormal condition of things.

Larynx, Bronchia, and Chest.—Unpleasant sensation of heat about the fauces and larynx.—(*Freligh.*) Irresistible disposition to sigh. Short, dry, cough, and scanty expectoration of white mucus in the morning. Oppression of the chest on waking.—(*Marcy.*) Sense of oppression about the epigastrium and chest. It was difficult to breathe enough to speak at times.

Clinical Remarks.—Eclectic physicians use it constantly as an expectorant. They expect the same effects from it which the allopath gets from his Ipecac, Squills, or Tartar Emetic. It undoubtedly increases the natural secretions of the bronchial surfaces. Such hints may be made useful. It indicates that we may use it in *hoarse, loose coughs*, with heat of the fauces; or cough with oppression of the chest; or short, dry cough, with scanty expectoration. Accompanying hydrothorax, and even ascites, we generally find a short, dry cough with oppression, and in such cases Apocynum is doubly indicated, both for the cough and dropsy. It has cured many cases of hydrothorax, and relieved many cases of dropsy from heart disease. As it causes the pulse to be slow, it probably quiets the action of the heart—a very important desideratum in hydro-pericardium.

Back and Extremites.—Unusual heaviness of the head, with dull, aching pains in the small of the back and limbs. There was no tenderness of the region of the kidneys on pressure, but a slight soreness of the parts when bringing the muscles into action, thus indicating the muscles as the seat of the pains.—(*Marcy.*) Hard aching was felt several times in both knees, sufficiently severe to make me fear that an attack of inflammatory rhematism was coming on.

Clinical Remarks.—It may be found useful in some rheumatic affections, but probably more for the other effects, as œdema. In synovitis, after the acute stage has passed, it will probably help to cause absorption of the effused fluid. It has been found useful in œdema of the feet and ankles remaining after typhus.

ARUM TRIPHYLLUM.

(*Indian Turnip, Jack in the Pulpit.*)

The A. triphyllum of the United States corresponds closely with the A. maculatum of Europe; both have very similar effects. Our native species is found throughout North and South America, growing in rich, shady woods and swamps. The *cormus* is an inch or two in diameter, and covered with brown, wrinkled epidermis, and internally white, fleshy and solid. The whole plant, when recent, has a peculiar odor and violent acrid taste; the root, when chewed, causes an insupportable burning and biting sensation in the mouth and throat, continuing for a long time. This acrid principle is very volatile, and is expelled by heat. Hence they are roasted and ate by the Indians. The acrid portion is not imparted to water, ether, alcohol, or olive oil. By drying, the root loses all its activity. The medicinal qualities of the root reside principally in this acrid, volatile principle. Owing to its unstable nature, it will be found very difficult to procure any preparation in which it will be retained. I would recommend, as the most probable way of preserving this volatile principle, that the juice of the fresh root, be rapidly triturated with sugar of milk, (according to the decimal scale) and the trituration kept in bottles sealed hermetically, and guarded from the light and heat.

The acrid principle has been called *Aroine*, and becomes an inflammable gas, by heat or distillation. Prof. Lee says: "The only way to preserve the active principles of the root is to bury it in dry sand, by which method it may be preserved for a year."

General Effects.—"The Arum may well be ranked among our most active alterants, for besides being a powerful local irritant, when taken internally, it stimulates all the secretions, particularly those of the skin and lungs. It also quickens the circulation and rouses the nervous energy, so that there is no organ or function but feels its influence."—*Lee.*

"It has been advantageously given in asthma, pertussis, chronic catarrh, chronic rheumatism, and affections connected with a cachectic state of the system."— *Wood.*

The fresh root grated, or reduced to a pulp, with three times their weight of sugar, is palliative to flatulence, cramp in the stomach, asthmatic and consumptive affections; and also in lingering atrophy, debilitated habits, great prostration in typhoid fevers, deep seated rheumatic pains, etc."—*Rafinesque.*

All writers agree that it is a remedy which may be used to advantage as a *stimulant.*

We have no proving, except that which relates to its local effects upon the mouth and throat. Its analogues are *allium sativa,* and cepa, *phosphorus,* capsicum, etc.

General Symptoms.—The fresh root, in doses of four or five grains, causes a sensation of burning heat in the stomach and œsophagus, which seems rapidly to spread all over the body. Then follows a quickening of the circulation, heat of the skin with warm perspiration, and some exaltation of the nervous energy. All the secretions are somewhat increased.

LOCAL EFFECTS.-**Mouth, Throat, Tongue, etc.**—The fresh root, when chewed, causes an insupportable *burning* and *biting* sensation in the mouth and throat, continuing for a long time. The sensation experienced in the mouth, throat, and tongue is absolutely indescribable. I never felt any sensation so tormenting and unbearable. The following narrative of the effects of the Arum *maculatum,* copied from the British Journal, Vol. XVI., p. 321, so nearly resembles the effects of the Arum tryphyllum, as I have observed and felt them, as to be nearly identical: "After chewing a young leaf-stalk for a few seconds, a very intense, prickling, stinging pain was felt upon the tongue and mucous membrane of the lips and throat, accompanied with a flow of saliva, which seemed to relieve the pain a little—the pains were as if a hundred little needles had been run into the tongue and lips. A friend, who followed my example, had, in addition to these symptoms, constriction and burning in the larynx, his tongue was swollen, and its papilla injected and raised. The mucus membrane of the throat and lips was inflamed. The pains on the tongue and lips were increased by pressure with the teeth. In two or three cases the leaves have been eaten by children, and have produced very distressing effects. In one instance, three children partook of them. Their tongues became swollen, so as to render swallowing difficult, and convulsions followed: one died in twelve, and another in sixteen days; the third recovered." Some cases of dangerous poisoning have been reported, as occurring from eating the A. tryphyllum.

CLINICAL REMARKS.—Although the local effects of Arum are very notable, yet we have no clinical experience to show its practical usefulness in cases of disease effecting the mouth and throat. Dr. J. S. Douglas recommends it in Quinsy and Angina. Dr. Hill, in his Surgery, proposes it in similar affections. If we could preserve the volatile, acrid principle intact in our preparations, we might expect good results from its use, perhaps, in cases to which it is homœopathic. It is indicated in the following affections: *Glos-*

sitis, when the swelling is *rapid* and accompanied with prickling and burning pains. *Stomatitis*, in its most acute form, with great tumefaction of the lips, mucus membrane of the mouth, etc., followed by superficial ulceration. *Œdema of the Glottis.*—The symptoms of Arum-poisoning present many points of resemblance to this fearful disease. The rapid tumefaction of the tissues, the pains and many other local symptoms, are very similar. It may prove more useful than Apis, Belladonna or Rhus, but we cannot expect much from any preparation of the Arum, unless it contains the acrid principle mentioned. *Mercurial or Idiopathic Salivation*, in some of its forms, may be met with this remedy; also, *Inflammation of the mucus follicles* of the throat, with exudation of mucus, constant "hawking," and profuse secretion from the diseased tissues. Acute and Chronic *Catarrh* of the fauces and posterior nares, may come under the curative range of this remedy. It has been used with advantage in enlargement of the Tonsils.

Respiratory Organs.—The Arum has a time-honored reputation in *Coughs*. In *dry* coughs the *dried* root is valued highly. It promotes expectoration and mitigates the paroxysms, and has even cured some obstinate cases. In *loose* coughs, occurring in children and aged persons, when there is inability to expectorate the accumulated mucus, this medicine is said to act in a beneficial manner. In this respect it resembles Squills, Phosphorus, etc. *Asthma humidum* has been relieved and notably palliated by the powdered dry root. In all these affections the lower triturations of the dry root will be the best preparation.

This is one of those peculiar remedies which can never come into extensive use, because of the evanescent character of its effects, and the difficulty of making a thorough proving of it. Its sphere of action is limited, being but a faint analogue of its great prototype Phosphorus.

ASCLEPIAS SYRIACA.

(*Milk-Weed.*)

This milk-weed is one of our common plants, growing by roadsides and in dry sandy fields, from Canada to the Gulf of Mexico. The stem is simple, and from three to four feet high, surmounted by numerous umbels, or balls of flowers, of a pale, purple color. The leaves are oblong, lanceolate, petiolate, pointed at the end and whorled, the under surface covered with a short matted hair; segments of the corona, five; petals and sepals reflex; corona erect. The seeds are enclosed in oblong, pointed, rough pods of from two and a half to three inches in length; each seed is attached to a mass of long, silky fibres, which can be made into a beautiful thread. The whole plant yields an abundant milky juice.

This plant has not been used much in the dominant school, but several eclectic physicians have claimed to use it successfully in dropsy, colds, catarrhs, and lung affections. They call it expectorant, diaphoretic, alterative, anodyne, &c. In acute rheumatism, Prof. Lee says it bears a close resemblance to cimicifuga. Of six cases of acute rheumatism which he treated with asclepias syr., the average duration was eight days; the inflammation confined to the large joints, with considerable pain and swelling. It had a remarkable effect in relieving the pain.

Dr. Pattee, a progressive allopath, has made some physiological experiments with the plant, which may be considered as a good "fragmentary" proving. It is to be regretted that *all* the symptoms were not noted.

He says: "Two ounces of the cold infusion, made from the fresh root gathered after the leaves had fallen; taken once every 4 hours, proved *diuretic;* two oz. of the warm infusion, taken every 2 hours, proved *diaphoretic;* 15 drops of the saturated tincture, taken once every 3 hours, had well marked *alterative* (?) effects; and one drachm of the saturated tincture, repeated once every three hours, until 8 drachms were taken, cause *headache*, *drowsiness* and *sleep*. In all the experiments, it increased the bronchial secretion.

"The first experiment was made upon myself. The *urine* for three days immediately preceding the experiment was as follows:

35 oz. per day; specific gravity 1019.7; solid matter 568 gr.; pulse 68.

After 12 oz. had been taken the first day, the quantity of urine passed in that time was 128 oz.; specific gravity 1020; solid matter 600 gr.; pulse 67.

Second Day. There was but a small increase of water. The specific gravity and solid matter about the same; pulse 66.

Third Day. (Quantity of medicine same as preceding days). Quantity of urine 130 oz.; specific gravity 1019.97; solid matter 608 grs.; pulse 63.

On the 4th, 5th and 6th days, the quantity of urine passed averaged 135 oz. per day, and the amount of solid matter 700 grs. each day; pulse 60. The diet and exercise were not materially altered from what it had been for a month past. The medicine did not seem to cause any derangement of the health; the urinary organs were not *irritated* in any way; the only perceptible effect it had upon the brain was to cause a calm, quiet feeling, perhaps a little drowsiness towards night."

"The subject of the second experiment was a young man 18 years of age, of good health; pulse 75. At 9 P. M., gave him 3 oz. of warm infusion; the young man in bed; in half an hour commenced sweating; in an hour he was sweating profusely, and continued to do so the rest of the night, the infusion being given every two hours.

The effect it had upon the brain was an agreeable sensation

at first; after that had passed off he expressed himself as "awful sleepy." When he awoke the next morning, said he had "slept rather hard," but felt no inconvenience through the day.

It produced the same effect the following night. The third day, I gave him one dram of the saturated tincture, made from the dry root, one every three hours, commencing at 6 P. M. At 9 P. M., said his head felt a little dizzy, and had some headache; slept sound through the night; skin quite moist; passed 4 oz. more urine than usual, in the morning. After continuing this for four more days, had to discontinue it on account of the derangement it caused to the system; he had but little relish for food; appeared dull and stupid; bowels had moved oftener than usual; the tongue was covered with a white fur; pulse 64. In a few days he was well as ever."

"In cases where the pulse had been from 50 to 60, they have increased to 65 and 70. Large doses in any form will produce nausea, vomiting, and, in some instances, *ardor urinæ.* If the medicine *does not produce diaphoresis, diuresis, or catharsis, violent headache will sometimes ensue,* but when given in medical doses and for disease, we do not see much headache." (The italics are my own. I will refer to the subject hereafter.—*H.*)

If this experimenter had understood the value of recording the characteristic symptoms evolved by the medicine, we should have a much clearer view of its pathogenetic action. As it is, however, the fragment is a very suggestive one, and we may draw some really valuable conclusions from it. Arranged after the Hahnemannian method, the symptoms would stand as follows:

General Symptoms.—Sensation of calmness and quietude of the whole system. In rheumatism, its action was very favorable. It had a remarkable effect in relieving the pain.

Skin.—Profuse sweating all night (from the warm infusion); in a low state of typhus fever it has produced a moist state of the skin, when other diaphoretics had failed, and convalescence was at once established. The milky juice that exudes from the stalk has been used externally for warts. A poultice of the fresh root, boiled, has considerable reputation for the cure of carbuncles, felons, and boils. (No *specific* effect is here produced—a poultice of *ulmus fulva* would do as well.)

Sleep.—Calm, quiet feeling, with drowsiness towards night. Great sleepines, with profuse sweating; sensation in the morning on waking as if he had "slept hard."

Fever.—It does not seem to cause febrile symptoms, as a primary effect, but it is said to cause the pulse to rise from 50 to 70, with increased heat of skin, *when it does not* cause diuresis or diaphoresis.

CLINICAL REMARK.—It would seem indicated in cases of fever from suppressed perspiration; with scanty urine, headache, and pulse at 75.

Head.—The only perceptible effect it had upon the brain of one of the provers, was to cause a calm, quiet feeling, perhaps a little drowsiness towards night. The other prover said it caused "an agreeable sensation at first," afterwards sleepiness; vertigo, with headache. When the medicine does not cause diuresis or diaphoresis, *violent headache* will sometimes ensue; dull and stupid.

CLINICAL REMARKS.—From the above it would seem to be homœopathic to sleepiness, which has followed upon any excitement of the brain of an agreeable nature; also, *headache with vertigo*. But it promises to be most useful in those cephalalgias which occur after suppressed perspirations, or which arise from the retention of effete matters in the system which ought to have been carried off through the skin or kidneys. It will certainly prove useful in nervous headaches, which are followed by profuse diuresis; in this respect it resembles ignatia, pulsatilla and gelseminum. Headache with dullness and stupidity.

Gastric Symptoms, etc.—Tongue covered with a *white* fur; had but little relish for food; bowels moved oftener than usual; diarrhœa with persistent nausea, and with vomiting.

Kidneys, etc.—The following table will best illustrate its action upon these emunctories:

	Quantity of Urine.	Specific Gravity.	Total Solids.	Increase of Urine.	Increase of Solids.
Normal Standard	33 oz.	1019.7	568 gr.		
Asclepias Syriaca					
First Day	128 oz.	1020	600 gr.	63 gr.	32 gr.
Third Day	130 oz.	1020	608 gr.	95 gr.	40 gr.
Fourth, Fifth and Sixth Days	135 oz.	1020	700 gr.	100 gr.	132 gr.

By this it will be seen that the asclepias syr. notably increases the *solid* matters of the urine. This is an important fact, for from the careful experiments of Dr. Hammond (Hammond's Physiological Memoirs), it appears that colchicum actually increases the organic and inorganic solids of the urine, while digitalis, squills and juniper increase *only* the inorganic matter. Now, as it is the *organic* matter which is generally considered as contaminating the blood in disease, it is evident they (digitalis, squills and juniper) exert no effect whatever in depurating the blood, but on the contrary are positively injurious.

CLINICAL REMARKS.—*Asclepias syriaca* then, is a congener of colchicum, and as such must be found useful in many diseases in which the latter drug has been successfully used.

In *Scarlatina*, when the head symptoms correspond, it may prove a useful auxiliary remedy.

In *Scarlatinal Dropsy*, I predict it will be found as useful as colchicum (which I have found one of our most important remedies), apis, apocynum, hellebore or arsenicum.

It is now fully established that the dropsy, which follows scarlet fever is caused by the scarlatinal poison which, in its passage into and through the kidneys, sets up an "acute desquamative nephritis."

Dr. Todd ("Urinary Diseases," page 120) says: "There are three conditions, which I imagine gives rise to the production of the dropsy. These are: 1st, a peculiar irritated state of the kidneys; 2d, an analogous morbid state of the skin; and, 3d, a certain depravity of the blood—by which I mean not only a deficiency in the amount of red corpuscles of that fluid, as well as of the solids of the serum, but also the unnatural presence of certain *poisonous matters* which interfere with its proper nutrient changes."

It is this "poisonous matter which irritates the skin and kidneys and causes the dropsy."

Now, it will be recollected, that the asclepias syr. causes "violent headache, increased rate of pulse, vertigo, dullness and stupor," when it did *not* cause *diuresis* or *perspiration*. That is, when the impression which the drug, after pouring into the blood, caused upon the nervous centres, did not react upon the kidneys and skin; the *brain* felt the force of the medicinal action. (Similar conditions occur from the use of alcohol.) Also, when the scarlatinal poison in the blood, is not carried off through the kidneys or skin, the brain and nervous system suffers, and convulsions more or less fatal ensue.

Asclepias syriaca, seems to be a more rational remedy for this condition than any other, not even excepting colchicum, and I predict that its use in scarlatinal dropsy will bear me out in my belief. It will also relieve, I think, those rheumatic pains which often occur after that disease. I would advise the patient to be placed in bed, and this remedy administered as follows: a few drops of the 2nd, 1st, or even the mother tincture, in an ounce of *warm* sweetened water; the dose repeated every hour, until the skin and kidneys begin to act *normally*. (Apis, Hellebore, Apocyc, or Colchicum, should be given in the same manner.) If more convenient, give a weak warm infusion—1 dram of the root to 1 pint water.

In Dropsy, especially when arising from suppressed perspiration, or some forms of renal disease, it will be useful. We do not know what are the peculiar pathological changes which it can cause in the kidneys, and we are equally ignorant of the pathological effects of Apis, Apoc. c. and most of our best remedies for dropsy. But it may be considered a general rule, that *a drug* which *primarily causes diuresis, will secondarily cause dropsy*. In proof of this, we may cite the provings of Canth., Apocynum c., Arsenicum, Apis., and all the so-called diuretics. They first excite the kidneys to *abnormal* action; then the reaction follows, and we have *suspension* of function, and consequent effusion.

Asclepias syr. then is truly homœopathic to renal dropsy. *Dr. Pattee* says: "It has in my hands certainly proved useful in the removal of dropsical effusions. *Dr. Smith* relates the case of a man of 80, who had general dropsy, caused by taking cold; he was enormously swollen; he commenced taking 2 oz of the cold infusion every two hours; in 24 hours he had passed over three gallons of water, and in a week, all the dropsical symptoms had disappeared."

I once treated a case of general dropsy from disease of the heart. In the advanced stages, after all the usual remedies had one after the other failed to give relief, I resorted to the Asclepias syr.; not having any tincture, I ordered an infusion—1 oz. to a quart of water—the fresh root was used; a tablespoonful of this preparation was given every two hours. Under its use the urine increased to nearly a gallon a day, and the breathing was much relieved. The patient was made comfortable by its use for many weeks, but finally died of the cardiac disease.

Dr. Pattee says, in large doses it will produce *ardor urinæ.*" The persistent use of small doses will have the same effect; in fact, all "diuretic" medicines have the same effect. By the continued irritation which they keep up in the urinary organs, inflammation is finally induced. This inflammation may lead on to organic disease, and consequent anasarca. Here we have the foundation for a general rule, viz.: *That all diuretics are secondarily homœopathic to the various forms of renal dropsy.*

Uterus, etc. In the case of dropsy from heart-disease, referred to above; the patient's menses had not appeared for 4 months; she showed no signs of pregnancy; indeed, it was deemed impossible, that such condition could exist. Such was the general œdema that no vaginal examination could be made.

About 24 hours after she commenced the use of the Asclepias syr.; and after diuresis had set in, she was taken with severe labor-like pains; pressing down from small of the back to the hypogastrium, with a scanty discharge of pale red blood. These pains increased with each dose, but disappeared a few hours after suspending the medicine. Upon resuming it, the pains again appeared. The experiment was tried several times with similar results. In her feeble state, it was not deemed prudent to carry the experiment further.

Clinical Remarks.—In this case, whether pregnancy was present or not, the Asclepias syr. manifested a decided specific action upon the uterus. It caused *intermitting*, bearing-down, labor-like pains, which but few drugs will do. (Macrotis, Caulophyllum, Uva ursi.) The uterine pains caused by Ergot, Tanacetum, and others of that class are more constant, *remitting.*

In domestic use it has some reputation as an emmenegogue, and abortivant. It has been employed in dysmenorrhœa and amenorrhœa by eclectic physicians with alleged success.

The above experiment would go to show, that it was homœopathic to dysmenorrhœa and threatened abortion. Especially when there is copious discharge of urine. Dysmenorrhœa is often accompanied by diuresis, in which case this remedy would be perfectly indicated.

ASCLEPIAS TUBEROSA.

(*Pleurisy Root.*)

The root of this variety of Asclepias is perennial, and gives origin to numerous stems which are erect, ascending, or procumbent, round, hairy, of a green or reddish color, branching at the top, and about 18 inches in height. (It rarely exceeds this, although it is stated to be *three* feet by some authorities.) The leaves are scattered, oblong-lanceolate, very hairy, of a deep rich green color on their upper surface, paler beneath, and supported usually on short foot stalks. The flowers are of a beautiful reddish-orange color, and disposed in terminal or lateral corymbose umbels. The fruit is an erect, lanceolate follicle, with flat ovate seeds, connected to a longitudinal receptacle by long silky hairs. This plant differs from other species of Asclepias in not emitting a milky juice when wounded. It flourishes from Massachusetts to Georgia, and when in full bloom, in the months of June and July, exhibits a splendid appearence. The root is the part used in medicine. This is large, irregularly tuberous, branching, often somewhat fusiform; externally brown, internally white and striated, and in the recent state, of a sub-acid nauseous taste. When dried it is easily pulverized, and has a bitter, but not otherwise unpleasant taste.

It is considered by the eclectic school and others to be diaphoretic and expectorant, and in large doses cathartic. It is employed in regular practice and domestic use, in catarrh, pneumonia, pleurisy and consumption. It is held in high estimation in dysentery, rheumatism, and in cardialgia from flatulence or indigestion.

The following proving, if such it can be called, was communicated to the Jour. de la Societe Gallicana de Med. Hom. by A. Savery, M. D., who, it seems was a pupil of Dr. B. Mure, of Brazilian provings "notoriety."

I insert the "proving," in order that no accusation of unjust bias can be made against me. At the same time I must enter my honest protest against the manner in which the experiment was made; and state my conscientious belief of the utter worthlessness of the proving. I will state the grounds of my objections.

Only *two* drops of the tincture was taken; no repetition of the dose was made, and *all* the symptoms, sensations, &c., felt by the prover, for the ensuing *forty* days were recorded. It is stated that at the commencement of the proving, the prover was sufferring from irritation of the *respiratory* organs and *stomach.*

Now when we consider that the Asclepias is a mild, unirritating medicine, except in large doses, much milder in its action than Ipecac, or Apocynum; that in domestic practice it is common for those having catarrhs, fever, or any simple ailment, to drink a pint of the decoction, and feel no other effects than gentle diaphoresis, and complain of no *after* symptoms; that eclectic physicians use it in almost every disease, in large doses of the fluid extract, or even the active principle *asclepin,* and note no bad effects; and finally, when I state that I have taken the tincture in 10 and 20 drop doses four times a day and never noticed any unpleasant effects—any such symptoms as Savery records, it seems incredible that the long list of serious symptoms should be caused by only *two* drops of the tincture.

We must remember, too, the admission that the experimenter had "respiratory and gastric irritation," when he took the first dose, and this alone should lead us to look with suspicion upon the proving.

It is with a good deal of hesitation that I have admitted this "proving" into the volume, for it is a very grave and important matter to give a proving, which may be instrumental in determining the life or death of a patient.

Suppose the proving of Veratrum alb. had been unreliable and false? How many thousands of cholera patients would have gone down to the grave without an administration of the proper remedial specific. We hold in our hands, oftentimes, the lives of our patients, and it behooves us to be solemnly conscientious in the selection of those remedies which we use at the bedside of the sick. We should neither be swayed, by theory, prejudice, or the *dictum* of other men, but carefully weigh the value of a pathogenesis by the light of reason and experience.

I copy the proving as it was translated and arranged by Dr. Rhees, and published in the Amer. Hom. Review, vol. 2, and will not offer any clinical remarks of my own *with this* proving, but let it stand by itself, and if any physician sees fit to accept the pathogenesis as a reliable one, let him do so upon his own responsibility. The symptoms enumerated bear some resemblance to those which have been cured by asclepias tuberosa; but throwing aside all other circumstances, this proving should be substantiated by others before it could be received. I fully agree with Prof. Small, that the true test of the reliability of all provings is the multiplicity of experiments. If they all evolve the same or similar symptoms, we cannot hesitate to accept them. (The numerals indicate the days after taking the medicine.)

DR. SAVERY'S PROVING.

General Symptoms.—Sensation of numbness in the whole body. Excessive weakness in the morning in bed. Walking seems impossible. Sensation while walking as if he run but forward toward the left side. Aching in the bones, and rheumatic pains in the extremities, principally in the joints; those pains appear in one arm and in the opposite leg at the same time; thus if the left arm is affected the right leg suffers in sympathy, and the left leg with the right arm; this circumstance was almost constant. Quivering and twitching of the muscles in different parts; emaciation.

Skin.—Pimples, vesicles or pustules began to appear on the 15th day, and spread gradually over almost the whole body, but particularly on the arms, legs, and in the face; they are very painful and itch excessively, and continue more than eight days. A red inflamed spot on the upper part of the right thigh, as large as a dollar, painful and itching, continuing several days, and leaving a dark stain (23). Many vesicles on the lips (23). Pock-like pustules on the arms.

Clinical Remarks.—We believe it be a powerful anti-psoric, useful for cutaneous eruptions.—Savery.

Sleep.—Difficult and late sleep at night, with great sleepiness in the morning, and through the day. Confused and anxious dreams.

Fever.—Feverish the first day, the pulse being at first 55, afterwards 70. Sometimes much thirst, sometimes none. On the eighth day, pulse 92. Pulse thready, 65, during diarrhœa.

Mind and Sensorium.—Excessive dejection (15). Weakness of memory (2). Difficulty of thinking, collectedly. Feeling of drunkenness after smoking very little, with weakness of vision.

Head.—Pain in the forehead with a feeling of heaviness in the side, continuing the whole day, (1). Headache is present almost daily, generally more severe early in the morning. Headache in the morning, while rising, with weakness, that he must lie down again; it continued the whole day, and all the following night, (7). Pricking as with nails in the head, and at the same time in other parts, (2). Pains in the scalp, in the left side of the occiput, like touching a pustule, (16). Falling of the hair, (39).

Clinical Remarks.—It has proved useful in Cephalalgia; gastric headaches, neuralgias.—S.

Eyes.—Transitory pain behind the left eyeball, in a few minutes. Broad dark spots before the eyes, with slow pulse of 55, (1). Itching in the angles and lids of the right eye, (3). Inflammation of the conjunctiva for many days; (this, however, is not an unusual symptom with the prover). Pain in the eyes, by gaslight. The eyes look lanquid and fatigued. Feeling as if sand were in the eyes. The lower lids are painful as if ulcerated.

Face.—Yellowness of the face, (15) Facies hippocratica (after violent diarrhœa on the 15th day). Yellow coating on the teeth. Pain in the right inferior molars, (24).

Mouth.—Itching of the lips. Lips inflamed and covered with herpetic vesicles. Gums very pale and almost yellow; they bleed easily and repeatedly. Yellow, tough coating on the tongue, putrid taste.

Pharynx.—Transitory constriction and stinging in the throat, extending to the larynx, (1). Pains in the throat. Soreness of the throat, (26).

Appetite, &c.—Deficient appetite, especially in the morning, insatiable hunger, (2). Eructations on the first day, less frequent on the second. Nausea in the morning on rising, (17). Taste of blood in the mouth.

Stomach.—Burning in the stomach (after 25 minutes). Pains in the stomach; nervous, even amounting to violent gastralgia; also cramp-like. Sensation as if the stomach would burst, while laughing. The pains in the stomach continue, almost without a day's intermission until the 42nd day.

Clinical Remark.—Gastralgia.—S.

Abdomen.—Throbbing in the left hypochondria. Pains in the intestines, (after 20 minutes) subsequently attended with burning in the right hypochondriac region and stomach. Much flatulence, smelling like the medicine, with colic-like pains, with a sensation when walking as if the belly would drop. Violent pain in the hypogastrium as if the region were ulcerated with tenderness to pressure. Colic, while going up stairs; while walking; after one o'clock, (8-14) and also in the morning, during each stool.

Clinical Remarks.—It is indicated and useful in enteritis. (Jaundice), etc. Savery.

Stool.—Fluid, painful stool (2) of very strong smell (37). Clammy stool, of green color, and smelling like spoiled eggs, followed by pain in the arms. On the 14th day, at 1 o'clock at night, a painful and copious stool with violent colic, and a sensation as though the bowels would come out; half an hour afterwards, small but very painful stool; at 2 o'clock the same kind of stool, but with increased pain, (Verat. 8, relieved the pain). At 11 o'clock, another stool almost black in color, clammy, with many ascarides, and yellow spots like fat, attended with a feeling as if a stream of fire passed through the abdomen. In the afternoon, a stool of intense yellow color, with green and yellow flakes. In the evening, a stool exactly like the white of an egg, with no fœcal matter whatever. The following day the fœces are entirely enveloped in froth. Tenesmus.

Clinical Remarks.—We have found it curative in acute enteritis; and it is indicated in dysentery, diarrhœa, etc. *

Urine.—During the first 12 days the urine is red to saturation. On the 17th day it looks as if mixed with blood; after standing a short time, small, dark red, almost black points of the size of a pin's head rise on the surface, and much mucus is deposited on the bottom of the vessel. The urine is more red than normal all the time.

Male and Sexual Organs.—Painful stitches in the urethra, repeatedly. Ulcerous excoriations on the glans, resembling chancre, with a pus-like secretion, (disappearing in a few days from washing in urine.) [The prover had chancre 10 years ago. One year ago, while proving this medicine, on the 3d day a chancre appeared on the left side of the prepuce, then on the right, lasting two days. Copious perspiration of the genitals.

Clinical Remarks.—We have employed this medicine with uniform success in constitutional syphilis, and it is indicated in venereal diseases. *

Catarrhal.—At first dry, then fluent coryza during the first few days, with much sneezing. Subsequently a blowing out of some blood from one nostril for several days.

Clinical Remarks.—It may prove useful in asthma and affections of the nose. *

Larynx and Chest, Heart.—Pain in the larynx. The breath smells like pepper. Necessity to inspire hurriedly, followed by a sensation of oppression. Want of breath like asthma, often very great, particularly after eating and smoking. Pain in the right lung. Pricking pain in the region of the heart. Contracting pain in the heart.

Clinical Remarks.—We have employed it successfully in cases of phthisis and asthma. It seems indicated in carditis. *

Back and Extremities.—Stinging, transitory stitches between the shoulder blades. Pain in the loins like lumbago. Pain in left shoulder, soon after, in the right, like rheumatism. Pain in bones of left arm. Rheumatic pain in fore arm down to fingers. Numbness of right hand. Violent itching in hands and fingers. Pain in hips like coxalgia. Rending pain in knees up to the hips, when walking and rising. The ankle feel as if sprained. Pain in bones of left ankle, drawing in soles and in the toes. Violent itching on the legs up to the knees.

Clinical Remarks.—It seems to be indicated in articular rheumatism and bone pains. Lumbago, &c. *

Remarks.—It is to be regreted that the foregoing experiment was not conducted differently. Had the dose (2 drops) been repeated every 4 or 6 hours, and other persons joined in the proving, something reliable might have been evolved; but in this case we are at a loss to know whether any of the symptoms resulted from the medicine, or whether the "gastric and respiratory irritation" which the prover had when he commenced, was not the cause of the long array of symptoms.

I am free to admit that the symptoms of the stomach, chest and bowels, are similar to those which I know to be caused by asclepias tuberosa, but we should have further provings before we blindly accept this one. I will briefly mention the conditons for which I have prescribed the asclepias tub. with apparent benefit.

Generally, it is very appropriate in diseases of children. In this respect it resembles Ipecac, also in asthmatic persons, and those subject to catarrhal affections; and many diseases which owe their origin to cold and damp weather.

(a.) It is useful in the coughs and colds of children; in a loose rattling cough with difficulty of breathing; in those nasal catarrhs which children suffer from ("snuffles"). I have known a child cured of hoarse croupy cough, tightness of breathing, and fever with hot but *moist* skin, by half a teaspoonful of weak infusion, administered by the mother, every hour; no vomiting or nausea was caused. (The dose in this case was about equal to a drop of the 1-10 dilution.) I once treated a case of pleurisy in a child 12 years of age with *Asclepias t.* 2nd; the symptoms were much pain of a cutting character in the left side, during inspiration; some dyspnea, fever, and hacking cough. No other medicine was given and on the fifth day the patient was convalescent.

Such confidence have the country people in this remedy, that I have known parents treat their children for catarrhal fever, pneumonias, etc., with this plant, giving it in warm infusion, rather than run the risk of placing them under the care of allopathic physicians. It is not necessary to induce its nauseant action, in order to get its beneficial influence on the organs of respiration. This fact the eclectic school now acknowledge, as does the allopathic school in relation to Ipecac and Tartar emetic. There is certainly a large amount of testimony in favor of the specific action of Asclepias tuberosa, upon the respiratory organs. We will quote some of the most important authorities.

Dr. Wood says, "it has long been employed in catarrh, pneumonia, pleurisy, consumption and other pectoral affections, and appears to be decidedly useful if applied in the early stages.

Dr. Bigelow writes, "I am satisfied of its utility as an expectorant medicine, and have seen no inconsiderable benefit arise from its use as a palliative in *phthisis*.

Dr. Beach declares, "its action on the lungs is specific, assisting suppressed expectoration, and relieving the difficult breathing of patients who are laboring under attacks of pleurisy, which circumstance has obtained for it one of its popular names." It relieves difficulty of breathing in general, together with pains in the chest.

Several writers have stated that they "have used it in many cases of pleurisy and pneumonia with the most marked advantage, and this too, in nearly every stage of these complaints. * * It not only operates favorably as a diaphoretic, but is an expectorant of trancendent value, invariably increasing the freedom of breathing, and exerts a specific control over inflammation of the thoracic viscera." "It has been used with benefit in asthma," etc.

(b.) I have found it useful in vomiting of mucus, and gastic debility. *Pro. Lee* says, "It is useful in atonic dyspepsia, restoring tone to the stomach, and relieving gastric pains and flatulence." Any drug which is capable of causing irritation of the stomach, induces weakness of that organ; deranges the digestive function, and thence dyspepsia. *Asclepias tub.* then cures this condition in small doses because it causes it in large.

(c.) In the colic from flatulence, or from intestinal irritation, in children or adults, or in catarrhal diarrhœa, this remedy will be found useful. In this respect it resembles Chamomilla. I have found it useful in the dysenteries occurring in the autumn months, when the nights are cold and damp. Dr. Parker, of Mass., employed it for 25 years in dysentery, and had the greatest confidence in its powers. I have known it to cure in a few hours, severe rheumatic pains from a cold, with chilliness alternating with heat. I have generally used the tincture in doses of two or three drops, or the 1st or 2d dil., in same doses. I have no doubt but the higher dilutions would act equally well especially in young children.

BAPTISIA TINCTORIA.

(*Wild Indigo. Horsefly-Weed.*)

This plant is indigenous, growing in most part of the United States, in dry and poor soils, in woods and on hills. It blooms in July and August, having bright yellow flowers, in small loose clusters at the end of the branches. It resembles a shrub, and grows from one to two feet high. The fruit is an oblong pod of a bluish black color. It contains indigo, tannin, an acid, and baptisin. When the whole plant or any portion of it is dried, it becomes black and affords a blue dye, inferior to Indigo. In some parts of the country the young shoots are used as a substitute for asparagus, to which they bear some resemblance, and they occasionally cause drastic purgation, especially if eaten after they assume a green color. Alcohol and water will take up its active properties. Its medicinal virtues reside principally in the bark of the root. This agent promises fair to become one of our most powerful and valuable polychrets. We have several provings of it, made by Drs. Burt, Hill, Douglas, Thompson and others. But the proving of Dr. W. H. Burt, is the most thorough and suggestive. Dr. B. is one of the most correct and enthusiastic provers in the homœopathic ranks. Eclectic writers utter their usual indefinite phrases, in relation to this agent. Without any clear idea of its physiological action, they assert it to be anti-septic, astringent, tonic, emetic, cathartic and alterative. One only wonders that they did not use all the rest of the terms found in Materia Medica. Not a few of that school consider it a "febrifuge," and many deem it to be powerfully "depressant" in its action over the nervous and vascular systems, while King says it is a "stimulant." It is only by a study of the general and special symptoms elicited by our provings, that we can arrive at any correct conclusion as to its real effects upon the healthy organism. There is one property which the physicians of the eclectic school allege the Baptisia to possess, which should command our attention and investigation. I allude to its asserted *anti-septic* power. Applied in the form of a wash, to ulcers, mucous surfaces, etc., when there is a tendency to putrescency of the fluids and solids, gangrenes, fœtid discharges, etc., it is said to correct the conditions alluded to, in a very prompt manner. It is therefore advised in "malignant sore mouth and throat, mercurial sore mouth, scrofulous or syphilitic ophthalmia, erysipelatous ulcers," etc. My experience, and that of some of my colleagues in the homœopathic school, would seem to verify some of these assertions. Its action seems to be somewhat analogous to the chlorine compounds.

General Symptoms.—"If given in very large doses it causes a very disagreeable prostration of the whole system."—(*King.*) Lying in one position for a few minutes, as upon the back, caused the sacral region to become exceedingly painful, as though I had lain on the hard floor all night, and inducing the conviction that a short continuance of the same position, would cause bed sores. When turning on the other side, the same sensation was produced on the hips, obliging me at last to turn on my face to relieve those parts. (D) (Arnica causes the same symptom, and it is very commonly met with in typhoid fever.—*Hale.*) Intolerance of pressure on all parts upon which pressure was made. Felt weak and tremulous, as though recovering from a fit of sickness. Incapable of making any vigorous mental or physical exertion. An indescribable sick feeling all over, with great languor. Stiffness of all the joints as though strained. Rheumatic pains and soreness all over the body.

Clinical Remarks.—All these symptoms, indicate clearly that the Baptisia is an analogue of Rhus, Mercury, and even some of the "nervous-sedatives." It powerfully lowers the vitality of the organism.

Characteristic Symptoms.—All the symptoms increased by taking a glass of beer. The pains are of a pressive, drawing character; aggravated by motion, relieved by rest and excitement. The right side of the body is most affected.

Nervous System.—The hands felt large and were tremulous, with a peculiar thrilling sensation through both hands and feet, somewhat like "going to sleep," a want of circulation. Intolerance of pressure on all parts of the body—it caused soreness. (D) Arms and legs tremble. Numb sensations all over the body. Sensation of paralysis of the eye-lids. The *general* action of the Baptisia, upon the nervous system, is that of a *sedative.* It seems to cause a degree of paralysis, both of sensation and motion. In this it resembles Rhus, Aconite and Gelseminum. It may cause a peculiar *erethism*, of the nervous system, but this condition is due to *debility* and not *stimulation.*

Lymphatic System.—Swelling of the inguinal glands. Swelling of the tonsils.—(*Burt.*) Like Mercury and Phytolacca, the Baptisia seems to stimulate or rather *irritate*, the glandular system. Allopathic writers decree that Mercury is a stimulant to the lymphatic and glandular system, although it depresses all the other functions of organic life. This is the general belief of the adherents of that school. It is not a *healthy* stimulation, but rather an *irritatiou.* Phytolacca and Baptisia have the same action. They are therefore homœopathic: *primarily*, to irritation of the glandular system, and *secondarily:* to indolent atonic states of that system. It may be as well in this place to quote the testimony of eclectic writers, as to the specific action of Baptisia upon the glands. "It acts powerfully upon the glandular systems, increasing all the glandular secretions. The leaves applied in fomentations have discussed tumors and swelling of the female breast, resembling schirrus."—(*King.*) "It has been used with advantage as a deobstruent, in visceral obstructions and engorgements." (J. & S. Mat. Med.) "Baptisia is a sure and powerful *alterative*, and may be employed with confidence in all affections of the glandular system. In scrofula and cutaneous disorders few remedies are more beneficial."—(*Coe.*) I have khown it used in phagadenic ulcerations of glands with excellent results. In several cases of ulceration of the tonsils, after scarlatina, or in diphtheria, it has, in my hands, surpassed my expectations. I used it both internally and locally.

Mucous Membranes.—By examining its special effects as recorded in the proving, it will be seen that the Baptisia causes ulcerations, of many mucous surfaces, particularly of the buccal cavity. In this respect it resembles Mercurius, Nitric acid, Phytolacca, and Cornus cir. It is specifically indicated in discharges from mucous surfaces having a fœtid odor, and a sanious excoriating character. The particular indications for its use will be given under appropriate headings.

Vascular System, Fever, etc.—Feeling of greatly increased compass and frequently of the pulsations of the heart; pulsations seem to fill the chest; the pulse (usually but little over 70) 90, full and soft. Uncomfortable burning heat of the whole surface, especially the face. Tongue felt dry, smarted and felt sore, as if burnt. The heat compelled me to move to a cool part of the bed, and finally to rise and open a window, and wash my face aud hands;

with these symptoms there was a peculiar feeling of the head, which is never felt except during the presence of fever; a sort of excitement of the brain which is the preliminary, or rather beginning of delirium. For a short time, slight febrile, chilly horripulations on the lower limbs and back. (D) Burning sensation over the body, followed by perspiration, vomiting, and diarrhœa with dark stools, debility slow, round, full pulse. (Beckwith.) Thirst and flashes of heat over the face. General heat after going to bed. Heat and burning in the lower extremities, so intense as to prevent sleep. Chill all day with fever at night, with rheumatic pains and soreness all over the body. Pulse at first accelerated; afterwards became very low and faint. Surface of the body chilly.

Clinical Remarks.—The careful investigator, cannot fail to be struck with the evident fact, that Baptisia, if long continued in large doses, would be capable of inducing a condition of the blood similar to the "typhus crasis"; and a state of the fluids of the body, nearly identical with that occurring in low fevers. Its action on the nervous system also would tend to set up a typhoid erethism, and its effects upon mucous surfaces would indicate its power to cause those peculiar intestinal lesions which constitute the characteristic of typhoid fever. Before giving the experience of our school in the use of Baptisia in fevers, I will present the testimony of eclectic physicians. *King* says it is indicated in typhus, and all cases when there is a tendency to putrescency. He uses it in the low stage of typhoid fever, and in all typhoid conditions, occuring in other diseases. *Jones* asserts, that it has been used successfully in cases of typhoid and typhus fever, whenever there is a tendency to putrescency. It is resorted to by eclectic practitioners in low fevers, with the same confidence, that we administer the mineral acids, Rhus, Bryonia, etc. Under its use, they claim that the disease is materially shortened in duration, and robbed of its intensity; but they unluckily compound it so often with other drugs, that we must look to homœopathic authority for clear proof of its usefulness. The following cases, related by Dr. Hoyt, in the North Amer. Jour. Vol. 6, p. 226, were the first to bring the Baptisia to the notice of the profession. It was used by many physicians however, before the cases alluded to were published: *Case* 1.—Mrs. C. was taken with typhus fever, and treated allopathically. She became so reduced that her life was despaired of, and after the continuation of the fever for thirty-one days, as a last resort, Mr. C. prepared a decoction of the Baptisia; taking a piece of the root about three inches long, and ⅝th inches thick, steeping it in ½ pint of water. He commenced by giving her 5 or 6 drops of the decoction once in 15 minutes, increasing till he gave nearly a teaspoonful at a dose. In about one and one-half hours the surface of the patient presented an appearance as though she had been literally scalded, so red was the skin, accompanied with a most intense superficial heat; at the same time noticing large drops of sweat standing on he forehead, the medicine was discontinued. In a few moments a profuse perspiration appeared all over the body, which continued for nearly 12 hours, or till she was bathed freely with brandy and water. From this time she began to improve, and with the occasional administration of a drop or two of the remedy, got well, without any febrile symptoms. It is worthy of remark that immediately upon the administration of the remedy she became quiet and fell asleep; she had been restless and delirious for three weeks previous. *Cases* 2 and 3.—Mr. and Mrs. S. being very unwell, I was called, and found them suffering with symptoms of continued fever. After prescribing Aconite, Rhus tox, etc., without much effect, and my patients growing rapidly worse, I was induced to use the Baptisia in decoction, as in Case 1. I remained to watch the operation of my remedy. To my great surprise in about an hour, the perspiration appeared upon the foreheads of my patients, and it gradually covered the entire surface. In about six hours they were thoroughly bathed with tepid water, and the next morning scarce a vestige of the fever remained, and a rapid recovery followed. *Case* 4.—Mr. R. was taken with typhus fever, and had the usual homœopathic remedies for several days. An unfavorable prognosis was given, and the Baptisia was decided upon. It was administered and its effects watched. In this case, drop doses of an alcoholic tincture were used. The fever was reduced more than one-half in a few hours, and by a continuation of the remedy he was saved. A fierce delirium was present in this case, but it rapidly gave way under the action of the medicine." Several other cases of undoubted typhoid fever have been reported as *arrested*, by the use of Baptisia. Indeed some physicians are so enthusiastic that they assert its power to "break up" a continued fever, in any of its stages. Were it necessary to substantiate the value of Baptisia in continued fevers, with typhoid symptoms, I could record the testimony of scores of homœopathic physicians, who have related their successful experience with this remedy. I have used it for nearly six years in my practice, and consider it equally important with Rhus, Phosphoric acid, and Arsenicum, when indicated. The following are, in brief, the characteristic indications for its use: Chilliness all day; heat at night; chilliness with soreness of the whole body; heavy, dull, bruised sensation in the head, stupefying headache, confusion of ideas, delirium at night, heavy sleep with frightful dreams, dry red tongue, or brown coated tongue, sticky mouth, fœtid breath, fœtid sweat, and great fœtor of the discharges, (urine and stool), great debility and nervous prostration with erethism; ulcerations of a bad character, etc. I usually use the mother tincture, or the lower dilutions a few drops in water, every one, two, or three hours. It acts well, when alterated with phosphoric or muriatic acid, and may be used with benefit in nearly all the stages of a typhoid, and even in the premonitory or forming stage. I am certain, that its timely use has prevented the establishment of the fever, if given when the first symptoms of languor, chilliness and soreness of the whole body begin to appear. It is doubtful if Baptisia is indicated in all *fevers*. It is one of the misfortunes of all schools of medicine, that when a new remedy comes up, it is seized upon by certain enthusiastic members of the profession, and they, losing sight of its specific indications, proceed to laud it in the most extravagant terms, as a panacea in all diseases. This has been the case with several new remedies lately introduced in the homœopathic materia medica. *Rumex crispus*, a really valuable remedy for pulmonary affections; an analogue of Phosphorus; was so highly lauded, that physicians, not finding it equal to the task of curing every kind of cough, threw it aside, and is now too much neglected. Some practitioners like Dr. Wolf, have gone stark mad about *Apis mel.*; others upon Aconite, Gelseminum and Atropine. Such has been the fate of Baptisia. Dr. Hill, does not hesitate to recommend it in nearly every type and variety of fever. (See "Epitome.") This wholesale recommendation, has been an injury to the reputation of the medicine, and indirectly an injury to our school, and our patients. The range of action of Baptisia is as limited as any other fever-remedy. It may sometimes be indicated in *catarrhal*, *bilious*, *rheumatic*, or *congestive* fevers; occasionally in the exanthematous fevers, when they assume an adynamic type; *but only when the symptoms and conditions resemble those caused by the medicine.*

Mind.—Restless, uneasy, frightful dreams—gloomy and cast down for several days."—(*Burt.*) "Troublesome dreams, mental excitement bordering on delirium." Indisposition and want of power to think; unhappy; mind seems weak. (D.)

CLINICAL REMARKS.—The above symptoms are similar to those which precede a typhoid fever. I have often given the Baptisia one-tenth in these premonitory states, with the apparent effect of preventing the establishment of the fever.

Sleep.—"Slept two or three hours and waked with difficult breathing, a kind of night-mare, dreams of laboring hard in the snow, suffering with heat from the exertion and finally being smothered in the snow; unusually sound sleep, dreams about fighting and disputation, always come off second best."—(*Douglas.*) Drowsy, stupid, tired feeling. Very restless after midnight. Restless night with frightful dreams. Restless until 2 A. M., then sleep with frightful dreams. (B.) Dreamed of being bound down with a chain across the mouth.

CLINICAL REMARKS.—The symptoms above noted bear a close resemblance to those occurring in typhoid fevers. The restless nights, with delirium, and frightful dreams, all point to its specific applicability in many low fevers.

Head.—"Feeling as if the skin of the forehead would be drawn to the back part of the head, great tightness of the skin of the forehead, with pain in the right eye, frequent pressive pain in the right temple. Sharp pains in both temples, dull pressive pain in the forehead, feeling as if the forehead would be pressed in, dull heavy, pressive headache, very much aggravated by motion. Feeling as if the head was too heavy, numb feeling of the head and face."—(*Dr. Burts Proving.*) Dullness of head. Vertigo. Confused feeling in the head, swimming sensation very like that one experiences before the operation of an *emetic.*" (*Dr. Thomson's proving, N. A. J. Vol. V. page* 547. "Peculiar feeling of the head, which is never felt, except during the presence of fever, excitement of the brain, such as precedes *delirium*. Dull feeling in the occiput with slight pain and fullness, vessels of head full, head feels large. Dizziness, severe frontal headache, heat in forehead, soreness in front part of head, soreness in the brain, worse when stooping. "Brain feels numb with occasional stitches or shocks in various parts of the head, bruised feeling in forehead. Vertigo. Sharp pain over right eye, then over the left, dull pain in both temples, growing more intense, dull stupid feeling all over the head with severe pain in the occiput. Head feels heavy as though I could not sit up, headache day and night, causing a sensation of wildness, noise increases the headache."—(*Provings by Prof. Douglass,* and *Beckwith*, Messrs. *Rowley, Smith, Hoyt* and *Sapp, N. A. J. Vol. VI., pages* 228 and 234.

CLINICAL REMARKS.—The head-symptoms of Baptisia resemble those caused by Bryonia, Gelseminum, Arnica and Muriatic acid. It is indicated in the headache which precedes and accompanies typhoid fevers; and is useful in some bilious, nervous and rheumatic cephalalgias. I have often given it in the febrile paroxysm of an intermittent, when the headache was similar to that caused by Baptisia. In such cases it not only relieved the head, but often hastened the critical perspiration and shortened the hot stage. My former pupil Dr. Rogers, of Laporte, Ind., thinks very highly of it in similar instances. He prescribes it at the commencement of the cold stage, and continues it through all the stages, and claims that it modifies the paroxysm, but has no anti-periodic power, in preventing further attacks. He claims also to have used it with benefit in his own case, during an attack of "cerebro-spinal fever," which was epidemic in his locality. The Baptisia has many symptoms which resemble very much, those which are said to occur in the so-called "spotted fever." We would suggest to our colleagues a careful comparison of the symptoms of this dreaded malady, with the proving of Baptisia. It may be found to be a valuable remedy in the treatment of that fatal epidemic.

Eyes.—"Feeling as if the eyes would be pressed into the head with great confusion of sight; cannot place anything till after looking at it a few seconds; everything seems to be moving. Vertigo attended with sensation of paralysis of the lids, eyes smart and ache severely." (B) "Bloated feeling of the eyes; eyes unusually glistening; disposition to have the eyes half closed; soreness in front part of head upon moving the eyes or turning them upward; soreness of eyeballs, eyes feel swollen with burning and slight lachrymation; congestion of the vessels of the eye, they look red and inflamed."—(*Doug. et al.*)

CLINICAL REMARKS.—Many of the eye-symptoms of this medicine are similar to those caused by Gelseminum and resemble those sensations which in the eyes are premonitory to typhus. It is evidently homœopathic to some varieties of ophthalmia. *King* and others recommend it internally, and as a "wash," in scrofulous and purulent ophthalmia.

Nose.—"Thick mucus discharge from the nose." (T) "Severe drawing pains along the nose." (B) "Catarrh, dull pain at the root of the nose." (D.)

Clinical Remarks.—Internally it may be found useful in some forms of catarrh and ozæna, as a topical application. I know the infusion, or dilute tincture to be serviceable in obstinate fœtid discharges from the nasal passages.

Face.—Burning heat of face, face flushed and hot; external vessels of face distended and full, flashes of heat over the face, feels flushed and very hot, cheeks burn." (D)

Ears.—Deafness, or dullness of hearing. Roaring in the ears, with confusion of the mind.

Clinical Remarks.—Dullness of hearing is a common symptom of debility, particularly the debility of typhoid states. Baptisia is indicated when deafness occurs during a low fever. It is useful as an injection in fœtid, corrosive otorrhœa.

Mouth, Tongue. etc.—"Profuse flow of saliva; well developed ulcers in the mouth; long, continued flow of saliva. Tongue feels as though it had been scraped." (T) "Tongue coated yellow along the centre; flat bitter taste in the mouth." (B) Tongue feels dry on rubbing it against the roof of the mouth, smarted and felt sore as if burned, slight, dry burnt feeling of the tongue. Saliva abundant, somewhat viscid and flat tasting, appetite somewhat impaired, food does not taste quite natural. Filthy taste with flow of salivia loss of appetite, slight yellow coat on the tongue; two days afterward, tongue coated whitish and slightly congested. Tongue coated, at first white with reddish papilla here and there, followed by a yellowish brown coating in the centre, the edges being red and shining; tongue feels thick and swollen, numb pricking sensation of the tongue, bad taste in the mouth. Teeth and gums feel sore. Oozing of blood from the gums.

Clinical Remarks.—The above symptoms of the buccal cavity, afford excellent proof of the law of "Similia" as a law of cure. They show that the Baptisia will cause conditions of the mucous membrane of the mouth, etc., similar to those for which it is so much used in eclectic practice. An exhaustive proving would undoubtedly develop symptoms of a more aggravated character, as putrid ulcerations, etc. *King* speaks highly of the Baptisia as a wash to malignant, ulcerous sore mouth; mercurial sore mouth, and many other pathological conditions of the buccal cavity. It causes salivation and ulceration; I have used it for many years in chronic, mercurial sore-mouth, when the gums were loose, flabby, dark red or purple, and the breath was intolerably fœtid. Next to chlorate of potash, it is the best remedy we have to remove and palliate that disagreeable condition. It is indicated in stomatitis materna; cancrum oris; and nearly all diseases of the mouth and tongue, characterized by ulceration, putrescency, etc. But in all these diseases, it should be used topically as well as internally. Like chlorate of potash, the mineral acids, hydrastus, etc., the cure is materially hastened by the local application of the diluted tincture, or watery infusion. I usually prescribe it as follows: Baptisia root one drachm, hot water one pint, or, Tincture Baptisia one drm.

cool water four oz. This may be used as a wash, gargle, or local application in any form, when it is indicated. At the same time, the tincture or the dilutions may be given internally, at suitable intervals. In typhus conditions we find many of the above pathogenetic symptoms, in nearly every case. They afford special indications for the selection of this medicine.

Throat.—"Soreness of the throat with scraping and burning. Raw sensation in the pharynx with a large amount of viscid mucus Constrictive feeling in the throat, causing frequent efforts at deglutition. Pricking sensation in the upper part of pharnyx. Slight angina, throat feels swollen or full; tonsils and soft palate injected with pain in the root of the tongue when swallowing.

Clinical Remarks.—The action of Baptisia upon the throat is quite marked. It irritates the tonsils, uvula, and follicular glands. It is homœopathic, and has been found curative in ulcerating sore throat, suppurating tonsils, catarrhal angina, etc. If the angina tends to assume a putrid character, the ulcers dark, and breath fœtid, the Baptisia is particularly indicated. Many of my colleagues as well as myself value it very highly in the treatment of diphtheria, as an auxiliary to Merc. iod, Kali bichrom. or Kali bro. It is indicated when putrescent symptoms appear, when the nervous system becomes depressed, and there is much prostration. The premonitory symptoms of diphtheria, bear a strong resemblance to many of the symptoms of Baptisia. It should be used as a gargle.

Stomach.—"Good deal of distress in the stomach, severe pains every few moment in the cardiac region of the stomach; disposition to vomit, but no nausea. Dull pain in the epigastric region, frequently recurring and aggravated by turning over, constant pain in the epigastric and hypochondriac regions aggravated by walking; burning distress in the epigastrium" (B.) "Frequent eructations of flatus; nausea" (T). "Gone," empty feeling of the stomach. Slight nausea, followed by vomiting; pain in the stomach; pains and cramp in the stomach; feeling as if there was a hard substance in it. Stitching pain in cardiac extremity of stomach. Slight nausea with want of appetite and constant desire for *water*." (*Doug. et al.*).

Clinical Remarks.—Typhoid and bilious fevers are ushered in by symptoms which resemble those above given. Baptisia seems to act specifically on the gastric mucous membrane. It is highly probable, that it causes the same lesions in that tissue, which it causes in the mouth and fauces, namely, inflammation and ulceration.

Dr. Coe, says he found it very servicable in certain forms of dyspepsia, particularly those cases accompained with irritability of the stomach, acid eructations, griping pains and looseness of the bowels, with frequent, small, and offensive stools.

Abdomen.—"Constant pain in the right hypochondriac region; sharp shooting pains all through the bowels. Severe colicky pains in the umbilical and especially in the hypochondriac regions; the pain comes on every few seconds, with rumbling in the bowels and desire for stool. Constant dull pain in the umbilical region; shooting pain in the umbilical region," (Burt). "Pain in the abdomen on pressure; dull heavy aching pain in the lumbar region on going to bed at night. Loud borborygmus, with diarrhœa, fullness of the abdomen, flatulence. Pain in the hypogastrium, soreness of the abdominal mucles as if from cold or coughing severely," (*Doug. et al.*) "Distension of abdomen, feeling as though it would be a relief to vomit, rumbling in the intestines" (*T*). (In a cat, poisoned with Baptisia, Dr. Burt found the small and large intestines congested and filled with bloody mucus).

CLINICAL REMARKS.—It is highly probable that the Baptisia causes similar intestinal lesions to those observed in typhoid fever. It is a drastic cathartic, and is homœopathic to profuse, dark, fœtid diarrhœas, sub-acute enteritis, colics, and other bowel affections.

Liver, &c.—Pain in the right hypochondriac region, aggravated by walking; constant dull pain in the region of the *gall-bladder;* pain extends to the spine. Soreness in the region of liver, pain in the liver.

CLINICAL REMARKS.—*King* says it arouses the liver to a normal action. *Coe* declares that in hepatic derangements it will be found a valuable *auxiliary* to other remedies. Dr. Burt found the *liver congested* in a cat poisoned with Baptisia. Its pathogenetic symptoms show that it is homœopathic to some disorders of the liver, the exact nature of which, further provings, and clinical experience can only decide.

Stools and Rectum.—Rumbling in the bowels and desire for stool, soft, papescent stool with a good deal of mucus, soft mushy stools with rumbling in the bowels, "constipation, severe constipation with hemorrhoids, diarrhœa two days before, bowels loose which is uncommon with the prover. Bowels costive for two days. Vomiting and diarrhœa with dark stools. Bowels constipated during whole proving." (*Douglas et al.*). [A cat poisoned with Baptisia had bloody mucus stools. The intestines were found congested and filled with bloody mucus.] In large doses Baptisia is a drastic cathartic; and in smaller doses a laxative. The stools are generally dark, offensive, mucous, and even bloody. In quite small doses it rather constipates. This, however, is an effect of all cathartics when given in small quantities. Baptisia then, is *primarily* homœopathic to diarrhœa, dysentery and acute mucous enteritis; *secondarily*, to constipation, with indigestion, torpor of liver and hæmorrhoids. *Coe* says, "in the treatment of ulcerative inflammation of the bowels and stomach, and chronic diarrhœa, and dysentery, its use should never be omitted; also, that it is useful in "acrid fæcal discharges, and "frequent, small and offensive stools." Thus it is that both allopathic and eclectic schools of medicine, use remedies successfully for the very symptoms they cause, thereby unwittingly treating their patients homœopathically. It is indicated particularly in adynamic diarrhœa and dysentery, with the general condition of the system usually present. But it has been found useful in those affections even when sthenic in character. In its action on the bowels it resembles Leptandria, Arsenicum,

Nitric Acid and Rhux-tox. Dr. Burt, one of the provers of Baptisia, thinks highly of it in dysentery. He reports the following: *Case 1st.* A pregnant woman was attacked with dysentery. It brought on labor, after which the dysentery grew worse. A council was to he held at noon, but on the morning of the same day Baptisia, (4 drops of the tincture every hour) was given; at noon she was much better, and her convalescence was rapid. Her symptoms were violent colic-like pains before every stool, and great tenesmus. Stools every five or ten minutes. They were pure blood, with a very little mucus, pulse 20, soft and full. *Aconite*, *Bry*, *Colocyuth*, *Merc. Veratrum alb.* were given for four days without any benefit, while the *Baptisia* cured her perfectly in four hours." In ten cases of dysentery I have never seen medicine act better. They all had violent colicky pains in the hypogastric region before a stool, the stools were mucus and blood, great tensemus which was relieved by the Baptisia in two or three hours, better than by any remedy I have ever used; the cases were not generally attended by much fever.

Urinary Organs.—Urine high colored, not very copious, but of dark red color. A sort of burning when urinating" (*Doug. et al*). Shooting pains in the region of the left kidney. The urine increased in quantity during the proving, and continued acid throughout.

Female Genital Organs.—Increased menses. Menses too soon and too profuse. Abortion.

Clinical Remarks.—This medicine has not been proven upon the female organism. But it has been known to cause the above symptoms. Its real action upon the uterus, ovaries, etc., has yet to be accurately determined.

Dr. Coe, says, "Baptisia is possessed of more energetic emmenagogue properties than the plant has generally been accredited with. We have employed it with gratifying success in the treatment of dysmenorrhœa and defective menstruation. Also in cases of vicarious menstruation, in combination with Podophyllin, with signal success. In the treatment of vicarious menstruation, particularly those cases accompanied with periodical diarrhœa, we have found the following combination entirely successful when administered during the intermenstrual period: Baptisia grs. xx, Podophyllin grs. x. Caulophyllin grs. xx. Mix and divide into ten powders. Give one every night or every other night according to the condition of the bowels."

One of the most ridiculous things in the old school practice, is the custom of prescribing a farrago of drugs like the above, and then giving to *one* of them the credit of curing the malady. Who knows which drug was the curative agent? If Baptisia is a specific for vicarious menstruation, its administration simply will prove its virtues. *Coe* adds that it "should not be used during the period of utero-gestation, as it is capable of producing abortion, for which purpose we have known it to be used by quacks and empirics. The danger to the general health is very great, when used in sufficient quantities to produce this result." It follows, then, that Baptisia is homœopathic to abortion when occurring as a consequence of debility, physical or mental depression, nervous prostration, etc, as in typhoid fevers, and other adynamic conditions. It is a useful application, in the form of injection, in cases of virulent leucorrhœa, ulcerations of the os uteri and vagina, with acrid fœtid discharges; also in unhealthy lochial discharges, and those peculiar putrid discharges which occur after an abortion, and depend upon the presence of shreds of membrane, or pieces of the placenta, remaining in the cavity of the uterus. In these cases the Baptisia, injected in the form of infusion or dilute tincture, will remove the fœtor and prevent mischief from the acridity of the discharges. The chlorate of potash, or still better the permanganate of potash will prove more effectual in grave cases. As there is usually present in all these cases, a general debility of the system, and a sort of *crasis* of the blood, the *Baptisia* should be given internally, in the lower dilutions, in conjunction with a nourishing diet, wine, etc.

Larynx, Trachea, etc.—Hoarseness to such an extent as to require the utmost effort to be understood. Tickling in the throat, constantly provoking a cough. Great hoarseness. Complete aphonia.

Chest.—Difficult breathing, increased compass and frequency of the pulsations of the heart, pulsations seem to fill the chest. Difficulty of breathing, the lungs feel tight and compressed, cannot get a full breath. Tightness of the chest, feeling of want of power in the respiratory apparatus such as is felt during fever (*D*). "Constriction and oppression of the *chest*,' (*Burt.*) Oppressed respiration, sharp pains in the chest when taking a long breath, throbbing in the heart so as to be distinctly heard. Awoke with great difficulty of breathing, the lungs felt tight and compressed; could not get a full breath, felt obliged to open the window, to get my face to the fresh air.

Clinical Remarks.—It may prove curative in some varieties of *asthma*, also typhoid pneumonia. I am inclined to the opinion, however, that many of the symptoms of *oppression*, are due to nervous atony, and resemble the anxious oppression which occurs during the low stages of fevers.

Back.—Dull heavy pain in the lumbar region very much aggravated by walking; back and hips are very stiff and ache severely; chills up and down the back as if *ague* were coming on; dull heavy aching in the lumbar region on going to bed at night, flashes of heat from the small of the back in all directions," (*Douglas et al.*).

Upper Extremities.—Stiffness of the joints as if strained, twitching in the left deltoid, also in latissimus dorsi of left side. Soreness of the muscles of the neck, muscular debility, feeling of weariness especially in the right arm and shoulder, hands feel too large and are tremulous with a peculiar thrilling sensation, somewhat like going to sleep or a want of circulation," (*D.*) "Drawing pains in arms." (*B.*)

Lower Extremeties.—Dull drawing pains in the right groin and testicle. Drawing pains in the legs especially in the knee joints. Severe drawing pains in the calves of the legs; legs are very weak and tremble." (*B.*) "Burning heat of the feet with feeling of pulsation, sacral region and hips exceedingly painful; feet become painful from resting on the floor; dull pain in the sacrum, compounded of a feeling as from pressure and fatigue from long stooping, soon extending round the hips and down the right leg; weariness of the lower limbs especially the right. Aching in limbs, heat and burning in the lower extremities so intense as to prevent sleep most of the night. Soreness in the anterior part of the thighs worse after sitting awhile; darting pain in the left knee and malleolus of left side. Extremities feel hot except the feet which are cold," (*Douglas*). "Sensation of weakness in lower limbs with weak knees." Cramp in the calves when walking.

DR. BURT'S PROVING OF BAPTISIA.*

Oct. 12th. Am in perfect health. Took 10 drops at 10 A. M., at 12 M. feeling of tightness across the forehead, with pain over the right eye. At 3 P. M. severe pain every few minutes in the cardiac portion of the stomach. Took 15 drops, 4 P. M. Skin of the forehead is feeling as if it was drawn very tightly over the forehead, with sharp pain over the right eye; quite a number of times there has been sharp shooting pains all through the bowels. Took 20 drops, 8 P. M.—Frequent pain over the right eye of a pressive character. There has been constant pain in the region of the gall bladder, very severe when walking. Dull pain in the epigastric region. Dull drawing pain in the right groin, legs ache. Took 25 drops.

Oct. 13th. Slept well until midnight, then could not sleep any more. Frequent pain in the epigastric region, very much worse by turning over which I had to do all the time; dreamed of being bound down with a chain across the mouth; drawing pains in the arms and legs. Slight rumbling in the bowels. Tongue coated yellow along the centre. 7 A. M.—Took 30 drops, 10 A. M. Dull pressive pain in the forehead. Sharp pains in both temples; dull pain in the right hypochondriac region. Slight rumbling in the bowels with a mushy stool. Dull pain in the small of the back; drawing pains in the legs. Took 35 drops, 2 P. M. There has been constant pain in the epigastric and right hypochondriac regions, very severe when walking, the pain is of a drawing character. Took 40 drops, 9 P. M. Have suffered constantly and severely all day, with pain in the *liver* and stomach, the pain causes a numb feeling to pass all over my body. Dull pain in the forehead. Drawing pain in the calves of the legs. Urinated 40 oz. acid.

Oct. 14th. Had a very restless night, with frightful dream. Good deal of dull pain in the liver, stomach and umbilical region. Tongue coated yellow. 9 P. M. Have had constant pain in the umbilical region with slight rumbling of the bowels all day. Soft stool. Urinated 26 oz., acid.

Oct. 15th. Had restless night, with frightful dreams. 9 A. M. Feeling quite well. Took 40 drops. 2 P. M. Have had constant pain in the stomach and right hypochondriac region. Took 50 drops, 5 P. M. Skin of the forehead feeling very much contracted. Slight

*This proving was made with the mother tincture, and crude bark.

pain all day in the stomach and right hypochondriac region, the pain in the right side is very severe when walking. Severe drawing pains in the right groin and testicle and right foot. Took 60 drops, 9 P. M. There has been constant pain in the stomach and right hypochondriac region. The pain was of a dull aching character and extended to the spine, very much worse by motion. Took 60 drops, slept until 2 A. M., then could not sleep any more. Took 40 drops at 4 A. M. Had a good deal of pain in the epigastric region all night. Urinated 28 oz., acid.

Oct. 16th. Feeling quite well. Injected 10 drops under the skin of the left arm over the biceps. I first held chloroform on my arm for five minutes, it was more painful than the making of the incision through the skin; ten minutes after, the skin of the forehead felt as though it would be pulled to the back part of my head, with a numb feeling of the forehead and face; in fifteen minutes, feeling as if I would vomit but no nausea, with severe shooting pain in the left kidney and left side of the umbilicus. Thirty minutes, feeling as if the forehead would be pressed in. Slight pain in the stomach and right hopochondriac region and umbilical, frequent gulping up of air. At 10 A. M., slight pressive headache and dull pain in the loins. The part where the incision was made became so numb that I could cut the skin without the least feeling of pain. I can assure my readers that the most painful part is holding the chloroform bottle on the arm. Took 100 drops, 2 P. M. Dull heavy pressive headache; by spells sharp pains in the temples; heavy aching pain in the stomach and liver, with a very hot sensation in the same parts. Soft stool. Took 120 drops 9 P. M. Feeling very weak and tremble a good deal. Pressive pain in the forehead, constant dull aching pain in the stomach and liver. The pain in the liver extends from the right lateral ligament to the gall-bladder—it is almost impossible to walk it makes the pain so severe in the region of the gall-bladder. Severe drawing pains in the calves of both legs. Took 106 drops. Urinated 42 oz., acid.

Oct. 17th. Slept well until 2 A. M., then very restless until morning; frightful dreams. Dull heavy headache in the forehead, constant dull aching pains in the umbilical region, aggravated by a full inspiration. Dull aching pain in the lumbar region, very severe when walking. Tongue coated yellow along the centre. Flat taste in the mouth, 9 A. M. Took 150 drops, 12 M. Head feeling very heavy, sharp pains by spells in the right and left temples, constant dull pain in the region of the gall-bladder, very severe when walking. Took 200 drops, 3 P. M. Skin of the forehead feeling very tight, with sharp pain in the temples. Constant pain in the stomach and liver, quite sharp at times. Fearing that all the medicinal properties of the drug was not in the tincture I was using, I concluded to take the green bark of the root and chew it. Took 30 grs. Had a natural stool, 9 P. M., constant burning distress in the epigastrium, with severe colicky pains in the umbilical and especially in the hypogastric region, every few seconds, with rumbling in the bowels and desire to vomit, but no nausea;

soft stool; drawing pains in the right hip and calves of both legs. Urinated 31 oz., acid.

PROVING WITH BAPTISIN.

Oct. 18.—Slept until 3 A. M., could not sleep any more, but had to toss about constantly. Had a dull hard headache, very much worse by moving. Sharp pains in the temples very often. Constant aching pains in the umbilical region. Took 40 grs. at 4 A. M. Tongue coated yellow, flat bitter taste in the mouth. Tonsils congested. Drawing pains in the legs. 11 A. M. There has been great distress in the stomach and bowels all the forenoon, with desire to vomit. Soft mushy stool. Took 55 grs. 1 P. M. Eyes feeling as if they were being pressed into my head, with great confusion of sight, cannot place anything until I look at it for a few seconds, everything appears to be moving; partial paralysis of the eyelids, it is very difficult to keep them open; fauces and tonsils good deal congested. Great distress in the epigastric and umbilical region, with good deal of rumbling. Cramp in the calves of the legs whenever I move them; am very weak and faint. 8 P. M. Have had frequent pains in the right temple. Eyes smart and ache severely. Tonsils vere much congested, with frequent inclination to swallow which produces pain in the root of the tongue. Constant aching distress in the stomach and umbilical region, with great deal of pain in the region of the gall-bladder. Rumbling with desire for stool. Stool papescent with a large quantity of mucus, but no real pain. Am very faint and weak, legs tremble and ache. Urinated 33 oz., acid.

Oct. 19. Had a very restless night. Frequent pain in the right temple; dull heavy headache. Tongue coated yellow, with flat bitter taste. Tonsils and soft palate good deal congested. Dull aching distress in the bowels. Back and hips are very stiff and ache severely; drawing pains in the left leg. 4 P. M.—Tonsils and soft palate look very red, but do not pain any, good deal of distress in the umbilical region all day. Back aches severely, aggravated by walking. Frequent drawing pains in the calves of the legs. Urine is of a whitish color and does not change blue litmus, and has no effect on red paper.

Oct. 20th.—Slept well. Tongue coated yellow. Teeth and gums have been very sore for two days, by pressing on them with my finger, large quantities of blood oozes from the gums. Tonsils and soft palate congested. Slight back-ache. Had a natural stool this morning, but none yesterday. Felt very gloomy for several days. Bowels moved regularly once a day—perfectly natural.

Oct. 28th.—Feeling well. Took 4 grs. at 10 A. M. Had a severe pain in the region of the gall-bladder lasted one hour; constant slight pain in the umbilical region; natural stool. Took 6 grs. All the evening had a dull frontal headache, with smarting of the eyes and a drawing pain down the nose. Constant dull pain in the umbilical and hypogastric regions, by spells the pain in the hypogastric region was very sharp.

Oct. 29th.—Slept well. Feeling quite well. 10 A. M.—Took 10

grs. 3 P. M.—There has been constant dull pain in the umbilical region. At times drawing pains in the right wrist and left ankle. Took 14 grs. Constant dull frontal headache, and dull pain in the bowels all the evening.

Oct. 30th.—Slept well until 1 A. M. Awoke with severe cutting pains in the hypogastric region, with loud rumbling of the bowels, very restless after; had frightful dreams. Tongue coated yellow, along the centre; flat bitter taste. Soft papescent stools. The inguinal glands of the left groin are very much swollen, one of them as large as a common sized hickory nut. Is this an effect of the medicine, or the effect of a cold? I have no symptoms of a cold. They are very painful when walking, 10 A. M.

W. H. BURT, M. D.

CAULOPHYLLUM THALICTROIDES.

(*Blue Cohosh. Squaw Root.*)

This is a smooth, glaucous plant, purple when young, with a high round stem, from one to three feet high, simple, from knotted and matted rootstalks, and dividing above into two parts, one of which is a triternate leaf-stalk, the other bears a biternate leaf, and a racemous panicle of small yellowish-green flowers, which appear in May and June. Panicle small, darker than the leaves. *Pericarp* thin, caducous, dark blue, resembling berries on thick stipes. Seeds one or two about the size of a large pea, erect and globose. It is a handsome perennial plant, growing all over the United States, in low, moist, rich grounds, near running streams or on grounds which have been overflowed with water. The seeds ripen in the latter part of the summer and are said to form an excellent substitute for coffee, when roasted. The fruit is dry, sweet, insipid, and resembles that of the Vaccinium. The officinal part is the root, which is sweetish, somewhat pungent and aromatic, and affords a yellow infusion or tincture. The resinoid, active principle of this root, is called *Caulophyllin*, and may be used instead of the tincture in nearly all cases. In the following clinical experience, it will be stated which preparation was used in the prescription. In our school Caulophyllin has been most used. I believe I was the first to call attention to this remedy. The original article was published in the North American Journal, Vol. 6, p. 373; since which time it has been quite extensively used The first mention that I find of it, by any medical writer, is in the work of John Thomson—author of the so-called "Thomsonian Practice;" who, after mentioning its employment by the Indian females to expedite delivery, and to relieve uterine pain and spasm, reports a case of inflammation of the uterus, cured rapidly by a decoction of the root. It is also highly spoken of by Smith, Matison, Beach and other "botanic" writers; but the best description of the plant, and resume of its properties and uses, is to be found in King's Dispensatory. He says: "It is principally used as an *emmenagogue*, *parturient* and *anti-spasmodic*; but it likewise possesses diuretic, diaphoretic and authelmintic properties. It has been successfully employed in *rheumatism*, *dropsy*, *colic*, *cramps*, *hiccough*, *epilepsy*, *hysteria*, *uterine inflammation*, *etc.* It is a valuable agent in all *chronic uterine diseases*." Other writers, as Jones and Scudder (Mat. Med.) and Coe, (Conc. Org. Med.) give the same statement of its virtues. If I were to compare any of our well-known remedies with it, I should name Asa f., Platina, Secale, Murex, and perhaps Pulsatilla.

General Effects.—Sensation of comfortable languor and disposition to sleep. A fine prickling sensation all over the body. Increased mental and physical vigor. Tremulous weakness of the whole system.

Nervous System.—The action of Caulophyllum on the nervous system is similar to that of Cimicifuga. It is sedative to the nerves of *motion*, and is secondarily homœopathic to spasms, cramps and even convulsions—especially when they arise from reflex irritation, originating in the ovaries or uterus. Its primary action is antagonistic to Ignatia, Nux vomica or Secale. It causes, secondarily, conditions which those drugs cause primarily. The nerves of *sensation*, are not directly influenced by this remedy. It relieves pain by arresting the cramp or spasm by which the pain is caused, or by some specific influence over the pathological condition known as rheumatism. I have not known of its successful use in neuralgia, nor do I think it indicated in that disease when idiopathic. "*Eclectic*" writers class it with the "anti-spasmodics." It has an extensive reputation in that school, in *hysteria* and other nervous affections. "It appears," says Jones, "to impart a vigorous and healthful energy to the nervous system. It has been found useful in epilepsy, chorea, tremors, spasms of the stomach, bowels etc." (Ec. Mat. Med.) If homœopathic to epilepsy, at all, it must be in that form known as "Menstrual" or "Uterine Epilepsy." In *Idiopathic Epilepsy*, neither Caulophyllum or anything else is of much service; while in the *epileptiform* spasms which occur during or near the menses, or in *hysterical* convulsions, connected with dysmenorrhœa, the caulophyllum is the most appropriate remedy, and has been useful in such cases, in my own practice. Cimicifuga, (Macrotys) and Bromide of Potash are also suitable in such cases. In *Chorea*, it has proved as useful as its near analogue Cimicifuga. Several cures of that malady by the use of Caulophyllin, one-tenth have come under my own observation. Nearly every case occurred in young girls, and had their origin in some menstrual irregularity. One case, however, was of a decidedly *rheumatic* origin. It is useful in the *tremors* of nervous women, and drunkards; also in the *cramps* of pregnant females.

Mucous Membranes.—It seems to act upon the mucous membranes of the mouth, fauces and vagina. It has been found curative in *aphthous* conditions of those surfaces; also in leucorrhœa.

Muscular Tissues.—It appears to have a specific relation to the muscular and fibrous tissues, but, whether directly or through the nervous system, is not yet determined. Its efficacy in rheumatism is undoubted, but it is not used in that disease as much as the Cimicifuga; indeed it is hardly mentioned in relation to that affection in works on "eclectic" medicine. The homœopathic school, have used it successfully in certain forms of rheumatism, as the following cases will show:

Dr. P. H. Hale, of Hudson, Mich., reports as follows: "A plethoric man, of nervous temperament, was attacked with rheumatic swelling of both feet. In a few days the swelling shifted to the knees, and from thence to the wrists and hands. No perceptible benefit accrued from the administration of Pulsatilla, Bryonia, Rhus, or Aconite. One night about the third week of his illness, I was called in great haste to see him. The pain and tumefaction had suddenly left the extremities, and he was suffering from excruciating pain in the cervical and dorsal regions, with spasmodic rigidity of the muscles of the back and neck; could not bear to be moved, slight twitching of the muscles of the arms; paroxysms of quick, panting breathing; complained of great oppression of the chest; high fever, severe delirium, and great nervous excitement. The tincture of Caulophyllum was administered, 30 drops every half hour. In a few hours the symptoms rapidly gave way, and from that time the patient rapidly improved, and in a week was attending to his usual avocations. I have also found it useful in rheumatism of the uterus." Dr. R. Ludlam contributes the following interesting experience relative to the use of this remedy. "A clergyman had inflammatory rheumatism, which became fixed in the carpal and metacarpal joints of the left upper extremity. No remedy seemed to be of any benefit. The pain was severe and constant. Caulophyllin was administered and a rapid amelioration, followed by a prompt cure, was the result." "A young lady had inflammatory rheumatism of the hand, after using the usual remedies with unsatisfactory results, Caulophyllin was given, and a rapid subsidence of the disease was the gratifying result." *Rheumatism of the Uterus* is a common cause of dysmenorrhœa, and many other painful affections of that organ and its ligaments. Caulophyllin will be found very useful in such conditions. Cimicifuga is also indicated, but the former is more useful in rheumatic affections *when spasmodic symptoms are present;* that is the chief diagnostic difference between the two remedies.

Sleep.—More sleepy than usual during the day. Sounder sleep at night. Disposition to sleep in the evening. (Primary). Sleeplessness at night, from a kind of nervous relaxation. Wakes frequently during the night. (Secondary).

Clinical Remarks.—Some eclectic physicians decree the Caulophyllin to be *narcotic*, while others as *Coe*, deny that it has such powers. It has a calming effect upon nervous subjects, and the provings show that it disposes to sleep in healthy subjects. A remedy may cause sleep however, indirectly, by acting as a sedative to irritated nerves. Dr. Ludlam reported the following case, illustrative of the action of Caulophyllin to insomnia. I abridge the case from my pamphlet on "abortion," page 17. A lady aborted at the third month; she had terrible floodings, which so shattered her nervous system as to render her very miserable. Her pulse was feeble, threadlike, and at times imperceptible; skin cool, extremities, upper and lower, as well as her features, and cellular tissue generally, œdematous, and her nerves in the most pitiable condition imaginable; the most prominent feature of which derangement consisted in complete *insomnia*. She could not sleep. Night after night passed and not a wink of sleep. All the usual remedies were tried, but without avail. Apis relieved the œdema, and under occasional doses of Arsenicum, her pulse approached a normal state. Upon the recommendation of Dr. P. H. Hale, I gave her Cauloph. 2. A few doses sufficed to break the spell, and I have never since failed to procure her the most refreshing sleep with this agent.

Head.—Slight mental exhilaration, swimming in the head, a sort of vertigo, with dimness of sight. Sensation of fulness of the head, with pressure behind the eyes, and fulness of the temporal arteries.

CLINICAL REMARKS.—It is useful in rheumatic and neuralgic headaches, the latter, when dependant upon uterine disorder, or, spinal irritation.

Eyes.—Dimness of sight. Pressure behind the eyes.

Mouth.—Sensation of dryness in the mouth, or as if scalded. Heat in the mouth and fauces.

CLINICAL REMARKS.—*King says:* "Combined with equal parts of powdered Hydrastis, made into an infusion, and sweetened with honey, it forms an elegant and effectual wash for apthous sore-mouth and throat." Caulophyllum *alone* will cure aphthæ of the mouth, especially in pregnant and nursing females, and even in children. A weak solution of the tincture in water, used as a wash, and taken internally, will often prove curative in quite severe cases.

Stomach.—Heat in the stomach. Slight nausea. Fullness in the stomach. Empty eructations.

CLINICAL REMARKS.—I have found the Caulophyllum useful in some of those reflex affections of the stomach occurring in females, such as spasms, cardialgia, spasmodic vomiting, excessive nausea (when attending uterine irritation). *King* does not mention its use in gastric affections, nor does any other writer, except *Dr. Coe*, who asserts that "it is an admirable remedy in some forms of dyspepsia, particularly those cases attended with spasmodic symptoms. When there is gastric irritability with vomiting of food, it may be employed with advantage."

Abdomen, etc.—Distention of the abdomen. Fullness of the abdomen with some tenderness. Rumbling in the bowels. Constipation. Stool only every other day. It is said to expel worms.

CLINICAL REMARKS.—"Combined with drastic purgatives, such as Aloes or Podophyllum, it prevents tormina better than any other known drug."—(*King.*) It is said to relieve attacks of spasmodic and flatulent colic. Caulophyllum is undoubtedly applicable when there is spasmodic action of the muscular tissues of the intestines, arising from the irritation of the motor nerves, or from rheumatism.

Urinary Organs.—Copious emission of pale, or straw colored urine. Slight pain in the neck of the bladder after urinating.

Clinical Remarks.—This remedy is recommended in spasmodic retention of urine, such as occurs in nervous and hysterical females. Dr. Scudder says he has employed it with advantage in chronic nephritis, albuminuria, cystitis and urethritis, but we have only his bald assertion. He gives no cases to substantiate his testimony.

Female Sexual Organs.—Sensation as if the uterus was congested, with fullness, heaviness and tension in the hypogastric region. Drawing in the groins—(uterine ligaments.) Menses too soon—3 days. Labor-like pains. *Abortion* with little or no flooding. *Intermittent* uterine contractions. Relaxation of the os uteri. Profuse secretion of mucus from the vagina. Increases the *natural* pains of labor. Spasmodic pains in the uterus, broad ligaments and various portions of the hypogastric region.

Clinical Remarks.—It may be interesting to those unacquainted with this medicine, to read the statements of medical writers of the eclectic school, concerning it. I quote from the most prominent: "It is principally used as an emmenagogue and parturient, * * a valuable agent in all chronic uterine diseases, appearing to exert an especial influence upon the uterus, and has been found serviceable in uterine leucorrhœa, amenorrhœa, dysmenorrhœa, etc. When used for several weeks previous to the parturient period, it is said to facilitate that process. It acts as an uterine tonic. In the more common unhealthy conditions of this organ and its appendages—even passive menorrhagia and congested cervix, it is equal to, if not surpassing the Cimicifuga."—(*King.*) Dr. Kindleberger writes to Dr. King that he has used it with much advantage in *after-pains*, menstrual suppression, and in *dysmenorrhœa*, * * it is far superior to Ergot, both in its acting more mildly and with more certain results. "In neuralgia and rheumatism of the uterus it has frequently been administered with benefit. * * It expedites delivery in all those cases when the delay is owing to fatigue, debility or want of uterine energy ; the contractions it occasions, more nearly resemble the natural ones, instead of the continuous, spasmodic contractions effected by Ergot, * * When there has been a tendency to hæmorrhage from relaxation of the muscular fibres of the uterus, after delivery," it will cause firm contractions, and arrest the bleeding.—*King's Obstetrics, p.* 650). "*Amenorrhœa*—that is—simple amenorrhœa is successfully treated with Caulophyllum. If there be hepatic aberration alternate with Podophyllin ; if Anæmia—with Iron. In *dysmenorrhœa*, it is an admirable remedy, both for the relief of the present symptoms, and for the radical alteration of the derangement. It relieves the distress attendant upon dysmenorrhœa, and its continued use during the inter-menstrual period, and when the menses are present, with Erigeron, Trillium, or Lycopus. For the relief of *after pains* it will be found efficient in a large number of cases. As a *parturient*, it quiets and harmonizes the action of the uterus, and the nervous system generally, relieving cramps and other unpleasant symptoms. —(*Coe's Conc. Org. Medicines*). "We have used it often, and known of its being frequently used by others, for a few weeks, prior to confinement as a preparatory measure to the important changes which take place at that time, with great apparent advantage. In many instances, when the females have been invariably the subjects of tedious and difficult labors, by the use of Caulophyllum for two or three weeks before confinement, all the anticipated difficulty vanished, the labors were rapid and easy, and the recovery speedy, when compared with previous confinements. "Although it may be somewhat difficult to assign a satisfactory reason as to the effects stated, or in other words its therapeutic action may be difficult of explanation, yet the effects have been so apparent, that any one knowing the character of different labors, would be forced to ascribe the different results to the use of this remedy. We have known many highly intelligent ladies, who, after having used it once, could not be prevailed upon to dispense with its use in subsequent pregnancies. It has appeared to us to afford great relief in that restlessness, and disturbed state of the functions, which generally obtains in the advanced stages of pregnancy. It allays false pains, if we can rely upon the testimony of those who have had the greatest opportunity to test its virtues."—(*Jones & Scudders Mat. Med*). Bating a little for the enthusiasm which eclectic physicians have for indigenous remedies, the above is a pretty fair enumeration of the virtues of Caulophyllum. The testimony of the homœopathic school is decidedly in concurrence with the above, as the following reported cases will show. My own experience, during the six years which I have used this remedy, has been such as to entitle me to speak decidedly as to its curative virtues. A thorough knowledge of the physiology of the female organs of generation; the pathological changes they undergo; and the reflex disorders they often give rise to, when diseased, is quite necessary, in order to understand and appreciate the therapeutical powers of this medicine. The *uterus*, in its healthy condition, possesses the qualities known as normal *tone*, *contractility*, etc. But when that organ is diseased, we have either atony (arrest of function) or *abnormal irritability*, (resulting in painful cramps, contractions, etc). These purely functional derangements of the uterus may exist *with* or *without* organic changes in that organ. Caulophyllum causes *primarily*, increased action of the uterine-motor nerves. In healthy conditions of that organ any action beyond the normal contractility, as to force and period, is a diseased state. *Abnormal* activity of any organ is *disease*. The uterus then when aroused by Caulophyllum, takes on increased action, which manifests itself in the form of *painful contractions*, *congestion*, undue *irritability*, and many other conditions of irritation, which are not confined to that organ alone, but extend to those contiguous, and connected. This remedy is therefore *primarily* homœopathic to *dysmenorrhœa*, *uterine cramps*, *congestion*, *spurious labor-pains*, *abortion*, *premature labor*, *after pains*, when these diseases are caused by *exaltation* of natural function, or hyper-stimulation. When administered for these conditions, small doses will be found most applicable, (the 3d or 6th dilution or trit.) Prolonged stimulation may wear out the normal irritability of any organ or tissue; we then have atony, a condition simulating paralysis, or, *irritation* from atony, which closely simulates the irritation from hyper-stimulation. These latter conditions are caused by the secondary action of Caulophyllum. Hence it may be indicated *secondarily* in the above named disorders, from causes opposite to those named in connection with them, also in such affections, as menorrhagia and *metrorrhagia* from deficient contractility, as after abortion and labor; *habitual abortion*, from uterine debility, a variety of pains, cramps, etc., during pregnancy, etc. When administered for its *secondary* effects, the doses should be somewhat larger—(the lower dilutions). I have not found it as useful in *Amenorrhœa* as many other remedies, and am of the opinion that it is seldom indicated in that affection, unless accompanied by spasmodic action, or extreme atony. The following cases marked "H," were originally published by me in the N. A. Jour. of Hom.

"Miss N. aged 17, plethoric, nervous, lymphatic, menses suppressed two and a half months. When I called to see her, found her in spasms, evidently hysterical, but resembling epiliptiform spasms, affecting the chest, larynx and uterus. She was unconscious. For three hours, under the administration of Bell. Hyos. and Lobelia— (which latter relieved the spasm of the chest and larynx somewhat) and even chloroform, and the hot bath—she remained in those peculiar and frightful spasms. As a last resort, after giving no medicine for an hour, I gave Caulophyllum 1-10 one half a grain. In fifteen minutes the spasms ceased; the patient lay in a stupid condition, free from pain. In the course of the night the menses came on, and in a few days she was about the house," (H). The *Dauloph.* was eminently indicated in this case, and it evidently acted as a prompt curative agent. In my "Monograph on Abortion," page 18, Dr. R. Ludlam, of Chicago, gives his experience with Caulophyllum in menstrual irregularities.

"Still another indication for the use of this remedy will be found in menstrual irregularities, occurring subsequent to, and consequent upon miscarriage. They are frequent and sometimes very perplexing cases, when neither Puls. Secale, Sabina or other remedies appear to be especially indicated, and we have either of the following symptoms: Spasmodic, bearing down pains, with scanty flow; sympathetic cramps and spasms of neighboring organs, as of the bladder, rectum and bowels, or, the motor power of the uterus seems almost entirely gone, and when we may reasonably suppose the menstrual flow is retarded from a simple lack of the excito-motor force, either in the Fallopian tubes, on the parietes of the uterus itself; the Cauloph. will afford almost instantaneous relief. In a case of this kind, post-abortive, when the spasmodic pains were located in the right lumbar region, occupying a limited space, say about the size of a silver dollar, and there was almost a total suppression of the catamenia, the Caulophyllin, 3d, dec. trit., repeated once in three hours, afforded prompt and permanent relief. We know of no other remedy which is so efficacious under these circumstances. It seems in general practice, to be indicated in many cases of *suppressio-mensium*, approaching dysmenorrhœa in some of its features, being always accompanied by the above named characteristic pains and sufferings of a spasmodic nature. Our experience would render us very loth to attempt the treatment of these and kindred cases, without a frequent resort to Caulophyllin." In *Dysmenorrhœa*, the testimony in its favor is very large. My correspondence with homœopathic physicians convinces me that it is one of the most successful remedies, in that distressing affection, now in use. It should be given in appropriate doses, once or twice a day during the inter-menstrual period, and every few hours, in the attack. In *Menorrhagia*, it is indicated for about the same symptoms as Ergot and Cimicifuga, and under some circumstances is superior to both. Dr. Williams reports several interesting cases of flooding after abortion, when ordinary allopathic and homœopathic remedies had been used in vain, but were promptly cured by Caulophyllin 1-10. The hæmorrhage was passive, had lasted several weeks, and was probably due to deficient contractility, or profuse involution of the uterine tissues. When similar conditions obtain after labor, immediately as in part portem hæmorrhage; or more remotely, as in profuse lochia, and that form which comes on several weeks after confinement, after every exertion of the patient, I have found the Caulophyllin as useful as any other medicine. Its action is not as rapid as Erigeron or Sabina, but more permanent. Caulophyllin will cause abortion, in the later months of pregnancy. Of this, I have conclusive testimony. As a remedy in threatened abortion it has no superior. "Mr. S. has had several abortions at about the third month. Each preceded for a week or more by a sensation of weight and pressure in the pelvis. When I saw her, labor-like pains had already set in, and the os uteri was partly open. Gave Caulophyllum first, one drop every half hour. In a few hours the pains abated. She has since given birth at full term to a healthy child," (H). In *uterine pains during pregnancy*—"*false pains*," etc., there is no remedy upon which we can rely with more confidence than Caulophyllin. It has never failed to give relief, in my practice, and its effects are so apparent that my patients are unanimous in its praise. I usually give the 2d decimal trit. every three or six hours, as the case demands. It is equally useful in *too severe* and *spasmodic pain* occurring during parturition; also in *deficient* or *absent* labor-pains. In the former case, however, it should not be administered lower than the 3d, and even the 30th might be efficacious; but in the latter condition the one-tenth trit. frequently repeated, is the most advisable.

Deficient Labor.—Mrs. E., a primipara, had been in labor twenty-four hours—a midwife attending her. I found the os uteri about the size of half a dollar, (the membranes had broken during the first hours of pain,) hard, rigid and unyielding, vagina dry, the pains frequent and spasmodic. Gave Belladonna and Pulsatilla and ordered warm fomentations. Twelve hours afterwards there was scarce any alteration in the condition of the patient, except that she had some fever, and was a little delirious. Gave Aconite, 1st. Six hours of agonizing pain and no progress; by auscultation I discovered the child to be dead; it was alive twelve hours before. I began to fear for my patient. Ergot was plainly inadmissible owing to the yet rigid condition of the os. I therefore gave Caulophyllin, one half grain every 15 minutes. In one hour the os uteri had become soft and dilatable, the vagina relaxed and moist; fever abated, moist skin, pains less agonizing, but strong and expulsive, and in one hour more she was delivered of a dead child, weighing 10 1-2 lbs. The mother had a good recovery. I do not think any other medicine could have produced so favorable a change in so brief a time. As an agent for inducing premature labor, after rupturing the membranes, it is invaluable. It is always safer, and in many cases, superior to Ergot," (H). The chief danger, both to mother and child, when Ergot is administered, is the powerful *continuous* contraction which it causes. It has been the cause of rupture of the uterus and perineum, and death of the fœtus by pressure on the cord, etc. These casualties are avoided by giving Caulophyllin. In *Suppression of the Lochia*, with symptoms simulating inflammation, such as pain, cramps, distention, and some tenderness, the Caulophyllin aided by warm fomentations of Hops, or Polygonum (smart-weed) will restore the discharge in a short time. To sum up the curative properties of this medicine—I do not doubt but it is homœopathic, primarily or secondarily, to all the morbid states mentioned by eclectic authors. It only needs an exhaustive proving to establish the special indications for its use. I can bear testimony to its value as a preparatory remedy, in case of difficult labor. My experience with it in such cases has been very satisfactory.

Caulophyllin in Paraplegia.—During the session of the Western Institute of Homœopathy, held in Chicago, May, 1864. Dr. Burbank, of Illinois, related a remarkable case of Paraplegia which he cured with this remedy. The patient was a middle aged lady. On the sixth day after her confinement she was attacked with Metritis—so called by her Allopathic physician. Under the usual treatment of the old school, the affection apparently subsided, but left her nearly completely paraplegic. There was partial loss of sensation, and complete loss of motion; could not move the limbs in bed, or stand upon them. There was considerable emaciation, anæmia, and general debility. When Dr. B. first saw the case, two years had elapsed since the seizure, and she was growing worse. After consultation with some of the most eminent physicians of Chicago, he gave her Cocculus, Nux. vom., Citrate of Iron and Strychnia, and several other medicines. Upon examining the uterus it was found retroverted, congested and enlarged. The patient was put upon the use of Caulophyllin 2nd, and its use was persisted in *until the paraplegia was cured.* Improvement set in soon after taking the medicine, and in a few weeks she was able to move her lower extremities, and now—six months after the commencement of the treatment—is as well as ever. The uterus, even, has assumed its normal position and condition. This case is one that demands our careful consideration. It is probable that real *metritis* never existed at all. My impression is that it was originally a case of retroversion of the uterus, existing before the process of involution had taken place. After the retroversion, a certain degree of inflammation may have existed; the process of involution was arrested, and the uterus remained in a congested or engorged condition. The case was one of *reflex* paraplegia, and the abnormal state of the uterus its real cause. Such being the ease Nux. vom., and the other remedies given, were not appropriate, but Caulophyllin, by acting in a specific manner upon the uterus, restored it to a normal state, and the paraplegia disappeared of itself. I predict this remedy will be found a very useful one in many cases of paralysis of the lower extremities.

Male Organs of Generation.—This remedy does not appear to have been used in any of the diseases of the male genital organs. I can only find it recommended in one disorder—*Gonorrhœa.* But a remedy capable of affecting so profoundly the sexual organs of one sex, must assuredly affect those of the other. I predict that it will sometimes be found useful in some diseases of the testes, etc. Even if the Caulophyllin, like Ergot, acts upon these organs *through* the spinal cord, it would not affect the above conclusions.

Respiratory Organs.—No chest symptoms have been elicited in any of the fragmentary provings. It may prove useful in certain spasmodic affections of the the thoracic organs, idiopathic or reflex, such as hooping cough, hiccough, asthma, spasms of the chest and lungs, and even cardiac derangements.

Back and Extremities.—Pain in the small of the back, like those of labor; Weight in the region of the sacrum; General lame feeling in the whole length of the back. Lassitude and weakness of the legs; Trembling of the lower limbs; Aching in the joints. Cramps.

Clinical Remarks.—Dr. R. Ludlam reports two cases of inflammatory rheumatism of the joints of the hands, cured rapidly with Caulophyllum.

Note.—Since the above was prepared for the press, I received a proving of Caulophyllum, accompanied by the following letter.

Lyons, May 2nd, 1864.

E. M. Hale, M. D.—*Dear Doctor*; Having received no word from you since I last wrote, I have concluded to send you my short proving of Crulophyllum. I have taken it, until I have become so used to the drug, my system fails to give out any more symptoms. I think you will be surprised to see what massive doses I took for such a few symptoms. I do not like to make provings with the active principles, so-called. They never give me half as many symptoms as the tinctures do. This is the first proving I have ever seen of Caulophyllum,—I am disappointed with it. As it has such a great influence over the female organs of generation, I expected that it would affect the male organs also, but not so. My genital organs were not affected in the least. Please tell me, if my proving corresponds with the provings of others, if you have them. I could not get any of my female friends to prove it. All the symptoms produced were of a rheumatic character. It appears to arrests the secretion of bile in a marked manner. The watery stool I cannot account for. Truly yours, W. H. BURT.

DR. BURT'S PROVING WITH CAULOPHYLLIN.

April 28th, 1864. Am in perfect health; tongue not coated; tonsils are natural; good appetite; bowels move once a day; urine acid; temperament sanguine-nervous; age 27; weight 148 lbs.; pulse 75. 4 P. M.—Took 10 grs. of pure resinoid. 5 P. M.—Dull frontal headache, with a contracted feeling of the skin of the forehead; drawing pains in the thighs, knees, legs and ankles; very sharp pains in the left knee joint, inside; elbows and wrists ache. 5 40.—Very hard pains in the forehead, with a sensation as of needles being stuck into the forehead. 6 P. M.—Constant flying pains in the arms and legs, first in one part and then in another, remaining only two or three minutes at a time in a place. *Severe* drawing pains in the inside of the left thigh; very hard dull frontal headache; distress in the fauces that causes frequent inclination to swallow; dull backache in the lumbar region; every few minutes sharp stinging pains in the glans penis. 9 P. M.—Severe frontal headache; severe colicky pains every few minutes in the umbilicus; very severe drawing pains in the sterno-cleido-mastoid muscle, that draws the head to the left side; severe drawing pains in the joints of the arms and legs; the ankle and toes of the left foot are very painful; dull backache.

April 29th. Slept well until 3 A. M.; after that I was very restless; skin was hot and dry; severe drawing pains in my hips, knees, ankles and feet, wrists and fingers. Shutting my hand produced severe cutting pains in the second joints of all the fingers, they were very stiff; frequent colicky pains in the umbilicus, relieved by emissions of flatus; severe drawing pains over the left eye. 10 A. M.—Have the same symptoms. Took 15 grs.; had a natural stool at 7 A. M. 12 M.—Distress in the stomach and bowels, with drawing pains in the right hypochondrium; drawing pains in the fingers, legs and feet; the pains are very severe in the feet. 4 P. M.—Dull frontal headache, by spells there is a very severe pain in the temples that produces a feeling as if both temples would be crushed together; frequent slight colicky pain in the stomach and umbilicus; slight dull backache; drawing pains in the right side over the liver; severe drawing pains in the legs and feet, but more especially in the feet; drawing pains in the fingers; natural but dark stool. 2 P. M.—Took 25 grs. 6 P. M.—Dull headache; profuse flow of tears; drawing pains in the nose; good deal of pain and distress in the stomach and umbilicus; dull pains in the lumbar region; severe drawing pains in the ankles and feet; severe pain in the wrists and joints of the fingers. 9 P. M.—Slight frontal headache; good deal of distress in the stomach, and small intestines; constant and severe drawing pains in the wrists and *fingers*, ankles, *feet*, and *toes;* the left ankle pains very severely; took 30 grs.

April 30th. Had a restless night; there was so much pain in the joints of the fingers; they look red, and are very stiff; closing the hand is very painful; slight frontal headache; teeth all feeling sore and elongated; slight dull pain in the umbilicus when moving, relieved by emissions of flatus; drawing pains in the knees, ankles, feet and toes; walking produces severe pain in the metatarsal bones; natural but hard stool. 10 P. M.—Feeling quite well, excepting my knees are very weak when walking; another rather soft stool, followed by slight pain in the umbilicus; took 50 grs. 12 M.—empty eructations; sligh distress in the stomach; drawing pains in the knees and toes, very sharp by spells. 5 P. M.—Feeling weak and nervous; dullness of the head; slight burning distress in the stomach; slight drawing pains in the wrists and fingers, ankles, feet and toes; took 75 grs. 10 P. M.—Frequent gulping up of a very sour, bitter fluid; frequent spells of vertigo; slight burning distress in the stomach; drawing pains in the fingers, ankles, feet and toes, but more especially in the toes; knees feeling very weak when walking; eyes aching with a feeling of something under the lids; profuse secretion of tears.

May 1st. Slept well until 1 A. M., then awoke with a great rumbling in the bowels, and a very urgent desire for stool; stool mostly of water that ran a perfect stream from my bowels, passed a great quantity. There was no pain. 8 A. M.—Feeling quite well; tongue coated white; canine hunger; fingers are quite stiff; slight backache; drawing pains in the toes; want to drink a great deal of water. 8 A. M.—Frequent slight pain in the umbilicus; drawing pains in the elbows, wrists, fingers, knees, ankles, feet and toes; all of my joints crack frequently when walking or turning.

May 2d. Restless night; my fingers, ankles, feet and toes pained me so much; fingers are very stiff. 7 A. M.—Soft stool, very white showing a great deficiency of bile in the excretions.

REMARKS.—The urinary or genital organs were not affected in the least; the pulse remained about natural all the time; its great centre of action on myself was the small joints; (the fingers and toes; the carpal, metacarpal and phalangeal; tarsal, metatarsal and phalangeal joints.)

DR. HALE'S REMARKS.

I know of no more remarkable substantiation of the truth of the law of *Similia*, than the above graphic proving. How perfectly Dr. Burt describes the rheumatic affection, so similar in its character to that variety in which Dr. R. Ludlam found the Caulophyllum curative? I know of no coincidence in my experience which has ever given me greater satisfaction. To settle any possible cavil or doubt in the minds of the most suspicious, I will say that Dr. Burt did not know of the use of Caulophyllin in rheumatism, much less had he any knowledge of Dr. Ludlam's experience with the remedy in that disease. I append Dr. Ludlam's report of the cases.

CHICAGO, May 4th, 1864.

E. M. HALE, M. D.—*Dear Doctor:* Meeting my friend, the Rev. Dr. C——, socially in the autumn of 1860, he inquired if I had ever prescribed the Caulophyllum for rheumatism? I replied in the negative. He then told me that he had once suffered from a very severe and protracted attack of articular rheumatism, in which the pain and swelling finally settled in the wrist and fingers of one hand. The usual remedies were tried but without avail. His physician finally prescribed, as a *dernier ressort*, a decoction of the Caulophyllum. In a short time he was perfectly relieved. "I would not," said my friend, "spend a night without the Caulophyllin in my house for half the city of Chicago!" It so happened that I was at the time treating an inveterate case of rheumatism affecting the metacarpal joints of the left hand of a servant girl in the family of D. S—— Esq. The remedies which I had prescribed did little good, and all concerned were impatient the girl should be well and at work again. I gave her empirically two grains of the second decimal trituration of the Caulophyllin. She was ordered to take a powder of that size and strength every two hours until relieved. The poor sufferer had not slept for two or more nights. After taking the second dose she fell asleep, and her pain vanished from that time forward. There was no metastasis of the complaint, and in two days she was down stairs at work. While she remained in the family—two years—she had no return of the disease. Since the above result was obtained, I have frequently prescribed the Caulophyllin for articular rheumatism affecting the *smaller* joints, and several times with as signal success. It has however, appeared more effectual in case of females than of males, who were ill with this painful disease. Very respectfully, R. LUDLAM.

CHIMAPHILA UMBELLATA.

(*Pipsissiwa.*)

This plant, known also as Prince's pine, ground holly, etc., is a native of this country, but grows in many parts of Europe and Asia. It is found in moist, shady places, and in a loose sandy soil; it flowers in June. The dried plant has scarcely any odor, with a sweetish, somewhat astringent and pleasant taste. It yields its medicinal virtues to boiling water and alcohol. The *leaves* are the officinal portion, but it is probable the root has some virtue. *Chemical Analysis*:—Dr. Holff obtained from 100 parts of the plant, 18.0, *bitter extractive*; 2.04, *resin*; 138, *tannic acid*. The remainder was woody fibre, a small portion of *gum* and some *calcareous salts*. Its medicinal virtues are decreed to reside in the bitter extractive, resin and tannin; but it may be that some of its medicinal powers reside in the calcareous salts—said salts may consist of Calcarea,

Sulphur and the Phosphates, each of which are powerful curative agents. King says the plant contains an acrid aud volatile principle—*and saline substances.* The great reputation which this plant has in chronic scrofulous and psoric affections may suggest the idea that its curative properties in this direction may be due to the anti-psoric substances residing in the plants. I shall refer to this subject when treating of Rumex crispus.

General Properties.—Wood (Therapeutics, vol. 1, p. 133)—says—"The fresh leaves bruised and applied to the skin, are said to be rubefacient and even vesicating. Internally they are mildly astringent and tonic, with the property of somewhat increasing the secretion of urine, to which they probably impart some degree of remedial power. It is, I think, scarcely doubtful that their peculiar active principle, through which they stimulate the kidneys, passes off, either unchanged or changed, with the urine." "Pipsissiwa was much employed by the aborigines of this country, to whom it owes the name by which it is now generally designated. From the Indians the medicine passed into popular use, whence it was adopted by the profession. It was used chiefly in *scrofula, rheumatism,* and *affections of the kidneys, and urinary passages.* King says it is diuretic, tonic, alterative and astringent. *Jones & Scudder* decree it to be diuretic, tonic, astringent, diaphoretic and alterative. *Lee, Coe,* and other allopathic and eclectic writers entertain similar views.

General Therapeutic Effects.—It has been found curative in chronic diseases, among which is *Scrofula.* Prof. Wood says; "In *Scrofula* it is, I think, a valuable remedy. The late Dr. Joseph Parish used it very extensively in this affection, and had great confidence in its powers. I have myself been in the habit of employing it in cases of external scrofula during the whole period of my practice, and have found few remedies which have appeared to me more efficacious. * * * It has seemed to me to exercise a favorably alterative influence in scrofula, independently of its astringency and tonic power; but it is extremely difficult to discriminate, in affections of this kind, between the course of nature and the effects of remedies, so that it is proper to speak of the latter with some reserve. Fully aware of the necessity of this caution, I am still of opinion, as the result of considerable experience, that pipsissiwa deserves to rank next to cod-liver oil, and the preparations of Iodine and Iron in the treatment of Scrofula. In order that its full effects may be obtained, it should be long continued, with interruptions now and then should any considerable degree of fever supervene (?). In cases attended with ulcers of an indolent and flabby character, it may be used with advantage as a wash." These are the deliberate statements of one of the best authors in the allopathic school, and are entitled to some weight. They should stimulate us to make a thorough proving of this plant. It may become a valuable *anti-psoric.* Other writers give their testimony in its favor in scrofula. Prof. Lee quotes Wood, expressing his "entire confidence in the opinions so strongly set forth." He has advised this remedy for a long time in the same class of cases, both in city and country practice, and with marked success: "It is a tonic-astringent of peculiar efficacy in the whole class of cachexia." The late Prof. Mitchell, of New York, made it the subject of his inaugural thesis (Phil. 1863): "In Scrofula it has proved eminently useful, and with some practitioners is held in very high repute in the various forms of this disease, both before and after ulceration. Some have thought it possessed of specific powers and hence it has acquired the title in some parts of the country, of the '*King's Cure.*' Dr. Justice, of North Carolina. informs us that he "has known it to effect perfect cures in several obstinate cases of Scrofula, *without the aid of other means.*" (Jones & Scudder's Mat. Med.) This last assertion which I have italicized, is of great import to the homœopathic physician. The *true test of a remedy in disease, is its effects when given singly.* The Illinois Homœopathic Medical Association, and the Western Institute of Homœopathy, which held their sessions in Chicago this year (1864), each appointed a Bureau of Provings. The Chimaphila has been selected by this Bureau as a proper medicine to investigate, and obtain its pathogenesis. I am sanguine that the profession will gain a valuable remedy in the Pipsissiwa.

Fevers.—In several instances in which I have administered this medicine, the following symptoms have been observed: About half an hour after each dose (of the 1st dil.) *a flushing of the cheeks, with some general heat, and accelerated pulse.* Wood seems to imply a caution not to use the Pipsissiwa when fever is present. It may be homœopathic to some form of fever, probably those having a *hectic* character. "During the Revolutionary War it was used extensively by the army surgeons as a tonic and diaphoretic in typhus fever." (*Lee.*) Prof. Mitchell relates many cases of intermittent fever effectually cured by it.

Rheumatism.—As a popular remedy in this disease, i thas always been in high repute. It is chiefly in *chronic* rheumatism that its curative powers have been most noticed. A proving, however, is necessary to show the particular variety for which it is indicated.

Special Effects.—In the absence of any proving I shall not venture any theoretical suggestions as to its influence on special organs and tissues, or portions of the body. I deem it proper, however, to note the large amount of testimony given by the allopathic and eclectic schools, in favor of its specific action upon, and curative influence over disorders of the

Urinary Organs.—Dr. Wood says it has been chiefly used in *affections* of the kidneys and urinary passages: "Its diuretic powers have recommended it in *dropsy.* In cases of this disease attended with debility, but little reliance can be placed upon its efficacy; and at best it should be used only as an adjuvant to other more powerful diuretics." Dr. Lee says: "In Germany it has long been deemed one of the best remedies in abdominal and renal dropsies, increasing the urinarysecretion and the depurating function. We have employed it to a considerable extent for many years, especially in the treament of dropsical affections, in broken-down constitutions and intemperate subjects, and generally with manifest advantage. It has tended to carry off the dropsical accumulations, while at the same time it imparted tone and vigor to the digestive system. In *Albuminuria* also, its effects have proved decidedly beneficial. It ranks with *Buchu*, *Uva Ursi* and *Pareira Brava*, all tonics, and all exerting a specific influence over the genito-urinary organs. Dr. Barton extols it highly for its anti-lithic properties, and ranks it with Uva Ursi. It may, however, well be doubted, whether it has any specific powers of this kind." Dr. Coe says it is useful in *dropsy*, (especially *ascites*) *gonorrhœa*, *strangury*, *gravel*, and syphilis, when these affections are attended with torpor and debility. "It exercises a specific influence over the urinary apparatus, increasing the renal secretion, and at the same time it is thought by some to lessen the quantity of lithic acid, or lithates secreted. It is especially serviceable in chronic diseases of the genito-urinary mucous membrane, as in chronic catarrhal affections of the bladder; chronic nephritis, or urethritis, attended with a purulent or profuse mucous discharge. It is also beneficial in calculous and prostatic affections; diabetes; in the advanced stages of albuminuria; and in other disorders of the urinary organs attended with local debility. In atonic or passive dropsies it has been found useful." (Jones & Scudder Mat. Med.) The last paragraph contains, in my opinion, the best *resume* of the curative properties of the chimaphila, as regards its action on the urinary organs. I believe a proving will establish its homœopathicity to the affections named.

I will now give my individual experience in the use of this remedy. My attention was first called to it in a case which happened in the early part of my practice. A young woman applied to me for a distressing *dysuria* which had troubled her for several weeks. She was plethoric, hysterical, had disorders of the digestive organs, constipation, hæmorrhoids, and scanty menses. The urine was scanty, but was voided frequently, with much pain before, (passing), during (scalding, smarting) and after. (Vesical tenesmus.) The urine was high-colored and deposited a copious mucous sediment. I gave her Cantharis, Cannabis, Pulsatilla, Capsicum, Copaiva, Sepia, Terebinthina and many other remedies, which seemed indicated, for several weeks, but they only palliated the difficulty. Cool hip baths, the wet bandage, mucilaginous drinks, and Nux Vomica, Sulphur and enemas for the constipation, etc., were tried, without much effect. An examination of the vagina and uterus was instituted, but elicited only a tenderness of the anterior portion of the vagina (bladder) and urethra, some prolapsus, and slight leucorrhœa (uterine). At this juncture, an old nurse proposed the use of the "Prince's Pine." I assented, having no prejudice against the plant, and hoping it might benefit my suffering patient. A decoction of the plant (of uncertain strength) was prepared, and a wine-glassful administered three or four times a day. In a week I called to see what the effects of the medicine had been. To my surprise, I was informed that improvement had set in the next day after the remedy was commenced. Not only was the *dysuria* nearly removed, but the sediment had almost disappeared from the urine; and, stranger still, the *constipation was cured,* and the digestive organs were in a normal condition. In two weeks she was as well as ever. The prompt cure which the Chimaphila effected in this case led me to use it in many cases of strangury, catarrhal affections of the bladder, etc., and in many instances I found it act certainly. It failed in some cases, probably because it was not truly indicated. I was once called in counsel to a case of chronic renal and vesical affection, in which the amount of sediment of a thick, ropy, character, and a pink color (the color was found to be owing to blood) was really enormous in amount. The patient, a young man, was debilitated, anæmic, dyspeptic, had hectic fever and night sweats, and altogether was in a bad condition. Various remedies, including China, Phosphoric acid, Cannabis, etc., had been given. Uva Ursi was tried with good results for a time. At my suggestion the Chimaphila was used, a few drops of the fluid extract in a glass of water, a spoonful every two hours. He improved rapidly under its use, and in a few weeks was able to resume his usual avocations. A relapse occurred after six or eight months. He was again benefited by the medicine, since which time I have not heard from the patient. It has one generally uniform effect, namely: *to cause mucous sediment to disappear from the urine.* I believe it will be found curative in *albuminaria,* as well as catarrhal affections of the urinary organs. In that distressing symptom, *vesical tenesmus,* occurring from prolapsus or retroversion, it is an excellent palliative, before the uterus is replaced; and *curative* after that operation.

I have used it successfullyin two cases of long lasting *gleet.* Under its use the discharge disappeared, and the general health improved. I have noticed the following *pathogenetic* symptoms from its use:

Copious discharge of clear limpid urine.

Frequent and profuse urination.

Urging to urinate after voiding urine.

Pressing fulness in the region of the bladder.

Loose stool, three or four times a day.

For the above symptoms, which are *primary effects,* I have found the 6th attenuations most useful. In chronic disorders and catarrhal affections of these organs, the lowest dilutions seems to act more beneficially. I have not tried the *high* potencies.

Case illustrating its value in irritable bladder:—

A married lady, aged 34, had been troubled for many years with prolapsus uteri, leucorrhœa, ulceration of the neck, etc., but who is now somewhat better of those difficulties, applied to me for the relief of an obstinate vesical irritability. Her symptoms were as follows:

Frequent desire to urinate during the day. At night the urging was so constant as to deprive her of all sleep. She had to get up and urinate as often as every hour. The urine was high colored, deposited a copious light-colored sediment (mucous), and there was considerable smarting, burning and pricking pain during its emission. The quantity of urine voided was not larger than normal. The patient was constipated, an evacuation only every third day. Some tenderness over the hypogastric region. She had a severe, racking, dry cough, but no indication of pulmonary difficulty. The prolapsus was aggravated by the cough.

April 2. Inserted an India rubber inflatable pessary. This relieved the prolapsus, and *stopped the cough altogether*, but the vesical irritation was not alleviated, at the end of five days.

April 6. Gave *Cannabis* 1st (4 pills No. 5, dry,) every four hours. The effect of this remedy was prompt in relieving the irritation, and indirectly causing sleep. She declared it acted as a direct *anodyne*. This improvement continued for five days, when the medicine ceased to give any relief, and she grew worse than before.

April 11. Gave *Chimaphila* first decimal dilution, 10 drops in a spoonful of water, every four hours. For several days no effect was noticeable, except a *flushing of the cheeks for about twenty minutes after each dose.* On the fourth night, however, she was able to sleep all night, and next day she noticed that the usual copious sediment was notably lessened, and the dysuria and frequent urging rapidly gave way. The bowels began to act regularly; the tenderness of the bladder disappeared, and at this date, April 20th, she is more comfortable than for many months previously.

Several things relating to the action of this remedy are worthy of note:

1. The pathogenetic symptoms mentioned above.
2. Its power in relieving dysuria.
3. Its influence in lessening the sediment (there was an evident *vesical catarrh.*)
4. Its curative action in constipation.

CIMICIFUGA RACEMOSA.

(*Macrotys racemosa. Black Snake-root.*)

This powerful medicinal plant has been used more or less since the settlement of New England by the whites. It was much used by the Indians, under the name of Black Cohosh or Squaw Root, for rheumatism and diseases of their women. It thus became introduced into domestic, and finally, to some extent, into regular practice. Still it has always been most in use among the eclectic school, who value it as we do our Bryonia and Pulsatilla. It is a tall and stately plant, growing in shady and rocky woods, rich grounds, from Maine to Florida, flowering from June to July. The root is the part generally employed in medicine, though probably the seeds will be found active; the root should be gathered early in the autumn and dried in the shade. It consists of a thick, irregularly bent, or contorted body or caudex, from one-third of an inch to an inch in diameter, often several inches in length, furnished with many slender radicles, and rendered extremely rough and jagged in appearance by the remains of the stems of successive years. The color is externally, dark brown, almost black; internally a yellowish-white; the odor is feeble and disgreeable, and the taste bitter, somewhat astringent, leaving a slight sense of acrimony. It yields its virtues partially to boiling water, but wholly to alcohol. The taste of the tincture reminds one strongly of that of laudanum. From the root is obtained the concentrated principle *Macrotin*, which contains most of the essential properties of the plant, and is often used in the place of the tincture. The *stem* is simple, herbaceous, smooth, furrowed, from 4 to 8 feet high. The *leaves* fine, alternate, one nearly radical, large, decompound, and tripinnate; upper one bipinnate. The *leaflets* are ovate, oblong, sessile, opposite, three to seven, incised and toothed. The *flowers* are fœtid, white, in a long terminal raceme, with oftentimes one or more shorter ones at base. The *fruit* or capsule is ovoid, dry, with one cell, containing numerous flat, smooth *seeds*, which are packed horizontally in two rows. In the late autumn, and winter, any motion of the plant, causes a rattling of the seeds, so much resembling the alarm of the rattle snake as to cause the hunter to start—hence the country people call it *Rattle-weed.*

The following pathogenesis which is pretty complete, is made up of the provings of Drs. Marcy, H. M. Paine, Hill, Douglas and others. The provings were made with doses of the crude tincture, the dilutions, (3d and 6th) and many of the symptoms are from its poisonous effects. Altogether it is probably as reliable a proving as any of our polycrests, and I predict that in a few years it will rank as high in the estimation of our school, as any remedy we possess. I have taken pains to collect all the reliable clinical facts which have appeared in the records of any school, in relation to its curative action in disease. My own experience with it has been large.

General.—Feels very tired. Nervous weakness during the afternoon. Great sensitiveness to the cold air, which seemed to penetrate the system. Continual restlessness in the afternoon, desire to move about, not knowing what to do or where to go. General feeling of illness; weak, trembling exhausted sinking feeling, with slight nausea. Easily fatigued, as after great exertion. Miserable dejected feeling. Tremors; so weak and trembling as not to be able to go out or study; believes the condition to be but one remove from *mania a potu.* Desire to lie down and close the eyes. General bruised feeling as if sore. Sensation as from severe muscular exercise, especially in the small of the back. It effects the *left* side most. Feeling which only those know who "spree"—or watch all night with the sick. Soreness and stiffness of the whole body, as after hard labor.

Clinical Remarks.—No particular indications are proper under this head. The general symptoms of a drug may be primary—as when the nervous system is profoundly impressed—and the local affections, the result; or, they may be secondary, as when particular organs are first affected, resulting in constitutional disturbance. I would classify its general action as follows :

Nervous System.— *Wood* classifies it with the "Nervous Sedatives," and I am inclined to think its primary action in pathogenetic doses is in that direction. *How* it effects the nervous system is beyond our ken. We know that it causes all those symptoms known to the profession under the name of "nervous prostration," and even extreme conditions which resemble *dilirium tremens.* This malady is defined by *Watson* to consist essentially of a state of "nervous irritation." He thinks this is as good a name as any for a state which we know exists. He contends that the nervous system can be *irritated,* as well as any organ in the body. It is also proper to designate certain conditions as states of "nervous exhaustion"—"nervous excitement." Cimicifuga seems to cause all these states of the nervous system. When given to a healthy person it causes first nervous excitement, which soon leads to *irritation* and finally *exhaustion.* Some observers have the folly to state that "very large doses cause no alarming effects." I have seen not only alarming, but *dangerous* effects arise from dram doses of the "fluid extract." administered to a girl, by a botanic quack.

Nerves of Sensation.—It seems to exercise considerable control over this system, independently of its action on the vascular system. It cures many of those purely neuralgic pains to which females are liable. Our provings show it to be capable of causing various aches and pains of a similar character.

Nerves of Motion.—It causes "nervous tremors"— with great restlessness—(See general symptoms.) It seems to exert a peculiar and specific action upon some of the diseases of the nerves of motion, especially in *chorea.* Not only in that variety which arises from *rheumatic* irritation, but when arising from other causes. A great number of cases of chorea treated successfully with this remedy have been reported, a few of which we collect.

Case 1st. A boy aged 11, had had Chorea for four months; one side was affected, and in almost constant motion, except when asleep; he had been under medical care all the time without avail. He then took one teaspoonful of pulv. black snake root every morning for three days, then omitted it three, then resumed it again until he had taken it nine times. When he had taken six doses he was almost well; when he had taken nine doses he was perfectly well, and remained so for at least four years.—*Dr. Young.*

Case 2nd. A girl sick with Chorea for a month; after taking three doses she was very much improved; six doses cured her entirely. It caused *pricking* all over every time it was taken.—*Ibid.*

Case 3rd. A lady, aged 19 had Chorea for two weeks; her left side was almost constantly in motion; it did not prevent her sleeping; her general health was perfectly good, and no cause could be detected. She was dosed with Calomel, Jalap, Tartar emetic and Cream Tartar, for seven days, when Dr. Young was startled, for he found that the Chorea had extended to the right side and was tenfold aggravated. Her arms, legs, head, face,, tongue and every muscular part, was in continual and irregular motion; she could with great difficulty speak intelligibly. The power of swallowing was lost to a great degree, she could not walk one step, nor stand up without support, nor could she sleep day or night on account of the constant twitching and jerking of the muscles. A teaspoonful of the powdered root of Cimicifuga was given three times a day; in five days she was much better, could walk 300 or 400 yards, could speak and swallow as well as ever; slept well at night; her legs had but little irregular motion, her head was steady, and the muscles of her face scarcely agitated; her arms were more affected than any other part. In seven days more she was quite well. It neither vomited, sweated, purged or acted on her kidneys; the only sensation she had was an uneasy sensation, almost amounting to an ache, through all her limbs, after every dose, and continuing three or four hours. Dr. Physic cured several cases with ten grain doses every two hours. Dr. Wood cured a case after the failure of purgative and metallic tonics; also a case of periodic convulsions connected with uterine disorder.

Case 4th. A girl aged 9, whose mental faculties were much disordered, and who had lost nearly all power over the left arm and leg; bowels irregular, headache, and pain frequently shooting down the left arm. Was cured quickly. A very intractable case was cured by Dr. Otto. A girl aged 18—Chorea with considerable gastric derangement, with suppression of menses for five months. Five grains of the pulv. root every 3 hours; no improvement for nearly a week; then improved rapidly and was well in three weeks. Dr. Davis says we can no longer doubt its efficacy in Chorea, in all cases arising from undue irritability or mobility of the nervous system, especially when induced by exposure to cold; in short, when Chorea arises from a rheumatic irritation of the motor nerves, and muscles, or of the anterior column of the spinal marrow. In the various Eclectic Journals, there have been reported from time to time very many cures of Chorea, made with Cimicifuga. In some cases the powdered root was used; in others the tincture, resinoid (macrotin), or the fluid extract. According to my experience it is most useful when the disease occurs in females, is aggravated at the menstrual periods, and seems to be somehow *connected with derangement of the generative functions.* The first decimal of the pulv. root seems to act more promptly in these cases, although the first dec. dilution is quite reliable. Physicians are in duty bound to report their *failures* as well as their cures. I have given the Cimicifuga in some cases without deriving any benefit from its use. One case was a child about 10 years of age. The first symptom was a "catching" of the lower limb, like the disease called "spring-halt" in horses; afterwards came twitching of the mouth, arms, fingers and feet. Cimicifuga 1st or 3d trit. did not cause any improvement in ten days. Agaricus was tried a week; but Nux vomica 2d. dil. five drops three times a day arrested the malady. A similar case also resisted its action, probably because it was not strictly homœopathic, but when the citrate of Iron and Strychnia was given, a rapid recovery was the result. This last medicine was selected because of the anæmia which indicated Iron, and the peculiar spasmodic symptoms called for Nux vom. One grain of the first decimal was given three times a day. Improvement immediately set in, and continued until the recovery was complete—about four weeks.

Fever.—Chilliness during the forenoon. Occasional cold chill. Coldness and chills, particularly of the arms and feet soon after waking. At 3 A. M., the whole surface became cold. Slight cold perspiration, and sensation as if it would become profuse, continuing for an hour, accompanied by lancinating pain along the cartilages of the false ribs, left side, increased by taking a long inspiration. Disposition to perspire at night for three weeks; irregular, usually three or four times a week, occurring about 3 A. M., commencing while asleep, and disappearing a few minutes after waking, never profuse. During the first week the surface was cold with the perspiration, but during the last ten days the perspiration was accompanied by heat rather than coldness; pulse too slow, every third or fourth pulsation intermitting. In three quarters of an hour, increased heat of the face; slight inclination to sweat; pulse rather full, 90 in the minute, it being 80 before taking the drug. In three quarters of an hour after taking the second dose, pulse weaker and very irregular, 80 in the minute. At the end of an hour pulse 80 and *irregular*. Pulse quick and weak. In morning pulse feeble, with weakness and trembling. Drowsiness, with creeping chills upon the back during the evening, followed by frequent wakings during the night, and desire to throw off the bed clothes, although the thermometer was below zero.

Clinical Remarks.—The febrile symptoms developed during a proving of Cimicifuga are very slight. Careful observers have almost uniformly found it to lessen the force and frequency of the pulse, at the same time soothing pain and allaying irritability. Dr. Davis says, it causes a depression of the pulse, which remains for a considerable time. Dr. Marcy says: "Like many other drugs which exercise a specific action upon the nervous system, the primary effect of actea, when given in small doses, is slightly stimulating to both the nervous and vascular systems, causing a slight increase in the force and frequency of the pulse, and followed speedily by a permanent depression of the circulation. When administering it for mild attacks of rheumatism, we have in several instances observed this primary and secondary action. Among the secondary effects which are strongly marked, are, diminished nervous irritability, and disposition to sleep." In *Rheumatic fever*, it is a valuable remedy. It will sometimes act promptly in reducing the force of the pulse, and bringing on a healthy perspiration. Some severe acute attacks of inflammatory rheumatism have been cured with Cimicifuga in a very short time. But it has been usually given in too large doses, by the dominant school, (30 to 60 drops of the tincture every two or four hours). Such doses are useless and injurious. I have succeeded with five drops of the first dilution, and rarely resort to the tincture. Five drops every hour should be the maximum dose.

In *Yellow fever*, it is recommended by some writers. It would seem to be somewhat homœopathic to the severe and peculiar "pains in the bones," as sufferers term it, but probably bears no relation to the real condition present. In nearly all fevers it may be indicated for certain conditions which may arise. Thus in many fevers, the nervous system, the brain, may and does become very irritable and irritated, and a train of symptoms, such as will be found under the head of "Brain," will arise. In such cases small doses will remove the symptoms, and permit remedies more appropriate to the general condition, to act untrammelled. Although this remedy is to a certain extent an analogue of aconite, yet it does not seem to control febrile diseases as promptly.

Skin.—Eruptions of white pustules over the face and neck. Sometimes large, red, papular.

CLINICAL REMARKS.—The above is a *curative* symptom, although it has been recorded in some of our works as a pathogenetic. So far in our experiments we have failed to develop any skin symptoms. It is indeed doubtful whether it is an eliminator like arsenicum, or a cutaneous irritant like sulphur. Dr. Hill, in his Epitome, highly recommends its use in Small Pox, but his indications are not based on any relation it has to the eruptions, but to the *peculiar pains, etc.*, which accompany the fever. Dr. D. S. Smith, of Chicago recommends it very highly in Variola and Varioloid, and asserts that it decidedly modifies the disease, preventing pitting, and even the development of pustules. It may prove useful, indirectly, in some exanthematous diseases. Thus: Urticaria often depends upon rheumatic irritation of internal organs; some eruptions are excited by menstrual derangements. Cimicifuga being homœopathic to the exciting causes, will, by removing *them*, remove the cutaneous irritation. Dr. Lee says, "it sometimes appears to have a specific action on the skin, causing a sensation of prickling, itching and heat on the whole surface." This may be (by its action on the terminal nerves) attended sometimes by a slight eruption.

Sleep.—Very restless at night. Restless at night after three or four hours of good sleep. Restlessness early in the morning, continuing for a week. Disturbed, restless, unrefreshing sleep, from 3 to 5 A. M., with disposition to fold the arms over the head; unpleasant dreams of being in trouble, of being in a sad plight; Somnolency.

CLINICAL REMARKS.—The sleeplessness and nightly restlessness caused by this drug belong to its power of causing nervous irritation. In *delirium a potu*, sleeplessness is one of the most troublesome symptoms, one which the dominant school try to subdue with enormous doses of opium. Opium is sometimes homœopathic to this condition, also Cannabis ind., Coffea, Arsenicum, etc., but none more so than Cimicifuga, unless it be Digitalis, which latter medicine is just now used with such success in delirium tremens. In typhoid states, hysteria, and those conditions brought on by mental excitement and labor, we have to deal with insomnia of an obstinate character. In many of these instances this remedy will assist us in our treatment of the difficulty. I have given it in the sleeplessness of children during teething, or when no apparent cause for the symptoms existed. A few pellets of the 3d, seemed to palliate as well as Coffea.

Mind and Sensorium.—Not disposed to fix the attention on any subject; vertigo; impaired vision; dizziness; dullness in the head; vertigo; fulness and dull aching in the vertex; ten minutes after taking the third decimal dilution, a sort of delirium, with an inclination to run over the subject on which he was reading. Miserable dejected feeling; mind dull and heavy. Feels grieved, troubled, with sighing; next day a feeling of tremulous joy, with mirthfulness, playfulness and clear intellect. Considerable exhilaration. Pleasurable excitement. Cimicifuga soon shows its action on the sensorium, when administered to sensitive persons. Dr. King made casual mention in his dispensatory, that this drug had caused symptoms simulating *delirium tremens.* To get at the real history of such action I wrote to Dr. King, who kindly favored me with the following statement: * * "I did not pay that attention to the symptoms as one of your school would have done, but merely noticed them in the aggregate. In the cases referred to, I gave the tincture for the cure of rheumatism, in ordinary doses of 20 to 30 drops, every hour, but finding the symptoms resulting therefrom to be similar to those of delirium tremens, I omitted the medicine until they had disappeared, and again administered it, but in smaller doses, and so continued until I found that even two or three drops would be followed by the same symptoms, and was therefore compelled to cease its use altogether in such cases. I have not met with this effect in but three cases, and in the first one that occurred, so positive was I from the symptoms of the patient, that his wife had allowed him the use of some liquor, that I came very near being discharged on account of the scolding I administered to both the patient and his wife. In fact, I did not believe in that case that the tincture produced the effects, nor until I met with the other cases. As near as I can recollect there were nausea, retching, dilated pupils, tremor of the limbs, incessant talking and changing from one subject to another without any order, though perfectly sensible when the attention was aroused by any person addressing them, or conversing with them, but soon relapsing into their vagaries when not disturbed; great wakefulness, imagining strange objects upon the bed, and in the room, as rats, sheep, etc. Sometimes arousing from their incoherent talkativeness as if startled, and inquiring regarding persons present:—'Who is that man?' 'What does he want here?' 'Tell him to go home,' etc. With quick, full pulse, a wild look of the eyes, and the peculiar indescribable expression of face commonly observed among those who labor under delirium tremens." I can corroborate Dr. King's experience with the Cimicifuga. I once gave the tincture to a girl who had dysmenorrhœa. I ordered her to take one drop every two hours during the premonitory stage, and when the pains, which were intense, painful, like labor-pains, and extended to the hips, thighs and ovarian regions had become severe, to take one drop every half hour. By some misunderstanding she took *five* drops every half hour for six hours. When I saw her she had *no pains,* but said her head felt "strange and wild;" her pupils were dilated, she talked incoherently, and exclaimed that she saw rats, mice, and insects, on the bed and on the floor and ceiling. She also complained of a *roaring* in the head, very distressing.

Clinical Remarks.—In its effects on the sensorium, (brain) Cimicifuga is analogous to Arsenicum, Belladonna, Hyoscyamus, Opium, Stramonium, and a few other drugs, but it has important points of dissimilarity which should be considered in the selection of the drug. I treated one mild case of delirium tremens with this remedy. It seemed to remove the condition. When the symptoms above narrated occur in typhoid, or hysteric states, the Cimicifuga will act beneficially. A few drops of the 3d dilution in water every hour seems the most appropriate method of administration.

Head.—Heaviness and dullness of the head; slight fulness of the head; slight dull pain in the head; acute pain generally through the head during the day, at times more severe on the left side; slight pain in the head in the evening; remittent headache of long standing, more or less severe every day, but increased every second day; dull pain deep in the forehead; dullness of the head and pain in the forehead and occiput; dull pain in the forehead in the afternoon; dull, boring pain in the forehead, over the left superciliary ridge, continuing for two hours, from 10 A. M; pain in the forehead and occiput, with heaviness of the head after one hour; pain from the eyes to the top of the head, which seemed as if the nerves were excited to too much action, lasting three hours—under large doses, it lasted six hours; pain over the eyes; pain over the left eye, extending along the base of the brain to the occiput; slight pain in the forehead; dryness of the pharynx; aching in the eyes, apparently between the eyeball and orbital plate of the frontal bone. At 10 P. M. occasional transient pain in the forehead, over the right eye; dull pain in the head; fullness in the forehead, over the eyes; severe pain in the head, particularly in the forehead and eyeballs; severe pain in the forehead over the right eye, and extending to the temple and vertex with fulness, heat, and throbbing, and when going up stairs, a sensation as if the top of the head would fly off; fulness in the vertex; aching pain in the vertex and occiput in paroxysms, at times quite severe, immediately after rising. Pain in the vertex during the afternoon and evening; sensation as if the temples were compressed occasionally through the day; dull, heavy headache, more in the left temple; slight pain in the left side of the head; aching pain in the head, particularly in the occiput, experienced only while indoors, relieved by the open air—it increased during the afternoon, and was quite severe in the evening; about 9 P. M., it disappeared entirely after a walk in the open air; constant dull pain in the head, particularly in the occiput, and extending to the vertex, during the forenoon and part of the afternoon. The pain in the head is always relieved by open air; dull sensation through the head as though he had been on a "spree" and was getting over its effects. Brain feels too large for the cranium; brain feels compressed. Awoke at 2 o'clock A. M., with excruciating, though dull pain in the forehead, extending to the temples, with coldness of forehead; pain in the eyeballs. Dull pain in the region of moral organs—a pressing outward and upward, as if there was not room enough for the upper portion of the cerebrum. This pain was very oppressive and intolerable; it began about 5 o'clock P. M., after taking the second dose, and continued unabated till morning, when it was relieved in thirty minutes by a dose of Bryonia.

CLINICAL REMARKS.—There is no remedy in our Materia Medica which so promptly and uniformly causes headache as the Cimicifuga—with the exception of Glonoine. It is homœopathic to a variety of headaches, particularly the nervous, rheumatic and menstrual. It effects the brain in a manner similar to Digitalis. Some of its symptoms resemble Nux., Ign., Glonoine, Spigelia and Belladonna. It has cured a headache with "severe pain in the eyeballs, extending into the forehead, and increased by the slightest movement of the head or eyeballs," also "dull pain in the occipital regions with shooting pains down the back of the neck."

Case 1st. A lady aged 35, has suffered from dyspepsia for several months, and for nine days past from severe pain in the forehead over the right eye, and extending to the temple and vertex, with fullness, heat and throbbing, and when going up stairs a sensation as if the top of the head would fly off. Coldness and chills, particularly of the arms and feet; faintness in the epigastrium; pain and regurgitation of food after eating. Cimicifuga first, three drops three times a day, afforded prompt and permanent relief.—*Paine.*

Case 2nd. Mrs. W. aged 47, has not yet passed the critical period, and suffers from various neuralgic pains incident to that time. Now suffers from severe pains in the head, particularly in the forehead and eyeballs. Cimicifuga second, afforded prompt relief in a few hours.

Case 3rd. Dull pain in the head; fullness in the forehead and eyes; pain in the eyeballs, increased secretion of tears; fluent watery coryza; frequent sneezing; soreness of the throat; cough at night, caused by tickling in throat—cured in two days by Cimicifuga 2. (Dr. Paine). This is a well marked case of *catarrhal* headache. I have found it useful in similar cases. Dr. B. L. Hill states that the pains in the head caused by Cimicifuga are all *from within outwards.* It is particularly useful in headaches of delicate, nervous and hysterical females, when the headaches occur at or near the menstrual periods, during pregnancy, and at the change of life. ("Sabina.") It is useful in the headaches of drunkards, occurring after a debauch; in the headaches of students and literary men, after mental labor, and that peculiar heaviness, dullness and gloominess which results from want of sleep. (Nux.) Children, during teething, or in the course of many diseases, frequently show symptoms of *irritation* of the brain. This is denoted by peevishness, wakefulness, flushed-face, injected eyes, etc. In such cases eclectics claim the Cimicifuga has a calming influence, and prevents cerebral congestion, spasms, etc.

Eyes.—Aching of the eyes, at 10 A. M. Heaviness of the eyes, as if caused by cold. Dull pain in both eyeballs. Pain in both eyeballs. Pain in the centre of the eyeballs, and also sensation as if pain were situated between the eyeball and the orbital plate of the frontal bone, in the morning, on rising, continuing all day, but not severe as in the morning; aching pain in the centre of both eyeballs, rarely in one alone, continuing for three weeks after discontinuing the drug; aching pain in both eyeballs through the day; aching in the eyeballs, in the evening; on going up stairs, eyeballs painful for a short time; pain in the eyeballs; increased secretion of tears; pain in the eyeballs, in the left more than in the right, and sensation as if they were enlarged—most severe in the morning; severe aching pain in the right eyeball, after retiring at night; constant dull aching pain in right eyeball, and across the forehead, accompanied with nausea. Pain extending from the right eyeball through to the right side of the occiput, slightly affecting the ear, at night; Stinging in the eyelid, stinging in the eyelids, an hour after taking the drug; stinging of the eyelids, dulness and heaviness of the head and eyes, as if produced by cold; inflammation of both eyelids; sensation of swelling of right eyelid, with heat as if inflamed, after four hours. Pain in the right eyelid when closing it, in the afternoon. (The above is from Marcy's proving.) Redness of face and eyes; eyes feel as if swollen; black specks before the eyes. Myopia increased. During the headache the eyes were so congested as to attract the attention of every one, although there was no disagreeable feeling in them. (Hill's proving).

Clinical Remarks.—Few medicines cause such intense and persistent pains in the *eyeballs*. The pains are principally *aching*. (Bell., Digit., Merc., Hepar., Cupr., Crocus., Cocc.) The pains caused by this drug simulate *rheumatic* and *neuralgic* affections of the eyes. It will probably be found useful in "ocular hyper-æsthesia" —a condition of irritation and over-sensitiveness of the optic nerves. It appears to effect the eyes in a manner somewhat similar to *Spigelia* in causing intense pains in the eyeballs. A young lady aged 20, of light complexion, had suffered for several weeks from ophthalima, pain in the eyeballs—a sensation as if they were enlarged—most severe in the morning; prickling in the inner canthus, aggravated by reading; inflammation of the eyelids; slight secretion of mucus early in the morning; sore throat; reading causes headache. Cimicifuga first, three drops, three times a day, entirely removed all the pains in the eyeballs and head. (Paine.) It seems to be indicated in *Amaurosis*, but we have no clinical experience in this disease. Dr. King (eclectic) says, "In doses of one dram of the tincture every hour, it has effected thorough cures of ophthalima conjunctiva, without the aid of any local application."

Nose.—Stinging sensation in the nose in the evening; obstruction of the left nostril, in the evening; inclination to sneeze twice in the afternoon. Frequent inclination to sneeze, in the afternoon; sneezing; headache; sneezing several times, at 10 A. M.; frequent sneezing and fluent coryza during the day. Fluent coryza; fluent coryza of whitish mucus during the day; constant coryza, during the day; abundant watery coryza; copious coryza; copious coryza during the forenoon; fluent coryza; aching and soreness in the nose during the day. Fluent watery coryza; frequent sneezing; soreness in the throat, causing difficulty in swallowing. Profuse coryza in the forenoon; aching pain in the head; pain in both eyeballs, many times through the day. Very profuse greenish and slighty sanguineous coryza, after rising; fulness of the pharynx, and constant inclination to swallow; dulness of the head, and pain in the forehead and occiput; fluent coryza, more so than for many weeks, as if caused by cold; dryness of the pharynx; sneezing, at 4 P. M. (Payne's proving). Stuffed condition of the nostrils, which was soon followed by an open moist condition, with great sensitiveness to cold air, as if the base of the brain were laid bare, and every inhalation of the brain brought the cold air in contact with it. (This is exactly similar to that produced by a sudden change of weather in winter, from cold dry, to damp thawing, as by a south wind which melts the snow). (Hills proving).

Clinical Remarks.—Some authors say that they have never known it to produce a perceptible increase of any of the secretions; others again say that it operates powerfully upon the secreting organs and absorbents, and that it is expectorant and diaphoretic. From the above symptoms it would certainly seem to have a specific affinity for the nasal mucous membrane, and causes a real catarrhal state. In acute rheumatic-catarrhal attacks, with pains in the limbs, head, face, eyeballs, chilliness, heat, and fluent watery coryza, it is certainly indicated; and in one epidemic influenza I found it useful for such conditions, also in the cough and sore throat by which it was accompanied.

Face, Jaws and Teeth.—Severe pain in the left jaw. Heat on one side of the face, with lassitude all over. Very severe pains in the face, more in under jaw, lower teeth, and articulations of lower jaw. The pains in the head and face constant, and very severe. Pain in the right superior maxillary bone, and teeth.

Clinical Remarks.—The above are just such pains as are nearly always present in catarrhal-rheumatic attacks in the winter and spring. I once took five drops of the first decimal for similar symptoms occurring in myself. The one dose seemed to cut short the attack, at least it mitigated the pains.

Mouth.—Offensive breath; dryness and soreness of the lips; dry lips; small ulcer on the inner surface of the lower lip. Unpleasant taste in the mouth, accumulation of thick mucus upon the teeth; spitting of thick saliva which seemed to stick to the mouth and throat, and to be detached with difficulty. Mouth dry in the morning. Swelling of the back part of the tongue. Root of tongue and fauces swollen.

Clinical Remarks.—In many cases of rheumatism, the gums and buccal mucous membrane became swollen and tumefied. In such cases this remedy may be found useful, used as a weak wash to the inflamed surface.

Throat.—Dryness of the pharynx; sneezing, at 4 P. M.; dryness of the pharynx and inclination to swallow, during the night; fulness of the pharynx and constant inclination to swallow; soreness of the throat when swallowing; sensation of fulness high up in the throat with fulness in the vertex and stiffness of the neck; sensation of rawness in the throat; slight difficulty in swallowing; hoarseness, which increased towards night; constant unpleasant fulness in the pharynx. Palate and uvula red and inflamed. Inflammation of the uvula and palate, fifth day more severe than the day before; copious coryza. Hoarseness, roughness and scraping in the throat; roughness and dryness of the throat, with thirst; dryness and soreness of the throat on swallowing, and on pressure worse on the left side.

Clinical Remarks.—It has cured Chorea when attended with almost complete loss of the power of swallowing. In sore throat, and cynanche maligna a decoction of the root is recommended by Dr. Barton. Dr. Marcy says it is an excellent remedy against dryness of the throat, or a dry spot in the throat causing cough (*Lachesis*), also in dry coughs proceeding from irritation and tickling at the lower part of the larynx. In a late number of an Allopathic Journal, it is highly recommended by a Boston physician as a most excellent remedy in Diphtheria, used in decoction as a gargle.

Appetite and Stomach.—Eructations tasting of the medicine; eructations and slight nausea, immediately. Pain and regurgitation of food after eating. Loss of appetite; no appetite for supper; repugnance. Nausea for fifteen minutes half an hour after taking the drug; nausea with loathing, soon after the dose; sense of internal tremor in the stomach, after breakfast; sensation as if too much food had been taken into the stomach; acute darting pain in the epigastrium, after a light supper; slight pain in the epigastrium, extending to the left hypochondrium, with faintness and sensation of emptiness; faintness in the epigastrium, with repugnance to food, which, however, did not prevent his partaking of a moderate breakfast; faintness in the epigastrium, generally in the morning before eating, particularly if the medicine had been taken over night, not preventing eating, which was followed by a sensation of repletion, as if too much food had been taken; faintness of the epigastrium; faintness of the stomach; slight faintness in the epigastrium, during the forenoon; faintness of the stomach two or three times, of short duration; violent retching and vomiting, with pain in the head. In a "proving," which Dr. Hill reported to the N. A. Journal of Homœopathy, he copies the above, with a few additions, and appropriates them to himself. The fact is, that proving (in vol. 7) is nearly all taken from Dr. Paine's original proving. Hill and Douglas also state that in their proving "all the stomach symptoms were produced on females; the drug producing no disturbance in the stomach of males." But in Dr. Paine's provings, men and women were alike affected with nausea and vomiting. The statement of Dr. Hill, reiterated in his "epitome," is therefore unreliable. It was probably originally put forth to favor the idea that Cimicifuga was specific to nearly all diseases of females, morning sickness, etc.

Clinical Remarks.—That Cimicifuga may cause sympathetic nausea and vomiting, by its irritating influence over the female organs of generation, I do not deny. But it is by no means a specific in "morning nausea" of pregnant women. If the uterine and general symptoms correspond, the remedy may be found useful for that distressing symptom. I have in a few cases found it useful, but no more so than Nux vom., Ipecac, Puls., or Oxalate of Cerium. Like its analogues—Digitalis, Belladonna, Opium, etc., this medicine may cause vomiting through its irritating effect upon the brain. Powerful vomiting is often the first symptom of Meningitis, Hydrocephalus and other brain diseases, and the so called "nervous sick headaches," which are accompanied by severe vomiting, probably consist eventually of cerebral irritation. It is in this type of "sick headache" that Cimicifuga is useful and *not* in the headaches which proceed from derangement of digestion.

Abdomen.—Flatus; rumbling in the lower part of the abdomen, at 10 A. M. Flatulence, causing a sensation of fulness in the abdomen, rumbling of flatus below the umbilicus, at 10 P. M. Fulness and pressure in the lower part of the abdomen. Increased pressure in the lower part of the abdomen with some pain. Acute cutting pain in the umbilical region, which, although acute, was not so severe as to prevent attending to his usual business; uninfluenced by eating and continuing during the afternoon; wandering pain in the bowels, slight pain in left iliac region; afterwards severe pains in the bowels, mostly below the umbilicus, with weight and pain in lumbar and sacral region; soreness of abdominal muscles, on taking full inspirations. Dull griping, twisting at the umbilical region, more towards the left. Pain in the left hypochondriac region, worse on motion, and on taking a deep inspiration. Periodic colic with inclination to bend forward, relieved after stool.

Clinical Remarks.—There are three diseases of the abdominal structures, in which this remedy may prove useful: (1) Rheumatism of the muscular structures; (2) Neuralgia; (3) Peritonitis, especially puerperal. I have found it useful in the *first* and *second*, but have never used it in the *third*, nor have we any clinical experience of its use in that affection.

Stool.—Evacuation regular and natural during the proving, but for a month afterwards, alternate constipation and tendency to diarrhœa; disposition to diarrhœa, in the evening; slight disposition to diarrhœa, after rising. Constipation; fæces hard and dry. Large papescent stool with general indisposition. Scanty diarrhœa with tenesmus. Copious papescent stool in the morning.

Clinical Remarks.—We have no proof that this drug has any laxative or cathartic effect. It cannot be homœopathic to abnormal intestinal discharges, at least we have no clinical testimony to that effect.

Urine.—Disposition to frequent urination. Increased flow of urine. Increased secretion of pale urine; retention of urine for eighteen hours followed by frequent micturition. Profuse flow of pale watery urine. Stitches in urethra in the morning.

Clinical Remarks.—The dominant school assert the Cimicifuga to be a diuretic. It does increase the quantity of urine, but probably not from any influence it has over the kidneys primarily. All drugs which bring on depression of the nervous system, will cause something akin to "nervous diabetes." In hysterical states, and many forms of uterine disorder, we find this condition:—a profuse flow of watery urine, with nervous prostration; sinking sensation at the stomach, chilliness, headache, *over* the eyes, *in* the eyes; lowness of spirit, and sometimes aching pains in the limbs. With this state of the system, it is supposed by physiologists, there occurs a waste of phosphorus—which is eliminated by the kidneys in the form of phosphates. Loss of phosphates indicates innervation. Dr. Lee says, "In some instances it acts as a renal hydragogue, increasing to a considerable extent, the amount of urinary secretion; but, in a majority of cases, this result cannot be anticipated with any considerable degree of confidence. We are rather disposed to regard it in the light of a renal alterative; increasing generally the amount of *solids* in the urine, without any great increase in the amount of water. To eliminate solid matters from the blood, whether lithates, phosphates, or animal matters, the cohosh, with the free use of diluents, may rank among our most efficient agents. Cimicifuga, has a similar action, over the renal organs, to Aconite, Asclepias syr. and Colchicum, all of which increase the solid constituents of urine. This condition is admirably met, by the dilutions of the remedy. It may be found useful in spasmodic retention of urine, from a cold, mental emotion, or as a symptom of rheumatism.

Genital Organs of Men.—Pain and retraction of the right spermatic cord; drawing pain along the right spermatic cord; pain and tenderness of the testicles.

CLINICAL REMARKS.—It is said to cure old standing cases of gleet and spermatorrhœa.

Genital Organs of Women.—Leucorrhœa; menorrhagia; suppression of the menses; feeling of heaviness; weight bearing down in the uterine region, with feeling of heaviness and torpor of the lower extremities; appearances of the menses eight days before their time; labor-like pains during pregnancy; abortion in the fourth, eighth and twelfth weeks of pregnancy; cold chills and prickling sensations during the day—in the mammæ; prickling sensations in the breasts.

CLINICAL REMARKS.—No remedy stands higher in the estimation of the eclectic school, for the treatment of diseases peculiar to females, than the Cimicifuga, and its concentrated principle—Cimicifugin. It is used by them in all uterine diseases, of the most opposite character. Dr. King, one of their highest authorities, says (Amer. Eclec. Disp.) "it is useful in amenorrhœa, dysmenorrhœa, leucorrhœa and other uterine affections. As a partus accelerator, it may be substituted for ergot. It brings on expulsive action of the uterus speedily and powerfully. After labor it will be found effectual in allaying the general excitement of the nervous system and relieving after-pains." In "King's Amer. Obsts." he recommends it, in addition, for menorrhagia, amenorrhœa, prolapsus uteri, etc. "It does not produce the powerful and continuous contractions of the uterus which follow the use of ergot, and, consequently, is not as dangerous to the child; neither does it lessen the susceptibility of the organ to subsequent doses, as is apt to be the case with ergot; it appears to excite the uterus to a normal activity only." Jones and Scudder, in their "Mat. Med.," reiterate the above recommendations. The writings of that school are full of clinical experience relative to the usefulness of this remedy in diseases of females. The homœopathic school are beginning to realize the value of this agent in similar affections, and although the pathogenesis which we have is meagre, and the recorded symptoms of the drug, so far as relates to its action on the reproductive organs, few in number, yet those who have used it much, upon the indications derived *ex uso in morbis*, are enthusiastic in its praise. I will proceed to give what I conceive to be its peculiar sphere of action, and point out the indications for its use in the various affections arising from derangements of the organs of generation. *In amenorrhœa*, or delayed appearance of the menses in young girls, from deficient nervous energy in the ovaries, and when the abnormal nervous influence is directed to other organs, giving rise to chorea, hysteria, nervous headaches, etc., the Cimicifuga will restore the functions of the reproductive organs to a normal state. Should there be, at the same time with the above conditions, a chlorotic state, Helonias or Ferrum should be alternated with this remedy. *In suppression of the menses* from a cold, mental emotions, and febrile symptoms, when rheumatic pains in the limbs, or intense headache, or uterine cramps, are present, this remedy will be found very useful. *In dysmenorrhœa*, the Black Snake root has been used successfully by all schools. The eclectics consider it a sort of panacœa. Many of our own school speak highly of its value. Dr. Hill, in his "Epitome," advises it in *all* cases, and in alternation with Caulophyllum. It is not a general specific, yet will benefit a majority of cases. It is most useful in rheumatic and neuralgic cases, but is often of benefit in congestive, dysmenorrhœa, when alternated with Veratrum viride, or Belladonna. The best method of administration in these diseases, is to give Cimicifuga, first decimal or one hundredth, three or four times a day during the inter-menstrual period, and every hour or thirty minutes during the severity of the pain. The Cimicifugin, second or third decimal trituration, will in some cases act more satisfactorily than the tincture. Several of my colleagues have reported cases of dysmenorrhœa cured or very much relieved. Dr. Ludlam thinks more highly of the Cimicifugin in the neuralgic type, than of Caulophyllum. The latter is more indicated in cases complicated with uterine spasms or general hysterical convulsions. Dr. Williams sends me the record of two severe cases of dysmenorrhœa, probably of a rheumatic origin, which were apparently cured under the action of Cimicifugin, first. I have treated many cases of difficult and painful menstruation, arising from various causes, and while in all there was improvement, in many the morbid condition seemed to be permanently removed. I consider the following symptoms as indicating its use: *Before* the menses the peculiar headache, similar to that caused by this medicine; *during* the menses, aching in the limbs, severe pain in the back, down the thighs and through the hips, with heavy pressing-down, labor-like pains, weeping mood, nervousness, hysteric spasms, cramps, tenderness of the hypogastric region, scanty flow of coagulated blood, or profuse flow of the same character; *between* the menses debility, nervous erethism, neuralgic pains, tendency to prolapsus, etc.; in *menorrhagia*, when the flow is profuse, but more of a passive character, dark, coagulated, and accompanied by the above mentioned pains. The Cimicifuga does not primarily cause hæmorrhage, like Sabina, Erigeron or Crocus, but secondarily, by impairing the tonicity and normal vitality of the uterus. In *Leucorrhœa*, the eclectics speak highly of its efficacy. The late Dr. Morrow, to whom is mainly due the introduction of the remedy into that practice, gained much celebrity by his treatment of leucorrhœa, with the internal and local use of the black cohosh. He gave it until it produced and kept up its peculiar action on the brain in a slight degree; a decoction of the root was to be used as an injection every day. Leucorrhœa may be vaginal, cervical, or uterine. In the present state of our knowledge of the action of the drug, we cannot point out accurately the particular form of leucorrhœa for which it is indicated. It may be beneficial in all varieties; the general symptoms of the patient must, to a great extent, be our guide. Dr. Hill mentions a "leucorrhœa of long standing cured during a week's proving," and another case of "leucorrhœa, and chronic inflammation and congestion of the uterus, cured during the proving, while no other symptoms were observed on the provers until the disappearance of the uterine disease." Believing in the *local*, as well as general action of a drug, I would advise it to be used both topically and internally. The lower dilutions seems to act most beneficially. It is now more than sixty years since it was claimed by *Stearns'* in the American Herbal, to have an especial affinity for the uterus, particularly over the menstrual function, and Dr. Tully regards this claim as well established by the experience of New England practitioners. As a parturiefacient, it was in general use among the Indians in the early settlement of this country. Bigelow speaks of it as an active agent in facilitating parturition; and Tully says he has known many cases where it has produced abortion in pregnant females, when prescribed for a cough. The evidence on this head is far more full and satisfactory than in regard to its emmennagogue properties. *Prof. Lee* says: "It is believed to exert a specific influence on the uterine contractions lasting longer than that of ergot, and followed by less torpor and greater susceptibility and capacity for action in the uterus than before its employment. Its operation, also, is not attended by that deleterious and stupefying influence on the fœtus which often follows the administration of spurred rye." It is doubtful if the ergot acts medicinally upon the fœtus at all. It is the continued, unintermitting pressure of the uterus upon the child, or the cord, which causes the coma or asphyxia in the infant, before birth. "After delivery, also, it has been extensively used for the purpose of inducing firm uterine contraction, expelling the placenta, and checking post-partem hæmorrhages. For this purpose a drachm of the saturated alcoholic tincture should be given every half hour, or oftener, until the desired effect is produced." This knowledge of the uterine-motor action of

Cimicifuga should be appropriated by homœopathists. They are capable of making much more valuable use of such knowledge than the adherents of other schools of medicine. The homœopathic school gladly avail themselves of the use of ergot, in slow and difficult labors arising from an atonic condition of the uterus, or perverted function. I cannot give my assent to those mythical relations of the effects of Secale third or thirtieth, in causing uterine contractions when deficient during labor—the proof is not sufficient. I consider the Cimicifuga, as well as Secale, Caulophyllum and other drugs possessing similar powers, as being *secondarily* homœopathic to conditions of uterine inertia. To explain: The *primary* action of ergot in moderate medicinal doses is to cause contractions, more or less persistent of the muscular tissue of the uterus. Under the continued action of the drug these contractions will become more intense and firm, until, from over-stimulation, an opposite condition or muscular atony obtains. Now, this latter condition, with its accompanying symptoms, is a secondary effect of the drug, as much due to pathogenetic action as was the primary. When, in practice, we meet with similar conditions, *i. e.*, when the uterus, after vain and powerful efforts, becomes exhausted, ergot is the proper remedy, if the *primary* symptoms corresponded with those of the drug, viz., persistent and unintermitting contractions. But if the uterine atony be caused by ergot, then that medicine will not answer our purpose, and we must resort to Cimicifuga, Caulophyllum, Uva ursi, or galvanism. Secondary states of uterine muscular atony may be brought on by all the last named agents, and for this reason they will all be found useful in similar morbid conditions. The *dose* which should be used in such cases should be as large as can be given with safety to the patient, and just large enough to arouse the torpid muscular tissue. My theory of *dose*, and which experience strongly substantiates, is, that for symptoms which simulate the primary effects of the medicine selected as the remedy, minute doses should be administered; but larger doses for symptoms simulating its secondary effects. In resorting to the Cimicifuga, in atonic labors, we need not give the massive doses of the eclectic school—doses which tend to bring on secondary exhaustion. I have found five to ten drops of the mother tincture, every fifteen or twenty minutes, to be amply sufficient to bring back or arouse the deficient vitality of the uterus. But there is an opposite condition of the uterus which sometimes obtains during labor, a state of hyper-excitation, in which the normal uterine contractions are spasmodic, painful, and intensely powerful, but *intermitting*, sometimes with cramps in the extremities, and a tendency to general convulsions. Here the Cimicifuga is *primarily* homœopathic, and a small quantity of the third or sixth attenuation will suffice to restore the normal parturient action. This medicine will be found useful after labor, in producing firm contraction of the uterus, expelling the placenta, or checking post-partem hæmorrhage. But I think for this purpose the Secale is to be preferred, because of its power to cause firmer and more *persistent* contraction. *After-pains* are often readily relieved by small doses of Cimicifuga second or third, or Cimicifugin third. I have used it with signal benefit in those cases which seemed to be kept up by a neuralgic disposition, or mental and nervous irritability, and the patient was sleepless, restless, sensitive and low spirited.

Suppression of the Lochia is treated successfully with this remedy. When from a cold or mental emotion the discharge is arrested, uterine spasms and cramps in the limbs sometimes occur, accompanied with headache, and even delirium. A case of this character which came under my treatment, was relieved in a few hours by Cimicifuga second trit., two grains every half hour. Warm fomentations were applied to the abdomen and vulva, as should always be the practice in such instances. It is useful to relieve those bearing-down pains, indications of prolapsus, which women frequently suffer after severe confinements. It is eminently homœopathic to a tendency to *abortion.* It has caused abortion in many instances, and is commonly resorted to for that purpose by reckless women, and advised by still more reckless physicians. It has been used successfully in those instances of "habitual abortion," with the result of preventing the usual miscarriages in the second and third months. But unless the general symptoms correspond, Caulophyllum, Sabina, Tanacetum or Helonias will have to be selected. When the chill, uterine pain, tenderness of the hypogastric region, and flooding have already set in, and the loss of the fœtus becomes imminent, the Cimicifuga, in small doses, may arrest the progress of the morbid process, provided the membranes have not become extensively detached. If the separated portion be slight, and the patient be kept quiet, and the proper remedy given, I believe it possible to prevent a further separation. If all hope of saving the fœtus be abandoned, and the uterus is deficient in expulsive power, then this medicine may be given, as recommended for uterine atony in labors. But no physician should rely alone upon medicinal action in such cases. The placental forceps and blunt hook should be used early and efficiently, to effect the entire removal of the contents of the uterus. In *prolapsus uteri*, the Cimicifuga is recommended by all eclectic authors. But here, as in other diseases, it can be no general specific. When the prolapsus is due to congestion, general or cervical, cervical leucorrhœa, or comes on as a result of abortion, or getting up too soon after confinement; and when a deficient innervation seems to lie at the root of the difficulty, then this medicine will be found an excellent remedy. Dr. Morrow, who probably used this agent more than any other physician in this country, was very successful in the treatment of prolapsus by its internal and local application. It already stands high in the homœopathic school in the treatment of uterine displacements. (Podophyllum, Caulophyllum, Helonias and Asclepias tub. will also be found useful). In *Ovarian diseases*, it will undoubtedly be found valuable. A medicine which exercises such profound influence over the reproductive organs must of necessity influence powerfully the ovaries. Dr. Cleveland recommends it for Ovaritis, and *spasm of the broad ligaments* (in the latter affection Caulophyllum and Magnesia mur. are specifics). In *irritable uterus*, next to Platina,

Sabina, Aconite or Caulophyllum, it will be found the most useful remedy we posses. Some writers recognize a variety of *epilepsy*, having its origin in uterine disorder—the epileptic convulsion being due to reflex action. This form of epilepsy generally occurs at or near the menstrual period. In such cases Cimicifuga has effected cures. It has also broken up the tendency to hysterical attacks occurring during the menses, also hysterical spasms due to uterine displacements after the womb has been restored to its normal position.

In *puerperal mania* it has been found curative. In part 43, Braithwaite's Petrospect, Prof. Simpson reports a case of Puerperal Hypochondriasis treated with tincture Cimicifuga. "A lady, the mother of several children, was twice the subject of the most painful mental despondency a month or two after delivery. On one of these occasions she was confined in London, and had the advice of several eminent physicians; but the disease took a very long and tiresome course, seeming to defy all remedies, and gradually and very slowly terminated. On the last occasion on which the attack occurred, this patient was confined under my care here, and went home to England some weeks subsequently, perfectly well. She returned, however, in about a month, to Edinburgh, in the lowest possible state of depression, a perfect picture of mental misery and unhappiness. I tried many plans to raise her out of this dark and gloomy state. All failed. At last, fancying from some of her symptoms and complaints that there might be a rheumatic element in the affection, I ordered her fifty drops of tincture of Actea, thrice a day. After taking one dose she refused to continue it, as the drug had a taste so similar to Laudanum, and as all opiates made her worse. On being reassured that there was no opiate in the medicine, she recommenced it, without any faith, however, in the results, as she had in a great measure lost faith in all medicinal means. When I saw her next, some eight or ten days afterwards, she was altered and changed in a marvelous degree, but all for the better. On the third or fourth day, as she informed me, the cloud of misery which had been darkening her existence suddenly began to dissolve and dispel, and in a day or two more, she felt perfectly herself again, in gaiety, spirits, and energy. But nothing would induce her, to give up the Actea for six or eight weeks longer; and the last time she passed through Edinburgh, she told me that she had prescribed her own remedy to more than one melancholic subject with nearly as great success as she had used it in her own case." The successful treatment of this case was rather a piece of *luck* than otherwise. It is doubtful, first, whether there was any "rheumatic element" in the case at all; and second, the medicine did not cure by anti-doting any "rheumatic element," but by virtue of its power of causing a similar state of the brain, and of inducing similar symptoms. This medicine has always had great reputation, not only as an accellerator in childbirth, but as a preventive of painful and difficult labor. Wishing to test its value in these cases, I have often given it to ladies whose previous labors had been slow and difficult, and generally with excellent results. It is best to begin three or four weeks before the time of the expected confinement, and have the patient take a few drops of the first or second decimal dilution, or trituration, three times a day. During the last week, the doses may be given every four hours. One case will illustrate the success attending its administration, as it is the type of many others. A lady, the mother of three children, expressed great anxiety regarding her expected confinement. She was in the eighth month of pregnancy. Her previous labors had been unusually severe, very tedious, painful, and accompanied by fainting fits, cramps, agonizing pain, etc., before the birth, and flooding, syncope, and many unpleasant symptoms after the expulsion of the placenta. She took for nearly three weeks, about *ten* drops of Cimicifuga first dec. dil. four times a day. Labor came on at the proper period, lasted only six hours; was not painful nor difficult; there was no flooding, no fainting, and no cramps, and both patient and friends were agreeably surprised. She got up in nine days, and had a better convalescence than ever before. If this remedy was useful in this condition alone, it would still be invaluable to the profession. The editor of the London Lancet, writes: "We are disposed to admit the correctness of the observations of American Physicians who allege that it has a peculiar action on the uterus. In the irritable condition of that organ, often observed in patients for some time after menstruation has ceased, or irregular when about to cease, and marked by pain more or less periodical in the lumbar region, Cimicifuga affords rapid relief. In neuralgic pains, often met with in such patients in other localities, it is equally beneficial. Females at the period of life we are speaking of, frequently suffer from a distressing pain in the upper part of the head, recuring with greater severity at night. These cases are very satisfactorily met by this remedy. Pains in the mammæ also, whether referable to uterine disturbance or to pregnancy, are relieved by the Cimicifuga very speedily."

In *phlegmasia alba dolens*, I would advise it on theoretical grounds; not having used it in that disease. Some of the symptoms of the drug simulate that disease very closely.

Larynx.—Hoarseness, after rising; hoarseness; unpleasant fulness in the pharynx; constant inclination to cough for half an hour, caused by a tickling sensation in the larynx, at 7½ P. M. An attempt to speak is followed by an inclination to cough; slight dry cough four or five times, produced by tickling in the larynx; hoarseness in the evening; short dry cough, several times during the evening, caused by tickling in the larynx; fluent coryza; cough, particularly at night, caused by tickling in the throat; very troublesome, hacking cough, of some month's standing.

Clinical Remarks.—The two last symptoms mentioned above are marked "curative" in one of the provings. In my experience it has been used beneficially for coughs. It is well known that many laryngeal symptoms result from uterine irritation. The morbid excitation is transmitted through the medium of *reflex action.* The Cimicifuga is especially indicated in such cases, or when cough arises during pregnancy, or from amenorrhœa, etc. It is also useful in those spasmodic actions of the larynx occurring in hysterical females.

Chest.—The pain in the head continued for ten days, followed by coryza, with sore throat and a gradual extension of the disease to the bronchial mucous membrane; dry, short and hacking cough, night and day, continuing two weeks, which is uncommon, the prover not having had a catarrh or cold for several years; acute pain in the right lung, extending from apex to base, about two inches to the right of the sternum, aggravated by every inspiration, continuing for two hours, and gradually diminishing in intensity until after retiring; similar pain the next morning for half an hour, but much less severe; lancinating pain along the cartilages of the false ribs, left side, increased by taking a long inspiration, soon after waking at three P. M. The same pain, very severe and piercing, so as almost to prevent inspiration for a short time, immediately after retiring, between ten and eleven P. M., and continuing for half an hour; soreness of the chest; cold chills and prickling sensations during the day, in the (female) mammæ; prickling sensations in the breasts. Dr. Tully says it causes cardiac palpitations, which, though transient and fugitive, are often quite severe, with neuralgic pains through the chest. In Drs. Hill and Douglas' proving, we find—Stitches in the region of the heart, or in the heart; pain in the left side of the chest.

Clinical Remarks.—Dr. Lee says "the Cimicifuga has been found a useful remedy in certain chronic affections of the pulmonary organs." Dr. Garden, of Virginia, was the first writer who called the attention of the profession to this article in this class of cases. Having observed its utility in domestic practice, he was induced to resort to it in his own case, which he considered one of "gastro-hepatic, or dyspeptic phthisis," though the physical signs are not given. The principal symptoms were: a pulse of one hundred to one hundred and twenty, harrassing cough, purulent expectoration, pain in the right breast and side, hectic paroxysms, loss of flesh and strength, frequent hamoptysis, and great derangement in the functions of the stomach and liver. No other medicine was taken except the Cimicifuga, and to this, aided by a suitable regimen, the cure, which was completed within a few months, was wholly attributed. Other cases of tuberculosis are given where striking benefit was derived from its use, and where the disease was evidently arrested by it. Dr. Garden used it in his own and other cases in doses of "an ounce or two of the tincture of the root once or twice a day. The tincture was prepared with good rye whisky." He considers its effect on the head is the test of the extent to which it should be carried. Such gross abuse of a valuable remedy is worse than foolish. Just in the same manner does the dominant school advise Quinine to be given until it effects the head unpleasantly. But it is as unnecessary in the one as in the other. A few drops of the mother tincture, or lower dilutions, frequently repeated, will have a better and more lasting effect. Dr. Hildreth (allopathic) says: "In nearly every instance the pulse was reduced to near the natural standard, the hectic symptoms disappeared, and with it the cough and

16

other signs of phthisis." In acute phthisis, uncomplicated with much inflammation, Dr. H. states that he has often seen the most prompt action from the decoction, in throwing off febrile excitement, or the hectic paroxysms, allaying cough, reducing the rapidity and force of the pulse, and inducing gentle perspiration; also, he has found it of the greatest benefit "in those intermittent congestions and inflammations, so frequent in the second and third stages of phthisis from atmospheric exposures." Prof. Lee says, "there is every reason to place considerable confidence in Cimicifuga in the early stages of tuberculosis, when there is a frequent hacking cough and other signs of the malady. We have used it for many years in such cases with much benefit, and have come to regard it as possessing almost specific power in allaying pulmonic irritability, thus abating cough, while it proves invigorating to the digestive organs. It speedily checks the diarrhœa and night sweats of phthisis." Dr. Wood thinks it proves useful in pulmonary complaints only by its allaying irritation through its sedative properties. Prof. Chapman has ranked it under the head of expectorants. This is all old school experience. But we have good reason, judging from our provings, to expect much from this remedy in some pulmonary complaints. It cures cough, pains in the chest, dyspnœa, fever, night sweats, and even diarrhœa. My own experience with it in this class of diseases has not been extensive, yet I have cured some harrassing coughs, with pains in the chest, difficulty of respiration and general debility, with the lower dilutions. In diseases of the lungs, bronchia, etc., it ranks with Aconite, Bryonia, Arnica, and Veratrum viride. In *pleurodynia* it has been used successfully in many cases. A student came to me complaining of a severe stitch between the sixth and seventh ribs of the right side. It had seized him suddenly and was agonizingly intense. He stated that such attacks generally laid him up several days. He had usually taken Bryonia for it. Cimicifuga, first decimal, ten drops every half hour, effected a cure in twenty-four hours. For those obstinate *pains in the left side*, which females so often complain of, this remedy is as nearly a specific as anything can be. Dr. Simpson (Obstetric memoirs, vol. 1. p. 27) in a paper on the diagnosis of uterine diseases, mentions those "sympathetic pains in different and distant parts of the body, "which are really *reflex* pains or neuralgias, caused by uterine irritation. Among these reflex pains are—"pain in one or both mammæs"—"pain under the left mammæ and upon the edges of the rib on that side"—"pains in the right side"—pain in some of the vertebræ of the back—pain in the sacral and lumbar regions—pains in the abdominal parietes —and pains in the joints extremities, head and face." For all these reflex pains, when dependent on uterine or ovarian disorder, there is no more useful remedy than Cimicifuga. But it is peculiarly useful in the "pain under the left mammæ." It occurs more commonly in unmarried females, and is probably as frequent in cases of uterine affections, as pain in the shoulder is in cases of hepatic affections. The pain is sometimes diffused along the side, but more usually it is limited to a small spot not larger than a half-dollar. When it is not severe it is not affected by the act of respiration, but in more severe cases it is increased by deep inspiration, and many a poor patient has been bled, blistered, leeched, etc., over and over again, under the idea that it was an indication of pleuritic inflammation." Dr. Simpson used the Cimicifuga in some of these severe and obstinate cases, and the pain rapidly subsided under its use. *Diseases of the heart* may be cured or greatly palliated by Cimicifuga. The functional disorders of that organ, the palpitations, irregular action, etc., dependent on rheumatic or uterine irritation, are benefited by this remedy. In cases simulating *angina pectoris* I have found it useful. In one instance, the pain, or rather intense anxiety about the heart, with pain in the shoulder (left) and extending down the left arm, (the shoulder and upper arm feel as if "bound to the side")—all subsided under its action after taking three drops three times a day for a week. It has occasionally appeared since, but promptly disappears after a single dose of Cimicifuga. In one case of pericarditis following an attack of inflammatory rheumatism, Dr. Marcy observed excellent effects from the use of the third dilution. It is better than Digitalis in heart affections, for while it controls abnormal action it invigorates the nervous system and the general dition of the patient. It does not interfere with digestion as does Digitalis.

Back.—Stiffness of the neck; drawing pain in lumbar region; pulsating pain in the lumbar region; in the morning, on bending the neck forward, he experienced a severe drawing, tensive pain, at the points of the spinous processes of the three upper dorsal vertebræ, which continued for several hours; trembling and weakness in the back; weak trembling; pain in the small of the back; same tired feeling in the back, extending from the region of the kidneys to the sacrum, relieved by rest and increased by motion; dull, heavy aching in the small of the back, extending to the sacrum; dull pain behind the right scapula; stitches in the back, below the right scapula; dull pain in the region of the lower dorsal and upper lumbar vertebræ; pain below the left scapula; pains as of boils on the back and extremities; cramping in the muscles of the neck on moving the head, first in the left, afterwards in the right side; occasional slight pain in either scapula and right shoulder; weight and pain in the lumbar and sacral regions, sometimes extending all around the body, somewhat below the crest of the ileum; rheumatic pains in the muscles of the neck and back; a feeling of stiffness and contraction; feeling of weight in the small of the back; drawing pain in a single muscle between the right scapula and spine for some hours.

Clinical Remarks.—The Cimicifuga exercises an undoubted influence over the spinal cord, or its membranes, and for this reason is capable of curing many affections arising therefrom. In true *spinal irritation*, which is a functional disease of the spinal marrow, this medicine is of great value. In this disease the spinal tenderness, and all the painful symptoms, is accompanied by no organic change in the cord or the vertebræ. The *cause* of this disease, says Wood, is not well understood. It occurs most frequently in women, and especially during the menstrual period. It would seem, therefore to have some connection with the uterus. Of the exciting causes, changes in the weather are probably among the most frequent. Mental disturbance seems to be capable of inducing it. The most rational view of the nature of the disease, is, that the affection is seated essentially in the *ligaments* of the vertebra, and is generally of a rheumatic or gouty character. It is readily conceived that irritation may be propagated from this structure to the nervous tissue of the cord, or at least to the nerves which proceed from the cord, and receive as they pass an envelop of the diseased tissue." In this affection I use the remedy internally and externally. The Cimicifuga in drop doses of the first decimal—or Cimicifugin first decimal or one hundredth, and apply a lotion of one part of the tincture to ten of water. Dr. Cleveland considers it specific for that painful affection—*crick in the back.* This may be only a symptom of *lumbago*, but is in some cases due to a rupture of some of the fibres of those ligaments which connect the spinous processes. Dr. Simpson and the editor of the *Lancet* consider the Cimicifuga almost specific in lumbago. Our provings give us ample basis upon which to select this medicine. It causes nearly all the symptoms of lumbago, as well as rheumatism of the dorsal and other muscles of the back. It is homœopathic to that affection which Dr. Inman so correctly describes in his work on "Spinal Irritation"—a weakness (atony) of the muscles attached to the spinous processes, etc. With regard to the *dose* to be resorted to in these affections, I would advise the lowest attenuations, for the reason that the rheumatic or neuralgic affections are caused by Cimicifuga, secondarily. I have never received much benefit in those diseases from any dilution or trituration higher than the *third.* The physician should not hesitate in obstinate cases to resort to drop doses of the mother tincture. If we do get up a slight medicinal aggravation, it cannot do as much harm as the continuance of the disease we are trying to combat.

Superior Extremities.—Dull pain in the right arm, deep in the muscles, extending from the shoulder to the wrist, continuing during the next day; itching and redness of the dorsal surface of the right hand, in the afternoon, and especially in the evening; a single pimple on the dorsal surface of the left hand, secreting a little pus at the apex, disappearing in three or four days; itching of the dorsal surface of the left hand and wrist, particularly on the dorsal surface of the thumb, in the evening; small red papula first appeared, becoming, after slight irritation, a diffused redness, which disappeared in a few hours, but could be reproduced at any time by slightly irritating the surface. This symptom gradually disappeared in a few days. Dr. Tully says it causes neuralgic pains in the extremities. It has caused some pains in the arms, with a numbing sensation, as if a nerve had been compressed. These pains were first felt in the shoulder, and passed down the arm and then the forearm, producing a very peculiar, lame, numb, and sometimes cramping sensation, as in heart disease. Similar pains in the legs, but more severe and constant in the upper part of the thigh, about the hip joint and inguinal region. (Sciatica.)

Lower Extremities.—Stinging in the left great toe, for a moment, on the lower surface, and afterwards on the upper, in the afternoon; dull, aching, burning pain in the second joint of the right great toe, extending up the limb, continuing an hour, from eight to nine P. M.; the same pain, less severe, on the third evening.

CLINICAL REMARKS.—It has been used with benefit in *Sciatica*, and other rheumatic affections of the extremities. Dr. Marcy writes: "We have been in the habit of employing this remedy occasionally in rheumatic affections, during the past eighteen years. We have prescribed all doses, from the nauseous decoction of the old school, to the highest homœopathic attenuation, and good results have followed both forms of the medicine—although experience has long since taught us to rely upon the latter form. It is most serviceable in articular rheumatism of the lower extremities—with much swelling and heat in the affected parts, and pain on moving the parts. Like Bryonia, it exercises a special control over inflammation of serous membranes; but its range of action, and consequently its applicability in rheumatic affections, are decidedly inferior to this drug." The Cimicifuga may be inferior to Bryonia in its action on serous tissues, but it is far superior to that drug in its influence on *nervous tissues*, or rather the neurilemma or fibrous portion of nerve structure. Bryonia does not cause or cure rheumatico-neuralgic pains, while Cimicifuga *does*, in an eminent degree. Bryonia has no influence over reflex-nervous pains, cramps, etc., while Cimicifuga controls many such abnormal manifestations.

COLLINSONIA CANADENSIS.

(*Ox-Balm. Knot-Root. Hard-Hack. Stone-Root.*)

This plant is found in the Eastern and Northern States. It is herbaceous, with broad, cordate, ovate, smooth, opposite leaves; the flowers in terminal panicles of a yellowish violet color; flowering from July to September. The whole plant has a peculiar balsamic smell, which is milder and pleasanter in the flowers than in the root, this having a somewhat rank, disagreeable odor. It has a warm and pungent taste. The plant grows to the height of two feet, with a perennial, knotty root. It contains a volatile oil,—a resin, tannin, gallic acid, starch gum, sugar, and a peculiar, bitter, neutral principle, *Collinsonin*. "The medicinal virtues of this plant has been pretty extensively tested in domestic, if not in regular practice, and is regarded as tonic, astringent, diaphoretic, and diuretic. With some practitioners, it ranks very high as an alterative, especially in chronic affections of the genito-urinary organs, as cystitis, catarrh of the bladder, gravel, leucorrhœa. By the common people it is highly esteemed as a remedy for headache, colic, indigestion; while many cases of dropsy have been reported to have been cured by it. Its influence over the secernent and absorbent systems is strongly marked. Like all aromatics, it produces an agreeable feeling of warmth in the stomach, increasing the force and frequency of the pulse, and the warmth of the surface; while it diffuses a pleasant glow over the system, without any special influence on the cerebral functions. Its effects seem rather manifested on the organic and sympathetic systems and the capillary circulation."—(Prof. Lee—Allopathic.) This is about as definite as an old school writer usually writes about any medicinal agent. It leaves the student in a state of profound uncertainty as to the real nature of its action. Let us be sincerely thankful that Hahnemann gave us a system of drug-proving, whereby we may escape from the uncertainties of old medicine. I have not been able to get an extended proving of this plant, but have noted some characteristic symptoms from its use, and have collected a good many clinical observations, which may serve us as a guide until we obtain a good pathogenesis. "In the mountains and hills of Virginia, Kentucky, Tennessee and Georgia," says Rafinesque, "this genus is considered a panacea, and used outwardly and inwardly in many disorders. It is used as a poultice and wash for bruises, sores, blows, falls, wounds, sprains, contusions, and taken like tea for headache, colics, cramps, dropsy, indigestion, etc." It is therefore used much as the common people in Germany use *Arnica*, which it somewhat resembles in some of its general effects on the system.

Head.—Slight fullness of the head; throbbing in the head.

Clinical Remarks.—I am inclined to think it only useful in gastric and hæmorrhoidal headaches. In headaches from indigestion, I have known relief to follow promptly upon its administration.

Gastric Symptoms.—Vomiting (from small doses of the fresh root); vomiting, with pain and heat in the stomach; cramp-like pain in the stomach, with nausea; sensation as of flatulence in the stomach; rumbling in the stomach and bowels; agreeable feeling of warmth in the stomach, with general glow of the system; increases the appetite; excessive appetite.

Clinical Remarks.—In indigestion, from want of tone of the stomach, and associated with constipation and hæmorrhoids, it rivals Nux vomica. Both eclectic and allopathic physicians consider it a valuable remedy for the expulsion of flatulence and the relief of spasms of the stomach and intestines. *Coe* says (Conc. Org. Med.) "no better remedy can possibly be had for the relief of cramp in the stomach, flatulent and bilious colics, and all spasmodic affections of the stomach and back. Drs. Fowler and Carroll have found it promptly curative in many cases of indigestion, loss of appetite, etc.

Intestines, Stool, etc.—Constipation, with a good deal of flatulence; sluggish stool, with distention of the abdomen; heat and itching of the anus; hæmorrhoidal tumors; the hæmorrhoids re-appear while taking the medicine for pulmonary hæmorrhage; loose, papescent stool; diarrhœa, with nausea.

Clinical Remarks.—It has a really wide reputation in affections of the bowels and rectum. *Coe* says, "in diseases of the bowels and rectum it stands unrivalled. We have experienced its sanative influence in diarrhœa in our own person." It is useful in diarrhœa, dysentery, and cholera-infantum. The specific homœopathic indications for its use in intestinal disorders are about as follows: In *diarrhœa*, when the discharges are mucus, or papescent, or watery, with cramp-like and spasmodic pains in the bowels, also vomiting or nausea. In the diarrhœa of children, so apt to be accompanied with colic, cramps, flatulence, etc., it has proved an excellent remedy (in the 3rd dilution). In the so-called hæmorrhoidal *dysentery*, it has proved curative in the hands of many of my correspondents. The discharges are of bloody mucus, and are accompanied with tenesmus, spasmodic tormina, expulsion of scybala, coated with bloody mucus, heat and burning in the rectum. In *Constipation*, it has been used very successfully by some of our best practitioners. Dr. Carroll writes (N. A. Jour., vol. 5, p. 546,): "In cases of habitual constipation it is invaluable, producing not a mere transient relief, but correcting, apparently in a permanent manner, the morbid condition of the digestive system. I say apparently, for, although I have tested its virtues with success in a good many instances, I have only known of it for a year, and consequently cannot say how enduring its remedial action may prove. I may only say, that in my own case, having been for fifteen years suffering from the reactive effects of a series of cathartics administered with systematic cruelty during my infancy, I succeeded a little more than a year ago in overcoming, by a month's use of the Collinsonia, the existing condition of affairs, and since that time I have not been obliged to recur to it for aid." Indeed, it has so far proved invariably remedial in all troubles depending on constipation. *Dr. Fowler*, in Cases I, II, and III, recorded below, gives its excellent results in obstinate and habitual constipation, associated with hæmorrhoids. I have used it in several similar cases, and so far with the best results. "The most remarkable influences of the Collinsonia," says Coe, "are observable in hæmorrhoids and other diseases of the rectum. The most inveterate and chronic cases are relieved, and frequently cured, by this remedy alone. We have known it to act promptly in suppressing hæmorrhage from the bowels (?), and in relieving those distressing pains characteristic of hæmorrhoidal affections." We have also from homœopathic sources some valuable testimony relating to the curative power of Collinsonia in hæmorrhoids. Dr. E. P. Fowler (North Amer. Journal of Homœopathy, vol. 6, p. 80,) writes: "Some two years since I remarked to a friend and patient that I was honored with a number of cases of obstinate *hæmorrhoids*, and that I really wished that I possessed some means of curing them, without danger of entailing some more serious disorder. My friend replied that he could tell me of a remedy, and remarked that two or three years ago he was an absolute martyr, in fact crippled with hæmorrhoids." The remedy was Collinsonia, and this patient was cured by the following preparation: A small handful of the chopped root was put into a quart of water, and it was boiled down to a pint. This he took three times a day,—a small wine-glass full. He was cured in two weeks. This gentleman added that he "had made some most remarkable cures among his friends." Dr. Fowler adds: "Upon his description of the root, I remembered having in early boyhood gathered from the woods some of the same kind of root for an old gentleman, who was by its use fully freed from hæmorrhoids of over twenty-five years standing." Dr. F. reports the following cases:

Case 1. "Mr. J. E. J., whose sufferings from hæmorrhoids rendered his life almost a burthen, and completely disabled him from business. I gave him two or three handsful, and directed him to use it in the manner described to me by my friend. He commenced its use, but found that it acted as an emetic. I then told him to take a dessert spoonful twice a day. This he did without disturbance to the stomach, and in somewhat less than three weeks reported himself to us, to use his own words, 'the humble and grateful subject of a real miracle—cured.' About two months after he had a slight return of the old trouble, but after taking the Collinsonia four days, was again well. My attention was attracted to another feature in this case. For years the patient had been a victim of most resolute constipation, and never had relief without the aid of enemas; and as these could not be administered without irritation and pain, the consequence was, that about four or five days were allowed to intervene between each time. The patient said that he was not more surprised at the rapid cure of such an old chronic complaint as the hæmorrhoids, than by the fact that the remedy had established a free and natural daily action of the bowels, which continued after the use of the medicine was suspended. Before the second attack he became again constipated, and was again relieved as before. He also attributed a cessation of dyspeptic troubles and an increase of appetite, which was never more than indifferent, to the use of the drug. But, whether this may have been owing to the direct action of the drug upon the stomach, or whether it may have been a secondary effect from relieving the intestines, is, of course, difficult to decide."

Case 2. "Was a gentleman afflicted with 'flowing piles,' who had submitted to almost every kind of treatment, both local and that addressed through the system, and invariably leaving the successive doctors' hands in a more miserable condition than he entered them. He had, in fact, come to consider medicine as a downright humbug, and came to me in a state of incredulity, only by having heard of some of the cures that I had made with Collinsonia. This patient was troubled with alternate constipation and diarrhœa, and the hæmorrhage was incessant, though not profuse. He was light complexioned, thin, nervous, and dyspeptic. I put him on one tablespoonful of the decoction three times a day. For the first week the action seemed to be almost wholly confined to the kidneys, and just as I was upon the point of considering the case non-amenable to the remedy, the renal action ceased, and the hæmorrhoids began to be relieved. Gradually the bowels gained a regular, normal, peristaltic action, the appetite and power of digestion became improved, and at the end of eight weeks, the patient pronounced himself in every respect well—in mind, as well as body.

Case 3rd. "Was an engineer of extreme bilious, nervous temperament. He came to me for *Varicocele*, which was considerable, and at times irritable. He had extreme constipation, and from various indications I deemed his complaint consequent upon constipation, and having observed the effect of Collinsonia in this respect, I gave it to him in the same manner as I had done to the preceding cases. I do not remember the exact length of time that he was under my charge; it was less, however, than four weeks, the action of the bowels became regular and natural, and the varicocele disappeared. This was about a year ago and he has remained well since."

Case 4th. "This case was a lady who sufferred from a bad form of *hœmorrhoids*, also from terrible *dysmenorrhœa.* Gave her the Collinsonia, as I had given it to the others, and at the end of six or seven weeks the hœmorrhoids were gone, and she had been exempt from dysmenorrhœa. She has since had one or two slight returns of hæmorrhoids, but which have rapidly yielded to a two day's use of this remedy. In this case there was almost constant diarrhœa and loss of appetite; the diarrhœa ceased, and the appetite became, as the lady thought, 'quite indelicate'." Dr. Fowler found it "an excellent remedy for the tenesemus of dysentery." "So far as my experience goes, this root seems to be a prime remedy for *hœmorrhoids*, *dysmenorrhœa*, *constipation*, and *dyspepsia*, in fact it seems to be soothing to all inflammation of the lower viscera."

Urinary Organs.—"For the first week its action seemed to be almost wholly confined to the kidneys.—"(Fowler). Probably in increasing the amount of urine, as it is a *diuretic.*

Clinical Remarks.—*King* says, "it is used in *gravel*, *catarrh of the bladder*, and urinary disorders." *Jones & Scudder* record that it is esteemed *diuretic*, and has been used in dropsies, and chronic diseases of the urinary passages; it is reputed *lithontriptic*, but we doubt its capability of dissolving urinary concretions, although it may be serviceable in allaying the irritation caused by them." *Prof. Lee* says it is a "valuable alterative in chronic diseases of the genito-urinary organs." Some patients of mine have related to me some extraordinary cures by means of this remedy, of "gravel," of which they were once victims. What the real disorder was I could not determine, although from the description of the patients it must have been some chronic affection of the kidneys or bladder, in which calculi was present. We may safely deduce, from our actual knowledge of its virtues, that it will be found more useful in chronic than acute affections of the urinary organs. It will probably prove useful in chronic cystitis, urethritis and nephritis; also in affections of the bladder arising from diseases of the *rectum.*

Genital Organs of Women.—Dr. Carroll thinks that it is capable of producing abortion in the early months of uterine gestation.

Clinical Remarks.—It is said to be curative in some forms of leucorrhœa. It has cured, in the hands of homœopathic practitioners, leucorrhœa, prolapsus, dysmenorrhœa, etc., as the following cases will show. It will strike the critical reader, however, that nearly all the abnormal conditions of the uterine organs were really dependent upon disease of the rectum or bowels, as constipation or piles, and that when the Collinsonia removed the latter diseases, the uterine disorder disappeared. It is too often overlooked by the careless and unobservant physician, that a prolapsus or retroversion may be caused by constipation; a pruritus or leucorrhœa, by hæmorrhoids, and even a congested cervix by an acute or chronic dysentery. It seems very probable that it will be found curative in *vicarious menstruation*, when the substitutive bleeding is from the hæmorrhoidal veins. In *Amenorrhœa* from congestion of the uterus aud pelvic viscera, it may be found beneficial. In *menorrhagia* from the same cause, it will prove equally useful. *Abortion* may be prevented by it use, when that accident is impending, as a result of constipation, piles, etc. I am not prepared to believe, however, that its action on the uterus is direct. *Dysmenorrhœa.*—We cannot find any recommendation for the use of this drug in painful menstruation in the literature of the allopathic schools, but it appears to have been used successfully by homœopathists in that affection. Dr. A. L. Carroll, of New York, (N. A. Jour. of Hom. Vol. 5, page 546,) says: "In dysmenorrhœa its action is most powerful—so powerful that I am led to believe it capable, during the early periods of utero-gestation, of producing abortion. In no instance that has fallen under my notice, has it failed to relieve promptly this menstrual derangement, which is so common among all classes of women in our climate, and I am convinced that when more extensively known it will be found a specific in this form of disease." Dr. Fowler, "case four"—under the head of Hæmorrhoids reports a cure of dysmenorrhœa, complicated with piles, loss of appetite, and constant diarrhœa. Dr. Snelling adds his testimony to Dr. Carroll's, in regard to its efficancy in dysmenorrhœa. "There is no doubt," he remarks, "that it exercises a strong specific influence over the female organs of generation, as we have also seen distressing symptoms of *pruritus*, and *prolapsus of the womb* yield under its use. "A lady aged about 35, unmarried, had sufferred for a long time past with all the distressing symptoms of a uterine prolapsus, complicated with pruritus, dysmenorrhœa, and most obstinate constipation. She had been for some time under the care of a distinguished practitioner for the prolapsus uteri, who, after relieving the more urgent symptoms, and restoring somewhat the tone of her system, told her that her only safety lay in avoiding constipation; and to this end prescribed a cathartic pill, which was to be taken as occasion required. Under this course she was gradually but steadily retrograding. Each recurring menstrual period brought its days of acute suffering, and confinement to the bed. Every movement of the bowels was accomplished only by the aid of a strong cathartic, and this had come to be an act of suffering and dread from the painful prolapsus of the womb at these times. The bowels refusing to act, it became necessary frequently to repeat again and again the opening pills, before their torpor could be overcome, and then a quick succession of copious and debilitating liquid stools would leave her prostrate for days. She thus alternated between a state of absolute inaction of the bowels, with its train of attendant evils, and the exhaustion consequent upon hypercatharsis. April 3d.—She was put upon three grain doses of Collinsonia can. one quarter trit, three per diem, with directions to abstain from the use of the habitual cathartic as long as was possible for her to do so; no other change whatever was made. Twenty-four hours had elapsed since the bowels had moved. Slight pains at times in the back and uterine regions, with distressing pruritus. Appetite small, pulse normal. April 5th.—Natural movements of the bowels without other assistance. No other effects. April 7th and 8th.—Healthy movements from the bowels. April 10th.—Much improved in every respect; constipation entirely removed; symptoms altogether so marked better that the medicine was discontinued for one week. During this week the monthly turn passed over, with much less than the usual amount of suffering, though some imprudence in diet was followed by colicky pains in the abdomen; these, however, passed over. At the end of the week the constipation having somewhat returned the remedy was resumed, followed in twenty-four hours by a natural movement from the bowels. The medicine was continued for one week and then given up. The relief was complete and permanent. No subsequent symptoms made their appearance, and a few days since she expressed herself as perfectly and entirely well, "without an ache or a pain." During the course of the administration of the remedy, the pruritus, dysmenorrhœa, and symptoms of prolapsus uteri, were quietly and completely removed." It may be that Collinsonia does not act specifically and directly upon the uterus, but cures congestions, pains, prolapsus, etc., by removing diseased conditions from other pelvic viscera.

Genital Organs of Men.—It has proved useful in *gleet*. It is indicated in spermatorrhœa from hæmorrhoids and constipation. Dr. Fowler (case 3rd) cured a case of *varicocele* from the above mentioned causes.

Respiratory Organs.—We find no mention in Allopathic or eclectic tharapeutics, of the use of Collinsonia in affections of the pulmonary organs. It has, however, been used in the new school with success. The following case illustrating the use of *Collinsonia* in pulmonary homorrhage was reported by *Dr. Liebold*, of Newark, N. J., in the *North American Journal*, *vol.* 7, *page* 494. "On the evening of the 11th of August last I was called in haste to the bedside of Mr. G., an American about forty years of age, who had just the third attack of pulmonary hemorrhage under Allopathic medication, in the space of four days. He had lost about a pint of moderately fresh looking blood each time, but this time more than previously. The history of the case was, that he had "inflammation of the lungs" two years ago treated allopathically. Up to this day he was comparatively well, and could assign no cause for his present sickness. On the first day he got sick he passed blood per anum too, but not subsequently. With a short hacking cough, he raised almost without intermission, and spat very tough and dark coagula of blood, as large as a bean, enveloped in viscid phlegm. Of course he felt somewhat uneasy in his chest, but had *no pain*. I put him on *Hamamelis Virginica* for the next three days but the hemorrhage returned twice, on the 12th and 14th, although diminished; the spitting of blood remained about the same. Then I gave *Ferrum-aceticum;* for twenty-four hours, some hemorrhage. *Lycopus virginicus* for twenty-four hours.

August 16th. No better. Complains of great inconvenience from constipation. Gave *Callinsonia Canadensis* one-fourth, one powder every three hours (having in view only its gentle laxative power). The next morning I was greeted, "Well, Doctor, that is the right remedy, that will cure me," and so it did almost. I say almost, for notwithstanding he took it up to the 25th, "by and by at longer intervals," there appeared for the last four days, two or three times blood in his sputa. The cure was completed by *Conium* first, in two days. Saw him well to-day. The *Collinsonia can.* acted in this case not in the least on the bowels, more on the kidneys, but developed an admirable carminative power. So also said a lady who took it for dysmenorrhœa, and who called them only by the name of "wind-powders." Mr. G. never had hemorrhoids."

CORNUS CIRCINATA.

(*Round-leaved dog-wood. Green Osier.*)

This is a shrub from six to ten feet high, with warty branches, large, roundish, pointed leaves, waved on their edges and downy beneath, and white flowers disposed in depressed cymes. The fruit is *blue.* The bark, when fresh, is of a bright green color; when dried, is in quills, of a whitish or ash color; its taste is bitter, astringent and aromatic. The plant grows on hill-sides and banks of rivers. It flowers in June and July.

Wood, Lee, and nearly all the allopathic authorities make but slight mention of this variety of Cornus. With characteristic want of accurate knowledge, they assert that all the varieties of this plant possess the same medical virtues. The general effects of all may have a *general* resemblance, but each has a peculiar action of its own upon the human system.

Generalities.—Dark and bilious stools with griping and tenesmus; dysenteric symptoms; bowel complaints generally, with pains in the bowels before, during, and after the discharges; general debility, and impaired mental energy, with great drowsiness; bilious derangements; dull, heavy sensation in the head; shooting, aching, or throbbing pains in the head; disposition to perspire on slight exertion; nausea, loss of appetite, bitter taste, lassitude; symptoms resembling jaundice; cholera infantum; diarrhœa, with excessive debility and nervous excitability; chilliness, followed by flushes of heat and sweat; sleep unrefreshing, and disturbed by unpleasant dreams; diarrhœa, with great prostration of the whole body.

Clinical Remark.—Dr. Marcy found it curative in all the conditions mentioned above.

Skin.—Itching of the scalp, legs, and feet, increased by scratching or rubbing, and succeeded by a painful burning sensation; aggravation of an habitual scurfy eruption of the scalp; amelioration of a long standing herpetic eruption while under the influence of the drug; occasional paroxysms of itching of the skin of the back, legs, and feet, mostly at night; fine scarlet rash on the breast, attended with itching; itching in various parts of the body; burning sensation over the whole face; skin covered with a copious clammy perspiration; itching around the genital organs; itching and burning sensation over the whole body; pricking sensation in the arms and legs.

Clinical Remarks.—These symptoms would seem to bear out the popular belief that it is a good "blood purifier." Dr. Beach, a veteran of the Botanic school, says:—"it is valuable in salt-rheum, scrofula, cancerous humors, itch, and *all* cutaneous diseases." A sweeping assertion truly! It might be classed among our anti-psorics.

Fever.—Flushes of heat, followed by easy general perspiration; chilly sensations, succeeded by transient flushes of heat; congestion of blood to the head and face; throbbing pains in the temples and vertex; flushes of heat and coldness in alternation; followed by cold perspiration; soreness of the scalp; aching pains in the eye-balls; rumbling of wind in the bowels; stitches in the chest and under the scapula; sense of debility and fatigue; heaviness of the head; drowsiness; nausea; dull pain in the forehead and vertex; copious general clammy perspiration, succeeded by general chilliness; transient flashes of heat pervading the whole body, with shooting pains through the brain; heaviness of the eyelids; peevishness; aversion to meat and bread; and itching of the legs, thighs, and around the genital organs; head and face hot; coldness, followed by flashes of heat and perspiration; general itching of the skin; loss of appetite; drowsiness; and griping pains in the bowels.

Clinical Remarks.—In certain forms of bilious remittent fever, if the gastric and intestinal symptoms correspond, this medicine will be found useful. *Professor Ives* says this variety of Dog-wood, resembles the pale Peruvian Bark. (C. Lancifolia.) It is used in domestic practice as an anti-periodic. (See C. *florida*.)

Sleep.—Profound sleep during the night; drowsiness and lassitude; very great drowsiness, and disposition to perspire; sleep disturbed by frightful dreams; very sound, but unrefreshing sleep; very great disposition to sleep, with entire loss of mental and physical energy; sleep disturbed by fulness and pressure in the head; sleepy, and weak during the day, with dull pains in the head, back, and limbs; stupid and sleepy feeling with nausea, and burning of the face, hands and feet.

Clinical Remarks.—Those physicians who have had to deal much with bilious disorders, will recognize the above symptoms as bearing a striking similarity to those which precedes a bilious fever, hepatic congestion, jaundice, or even an ague. Should the totality of the symptoms correspond, it is quite likely that the use of the Cornus c. will prevent the establishment of either of those affections.

Mind and Sensorium.—Drowsiness; confusion of ideas; indifference with respect to subjects which usually interest; drowsiness, with entire disinclination to mental or corporeal exertion; depression of spirits; difficulty in fixing the mind, and in attending to ordinary business; mind confused, stupid, with inability to concentrate it upon any subject—worse toward night; lightness of the head; great depression of spirits, and petulence; very great disposition to sleep, with apathy and indifference; feeling of indolence, and loss of energy; lassitude, confusion of ideas, vertigo; giddiness, and lightness of head, worse on shaking it or on stooping; dread of making any exertion.

Clinical Remarks.—The suggestions offered under the preceding paragraph, are also applicable here; the stupor, indifference, etc., all resemble the premonitory symptoms of disordered conditions of the liver. In hypochondriasis it will be found curative, when arising from hepatic torpor.

Head.—Dull, heavy pain in the whole head, with drowsiness, the headache increased by walking, stooping or shaking the head; sense of fulness in the head relieved by a copious stool; dull pain in the forehead; aching pains through the temples, and on the top of the head; confused feeling in the head, and sense of fulness in the brain, with unusual heat in the head and face; congestion of blood to the head and face; throbbing pains in the vertex, and soreness of the scalp; heavy, aching pains in the head, with almost irresistible desire to sleep; drawing sensation (pain) from the back of the head to the nose; dull throbbing pains in the temples and side of the head; deep seated, pulsating pains in the occipital and parietal regions; deep seated, dull pains under the centre of the skull; dull pain in the back of the head; pulsations extending from the front to the back part of the head; Severe pulsative pains in the temporal regions, which passed off during the evening and night; heavy, confused feeling in the top of the head; slight, tensive aching pains through the whole brain; slight pain over the right supra-orbital ridge; dull pain in the forehead and vertex; flushes of heat in the head and face; heat in the top of the head; head feels light and giddy, worse on shaking the head, or on stooping; shooting pains through the whole brain; drawing pains in the back part of the head, and in the nape of the neck; sense of fulness and pressure in the head, preventing sound sleep.

Clinical Remarks.—Dr. Marcy found it curative in cases when there was—"Dull heavy sensations in the head; shooting, aching or throbbing pains in the head." It would seem to be indicated in various forms of bilious headache. One particular form of bilious cephalalgia is well represented in the symptom —"Sense of fulness in the head, relieved by a copious stool." Allopathic physicians, noticed long ago that some forms of headache were relieved by free evacuations from the bowels, occurring spontaneously. This led to the use and *abuse* of cathartics in head affections generally. I have treated many cases of habitual headache, which were relieved naturally, by diarrhœa, in which the pains in the head and the subsequent diarrhœa symptoms corresponded well with the above. In such cases it should be tested.

Eyes.—Aching pains through the eyeballs; heaviness of the eyelids; eyes sunken; yellowish tinge of the conjuctiva; hollowness of the eyes; dark circle under the eyes; sense of weight around the eyes; very dull sensations over the eyeballs; sense of contraction around the eyes; eyes dull and heavy, as after a debauch; sore pain in the eyeballs.

Clinical Remarks.—The "aching pains through the eyelids," are with some patients always premonitory of an attack of ague, or a bilious fever. We find it prevents a jaundice and bilious headache. The "yellow tinge of the conjunctiva" is often one of the first symptoms of jaundice. Dr. Marcy found it useful in "symptoms resembling jaundice." (See remarks under "*stool.*") Dr. Beach says it is useful for "inflamed eyes." This is about as correct an indication as Botanics usually have. *Theoretically*, I would strongly recommend it in ulcerations of the cornea; ulcers of the conjunctiva, from scrofula, or apthous ophthalmia; also for herpes of the eyelids. It should be used internally, and a wash or collyrium. (See remarks under the head of "mouth.")

Nose.—Itching of the nasal mucous membrane; coryza early in the morning; prickling sensation in the nasal canal; severe prickling sensation in the bony part of the nose.

Mouth and Throat.—Tongue covered with a thin, yellowish fur; insipid taste and clammy mouth; tongue covered with a whitish fur, with dry mouth and throat; pungent taste in the mouth; bitter taste in the mouth; smarting in the mouth and throat; bad taste in the mouth, with loss of appetite; white fur on the tongue, with desire for cold drinks.

Clinical Remarks.—The above symptoms are those found in bilious affections generally. But it is a little remarkable that no symptoms of ulceration, inflammation, or apthae of mucous membrane of the mouth were elicited in this proving. Perhaps stronger doses would have caused more decided lesions. During the early part of my practice I was surprised, and sometimes mortified, at the facility with which my patients would cure "sore mouths," with the decoction of the bark of the *green osier*, after I had vainly used mercury, nitric acid, sulphuric acid and other remedies laid down in our books. In *apthous stomatitis* of children, and even in *stomatitis materna*, I have known it to effect a prompt cure after all other means had been used in vain. Even in *mercurial salivation* it will arrest the diseased process, but not so surely and permanently as chlorate of potash. In *ulceration of the buccal mucous membrane* from a cold, or gastric derangement, and in that affection sometimes called "bilious sore throat and mouth," it has, under my observation, proved specific. Persons of a scrofulous habit are often troubled with frequently recurring ulceration of the tongue, gums, and mouth generally. Such patients I have known who always resorted to this remedy with a certainty of absolute relief. One patient in particular always carried some of the inner bark in his pocket, and chewed it as a substitute for tobacco, alleging that if he suspended its use the "sore mouth" very soon returned. Another patient had this "sore mouth" occasionally, alternated with ulcers on the *conjunctiva* and *cornea*. At my suggestion he used the cornus as a collyrium with the happiest result. It may prove one of our most valuable remedies in *all* ulcerations of mucous surfaces. The infusion is generally made by pouring hot water upon the bark, in the proportion of *one ounce of bark* to *one quart of water*. For homœopathic use, this method might answer in case the tincture was not readily obtained. A few drops of the mother tincture in half a teacup of water, would be about the proper proportion. I have rarely used the tincture, as the infusion is so easily made and readily administered. In order to test its virtues, in minute doses, I once gave a child, suffering under apthous ulceration of the mouth, the *cornus c.* prepared as follows: One drachm of the inner bark was placed in a vessel containing one quart of hot water. This was left standing one hour, then filtered. Nitric-acid, Chlorate of Potash, Borax, had been previously used internally and locally. In twenty-four hours after using the medicine the mucous membrane began to assume a healthier appearance, and in about a week, was quite well. The child was in ill health, and had had diarrhœa for weeks, and had become quite emaciated. Under the use of the remedy the diarrhœa ceased, and the general health decidedly improved. The dose was one teaspoonful of the above preparation every four hours. (No attempt was made to wash the mouth).

Eclectic writers call it an "Anti-scorbutic," and so far as my observation goes, it seems worthy the appellation. In this respect it is the analogue of the mineral acids, Baptisia, Kali Chlor., Mercurius and Hydrastis.

Appetite and Stomach.—Nausea, with bitter taste, and aversion to all kinds of food; empty feeling in the stomach, with tasteless eructations; aversion to food, and desire for sour drinks; burning sensation in the stomach, which lasted an hour and a half; flatulent distension of the stomach; nausea; bitter taste, and a gnawing, faint feeling in the stomach; heavy pulsations in the stomach, with nausea and impaired appetite; pain at the pit of the stomach during dinner, with distension of the stomach and bowels, relieved by a copious stool after dinner; nausea, with great debility and eructations; fulness and oppression in the stomach, with bad taste and dry mouth; nausea, with bitter eructations and loss of appetite; smarting and burning in the mouth, throat and stomach, with desire for stool; weakness of the stomach, with bitter taste and nausea; sensation of faintness in the stomach and bowels; drawing pains from the stomach to the lower part of the abdomen.

Clinical Remarks.—Many of the symptoms of this drug, especially the gastric, closely resemble those of Nux vomica. It stands somewhere between Nux and China in this respect. It has been used successfully in vomiting of pregnancy and dyspepsia.

Abdomen.—Slight griping pains in the abdomen, accompanied with rumbling of wind; the pains penetrated the whole abdomen, but were most severe in the vicinity of the umbilicus; pressing down pain in the rectum during stool; slight burning pain in the rectum during an evacuation; pressing pain in the rectum, and smarting at the anus in the morning, during and after a thin and scanty stool; tenesmus at stool, with griping in the umbilical region rumbling of wind and large discharge of offensive flatus; urging to stool, with fulness and uneasiness of the bowels; vague pains and general sense of uneasiness in the bowels; slight tenesmus, and considerable burning at the anus, after a bilious discharge; abdominal pains more acute during stool; urging to stool, (sensation in the rectum) in the morning, at five o'clock; on taking more of the drug, this bearing-down sensation extended to the bowels, increasing the disposition to evacuate. Stool accompanied with some tenesmus and burning at the anus; distension of the stomach and bowels with wind; constant working in the bowels, as if their contents were all in motion; shooting pains from the centre of the thorax to the lower part of the abdomen, the pains coming on severely at intervals, and then remitting; distension of the bowels with wind, relieved by a copious, dark and bilious stool; immediately after dinner; sense of weight in the lower part of the abdomen; burning sensation in the stomach and bowels, with same desire for stool; urging to stool very early in the morning, but unable to accomplish anything satisfactory, the discharge consisting of a few slimy lumps, with pressing and smarting at the anus; sensation of emptiness in the stomach and bowels; drawing sensation from the stomach to the lower part of the abdomen.

Clinical Remarks.—No drug, except, perhaps, mercury, presents a more formidable array of "bowel symptoms." Dr. Marcy says "its chief action appears to be upon the liver and intestinal canal. A marked influence is likewise exerted upon the brain, but whether the action of the drug is direct upon this organ, or whether the head symptoms proceed from the bilious derangement induced by it, is a question. We have found it curative in all the intestinal symptoms found under the head of "*Generalities.*" "It was first introduced into practice as a remedy for bowel complaints, by Prof. Ives, of New Haven, some thirty years ago. Its empirical use in the hands of this gentleman, proved it to be a valuable remedy in bilious diarrhœa, dysentery, cholera, infantum, and against the diarrhœas peculiar to abdominal typhus." If it so promptly cure ulcerations of the mouth and fauces, why should it not prove just as much a specific for the intestinal ulcerations, which are peculiar to this form of typhoid fever? The result most to be feared in all inflammatory affections of mucous surface—as in inflammatory diarrhoea, dysentery, abdominal typhus, etc., is ulceration. Had the experiment been carried far enough by the provers, we have no doubt this pathological condition would have occurred. The dysentric symptoms did not proceed so far as to cause *bloody* discharges, yet any physician who reads the above will perceive that it was only a question of *time;* blood evacuations would have soon been obtained if the drug had been continued in large doses, and if the prover had still persisted, *ulceration* would have certainly resulted. We cannot come at any other conclusion than that the Cornus cir. will prove as valuable in a certain class of diseases as Mercurius, Leptandria, Podophyllum, or Nitric acid. In one case of dysentery, in a child, when there was unmistakable ulceration of the mucous membrane of the rectum, the mother, by my permission, used enema of a weak infusion of the green-osier. After using it a few times the pus disappeared from the stools, and the child suffered less. It had not improved under the use of Merc. cor., 6th, and subsequently Nitric acid, 3d. Would it not be well to try this form of application, as well as internally, at the same time?

Stool.—Slightly loose stool in the morning, accompanied with slight pressing-down pain in the rectum; Stool, thin and scanty, with burning at the rectum, and at the anus, during the discharge; thin, scanty and slimy stool, attended with griping in the umbilical region; tenesmus, rumbling of wind, and large discharge of offensive flatus; copious, thin and bilious discharge, succeeded by some tenesmus and burning at the anus which lasted half an hour; dark green, thin, and very offensive stools, accompanied by copious emission of offensive flatus; bilious and slimy stool, with much wind, some tenesmus, and severe, burning pain at the anus, and a short distance within the rectum, whichcontinued after the motion; dark, thin and moderately copious stool, with some tenesmus, and a burning at the anus; frequent, small, dark and slimy stools with much offensive flatus; copious, dark stool of the natural consistence, attended with pressing-down sensation in the rectum; large emission of very offensive flatus; hard, dry and scanty stool, with pressing in the rectum; stool, consisting of a few thin and slimy lumps, with pressing and smarting at the anus. (See remarks under "*Abdomen.*")

Urine.—Urine, scanty and red or pale; sensation of fulness and weight in the region of the bladder; urine, scanty and high-colored, and frequent inclination to pass water.

Genital Organs.—Strange and persistent erections through the night; increased sexual desire during the evening and night, with diminished power.

Larnyx and Chest.—Stitches in the chest and back; stitches in the chest and under the right scapula; a fine scarlet rash upon the chest, attended with itching; sensation of dragging or bearing down on each side of the thorax, with accelerated pulsations of the heart; a sore, bruised feeling in the chest and back; shooting pains from the centre of the thorax to the lower part of the abdomen, severe at times and then remitting; choking sensation in the upper part of the thorax; smarting in the mouth and throat; frequent inclination to take a long breath.

Back.—Dull pain in the small of the back, with drowsiness and lassitude; stitches in the back and chest; pain in the lower part of the back; sore pain in the lumbar region, worse on bending forward or to either side; occasional paroxysms of itching in the back, especially in the evening.

Upper Extremities.—Burning and itching sensation in the hands and arms; coldness of the hands following a loose stool; prickling sensation in the arms; stretching sensation in the arms, mostly in the evening and at night; sense of weakness and fatigue in the arms.

Lower Extremities.—Weary feeling in the legs; itching in the legs; weakness and weary feeling in the legs; weakness and trembling of the legs; itchings on the legs and thighs, and around the labia; burning sensation in the feet; coldness of feet following a loose stool; tired feeling in the legs when walking or ascending stairs: prickling sensation in the legs; paroxysms of itching in the legs in the evening.

CORNUS FLORIDA.

(*Dogwood, Boxwood*).

Common throughout all our forests; conspicuous in spring-time by its festoons of large, white blossoms, and equally so during the autumn, from its clusters of scarlet berries; a handsome little tree, usually about fifteen to twenty feet high, is the Cornus florida of the United States. In this genus of *Cornaceæ*, there are about twenty species, of which America has, north of Mexico, eleven. The Flowering Dogwood is the most beautiful and showy plant of its genus. It is too well known to need description. The bark is officinal, though that of the root contains the greatest amount of the active principle. "The principle obtained from it is called *cornine*, and has all the properties of Sulphate of Qninine." This loose assertion must be taken *cum grano salis*, like all similar assertions of the dominant school. No pathogenesis of the *Cornus florida* has yet appeared. I propose, therefore, to collect what has been written of its therapeutic uses, and gather the few pathogenetic symptoms which are scattered through the pages of various authorities. We can, by these means, get some idea of its sphere of action, which will lay the foundation for rational clinical experience, and stimulate us to prove the drug, as Hahnemann did its great analogue, *China*. *Prof.* Lee (*Jour. of Mat. Med.*, vol. 1., p. 294,) thus speaks of it: "The physiological effects of the *Cornus* bark are similar to those of the vegetable bitter tonics generally, viz., increased frequency of pulse, exalted temperature, diaphoresis, sensation of fulness or pains in the head, and gastric derangement. Of these, the most strongly marked are the increased temperature of the skin, and the general perspiration. Some experimenters have observed a constant tendency to sleep, which has continued for several hours. This, as occurs in many other cases, does not indicate any specific narcotic properties, but is the result of the cerebral fulness." Dr. Blackie says that it causes "severe headache, quickens the pulse, and produces violent pains in the bowels." Other writers give testimony to the above statement. Here we have good evidence that the Dogwood will cause febrile symptoms of a peculiar character. Who can doubt its ability to cause a type of intermittent, bilious, or remittent fever, with gastric and intestinal irritation? Just such types of fever are found in the West, and may be treated successfully with *Cornus*. We have considerable testimony in favor of its value in intermittents. *Eberle* states that thirty-five grains of the bark are equal to thirty of Cinchona. Its effects are closely analogous to those of the cinchona bark, for which it may often be successfully substituted. *Lee* says: "Our own experience with this article has satisfied us that most cases of our periodic or miasmatic fevers will yield to its judicious use." *Prof. Barton* says: "That it may be asserted with entire safety, that as yet there has not been discovered within the limits of the United States any vegetable so effectually to answer the purpose of Peruvian bark in the management of intermittent fevers, as the Cornus florida." *Dr. Morton*, who experimented largely with the bark, declares that in an extensive practice of many years he used no other remedy in intermittent and remittent fevers." *Dr. Coe* writes: "Its anti-periodic powers render it of peculiar value in the treatment of intermittent and other periodic fevers. In such fevers we have employed it with much success. It is certain that *Cornine* has cured fever and ague when quinine has failed, and that in all cases when the latter cannot be employed, the Cornine answers as a substitute." In domestic practice, I have observed for many years that it was often more successful than quinine in certain types of ague. The country people generally make an infusion of uncertain strength, and drink of it during the apyrexia. If taken during the paroxysm, it causes an aggravation of the fever, headache, etc. From its known effects when taken in large doses, as well as certain observations of my own, I would lay down the following indications for its use in miasmatic fevers: Paroxysm preceded for days by sleepiness; sluggish flow of ideas; headache of a heavy, dull character; nausea; vomiting; loss of appetite; and sometimes bilious or watery diarrhœa; *chill*, with cold, clammy skin; nausea and vomiting, and violent pains in the bowels; *fever*, with violent headache; hot, but *moist* skin; stupor; "cerebral fulness;" pulse quick and hard; confusion of intellect, etc. *Apyrexia*—Debility, gastric irritability; painful diarrhœa. In bilious remittent, and even typhoid fever, it may prove a useful remedy. It seems to occupy an intermediate position between China and Podophyllum.

Lee admits that it will aggravate an existing febrile condition, but resorts to the usual false logic to explain its curative action: "A person in health may take the Cornus, as well as any of the other vegetable tonics, in moderate doses, and for a long time without any marked effects on any of the functions; but taken in the same manner and the same quantities, in certain pathological states, as a general lowering of the vital forces and nervous energy, independent of organic disease, or when miasmatic poison has caused a tendency to paroxysmal attacks, the therapeutical influence of Cornus will be promptly manifested in a general invigoration of the vital forces and suspension of the paroxysms. Here, as in regard to Cinchona, we must be satisfied with the result, for the manner in which it is brought about must ever *remain a mystery*. In certain morbid conditions, as hectic fever or great debility, attended with frequency of pulse, and cold, colliquative sweats, the *Cornus* would seem to possess the power of a *sedative*, as manifested in decided lowering of pulse, and abatement of perspiration. This effect is common to all neurotic tonics, in certain pathological conditions of the body. It depends on their imparting increased tonicity to the muscular fibres of the heart through the organic nerves, thus enabling the central organ of circulation to throw out a greater quantity of blood at each contraction. The cardiac irritability also is lessened by the temporary increase of tonic power and vital contractibility. On the contrary, if *Cornus* and other analogous substances be given in acute and sthenic conditions marked by those phenomena which are characteristic of inflammatory action, the circulation will be correspondingly increased by an *increase of inflammatory action;* in both conditions, however, acting as a stimulant." The above is open to much just criticism. We will take up a few of his propositions. 1. A person in health *cannot* take Cornus, or any other vegetable tonic, for a long time, without any marked effect. His own statement regarding the effects of Dogwood disprove it. Besides, the slightest knowledge of physiological processes teaches us that no tonic can be taken with impunity by a healthy person. We soon have an exaltation of function, then derangement of function, and, finally, more or less depressed condition of the vital powers. 2. We are *not* obliged to remain in mystery relative to the action of Cornus and Cinchona. Hahnemann discovered that the latter cured disorders like those it was capable of causing; and the *Cornus* acts in a similar manner. *Trosseau* and *Wood*—highest allopathic authorities—admit this virtually, but cloak the real fact, under the term, "Substantiation." 3. Cornus cannot be a *sedative*, and at the same time a stimulant. The terms are contradictory, and used in the manner above, causing no idea at all. The whole truth is, that the Cornus, like all other drugs, have two series of actions—*primary* and *secondary*. The *primary* action is, to cause exaltation of the functions of the vital organs, thence fever, congestion, inflammation. The secondary effects are nearly opposite, such as depression of the vital forces, loss of tonicity in the heart and muscular fibre generally, irritation of the various tissues, coldness, colliquative sweats.

Prof. Lee's facts are not to be disputed, but his theory of the action of the medicine is untenable. *Cornus* is homœopathic to both the primary and secondary symptoms above enumerated, in doses varied to suit the existing conditions; and it can cure such pathological states only by virtue of its power to cause similar ones. 4. Cornus and its analogues will *not* aggravate existing inflammatory conditions, if given in *proper* quantities. Administered in minute doses, it will promptly remove inflammations and congestions, if indicated by the symptoms, and if the quantity is small enough, no aggravation will follow its use. *Prof. Lee*, *King*, and other authorities assert that the tincture of Cornus will cause "violent pain in the bowels, purging, derangement of the digestive organs, vomiting, nausea, gastric derangement," etc.; yet all are equally free to admit, and even advise its use in similar conditions. They say, "It will promote the appetite and digestion, and is useful in atomic and enfeebled conditions of the stomach; and will act as an anthelmintic, by improving the functions of the alimentary canal, and correcting those conditions of the digestive organs which favor the production of worms." And yet, if it was suggested to these worthy writers that the medicine might act according to the law of *similia*, they would reject the proposition with contempt! It is just possible that many of the indications laid down for the *Cornus circinata* may be applicable to this medicine; to be exact we ought to have a scientific proving. But most Homœopaths are not aware that, although it is asserted by both schools that the varieties of Cinchona bark differ considerably in their action, yet our pharmaceutists use the C. augustifolia and C. lancifolia almost indiscriminately. To meet the demands of a perfectly scientific materia medica, *each* variety of Peruvian bark should be separately proven. It is quite suggestive, that authorities recommend *Cornus florida* in about the same cases and conditions for which Hahnemann used China, viz: general debility from loss of fluids, or in the convalescing stages of acute diseases; hectic fever, night sweats, indigestion, lientery, etc. A tincture made from the *berries* when ripe, is considered by some as being most efficacious in the above conditions.

Reports of cases of ague successfully treated by the late E. J. Bates, M. D., with Cornus florlda, will be found in *American Homœopathic Observer*, Feb. 1864, page 29.

Cornine.—This is the so-called *active principle*, of the *C. florida*, and stands in the same relation to the bark, as does Quinine to the Cinchona. Some prefer the *Sulphate*, as the best preparation. I have not used the Cornine extensively. In a few cases of debility from loss of fluids, when China, Quinine, and Phos. acid failed to act beneficially, I used the first trituration with apparent good effect. Those of the eclectic school who use it largely, declare it to be a prompt remedy for the cure of the usual types of intermittent fevers. They assert that it does not affect the head as do other preparations of the bark; nor does it cause gastric or intestinal derangements. Here let me call attention to one notable fact in relation to all these so-called "*active principles*," resinoid, alkaloid, or whatever they are called. While they retain to a considerable extent the specific properties of the drug, they are destitute of many of its more important virtues. Thus Quinine possesses not all the curative power of China; Macrotin does not represent all the properties of Cimicifuga; and Leptandrin has no such specific effect upon the brain as the tincture of Leptandria. So with *Cornine;* it represents only a part of the qualities of the original drug. These "active principles" ought to be subjected to separate provings. But we are partly justified in using them; for, it may be asserted with truth, that, *while they do not possess all the virtues of the tincture of the bark, etc., they do not* DIFFER *in their action.* They have lost something, but have gained no *new* qualities. Thus we may use the Cor*nine* in states of general debility, although the bowel symptoms which indicate the Cor*nus*, are not present. *Dr. Coe* says, "for *ague*, Cornine should be given in three to five grain doses every three hours, preceded by, or alternated with Leptandrin." I would advise the lower triturations instead, and know they are just as efficacious. The same writer teaches that, "although Cornine does not possess the power of neutralizing acidity of the stomach, yet it is of exceeding utility in those cases of indigestion, in which that symptom is a troublesome feature. It gives almost instant, immediate relief in that distressing symptom called "heartburn," and its continued use will prove a sure preventive of its occurrence, by restoring the tone of the stomach, and so obviating the tendency to fermentation.

CYPRIPEDIUM PUBESCENS.

(*Large Yellow Ladies' Slipper*).

There are eight varieties of Cypripedium indigenous to this country, but the C. pubescens from some cause appears to have been selected as *the* variety to be the most used in medicine. It is known by the common names of American Valerian, (this name is Smith's, applied to the Scutellaria,) Nerve-root, Yellow moccasin flower, etc. For minute description of this and other varieties see King's Dispensatory. The *root* is the officinal portion. The roots of all these varieties are undoubtedly collected, sold, and used, with the officinal article indiscriminately. Homœopathic pharmaceutists should therefore be very careful in the selection of the root. This plant has always been a favorite remedy in domestic and "botanic" practice. As a "true *nervine*," it meets a great many indications in the treatment of females and children, and its harmlessness commends it to general use. It is an analogue of Valerian, Coffea, Thea, Chamomilla, Scutellaria, Senecio gracilis, and Ambra-grisea. The Eclectic school thus estimates its properties: Dr. King says it is "Tonic, stimulant, diaphoretic, and antispasmodic. Useful in hysteria, chorea, nervous headache, and all cases of nervous irritability; has proved useful in neuralgia, delirium and hypochondria. Combined with nepeta, and scutellaria, it has permanently cured headache (nervous) not dependent on acid stomach. An infusion is said to be beneficial in the *pains of the joints following scarlet fever.*" Jones and Scudder, (Mat. Med.) write—"In numerous affections termed neuropathic, we have employed the Cypripedium with decided advantage. It equalizes and energizes the nervous powers, lessens excitement, allays nervous irritability, alleviates pain, and appears to invigorate both body and mind, leaving the patient more cheerful and lively than when any of the narcotics, or many of the anti-spasmodics are prescribed. The diseases in which it is indicated are hysterical affections, hypochondriasis, delirium tremens, epilepsy, chorea, hemicrania, neuralgia, ataxic or nervous fevers, etc. In low fever accompanied with morbid nervous excitability, or irritability, as manifested by ruthlessness, vigilance, watchfulness, with great sinking of the vital powers, the Cypripedium produces a calm or tranquil state of mind, invigorates the system, and favors sleep. It is not so important in the relief of spasms or convulsions as many other agents, yet its peculiar nervine and stimulant qualities admirably adapt it to the relief of that morbid state of the cerebro-spinal system, upon which spasms depend." Dr. Coe places about the same estimate upon the medicinal powers of this plant. He says: "As a substitute for paragoric, Godfrey's cordial, etc., it is most advantageously employed in alleviating the disorders of children, requiring the use of an anodyne. *It possesses, however, some narcotic power, and many times will be found as inadmissible as opium.*" This last admission is quite an important one, and throws some light on the action of this remedy. I have noticed this *narcotic* effect upon the persons of some of my patients who were in the habit of using this plant to excess. In country practice, it is not unusual for the practitioner to find persons who are as strongly addicted to the habitual use of the Cypripedium, as others are to the use of Opium. They are generally persons beyond the middle age, whose nervous systems have once been shattered by some serious illness, and they have resorted to the lady-slipper for palliative relief. Such individuals, under the influence of the drug, are lively and talkative, disposed to work, and are really capable of making unusual exertions without much fatigue. They are tranquil, feel no pain, and altogether very comfortable. But when the use of the drug is suspended they become irritable, irascible, fretful; their motions are hurried and uncertain; they are agitated by the least contradictory word, a noise, or any excitement of those around them; they cannot sleep, and even have jactitations, pains, and hysterical spasms. These are the primary and secondary states and symptoms which are directly caused by the pathogenetic action of the Cypripedium. I do not think the plant has any specific influence over the skin or mucous membranes.

Clinical Remarks.—My observations and experience with this remedy has given me the following impressions relative to its true sphere of therapeutic action. (1.) Its action on the *brain*, is similar to that of Tea, Coffee, Cannabis indica, Cocoa, and a few others of that class. Its pathogenetic action does not extend as far as that of Agaricus, Belladonna, Hyoscyamus, Stramonium, and others of that group. I do not believe its toxical effects go beyond the causation of *functional irritation*. It is therefore not homœopathic to congestion, inflammation, or apoplexy of the brain and spinal cord and its membranes, but only to conditions of *morbid irritability, or hyperæsthesia of the nervous tissues*. I do not doubt its ability to cause serious brain affection in young children, for the nervous mass in infancy is so delicate and sensitive, that any agent capable of causing simple irritation, (tea, coffee, bright lights, noise, fright, etc.,) may induce a condition, which readily runs on to serious disorder. In young children, *irritability of the brain* often appears many days or weeks before more serious disease sets in. Proper remedies will often arrest this condition, and prevent congestion and inflammation. Children thus afflicted are noticed to be more lively than usual, more inclined to laugh and play at unwonted hours, even in the night; will often laugh in their sleep, or are very wakeful and excitable. If the little ones are urged to play, are excited by light, noise and laughter—all these tend to fix the irritation more strongly upon the over-sensitive brain, and soon the child is attacked with spasms or convulsions, and a meningitis closes the scene. It is in these premonitary conditions, or states of simple irritation, that the Cypripedium and Scutellaria, as well as Coffea and Cannabis indica are really indicated; and in my hands, the first named remedy has acted admirably, and in a highly satisfactory manner. To very young infants I usually administer the third or sixth dilution in water, or pellets, as often as the case seems to demand. On the *Nervous System* generally, of children or adults, it acts as a pure hyperæstheseant; primarily, elevating the excitability and activity; and secondarily, decreasing the strength, and awakening a morbid irribility of a low grade. It is *not* therefore homœopathic to neurotic diseases due to inflammation, congestion, or any organic change, but to a peculiar irritability such as I have described above. In many cases of *Neuralgia*, "*the pain is the disease*." In such instances the Cypripedium will be found curative in many cases. The same observation will apply to chorea, epileptiform symptoms, hysteria, etc. I have used it with good effects in the watchfulness, and nervous agitation of low fevers; but only as a palliative, for the drug is manifestly not homœopathic to the pathological conditions which are present. In the treatment of diseases of females its use will give satisfaction to the practitioner who adapts it to the symptoms for which it is truly homœopathic. *The Dose* is to be graduated according to the age of the patient, and whether the symptoms are primary or secondary, ranging from the 6th dilution or trituration, down to drop doses of the mother tincture.

CYPRIPEDIN.

This is the active principle of the Cypripedium pub., and for all practical purposes, or until we have a thorough proving of the plant, may be used instead of the tincture and dilutions. I have used the triturations, and find this preparation curative in about the same conditions, and for the same symptoms, as the preparation from the crude root. It is, of course, much more powerful than the tincture, and the dose should be selected accordingly. I have never given it to children, but in adults it may be given in the *sixth* or *first* triturations, without fear of aggravation, if not too long continued, or inappropriately applied.

DIOSCOREA VILLOSA.

(*Wild Yam. Colic-root.*)

This is an indigenous plant, growing in most parts of the United States, but in most abundance in the West and South. It is a slender vine, growing in thickets and hedges, and along-side fences, flowering in June and July. The *root* which is the part used in medicine, is long, from two to four lines in thickness, woody and contorted. It is of a yellowish-brown color externally, a slight, not unpleasant odor when bruised, and sweetish, slightly bitter taste. Water and alcohol extract its medicinal qualities. *Dioscorein*, the active principle of the plant, is much used, instead of the crude preparations; but generally it is most successful when given in infusion, one ounce to one pint of boiling water. Of this, one to two fluid ounces are given at a dose. This is one of those remedies principally known for certain specific effects upon one organ or tissue. I will here give the estimate of the eclectic school concerning its properties, together with the theories concerning its *modus operandi*, in order that we may have the testimony before us, to aid in our further investigations. *Wood* does not mention it in any of his works, neither do other strictly allopathic writers. *King* calls it an anti-spasmodic, "successfully used by eclectics in bilious colic, in doses of half a pint of the decoction, repeated every half an hour or hour; in fact, no other agent seems necessary in this disease, as it gives prompt and permanent relief in the most severe cases. It will likewise allay nausea, also spasms of the bowels." Of the *Dioscorein* he says: "It is undoubtedly as much a specific in bilious colic, as quinia is in intermittent" (*i. e.* only specific to *some cases?*) "In a severe case of bilious colic, pronounced past hope by several physicians, four grains, rubbed up with a tablespoonful of brandy, afforded prompt relief, and a repetition of the dose in about twenty minutes from the time of taking the first, effected a cure. In ordinary cases one or two grains of Dioscorein may be administered every five, ten or twenty minutes." It is useful in cramp of the stomach, flatulence, and even uterine cramps. *Coe* (Conc., Org., Med.,) says: "The wonderful efficacy of this remedy in the cure of bilious colic, renders it an indispensible agent to every practitioner of the healing act. In this complaint it is as near a specific as any remedy can well be. The relief it affords is both prompt and certain. But its entire value does not relate to this disease alone, as it has been found useful in cholera morbus, nausea attending pregnancy, spasms, coughs, hepatic disorders, after-pains, flatulence, dysmenorrhœa, and in all cases where an anti-spasmodic is required." "In our experience of the management of cholera morbus, as well as vomiting from other causes, we have found that small doses, frequently repeated, will oftentimes control the symptoms, when large doses fail," (one-fourth grain of Dioscorein.) "In conclusion, we would reiterate the fact that Dioscorein is eminently anti-spasmodic, and diaphoretic, and that its power of relieving spasms, relates more particularly to the stomach and bowels, in the disorders of which it has become to be looked upon by many as nearly a specific. We speak of our own knowledge when we state it to be the most reliable remedy yet discovered for bilious and flatulent colic, and intestinal spasm and irritation generally. It is a safe and harmless remedy, *but in over-doses will produce vomiting.*" The italics above are our own. If it will cause vomiting in over doses, why may it not cause spasms, cramps, irritation, and other phenomena of bilious and flatulent colic, for which it is so specific? I do not doubt its power of inducing these affections, when long given in pathogenetic doses. "Jones and Scudder assert that it acts as "a very gentle diaphoretic, without exciting the action of the heart and arteries, or increasing the temperation of the body. It has been but little used, however, for this purpose, although it might undoubtedly to employed with much advantage. It appears to act as an anodyne and anti-spasmodic, and likewise as an anti-emetic, in the diseases in which it is principally employed. The only affection in which it has been used sufficiently to give it a fair test to its virtues, is *bilious colic.* In many instances it has appeared to act with great promptitude in allaying nausea and vomiting, and relieving the pain and spasmodic action invariably present in that disease. "In various cases of great severity, when other remedies had been faithfully and perseveringly employed, and when all had proved unavailing, the nausea and vomiting, severe pain and spasms continuing unabated, with a dry and husky state of the surface, the Dioscorea has afforded entire relief in every respect, in twenty or thirty minutes, and the patient has fallen into a comfortable state of repose, and slept quietly the first time since the attack." Of the Dioscorein, they add, "We have used it in bilious colic with much success; and as an anti-emetic in other cases. In the cholera-infantum of children, it is one of our most efficient agents; combined with Leptandrin, we have succeeded in curing cases which were considered hopeless. From our experience with this agent, and it has been somewhat extensive, we believe it has a specific action upon the liver, not only increasing, but changing the character of the bilious secretion." The above is better and more definite testimony than we usually get from allopathic sources. We can afford to laugh at the name "anti-emetic," when their own authorities admit that it *causes* vomiting. Yet they *will* not see that it cures according to the law of *similia.* Doubtless they would seek to explain its action upon some other hypothesis even if was known to cause intestinal spasms. Dr. I. G. Jones, late professor of practice in the Eclectic Medical College of Cincinnati, and author of an extensive work on Practice, writes concerning this medicine: "The remedy upon which I rely in the treatment of bilious colic is *Dioscorea villosa.* I have used it with entire success in all the cases that have come under my care. In one case that had been previously treated forty-eight hours with injections, fomentations, anodynes, and cathartics, without success, the patient was relieved in half an hour by taking one dose of *Dioscorea.* In another case, to which I was called in the night, the patient, who had been suffering severely for twelve hours, was perfectly relieved in a few minutes and soothed into a quiet sleep. It has never been known to fail, and I should rely upon it with entire confidence in all cases of this disease. The philosophy of its therapeutic action may not as yet be fully understood, or clearly explained. That it is eminently adapted to the case is very certain, and *that*, after all, is the main point in practice." It may be interesting to us to know what condition Dr. Jones calls "bilious colic." He think it does not depend on hepatic disturbance at all. The *symptoms* are gastric derangement; furred tongue; constant pain, aggravated by regular paroxysms of increased sufferings; pain located at first in the centre of, but gradually diffused over the whole abdomen; febrile reaction, vomiting, distended, tender and sensitive abdomen, etc. The clinical experience of the homœopathic school, with Dioscorea and Dioscorein is not extensive. In fact I find no published record, and can only give the statements of my intimate colleagues. Dr. P. H. Hale, of Hudson, Michigan, informs me that he has used the tincture and lower dilutions successfully in *cramps of the stomach, flatulent colic, bilious colic, and cholera morbus.* Dr. A. R. Smart, who administered the remedy at my solicitation in the same affections, writes me that it seems to act curatively in cases in which Colocynth, Nux vomica and Chamomilla are usually given. Dr. C. A. Williams, reports the following cases: "Mr. ——, aged 50, subject to severe attacks of cholera morbus, attended with vomiting, diarrhœa, painful cramps in the stomach, bowels and extremities, from which, under allopathic treatment, he would not recover for several days. I was called in the night to see him after the attack had lasted about an hour. He was suffering intensely from the above symptoms and supposed he was to have an illness of several days duration. Wishing to test the alleged virtues of Dioscorein, I gave him about two grains of the first trituration every fifteen minutes. After the third dose he became easier, and before the sixth dose, expressed himself as quite comfortable. He shortly fell asleep, and in the morning went about his usual avocations." To this I will add my own observations. I have used the 1st, 2nd and 3rd dilutions, and triturations, in the above affections. In *cramps of the stomach*, (Cardialgia) the first decimal dilution often acts more promptly and satisfactorily than Nux vom. In the dioscorea-gastralgia there is generally a great tendency to erucate, and the pain is paroxysmal. In *spasmodic colic*, it seems to be indicated when we usually give Colocynth and Chamomilla. In these cases there is usually much flatulence, rumbling, and paroxysmal pain. In the *colic of children*, accompanied or not by diarrhœa, and attended witb screams and cries, and emission of flatulence, the second and third triturations have been useful. The true sphere of its action, whether upon the *muscular or nervous* tissues of the abdomen, etc., cannot yet be defined. I am inclined however, to the opinion that it acts more specifically upon the former. Its action is probably confined to the stomach and intestines. If useful in after-pains, or hepatic disorders, it must be because they depended upon some intestinal derangement. I once treated a gentleman for several years, for an anomalous disease of the abdominal organs, of which I could never form any satisfactory idea. He had been troubled with it from early youth. The *pain*, for that constituted nearly the whole of the malady, appeared at irregular intervals, sometimes once a week, at others once a month, and lasted several days. I never prescribed anything, nor did any other physician, which seemed to give him any relief. Anodynes dulled the pain for a time, but gave no permanent benefit. It was a crampy spasmodic pain, commencing near the crest of the ileum, and extending to the lumbar region and hypogastrium. Physical or mental labor would bring on an attack. It would gradually increase for days and end in an attack of vomiting; or at other times affect the head. When it *did* leave, it was always *suddenly*. Lying on the left side and back, only, was endurable. My impression was that it was a spasmodic disease of the vermiform process, excited by some matters introduced into that portion of the intestine. A travelling "Spiritual Doctor," prescribed for him a medcine or compound which gave him more relief than anything he had ever used. The chief ingredient in this mixture was the Dioscorea. The clairvoyant insisted that the malady was "piles in the bowels." (?)—a disease which is not down in our nomenclature. I have been promised a proving of this unique remedy, but it has not come to hand. I know of no drug that would better repay a trial, and none that would aid more in establishing the universality of the law of *Similia*, if we got a pathogenesis *verified*, wherein we could see a picture of those painful affections, in the cure of which it has gained such empirical reputation. I have repeatedly taken the tincture and first dilution several time a day for several days, but never elicited any notable symptoms. I have also tried it in several patients, affected with other than gastric complaints, but with no better results than in myself.

If this work should be so fortunate as to reach a second edition, we hope to give a proving of Dioscorea. At present, we can only treat this, as we have many other drugs, namely: make such mention as will stimulate our co-laborers to investigate its pathogenetic powers, and curative virtues.

ERIGERON CANADENSE.

(*Canada Fleabane. Colt's Tail.*)

This plant is common to the northern and middle portions of the United States, growing in fields and meadows, by road-sides, and in waste places, and flowering in July and August. It is an indigenous, annual plant, with a high, branched, furrowed and bristly, haired stem, from six inches to nine feet high. There are several other varieties—as the E. annuum, E. strigosum, etc., all possessing similar properties. The whole plant is officinal and should be collected while in flower. It has a feeble but agreeable odor, and a bitterish, acid, and astringent taste, and yields its properties to water and alcohol. It may be prepared and used in the form of tincture, or the dilutions made from the volatile oil. In most cases the Oleum Erigeroni is the best preparation from which to prepare the dilutions. It is decreed to be "tonic, astringent and diuretic." *King* says it is useful in the form of infusion, in diarrhœa, gravel, diabetes, dropsical affections, dysuria of children, painful micturition, etc.—"The volatile oil, acts as an astringent, and may be used as a local application to hemorrhoids, bleedings from small wounds, etc., also in rheumatism, boils, tumors, and sore throat." But it is in *hemorrhages* that the *oil* has been most strongly recommended; and the testimony relative to its successful use in this condition is so large that we must accord some specific virtues to it. It is considered by the country people as being quite infallible in its power over hemorrhages. The usual practice is to apply the bruised fresh plant to the wound, binding it on with a compress. I have known it thus applied to arrest quite alarming arterial bleedings. In its general action, it is an analogue to Terebinthina. Its *primary* action is similar to Turpentine, in causing intense congestion of the kidneys, etc. It is primarily homœopathic to *active* arterial hemorrhages, with congestion, and even inflammation; secondarily, to passive hemorrhages, with relaxation, ulceration, etc. Large quantities cause a large stimulating effect, increasing the heat of the body and the force of the pulse.

Skin.—When the oil is applied to the skin it "causes a burning sensation, much resembling that produced by Capsicum, but will not vesicate. It is a powerful rubefacient, but we never remember to have seen it vesicate."—(*Coe*). Dr. White, however, says that it causes "slightly elevated, sharply defined vesicles."

Eyes.—Applied to the conjunctiva it causes redness, swelling, inflammation, with profuse muco-purulent discharges. Yet Jones and Scudder, 'Mat. Med.,' say that the infusion is useful, as a local application, in ophthalmia, after the acute symptoms have subsided. It will form a useful application to ecchymoses upon the eyeballs, or around the eye, from a blow, etc. It should be given internally, and a weak dilution of the tincture applied locally.

Nose.—It is a useful remedy in epistaxis. It may be applied locally by injecting a weak dilution in water, or saturating lint with it, and plugging the nostrils. But it is undoubtedly useful in epistaxis, when administered internally. A few drops of the first or second decimal dilution of the oil, given every fifteen minutes, will often arrest profuse bleedings from the nasal passages. When given for *active* hemorrhage from the nose, accompanied with congestion of the head, febrile action, red face, etc., it should be given in the third or sixth dilution, and in alternation Aconite, Belladonna or Veratrum viride. But, when the hemorrhage is *passive*, occurring in debilitated subjects, or is chronic, and associated with ulcerative catarrh, the one-tenth, or even the tincture, in drop doses, may be resorted to with benefit.

Mouth, Throat.—In bleeding from the gums, profuse bleeding from the cavity after a tooth has been extracted, it has been used, locally, with benefit. *Dr. Coe* says, "as an application to inflamed and enlarged tonsils, and inflammation and ulceration of the throat generally, the remedy has few superiors. It should be applied with a probang, of the strength of one dram to two ounces of alcohol. It should be applied externally to the throat at the same time." This recommendation will remind the practical physician of the popular use of Turpentine in similar cases. Indeed, it is quite certain that in the early stages of Tonsillitis, the latter remedy will arrest the disease, when applied to the external throat over the situation of the tonsils. Its local curative action is as strictly homœopathic as that of Nitrate of Silver, for either remedy when applied to the mucous surface will cause inflammation, and even ulceration.

Stomach, etc.—Nausea; violent retching and vomiting, with burning sensation of long duration in the stomach; sensation of heat in the stomach.

Clinical Remarks.—It should be useful in hæmatemesis. Vomiting of blood may be caused (a) by erosion of the mucous coats of the stomach, (b) inflammation of the stomach and consequent ulceration, (c) rupture of an artery, (d) cancer, (e) disease of the liver and spleen. In all these cases the Erigeron will prove a valuable auxiliary to such remedies as Hamamelis, Sulphuric acid, Ipecac, etc. When the vomiting is the result of acute inflammation the higher dilutions will be most appropriate, but when it proceeds from ulceration, rupture of an artery, or when the blood is black and grumous, then the lowest dilutions will prove most efficient.

Abdomen, Intestines, etc.—Cathartics, with burning sensation throughout the alimentary canal; thin, papescent stool, with burning in the bowels and rectum; burning in the margin of the anus. (The experiment of Dr. Burt, in which he injected the oil under the skin of a cat, throws some light on its action on the bowels. He got the following symptoms: Undigested stools of meat; stools loose and *streaked with blood*. Autopsy showed the colon and rectum much congested, and in which was dry fæcal matter, agglutinated to the surface so firmly as with difficulty to be removed. All these symptoms, and the pathological condition, point to an inflammation of the mucous coats of the colon and rectum).

Clinical Remarks.—It has been found curative in diarrhœa and dysentery. In some portions of the country it is considered a specific for "bloody flux." In domestic practice I have often known it to be used in the form of an infusion, with astonishing results. Taking the hint from this observation, I have given the lower dilutions in dysentery, with excellent results. Several of my colleagues bear testimony to its curative action in this disease. It is indicated when the urinary organs are sympathetically affected, and we find dysuria, or suppression of urine. The stools are small, streaked with blood, accompanied with tormina, burning in the bowels and rectum. The appearance of scybala (lumps of indurated fæces) in the discharges would be a further indication for the Erigeron. In *hemorrhoids*, especially in the bleeding variety, this remedy is specifically indicated. In profuse bleeding from the hemorrhoidal tumors, we should not rely entirely upon its internal use, but apply the diluted tincture locally. *In hemorrhage from the bowels*, the Erigeron will probably prove as valuable as Terebinth. to which it bears so close analogy. Both remedies are capable of causing inflammation and ulceration of the intestinal mucous membrane. In typhoid fever, dysentery, and several other diseases, ulceration occurs, resulting in copious and often fatal hemorrhage. The usual remedies are Nitric and Sulphuric acids, and Turpentine. These remedies arrest the bleeding, and heal the ulceration. Erigeron I believe to have a similar curative action, and should the above medicines fail, I should resort to the first or second decimal dilution in ten drop doses, repeated every hour, with a confidence in the result.

Urinary Organs.—The Erigeron has a specific affinity for the urinary apparatus. Dr. Burt found the cortical substance of the Kidneys, (in a cat poisoned with the oil) slightly congested. At first the urine was suppressed, then increased. In this its action resembles Cantharis, Cannabis, Copaiva, Turpentine, etc., when given in large doses. The pathogenetic symptoms in men are: (1) Complete suppression of urine, with pain in the region of the kidneys; urging to urinate, with emissions of only a few drops of burning urine (large dose). This condition was followed in a day or two by copious emissions of pale urine, smelling of the oil. (2). Small and repeated doses caused frequent urination, with burning in the urethra when urinating; discharge of mucus with urine.

Clinical Remarks.—Dr. Ring was the first to introduce this remedy to the homœopathic schools for the treatment of urinary affections. In the N. A. Journal of Hom., Vol. V., page 282, he writes: "Recently I have had two cases of dysuria in teething children, which yielded to no remedy until I made use of drop doses (two or three drops every two or three hours) of a tincture of the Erigeron c. The symptoms in the two cases were more particularly —pain so as to cause a great deal of crying on voiding urine, the calls for which were frequent. The secretion was abnormally increased, and had a very strong odor. The parts externally—both were female children—were in both cases very much inflamed, or irritated, with considerable mucus discharged. The children were very fretful at all times. Several remedies we tried in both cases without any benefit, but prompt relief followed the use of the fleabane." Nearly every writer upon indigenous remedies has recommended the Erigeron for similar cases, as well as for other affections of the urinary organs. *King* says it has been found efficient in gravel, diabetes, dropsical affections, *dysuria of children*, painful micturition, and also many nephritic affections. "It has been used with benefit in diabetes, nephritis, cysitis, and to subdue the irritation arising from the presence of calculi in the bladder; also, in gonorrhœa and gleet."—(Jones and Scudder). Several cases are reported in the Eclectic Journal of its successful use in hæmaturia, also in chronic vesical catarrh. *Coe* says he has used the Erigeron in gonorrhœa with the most marked and beneficial results: "It allays the scalding of the urine, and assists materially in cutting short the disease. It is of much service in inflammation of the kidneys and bladder." All this testimony is eminently suggestive to the homœopathist. In the study of a medicine, it is most important to ascertain its specific affinity for any particular organ or tissue. This inquiry settled, we may rationally prescribe it in affections of those structures, even before we know the *peculiar* pathogenetic *symptoms* which it causes *in* those organs. We have ample testimony that the Erigeron has a specific affinity for the urinary organs, as much so as Cantharis or Turpentine; and although its *characteristic* symptoms may differ from those medicines, yet we know it will prove useful in nephritis, cystitis, hæmaturia, dysuria, etc. A good proving should be made; but, if we can have such careful observations as that of Dr. Ring, we can be guided materially in our selection of the drug.

Genital Organs of Women.—*Uterine hemorrhage*, with violent irritation of the rectum and bladder; hemorrhage from the uterus and bladder; *abortion*, with profuse hemorrhage, diarrhœa, and dysuria—(from very large doses); scanty menses.

Clinical Remarks.—We have at command a large amount of clinical testimony, from the most reliable sources, both allopathic and homœopathic, as to its curative action in hemorrhages from the uterus, and other abnormal discharges from the sexual passages. *Beach* says (Mat. Med.): "The oil is an infallible remedy in hemorrhages, in doses of from five to ten drops." King (Obstetrics) says it "exerts a powerful influence in menorrhagia and uterine hemorrhage. From two to ten drops, on sugar, or dissolved in alcohol, and mixed in a little mucilage or sweetened water, repeated every ten or twenty minutes, usually acts promptly. It may possibly have some other influence in checking uterine hemorrhage than that of a mere astringent; for, without the muscular fibres of the uterus are caused to contract, I do not believe the hemorrhage after delivery can be checked." King's theory of the action of Erigeron is doubtless correct. In tympanitis, the gas cannot be expelled, unless there is a contraction of the muscular coats of the intestines. Turpentine has the same effect in tympanitis that Erigeron does in uterine hemorrhage, namely: causing contraction of muscular fibre; but Erigeron must have also the general power of causing contraction of the muscular coats of the arteries, else it could not be so specific in all forms of hemorrhage (arterial). *Coe* (Conc. Org. Med.) writes: "Although not a specific, it is undoubtedly the best agent we possess for the relief of uterine hemorrhage. The dose of the oil, in these cases, is from five to ten drops, repeated every thirty or sixty minutes. It will act more promptly, being rendered more diffusible, by being previously dissolved in alcohol. In addition to its internal administration, it may also be applied locally with the best results. A case occurred under the observation of the writer, over twenty years ago, in which the patient, from excessive loss of blood, was reduced to a comatose condition, and incapable of swallowing. A piece of cotton wool, saturated with the oil, was introduced into the vagina, and placed in close contact with the mouth of the uterus, when an instantaneous stop was put to the bloody flow. During the past season we were consulted in a similar case, in which we advised the adoption of the above plan, and with complete success." *Coe* says, "it allays the spasmodic pains accompanying leucorrhœa, and restrains, without suppressing, the menstrual flow when too profuse." Cases have come under my observation, however, where the Erigeron in small doses, has undeniably restrained the menstrual flow, when *not* too profuse. One cannot read the above testimony from Eclectic sources, without noting the similarity of its curative action with that of Sabina. In fact, it is a very near analogue to Sabina. Both cause, in poisonous doses, abortion, hemorrhage, etc. Both are indicated in nearly the same conditions. Like Sabina, it is capable in toxical doses of causing congestion, inflammation, and even hemorrhage from the kidneys and uterus. We have, in addition to the above, some reliable homœopathic testimony as to the specific curative action of Erigeron in uterine hemorrhage. *Dr. White* (Trans. Ill. Hom. Med. Ass., vol. 9, p. 55,) states: "I have used the volatile oil in the first, second, and third att., as well as the crude oil. In uterine hemorrhage, it is the first remedy I have recourse to. It has never failed me. I have given from one to ten drops of the 1st, and the same internally, as an injection into the uterus, in extreme cases." *Dr. Rogers* reports to me the following cases: (1). A lady, aged thirty-five, had an abortion, followed by profuse and alarming hemorrhage, which continued for six weeks, in spite of all the efforts of her allopathic attendants, who used all the astringents, etc., at their command. She became almost exsanguined, nearly catamose; could not move without flooding; and the case was given up as hopeless. Erigeron, 1st dil., was given in ten drop doses, every hour. A piece of cotton wool was wet in the same, and applied to the os uteri. No more hemorrhage took place after the first six hours, and under the use of appropriate nutriment, &c., the lady made a good recovery. (2). A case of profuse and alarming flooding after labor was promptly arrested by the internal administration of Oleum Erigeron 1st dil. Dr. P. H. Hale used it in a case of post-parturient hemorrhage. Cold applications, posture, etc., were tried without perceptible effect, but the flooding ceased soon after giving the patient the oil of Erigeron, 1st dil. in fifteen drop doses, every thirty minutes. I might add the testimony of a score of other homœopathic physicians, as to its efficacy in hemorrhage from the uterus, but enough has been adduced to show that it is a valuable and important remedy in such conditions. It will hereafter prove a powerful auxiliary to such remedies as Sabina, Trillium, Crocus, Secale, Platina, and others of similar virtues. The following may be considered a good *resume* of its curative indications in diseases of women: (a.) In profuse and frequent menses. (b.) In dysmenorrhœa with menorrhagia. (c.) In hemorrhage after labor, or after an abortion. (d.) In threatened abortion with flooding. (e.) In hemorrhage previous to labor. (f.) In profuse lochial discharges. (g.) In profuse uterine and vaginal leucorrhœa. It has been found useful in palpitation of the heart, when arising from uterine irritation. It is alleged to have been used "with remarkable success in those peculiar headaches which accompany defective menstruation."

Organs of Generation of Men.—(See Urinary Organs.) It has been found curative in gonorrhœa and gleet.

Respiratory Organs.—*Jones and Scudder* (Mat. Med.) say: "In coughs and chronic bronchial affections, when attended with copious mucus or purulent secretion, and in the incipient stages of phthisis attended with bloody expectoration, this agent, used in the form of a syrup or infusion, will be found to answer an excellent purpose. It is of value in hæmoptysis." King records his estimate of its value in hæmoptysis, also various other eclectic writers.

DR. BURT'S EXPERIMENT WITH ERIGERON CANADENSE.

Sept. 5. 4 A. M., injected five drops of the oil under the skin of the foreleg of a cat. Quarter of an hour afterwards *mews* constantly; runs about; appears restless, uneasy. 5 P. M., lies quiet, with eyes half closed. 7 P. M., injected thirty drops of oil. After half an hour appears in great distress. Profuse secretion of saliva. At 8 P. M. is quiet, with mouth open.

Sept. 6. Passed four stools, natural, during the night; the last slightly streaked with blood; has not urinated; refuses to eat. 9 A. M., injected fifty drops under the skin of the foreleg; followed by *great* agitation as before. 10 A. M., ears and legs very cold; excessive trembling. 4 P. M., has had two undigested stools, and urinated. 6 P. M., injected forty drops; one hour after unable to get up; trembling excessively.

Sept. 7. Appears quite natural; has passed stools and urine during the night. Injected thirty drops under the skin of side. 5 P. M., very weak; has been trembling all day. 7 P. M., injected fifty drops; tries to walk, but is unable to do so. 8 P. M., injected thirty drops.

Sept. 8. Just alive. Injected 30 drops. Ears and legs very cold. Died at 9 A. M.

AUTOPSY.—Nine hours after death, encephalic and thoracic *viscera* natural; liver much congested; also, the *colon* and *rectum*, which were filled with *dry, fœcal* matter, agglutinated to the intestines so firmly as to be removed with difficulty. *Kidneys*, cortical substance, slightly congested. *Bladder* much distended; other abdominal viscera natural.

ERYNGIUM AQUATICUM.

(*Button Snakeroot.*)

This plant is a native of the United States, growing in swamps and wet lands, from Virginia to Texas, and especially on the prairie lands. The root is the officinal part. Water and alcohol extract its properties. (For full botanical description, see King's Dispensatory). No proving of this plant has yet appeared, and the clinical experience is very scanty. King says: "it is very useful in dropsy, nephritic and calculous affections; also, in scrofula and syphilis; it is said to be diuretic, stimulant, diaphoretic, expectorant, and, in large doses, emetic. It has been recommended as a substitute for Senega." "The pulverized root, in doses of two or three grains, has proved very effectual in *hæmorrhoids*, and *prolapsus ani*. Two ounces of the pulverized root, added to one pint of good Holland gin, has effected cures in obstinate cases of *gonorrhœa* and *gleet* (one or two fluid drachms three or four times a day). By some practitioners this root is employed as a specific in gonorrhœa, gleet and leucorrhœa. Howard speaks of it as a powerful diuretic, and says he has cured asthenic dropsies with it. He has also used it with benefit in gravel. The only mention made of this remedy in the literature of our school, is to be found in Hill and Hunt's Surgery, page 400. In the treatment of *Spermatorrhœa*, after referring to various remedies, they propose the Eryngium, and give two "remarkable cures" made by Dr. Parks, of Cincinnati.

Case 1st. "A married man injured his testicles by jumping upon a horse; this was followed by a discharge of what was considered semen, for fifteen years, during which time he was treated allopathically and homœopathically. Dr. P. exhibited a number of the usual remedies without permanent benefit. He then gave a half-grain dose, three times a day, of the third decimal trituration of Eryngium aquaticum. In five days the emissions were entirely suppressed, and have not returned to this time (over two years). The emissions were without erections, day or night, and followed by great lassitude."

Case 2nd. "A married man, not conscious of having sustained any injury, was troubled for eight or ten years with emissions at night, with erections. The semen also passed by day with the urine. The loss of semen was followed by great lassitude and depression for twelve or forty-eight hours. There was also partial impotence. He had been treated allopathically. Dr. P. gave him

Phos. ac. for two weeks without material benefit. He then exhibited the Eryngium as above, with like excellent and prompt result."

It does not do as well in the hands of others, for several physicians have informed me they never found it of benefit in similar cases. I have tested it in several instances with like poor success. That the remedy has some specific affinity for the urinary and genital organs appears probable, but we want a pathogenesis to guide us in its selection.

EUPATORIUM AROMATICUM.

(*White Snake Root.*)

This is an indigenous plant, growing from Massachusetts to Louisiana. The root, which is the officinal part, has a pleasant aromatic odor, and a bitterish taste. "This species of Eupatorium (see Eclectic Mat. Med.) is anti-spasmodic, nervine, diaphoretic, and expectorant. It is esteemed a valuable nervine, and anti-spasmodic, and one peculiarly adapted to many cases of debility and irritability of the nervous system, such as hysteria or hysterical affections, chorea, tremors, convulsive, or spasmodic diseases, subsultus tendinum, restlessness and morbid watchfulness, etc., occurring in the advanced stage of fevers. It is diaphoretic and expectorant." The only mention of this medicine in our literature is the assertion of Dr. B. L. Hill in his epitome that it is a specific for apthous stomatitis in females and children. We can nowhere find that he has given any reason for this recommendation. Judging, however, by the *perfect reliability* of that gentleman's teachings, we should perhaps have all confidence in his dictum. Some of our physicians say that they have found it useful in nursing sore mouth and in apthæ of infants. It may be worth a proving, but so long as there are such drugs as Trillium and Leptandria to be proved, we shall not recommend it.

Dr. Wm. Huntington says: "My use of Eupatorium aromaticum is quite limited. I have derived considerable benefit from its use in alternation with Hydrastus c. in nursing sore mouth. It acts as a palliative only. I have also used it with good results in apthons affections of the mouth and throat closely resembling nursing sore mouth, but the most benefit that I have ever derived from its use has been in those cases of burning at the stomach so often met with in pregnant females for a few weeks previous to confinement. In such cases it seldom fails to give very marked relief."

Dr. Smith Rogers has found the Eupatorium aromaticum effectual in curing apthæ and nursing sore mouth without giving any other drug in connection with it. Dr. Lodge states that many other physicians have made similar reports.

EUPATORIUM PERFOLIATUM.

(*Bone-set—Ague weed.*)

There are at least sixteen species of Eupatorium in the Northern States alone. The *stem* of the Eupatorium perfoliatum is villous, hirsute, cylindrical; the *leaves*, opposite, connate, perfoliate, oblong, tapering, acute, senate, rough above, tomentose beneath, heads about ten-flowered. The *root* is perennial, horizontal, crooked, sending up many erect stems, which are simple at base, branched above, round, hairy, and of a greyish-green color. The whole plant is officinal. The whole plant is intensely bitter, having a peculiar flavor, but without astringency or acrimony. Its odor is but slight, and it yields its sensible and medicinal properties to water and alcohol. It is supposed to contain a resinoid *Eupatorine* which is said to contain the specific virtues of the plant.

General Effects.—It is decreed by the old school to be diuretic, diaphoretic, purgative, emetic, alterative, expectorant, and tonic. It proves *emeto-cathartic* when given in large doses. (Therefore, it is homœopathic to vomiting, *with* diarrhœa—bilious). Prof. Lee gives his testimony in favor of its successful use in intermittents, but doubts its asserted *anti-periodic* power. It was in general use among the aborigines of this country, on its first discovery, as a remedy for intermittent fever, and was accordingly adopted by the whites for the cure of the same disease. "Whether it proved successful or not depended very much on its mode of administration. Sometimes it would arrest the disease, if freely given in warm decoction just before the expected recurrence of the paroxysm, proving emetic, or emeto-cathartic, and in other cases it would prove successful if given in cold decoction, or the powdered plant, at frequent intervals between the paroxysms; but in a majority of cases it failed to subdue the disease" (because it was not homœopathic to a *majority* of the cases, any more than is quinine or any other medicine). Prof. Lee says: "With regard to the use of this plant in *Influenza*, whether sporadic or epidemic, we have proved it possessing great efficacy—relieving the pain in the back and limbs, as well as the general lassitude, with great promptness; for although in this disease the skin is often bathed in perspiration, yet it is of a morbid character—the surface being pale, and morbidly sensitive, and the excretion of a passive kind. When the secretions are of this morbid nature, and the pulmonary system is involved, the Boneset has proved in our hands a most valuable remedy, inducing a healthy and free perspiratory discharge, and replacing the chilly or febrile sensations with a uniform or healthy glow." (Yet the Eupat., in large doses, will cause the same *unhealthy* perspiration and state of the skin which Dr. Lee mentions, so that he uses it homœopathically after all.) "As it has but slight influence in augmenting the action of the heart and arteries, it may be employed with advantage in almost every variety of inflammatory action." "In the atonic forms of dyspepsia and general debility it is relied on by many practitioners as an efficient remedy.

In that form of indigestion consequent on the use of alcoholic drinks, it has proved highly beneficial, as well as in that of old people." "Its efficacy in certain forms of *dropsy* has been dwelt upon by some writers. Dr. Thatcher, who has tried it extensively in various diseases, says that in anasarcous swellings of the extremities, depending on general debility, it may be safely recommended as an excellent tonic." Dr. Zollickoffer thinks it possesses medicinal virtues which are admirably adapted to a variety of affections, and that in conjunction with sup. tart. potassa, it is one of the most valuable remedies in *tinea capitis.*

Dose.—In old school practice, the concentrated tincture or fluid extract is given in doses of one to four drachms. The Eupatorine in doses of two or three grains. The *Infusion*, (one ounce to one pint of boiling water) in doses of two to six ounces, the latter dose causing emesis and catharsis. In homœopathic practice, it has been used successfully in agues, in drop doses of the *first* dilution; also in ten-drop doses of the tincture; and teaspoonful doses of a cold infusion (vide Trans. Amer. Ins. of Hom.).

Fever.—Chilliness through the night, and in the morning, with nausea from the least motion; aching pain and soreness, as if from having been beaten in the calves of the legs, small of the back, and in the arms, above and below the elbows; nausea as the chill goes off; aching in the bones of the extremities, with soreness of the flesh; chilliness, with excessive trembling and nausea; chilliness in the morning, heat through the rest of the day, but no perspiration. The patient feels worse in the morning of one day, and in the afternoon of the next day. Nocturnal sweat, with chilliness, from motion, or removal of the covering. A greater amount of shivering during the chill than is warranted by the degree of coldness. Retching and vomiting of bile; vomiting after every draught; trembling in the back during fever; thirst several hours before the chill; chilliness from motion; pungent heat attending the perspiration at night; alternate chilliness and flashes of heat.

Clinical Remarks.—The Eupatorium is recommended by Drs. Jaynes, Neidhard, Gray, Williamson and Douglas, in intermittent fevers, quotidian, tertian, and quartan. The general and specific indications for its use are said to be: (a.) The paroxysm generally commences in the *morning. Thirst several hours after the chill—which continues during the chill and heat.* It has proved curative when the symptoms have been:—Chill at seven o'clock in the morning, preceded by thirst, and attended with moisture of the hands; *vomiting at the conclusion of the chill;* chill in the morning; heat during the rest of the day; slight perspiration in the evening; heavy chill early in the morning of one day, and a light chill about noon the next day, and so on successively; chill preceded by pain above the right ilium, with thirst and disposition to yawn; pain in the bones early in the morning before the paroxysm; the chill is induced or hastened by taking a drink of water; headache, backache and thirst during the chill; coldness, with a great deal of trembling, attended with nausea; coldness and stinging and pricking, as from pins, in both feet, at the commencement of the chill; aching in the bones of the extremities, in the latter part of the chill and in the beginning of the heat; stiffness of the fingers during the chill; aching pain, with moaning throughout the chill. (b.) Throbbing headache during the chill and heat; violent pain in head and back before the chill; distressing pain through the scrobiculus cordis throughout the day; chill and heat; flushed face and dry hot skin during the fever; fever, accompanied with sleep and moaning, and followed by slight perspiration; nausea and sickness at the stomach at the commencement of the heat, with violent throbbing headache; headache and trembling during the heat; fever in the forenoon, preceded by thirst early in the morning, but no chill; attended by fatiguing cough, and not followed by perspiration; great weakness and prostration during the fever, with faintness from motion; the patient cannot raise his head from the pillow while the fever lasts; the heat goes off with moderate perspiration, during sleep in the evening; the thirst continues during the chill and heat, with vomiting after each draught of water; vomiting of bile at the close of the hot stage; nocturnal perspiration, with coldness; fever, with despondency of mind, morbid sensitiveness of the skin and sleeplessness. (c) Loose cough in the intermission; cough in the night, previous to the paroxysm; thirst throughout the night, before the paroxysm, (in tertian ague).

"I have for many years applied the Eupatorium, in cases of intermittent fever, when there was *little or no sweat, at any time during the disease*; and consequently in those forms closely verging upon the remittent type."—(*Dr. Gray*).

The above clinical symptoms I select from the proving published in "Trans. of Amer. Ins. of Hom." They are there marked with an *, and are the result of the clinical experience with the remedy, contributed by Drs. Neidhard, Williamson, and others. The cases from which they were taken I give in full:—

Cases of Intermittent.—Dr. Neidhard has observed the most decided effects from the Eupatorium perfoliatum in the treatment of certain cases of intermittent fevers, in two of which the following symptoms were present: Violent thirst before the chill, and slight during it; nausea and sickness of the stomach (in one case vomiting) at the commencement of the heat, with violent throbbing headache; tastelessness of food; want of appetite; tongue coated yellow; the chills set in in the morning and lasted for one or two hours; heat during the rest of the day, and slight perspiration in the evening. Type certain. In one case the sulphate of quinine had been administered without preventing the recurrence of the paroxysms.

Dr. Williamson has exhibited it successfully in various cases of fever.

Case 1st: The chill generally began at nine o'clock in the morning, and lasted four hours from the time, when they commenced, and continued about seven hours, and was seldom followed by perspiration. The next day there was a lighter paroxysm, which usually commenced at twelve o'clock and ceased about the same time in the evening, as the heavier on the day preceding. The paroxysms continued to occur thus alternately with but little variation for the space of twenty-three days, notwithstanding my unceasing efforts to arrest them by the administration of a number of remedies. On the 12th of December the following symptoms were present: Chill commenced at nine o'clock in the morning, and lasted four hours, attended with a good deal of shivering and trembling; raging thirst before the chill, and during the chill, and heat; vomiting of whatever was taken into the stomach, and of bile, with distressing pain in the epigastrium; distressing headache during the heat; fever ceased about eight o'clock in the evening, and was followed by inconsiderable perspiration. Eupatorium perfoliatum first, in water, a teaspoonful every hour, in the apyrexia, cured the case, without the occurrence of another paroxysm.

Case 2d: Bilious diathesis; tertian ague; chill at nine o'clock in the morning, which lasted an hour and a half; thirst in the night before the chill; raging thirst during the chill and heat; violent headache throughout the paroxysm; some perspiration; retching and vomiting during the chill, immediately after drinking; vomiting of bile. Eupatorium perfoliatum first, five drops in as many teaspoonfuls of water, of which she took a teaspoonful every two hours on the alternate day. Early on the morning of the expected chill, Eupat. perf. tincture four drops, in eight teaspoonfuls of water, a teaspoonful every hour. The paroxysm did not return. This patient had been subject to frequent attacks of intermittent fever for several years, and had always suppressed them with sulphate of quinine, but since the above attack, now a period of four years, she had no return of the disease.

Case 3rd: A girl of fourteen years of age; tertian intermittent fever; thirst before the chill; became stretchy and looked pale at nine o'clock in the morning; felt cold and chilly, but did not shake; walked about the house crouched up; was very thirsty during the chill and heat, but took only a little sup of water at a time; headache and trembling during the heat; the coldness lasted one hour, and the heat about two hours, followed by very little perspiration. Eupat. perf. tinct. a few drops in water. Dose, a teaspoonful every three hours.

Case 4th: At eight o'clock in the morning was attacked with pain above the right ilium; thirst and a disposition to yawn; fingers became stiff, with slight coldness; upon taking a drink of water shuddering commenced immediately; chill lasted two hours and a half; headache, backache, and thirst during the chill; nausea as the chill was going off; the headache was increased, but the thirst was diminished during the heat; sensation of great weakness during the fever, so much so that she could not raise her head from the pillow; trembling in the back, with faintness from motion during the fever; the fever terminated by moderate perspiration during sleep in the evening. She felt pain in her bones early in the morning before the attack. Eupat. perf. tincture in water a teaspoonful every three hours.

Case 5th: Tertian ague, for two weeks, sickly, sallow countenance; chill at eight o'clock in the morning; thirst throughout the night previous to chill; thirst during the chill and heat, and vomiting immediately after each draught of water; vomiting of bile at the close of the hot stage, which was followed by inconsiderable perspiration. Eupat. perf. tincture, in water, a teaspoonful every three hours. No more chills.

"Nearly half a century ago, there prevailed throughout the United States, but particularly in the State of Pennsylvania, a peculiar Epidemic, which, from the constancy of the attending symptom of "pain in the bones," was called *break-bone fever*. The Eupat. perf., though a diaphoretic, so signally relieved the disease, notwithstanding *copious perspiration* was a frequent attendant, that it was familiarly called *bone-set*, a common name by which it is extensively known. "In all cases of typhoid disease, attended with hot, dry skin, it is reputed to be an estimable medicine." "It was used with great success in an epidemic of Influenza and lake-fever, which prevailed a few years ago in the neighborhood of Lake Ontario." "In miasmatic districts, along rivers, at fisheries, on marshes and their several neighborhoods, where intermittent and remittent fevers have prevailed epidemically, the Eupatorium has been a favorite remedy with the most successful practitioners, as well as a deservedly popular one in the hands of the people, very often superseding the necessity of calling in medical aid. In 1812, it was substituted for Peruvian bark, in the treatment of intermittent fevers, in the New York Alms House, and with uniform success." Dr. Williamson recommends it in gastric fevers, remittent fevers of typhoid character, bilious fever, etc. It is highly recommended as a *prophylactic* against agues.

Head.—Headache with a sensation of soreness internally, better in the house; aggravated when first going in the open air; relieved by conversation; pain extending from the forehead to the occiput, greatest in left side; *throbbing* headache; beating pain in the nape and occiput, better after rising; darting pains through the temples, with sensation of blood *rushing across* the head; *distress* on the top and in the back part of the head; *shooting* pains from left to right side of the head; *painful soreness* in the right parietal protuberance; *heat* on the top of the head, with pain, which is relieved by pressure; *thumping* in the side of the head, above the right ear; *soreness* and *beating* in the back part of the head.

Clinical Remarks.—Besides those symptoms which are *italicized* above, the Eupatorium has cured certain forms of *periodical* headache, namely: "A headache with nausea, every other morning, when first awaking, which continues all day, with loss of appetite during the day, but good appetite during the intervening day." Nux vomica will cure such headaches when they occur *every* day. Eupatorium has also cured a "pain in the occiput after lying, with sensation of a great weight in the part, requiring the hands to lift it." This kind of headache is common in ague patients.

Eyes.—Soreness of the eyeballs; intolerance of light; redness of the margin of the lids, with glutinous secretion from the meibomian glands; increased lachrymation; pain and soreness in left eyeball.

Clinical Remarks.—*Soreness of the eyeballs* is one of the most common and permanent symptoms of ague, and usually precceds an attack for several days; this symptoms would be a good indication for the selection of this medicine.

Face.—Sickly, sallow countenance; flushed face; redness of the cheeks, with dry skin; pale face.

Mouth.—Paleness of the mucous membrane of the mouth; tongue coated yellow; white coated tongue; sores in the corners of the mouth; dryness of the throat; soreness of the fauces with catarrh.

Appetite.—Insipid taste in the mouth; tastelessness of food. Want of appetite; distaste of food; nocturnal thirst for something cold; thirst for cold water; desire for ice-cream; great appetite.

Clinical Remarks.—When the Eupatorium is taken in small doses for a few days, the appetite is *first increased;* a still further continuance gives rise to unnatural hunger, accompanied by disorders of digestion, and finally to complete loss of appetite, and loss of taste for food. This remedy is homœopathic to the canine hunger which attends or precedes ague; also when arising from abuse of quinine. It is also indicated (secondarily) in the loss of appetite and indigestion from the same causes. It will be found useful in many forms of dyspepsia, anorexia of drunkards, loss of appetite, etc. (See general effects.)

Stomach.—Belching of tasteless wind, with a feeling of obstruction at the pit of the stomach; sensation of something in the stomach that ought to come up, without the ability to raise it. General shuddering proceeding from the stomach; sensation of fullness in the stomach; beating in the epigastrium—in the night; heat in the stomach; *nausea;* nausea and vomiting of food; vomiting of bile; vomiting of mucus and bile; *vomiting of bile with trembling, attended with pain in the epigastrium,* with nausea and extreme prostration, almost syncope; distressing disposition to vomiting; nausea and vomiting with free perspiration, and expectoration; qualmishness from odors, the smell of food, cooking, etc.

Clinical Remarks.—When a *warm* infusion or decoction of this plant is administered, it invariably causes profuse and long-continued vomiting, nearly always of *bile.* Hence its reputation as a domestic remedy for bilious affections and fevers of that type. Its use is resorted to with a great deal of confidence in the forming stages of a bilious fever, and it *seems* to have the power of arresting the attack. It is eminently homœopathic to vomiting of bile, of food, and even of drinks, as soon as taken.

Liver.—Soreness around the waist; tight clothing is oppressive. Soreness and fullness in the region of the liver; tightness in the left hypochondrium.

Intestinal.—Purging stools, with smarting and heat in the anus. Four or five watery stools in the day; tenesmus, with small discharge of loose stool; morning diarrhœa; constipation.

Clinical Remarks.—While the *warm* infusion causes vomiting only, the same preparation when taken *cold* acts as an active cathartic, causing profuse bilious watery stools, with nausea and severe colic, prostration and relaxation. *Catharsis* is a primary effect of Eupatorium, constipation the remote, secondary.

Urinary Organs.—Urine scanty and high colored; copious evacuation of limpid urine; dark, brown, scanty urine, depositing a whitish clay-like sediment; voided but once in twenty-four hours. Dark colored, but clear urine; itching of the mons veneris.

Clinical Remarks.—It seems homœopathic to the dark colored urine met with in bilious disorders; also the watery urine observed during intermittents. It is said to have been very successful in the treatment of a peculiar herpetic eruption, affecting the anus and adjacent parts, as the scrotum and thighs, and also extending its ravages to the rectum.

Catarrhal Symptoms.—Flowing coryza; sneezing; hoarseness, with roughness in the voice; hacking cough in the evening; cough with soreness and heat in the bronchia; cough aggravated in the evening.

Clinical Remarks.—The Eupat. per. has an extensive reputation in colds, influenza, and catarrhal fevers. In domestic practice it is usually given in small doses of the warm infusion, and produces copious sweating. Some physicians consider it almost specific in colds, etc. In homœopathic practice, it has cured, in small doses: "Hectic cough from supposed intermittent fever; nocturnal loose cough; hoarse rough cough with scraping in the bronchia; violent cough with soreness in the chest; cough with flushed face and tearful eyes—the patient supports the chest with the hands; cough preceding measles; cough following measles; disposition to cough with dyspnœa." The above are quite prominent symptoms, and show this remedy to have quite a specific action upon the bronchial mucous membrane. In eclectic practice it is highly esteemed as a "cough remedy." Its effects on the respiratory tract, seems somewhat analogous to Phosphorus, Tartar emetic, and Causticum. It has been found useful in epidemic *influenza*. (See General Effects.)

Chest.—*Difficulty of breathing*, attended with anxious countenance; perspiration, and sleepiness; *painful irritation* of the pulmonary organs with heat in the chest; aching pain under the left breast; inability to lie on the left side; soreness in the chest from taking a full inspiration; grating sensation in the chest at every deep inspiration.

Clinical Remarks.—It has been used successfully in asthma, bronchitis and even pneumonia. It has given relief in a case when the "Dyspnœa was very great, obliging the patient to lie with his head and shoulders very high," also the two symptoms *italicized*.

Back.—Weakness in the small of the back; deep seated pain in the loins, with soreness from motion; pain in the back as from a bruise; beating pain in the nape of the neck; *pain in back and lower extremities.*

Upper Extremities.—Soreness and aching in the arms and fore-arms; stiffness of the arms; painful soreness in both wrists, as if broken or dislocated; stiffness of the fingers with obtuseness of the sense of touch; *heat* in the palms of the hands, sometimes with moisture.

Lower Extremities.—Pain in a spot not larger than a pea, over the left hip, with soreness; pain with extreme sensitiveness in the left glutei muscles, passing around in front of the trochanter major; burning in the skin, on the inner side of the thighs of a female; flagging of the muscles of the left thigh, as if they were falling off the bone. The pains are worse from ten o'clock, A. M., until four o'clock, P. M. Pain and soreness of the upper part of the left foot, with increased sensibility of the left big toe; the pain in the foot is increased by standing on it. Stiffness and general soreness of the lower extremities when rising to walk; calves of the legs feel as though they had been beaten; soreness and swelling of both feet, when standing on them, in a gouty subject; pain in the first joint of the left great toe, which suddenly moves to the corresponing joint of the right one; pricking in the soles of the feet; aching pain in the right hip, while sitting; lameness in the right hip and lower extremity, when walking; soreness and aching of the lower limbs; throbbing in the right foot; rheumatic pains on the inside of the left knee; dropsical swelling of both feet and ankles; heat in the soles of the feet in the morning.

CLINICAL REMARKS.—Dr. Williamson considers it indicated in Rheumatic affections, accompanied by perspiration and soreness of the bones. Also in Gouty affections. It is said to have cured "Gouty inflammation of the left knee and right elbow." "Dropsical swelling of both feet and ankles," also symptoms recorded above.

EUPATORIUM PURPUREUM.

(*Queen of the Meadow. Gravel root.*)

This plant, known all over the United States by the common names above given, grows abundantly in low wet ground. It flowers in August and September, and the *root*, which is the officinal portion, should be collected in the fall. The active principle, *Eupatorine*, or *Eupurpurin*, as it is sometimes called, is said to contain, in a great degree, the medicinal properties of the root. Probably no plant has such an extensive reputation among the people in diseases of the kidneys and bladder, and such a popularity must be found upon some reliable foundation. In an extensive country practice for many years, I found it used successfully in the most obstinate cases of dropsy, gravel (so-called) and chronic renal and vesical diseases. It is from these popular uses that the eclectic physician has gained his empirical knowledge of this remedy. It is decreed to be diuretic, stimulant, astringent, tonic, and antilithic.

"There is no doubt but what this agent exerts a specific influence upon the kidneys, increasing the quantity of urine secreted, and to some degree the amount of solids excreted in it. It has been employed in atonic dropsies, chronic nephritis, catarrhus vesicæ, attended with ulceration; chronic irritation of the bladder, attended with increased mucous secretion. It has also been employed in hæmaturia, gleet, leucorrhœa, and other forms of female weakness, rheumatism and gout, with success. It is a popular remedy in gravel, and said by some to possess solvent powers; although we cannot award it any positive powers of that kind yet, as it increases the amount of water excreted, which is acknowledged to be the best solvent for stone, and always allays irritation of the bladder, we must consider it at least the equal of Uva ursi and Chimaphila. We have used the *Eupurpurin*, and consider it among our most efficient curative agents in diseases of the kidneys, bladder, and urethra. In one case of marked *albuminuria*, when other agents had failed to produce any relief, the continued use of this remedy for two weeks entirely relieved the patient. In two cases of *Diabetes insipidus*, its use was attended with the same results. We have also employed it in *incontinence of urine*, especially in children, with good effects. It is of the most importance, however, in allaying *irritation of the bladder;* in many cases of this kind caused by displacement or chronic inflammation of the uterus, or arising during, or after pregnancy, we have obtained more benefit from its use than from any other agent." (Eclec. Mat. Med.)

Dr. King says: "It is used with excellent effect in dropsical affections, strangury, gravel, and all chronic urinary disorders, hæmaturia, gout and rheumatism."

It is in the class of diseases just named, that I know it to be more useful. I have known it to remove symptoms of the urinary organs, that had resisted the use of Canth., Cann., Copaiva, Pulsatilla and Thuya. My experience with this variety of Eupatorium has been quite extensive, and my observation of its use are equally so. It seems to be a close analogue of Uva ursi, Cannabis, Chimaphila, Pulsatilla, and Copaiva. I have known it, when taken excessively, as it often is by the country people, to materially aggravate renal difficulties, and even give rise to the very symptoms for which it is so strongly recommended, and so really useful. To be more specific, I have cured with this remedy a severe case of *strangury*, in a female, due to uterine displacement; the usual remedies had been used without benefit. In a case of excessive irritation of the bladder, with large deposit of *lithates* in the urine, it removed all the symptoms in a week. Several minor cases might be mentioned. Next to Apocynum cann., I consider it the most powerful remedy we possess, for the alleviation, and even permanent cure of *Dropsy*.

It is even superior to that medicine, for its action on the kidneys is of a more pervading and profound character, *i. e.*, it is capable of modifying the various tissues of those organs, to a greater degree than the Apocynum. One of the most intractable cases of dropsy, due apparently to renal disease, that ever came under my care, I believe to have been permanently cured by the tincture of this root. I usually use the mother tincture, and lower dilutions; a few drops at a dose, every two or six hours, as required.

EUPHORBIA COROLLATA.

(*Go-Quick. Milk-weed. Spurge.*)

This plant is as yet but rarely used in Allopathic or Homœopathic practice, but our Eclectic colleagues have made extensive trials with it in disease for many years, and thus indirectly given us some valuable pathogenetic hints. But, much as it is used by that school, their literature contains but little in its reference to therapeutic power. With physicians of that school it supersedes the use of Lobelia or Ipecac, as an emetic or diaphoretic; and is substituted for the Podophyllum, Jalap, &c., as an active cathartic. But in the doses in which it is administered, it is often productive of unpleasant and even dangerous symptoms, and capable of doing much injury to the gastric mucous membrane.

I have never administered it in disease, save in a strictly homœopathic manner, but I have experimented upon myself, testing the effects of the dried root in grain doses; and I have often had opportunities of observing its immediate and remote effects upon the persons of the patients of eclectics.

The Euphorbia cor. belongs to the Nat. Ord. Euphorbiaceæ, with the Euphorbia off., of Hahnemann; and the Euphorbia ipecacuanha of American writers. There are two other varieties, the Euphor. maculata, and E. hypericifolia but as their effects are quite different from the former, they cannot properly belong to the same group of remedial agents.

The E. off., of which we have a proving by Hahnemann himself, is one of the most irritating and powerful agents known, in its action upon the skin and gastric mucous membrane. It is said to have an irritant effect upon the brain. It is seldom if ever used internally by the old school, because of its severity of action. Its principal use is externally as a rubefacient or vesicant. Hahnemann, although he does not give a picture of its general effects upon the skin, mentions its causing erysipelas of the face of a severe character. But its real sphere of action is more like that of Croton tiglium, than any other drug. It causes a most intense inflammatory eczema, which often puts on an erysipelatous appearance.

In Hahnemann's proving, sufficient prominence is not given to its effects upon the stomach and intestines, although he gives a few of the symptoms indicative of its peculiar action in that direction. The E. Ipecacuaha has been used by American botanic physicians, and by the country people in domestic practice, for many years, as a prompt and easy emetic. It is the mildest of this class, causing free and copious emesis and catharsis, with little pain, except when given in large doses. Yet the milky juice of *this* variety will, when applied to the skin, produce vesication and eczematous inflammation. It is used by the eclectics as an emetic, diaphoretic, expectorant, and epispastic. They claim that it is superior to Elaterium as a hydragogue in dropsy; that it will bring on the menstrual discharge when given in cathartic doses; and is useful in hepatic torpor, bilious colic. &c.

Probably it is not specifically indicated in any of these diseases but may prove homœopathic to some form of eczema, gastric disorder, with irritation of the mucous coat of the stomach and bowels. But it is the Euphorbia corollata which I prefer to consider, as being the more powerful remedy, and perhaps more capable of attaining a position in our Materia Medica, by the side of the E.-off. This plant is incorrectly termed by Wood, King, and other writers as the "large flowering spurge." In their botanical descriptions, the peculiarities of the different varieties are mingled together, so that I can nowhere find a correct description of the E.-Corollata. It grows in waste and sandy places all over Canada and the Northern States, flowering in July and August. It has several straight stems rising from a small yellowish root, which, when broken, yields a milky juice which irritates the skin when applied to it for a few minutes, creating a pustular eruption. The stalk contains the same juice, but of less strength. The bark of the root is the officinal part, and, together with the whole root, *inodorous and tasteless!* Its virtues are imparted to water and alcohol. The tincture of the powdered bark, or the bark itself, triturated with sugar or milk after the usual manner, is the best method of preparation. Being destitute of taste, it is easily given to children, should it be necessary to use the lower triturations. Pellets saturated with the mother tincture, the first trituration or the strong tincture, or powdered bark, should be used in provings. Its action on the system is intense and peculiar. It is called by the country people by the expressive name of *Go quick*, referring to its quick and prompt action. I am indebted to Dr. A. R. Brown, of Litchfield, Mich., for many interesting facts relating to its action. It is considered by those who use it, as the most powerful "revulsive agent" in their Materia Medica, in all cases of local congestion, especially of the lungs and head; also in inflammation of the pleura, lungs and liver, and it is used as a substitute for bleeding and Calomel. Its admirers allege that it will certainly *arrest* the progress of the above affections in a few hours, and break up all simple fevers. This is of course erroneous, but it reminds one of the Helleborism of the ancients, so graphically described by Hahnemann. In fact no drug with which I am acquainted so much resembles the Veratrum album. It will be seen that its near analogues are also Jatropha, Elaterium, Croton-tig. Arsenicum, Tartar-emetic, Verat. viride; and will undoubtedly prove as useful in practice.

Dr. Brown, who has repeatedly tested the pure effects of the root upon his own person, thus describes the action. After taking the dose (twenty-five grains of the powdered root) and while in good health no effects were noticed for about one hour and a half, when suddenly, with no premonitory symptoms of pain, a distressing sense of *deathly* nausea set in, accompanied in a few minutes by faintness; then sudden and powerful vomiting of, *first* the food, etc., in the stomach, then of large quantities of water mixed with mucus, then clear fluid like rice-water. In less than a minute after the vomiting commenced, great commotion in the bowels, followed immediately by copious watery evacuations, set in. This simultaneous vomiting and diarrhœa continued for nearly an hour, at short intervals, or intermissions, all the while accompanied by great anxiety, a death-like sense of faintness and exhaustion; cool-skin—covered with beaded sweat; cold hands, feet, and nose, and great weakness. In about two or three hours all these symptoms passed away, leaving only weakness as from hunger, no pain or distress, only a peculiar languor. During the height of its action the pulse sank to forty. After taking fifty grains the effects were much more intense, but lasted only a little longer. It resembled more nearly a severe attack of sea-sickness, or cholera morbus, than anything the doctor could imagine. Taken in doses of two or three grains every two or three hours, it causes languor, perspiration, and softness of the pulse.

King (Dispensatory), says, "fifteen or twenty grains of the powdered root will excite emesis, rarely occasioning pains or spasms, and giving rise to very little previous nausea or giddiness. Four grains given every three hours, will act as a diaphoretic. When given in large doses it is apt to induce inflammation of the mucous coat of the stomach and bowels, with hyper-catharsis. It causes distressing nausea with prostration."

Wood, (Therapeutics, Vol. II, p. 442). It is not like Ipecacuanha, safe in over doses, but when taken too largely acts with great harshness, causing much nausea, violet vomiting, hypercatharsis, and symptoms of general prostration. Other medical writers speak of it in much the same manner; but the most extended notice of its virtues which has yet appeared, is from the pen of Dr. Grover Coe, in a work on "Concentrated Organic Medicines." Were Dr. Coe a homœopathist, he would appear in a much better light in his essay on remedial agents, as it is, he makes himself obscure and sometimes ridiculous, by seeking to account for the *modus operandi* of certain medicines, upon vague and theoretic grounds, and by ignoring the law of *Similia.*

Of *Euphorbin*, the concentrated principle of the E.-corrollata, he says: "The Euphorbia is a reliable acquisition to our indigenous materia medica, and fulfills many important indications. In small, repeated doses it acts as a diaphoretic, inducing free perspiration, deterges the mucous coats of the stomach and bowels, stimulates the functions of the liver, and corrects the tendency to *colliquative diarrhœal discharges.*" (!!) "When administered as an emetic, it will generally vomit without exciting any previous nausea, while at other times considerable prostration of the muscular system with lingering nausea will be observed; paleness of the countenance, and cool, moist state of the skin, from which, however, the patient rapidly recovers, as soon as the medicine has operated on the bowels." "We deem the Euphorbia one of the most powerful and at the same time, safest revulsive remedies that can be administered for the relief of cerebral congestions. It excites powerfully the absorbent and venous systems, and is therefore frequently employed for the removal of dropsical effusions, removing them when other means fail." [This is all vague theory. It acts similarly to the Elaterium.]

After stating pretty fully its irritating action on the mucous coat of the stomach and bowels, this author, strangely enough, goes on to say: "We have found the Euphorbin of much ability in the treatment of cholera infantum, diarrhœa, and dysentery. (!) It seems to exercise a peculiar control over the glandular structure of the intestinal canal, correcting and giving tone to the action of the secreting vessels, and promoting the assimilation of nutritious matters." All of which is mere nonsense. It acts by virtue of its power to cause similar pathological conditions in healthy persons. Is it not strange that allopathic writers should labor so hard to cover up the real action of drugs, when the actual law of their remedial action is so apparent to every sensible mind? With a full knowledge of its power to cause "hypercatharsis with inflammation of the bowels, cramps, and vomiting," he says: "We (I) have administered it in cases of cholera infantum, when the alvine discharges were watery, copious, and offensive, and had, as the result of its operation, well-digested stools without fœtor." Then, to gloss this, to him incomprehensible power, he resorts to unworthy special pleading, thus: "We have been unable to discover that the Euphorbin acts as a special irritant upon the bowels, but, on the contrary, esteem it as a corrector of irritation." (In small doses.) "Our observations of its operation have led us to the conclusion that the irritation sometimes observable is the result of an increased activity on the part of the eliminating vessels of the alimentary canal, and the consequent depurition of certain morbid and acrid materials from the blood, which being brought in contact with the mucous surfaces, constitute an extraneous cause of excitement." This language reminds one of the obscure and foggy reasoning that our medical grandfathers indulged in a few centuries ago—a jargon of unmeaning phrases.

The Euphorbium-cor. causes, like the Verat.-alb. and its analogues, a decided and profound depression of the vitality of the nerves of the stomach and bowels, and an utterly relaxed condition of the intestinal capillaries. It induces a pathological and pathogenetic state, which presents a picture resembling with wonderful fidelity cholera morbus, cholera infantum, colliquative diarrhœa, sea-sickness, and many other forms of lesion affecting the digestive tube. It may act in large doses as a direct local irritant, in the same manner as Tartar-emetic; for the juice of the root will produce vesication and pustules upon the skin, and perhaps upon the mucous membrane. But it certainly possesses a dynamic power, which exercises a profound influence through the medium of the nerves.

Pathogenesis.—A resume of the *symptoms* after Hahnemann's method would be as follows:

Head, &c.—Vertigo; Swimming in the head, with faintness, dimness of sight, and prostration; everything seems to be whirling around; vertigo, with ringing in the ears; he fears he is going to die; death-like sensation, with anxiety of miud; no desire to live unless relief comes soon.

Digestive Tract, &c.—Burning in the mouth and on the tongue after taking the dry powder; vesicles on the lips and tongue after taking the fresh root; sudden nausea one hour after taking the powder, followed in a few minutes by sudden and forcible vomiting and diarrhœa of watery (rice-water) fluid, with sinking, anxious feeling at the stomach, faintness, slow and week pulse (40), cool skin, cool hands and feet, which become affected with painful cramps; profuse colliquative discharges from the bowels, like the evacuations in cholera, with painful spasms of the intestines; cold sweat on the body and extremities; spasms of the legs and feet.

Pathology.—I had intended to make some experiments on animals, with the view of showing its pathological effects upon the mucous membranes of the stomach and bowels, but have been unable to devote the necessary time. I hope to present the profession with the results of such experience soon. This article is published to call the attention of my colleagues to this important remedy, and ask their assistance in perfecting its pathogenesis. If we may be allowed to judge from analogy, we can safely affirm that its physiologico-pathological effects are similar to those caused by the Elaterium, Verat. alb. and viride, Jatropha curcas., and perhaps Aconite.

Clinical Remarks.—This remedy is perfectly homœopathic, judging from its pathogenetic symptoms and its known effect in disease, to many morbid conditions of the digestive tube; many serious and severe diseases of the stomach and bowels, as well as some affections of the liver, kidneys, and skin. In some forms of *aphthæ*, accompanied by vomiting or diarrhœa, and that condition of the alimentary mucous membrane characterized by any aphthous exudation extending from the mouth to the anus. This condition is often seen in children and nursing women, and vulgarly known as "*thrush.*" In this affection I should advise the lower dilutions of the tincture of the plant. After this, Hydrastus, Rhus-vernix, Borax, and Arsenicum or Tartar-emetic may be tried. In weakly subjects Phosphoric and Sulphuric acids will prove useful. Chlorate of Potash is an admirable remedy in some cases. *Sea-sickness* and the severe *vomiting of pregnancy* will be benefitted by the medium dilutions of the tincture of the dried root. It is useful in the vomiting which arises from fright, over indulgence in ices, fruits, etc., or from the effects of acrid matters in the stomach, such as large doses of Ipecac., Antimony, Lobelia, etc. In *cholera morbus* and *cholera infantum* we have abundant proof of its utility. I have known it to cure these affections after the usual remedies had entirely failed. In such conditions, if the evacuations be *acid* in their nature, the acidity should be corrected by small quantities of Carb. soda or Magnesia, otherwise the prompt curative effects of the Euphorbium will not appear. This is a point too often ignored by homœopathic physicians. Hahnemann taught that these chemically altered conditions of the fluids were the result of actual acid fermentation of the contents of the stomach and intestines, and must be met by remedies which act in a chemical manner. Many remedies, apparently well chosen, will not act beneficially in such conditions, but act promptly upon its removal, the acid in such cases antidoting, perhaps destroying, its medicinal principle. In *acute enteritis*, *gastritis*, and other inflammatory diseases of the gastric and intestinal mucous membrance, I should consider it admirably indicated, if the other symptoms correspond. In toxical doses it undoubtedly causes active inflammation of their structures, and then, instead of watery evacuations, we may have mucous and bloody discharges, accompanied by pain and tenesmus. In these diseases the higher dilutions would be preferable. The *colliquative diarrhœa* of consumptive and typhoid patients may be benefited by this remedy, as also those obstinate chronic diarrhœas which are prevalent among soldiers in camps, and are probably caused by bad food and worse water. It will undoubtedly prove useful in many of the diseases of children, such as sympathetic or irritative fever, worm fever; in fact, all febrile action when caused by irritation of the bowels. Dr. Coe says: "We value it exceedingly in the treatment of the indigestion of children, and for the removal of all that train of symptoms which is usually supposed to indicate the presence of worms. These are: loss of appetite, or it may be variable, voracious at times, and none at others; furred tongue; feverishness; fœtid breath; bloating of the stomach; constipation, or, on the contrary, a troublesome diarrhœa; emaciation; peevishness; wakefulness, etc." In such cases I had the best effects from the first decimal trituration of the root-bark, or the third trituration of the Euphorbin. But Santonine is the most reliable specific. Finally, it may prove useful in some of the exanthemas, such as eczema, pustular ring-worm, erysipelas, and milk-crust of children when associated with diarrhœa. I do not know whether its internal administration will cause its peculiar effects on the skin; my experiments were not carried far enough to test the matter. We may safely suppose however, that it may thus act, similarly to Croton, Rhus, and Tartar-emetic. In all affections of the skin, its external use as a lotion, Cerate, or Glycerole should accompany its external administration. I earnestly solicit a trial of its remedial virtues in the above mentioned diseases; and careful provings on healthy persons, and the lower animals.

GELSEMINUM SEMPERVIRENS.

(*Yellow Jessamine.*)

The Root is the officinal part, and yields its virtues to water and alcohol.

Description.—This plant is likewise known by the name of *Field Jessamine*, and *Woodbine;* it is the *Bignonia Sempervirens* of Linnæus, and the *Gelseminum nitidum* of Michaux and Pursh. It is named the Gelsemi*um* nitidum by some authors. It has a twisting, smooth, glabrous *stem*, with opposite, perennial lanceolate, entire *leaves*, which are dark above, pale beneath, and which stand on short petioles; the *flowers* are yellow, having an agreeable but rather narcotic odor, and stand on axillary peduncles; the *calyx* is very small, with five sepals; the *corolla* is funnel-form with a spreading border, and five lobes nearly equal; *stamens* five; *pistils* two; *capsule* two-celled, compressed, flat, two-partible; *seeds* flat, and attached to the margins of the valves. The berries are black.

This is one of the most beautiful climbing plants of our Southern States, ascending lofty trees, and forming festoons from one tree to another, and in its flowering season, in the early spring, scenting the atmosphere with its delicious odor. On account of its gorgeous yellow flowers, and the rich perfume which they impart, as well as the deep shade it affords, it is extensively cultivated in the gardens of the South as an ornamental vine. It grows in the North as an exotic. It begins to blossom about the first of March, and its blossoming season lasts until the end of May. The root is several feet in length, with scattered fibres, and varies from two to three lines in diameter, to nearly two inches. The internal part of the root is woody, and of a light yellowish color, the external part or bark, in which the medicinal virtues are said principally to reside, is of a light snuff color, and from half a line to three lines in thickness.

A vine, the root of which is sometimes gathered for the Gelsemminum, resembles it very much in appearance, though it is of a lighter color, and the outer bark is covered with white specks or marks somewhat similar to those on young cherry or peach limbs, and the lower part of old vines become rough and have small tendrils that fasten upon the bark of trees, and which are never seen on the Gelseminum. The bark of the vine is also more brittle, and the leaves are always on long footstalks, which are opposite, at the end of which are two opposite leaves, almost exactly resembling the Aristolochia Serpentaria. The root is almost white, very tough, straight, and about the same length of the medicinal root, and has a slightly bitter, disagreeable nauseous taste. I never saw any of the flowers, though they are said to resemble the others in shape, but are *snowy white*, with a slight, unpleasant odor. The vine is called the *White Poison Vine* and *White Jessamine.*

I am thus particular in giving a correct description of this plant, in order that there shall be no mistake about the matter.

Homœopathic pharmaceutists, above all others, should be scrupulously careful to prepare the medicines we use in their utmost purity. The Gelseminum, more than any other vegetable remedy, demands the most careful preparation. It is not known to me whether the leaves possess any medicinal qualities. But I should suppose from analogy that they possess as much comparitive power as the leaves, etc., of Aconite, or Veratrum viride. The tincture made from the flowers is comparatively inert.

Toxicological Effects.—We do not find any well authenticated report of any case of fatal poisoning from the use of Gelseminum, and do not know therefore what pathological changes it produces in the human body.

Case 1.—This is said by King to be the first known case of poisoning by Gelseminum; and that by it, the plant was first brought into notice. "A planter on the Mississippi, while laboring under a severe attack of bilious fever, which resisted all the usual remedies, sent a servant into his garden to procure a certain medicinal root and prepare an infusion of it for him to drink. The servant by mistake collected another root, (the Yellow Jessamine,) and gave an infusion of it to his master who, shortly after swallowing some of it, was seized with the following—

Symptoms.—Complete loss of muscular power; was unable to move a limb, or even to raise his eyelids, although he could hear, and was cognizant of circumstances transpiring around him. His friends, greatly alarmed, collected around him, watching the result with much anxiety, and expecting every minute to see him breathe his last. After some hours he gradually recovered, and was astonished to find that his fever had left him."—(*King's Disp.*)

In this case no treatment was reported to have been given, yet the man recovered perfectly, besides being rid of an obstinate fever. No one can compare the above symptoms with those of Catalepsy, without remarking the striking resemblance. It ought to prove a specific for that malady.

Case 2.—Several deck hands of a steamer on the Mississippi river, tapped a barrel of tincture Gelseminum which they supposed to be whisky. All who drank of it were more or less affected. The symptoms were about the same as in case 1. It was reported that two out of these three died, but Dr. H. H. Hill, who was present, says they were saved by the employment of Quinine and Capsicum in large doses, aided by external stimulation.

He makes the following report of these cases: "In the summer of 1853, late in June or early in July, I had five barrels of tincture of Gelseminum shipped from Vicksburg, Mississippi. The boat grounded on a sand bar on the Ohio river near night. I happened to see the barrels on deck, they having been taken out of the hold in shifting freight. I requested the mate to have the barrels lowered again as they contained medicine, and it was not safe in case the hands should get at them. The next morning another boat made its appearance, and the captain told us we had better get aboard of that boat as it was of light draught. As we were getting aboard, I heard two physicians say to the captain that some of his men had been drinking alcohol or some poison, and two or three of them were about dead. They told the captain to give them an emetic. Being well convinced what they had been drinking, I told him not to do so, as they were already too much relaxed, and that they needed stimulants. During the night they had opened a barrel and drawn a bucket full, as I learned from the men, and had drank it from tin cups, it was supposed from half a pint to a pint each. They looked very much like dead men, their eyes were closed; circulation very feeble; no pulse perceptible; and breathing so low that it could hardly be perceived at all. Two of the men were taken on board the other boat and the other three were left. I went up the river with the two men and gave them stimulants, and in less than two hours they were able to walk. They recovered. When I got to Louisville, I learned that there was a statement in the Louisville Journal that it was supposed that the three men who were left behind were dead, they having been left in an apparently dying condition. Some three days afterwards the boat got up, and another statement appeared in the paper that stimulants had been given to them and they had recovered."

Case 3.—A lady aged 24, suffering from Typhoid Pneumonia, took ten drops of Tincture Gelseminum; in an hour eleven more; and in two hours after twelve drops. Shortly afterwards appeared the following—

Symptoms.—She could not see any one in the room, although persons stood close by the bed. Her eyes were wide open, pupils dilated, pulse regular and full, skin natural and healthy in color, feet and hands cold. She seemed to know all that was going on; described her symptoms; said she felt faint; felt as though her blood had ceased circulating and that her head felt very light.

Treatment.—She was given a teaspoonful of Aromatic spirits of Ammonia in water, and repeated in fifteen minutes. At the expiration of half an hour she said *she felt perfectly well*, complained of no pain whatever; the fever was subdued, and in four days she was quite able to rise from her bed.—(*Dr. Lungren, of Franklin, N. C.*)

Case 4.—Dr. B———, a practicing physician in one of the upper counties in Georgia, while suffering from a severe nervous toothache, took what he guessed was about thirty drops of the tincture.

Symptoms.—In ten minutes he said, "I cannot see you." His eyes were wide open, pupil dilated; pulse eighty to ninety. He attempted to walk, and staggered like one intoxicated. (He was immediately given a dose of Ipecac, as an emetic). He wrote with a pencil on paper, for he could not speak, "I am very sick; wish to vomit but cannot." In a few moments he vomited, but the discharge passed through the nostrils. His hands and feet became icy cold, pulse regular, eighty to ninety.

Treatment.—Warm bricks were applied to his feet, his hands and ankles were chafed; strong Aqua ammonia was placed to his nose and upon his chest. In an hour he was able to speak. The next he complained of being very faint; took aromatic spirits of Ammonia, and the next day rode home a distance of twenty-three miles. It is needless to say the toothache left him—[Ib.]

Case 5.—A convict in the N. H. State Prison swallowed *one-and-a-half* ounces of the fluid extract, with intent to poison himself. The effects were, great prostration, nausea and vomiting, dilated pupils, inability to speak or move, coldness of the surface, feeble pulse, etc. The effects passed off, with proper antidotes, in about twenty-four hours.—(*Dr. Pattee, in Tilden's Journal.*)

In this case we observe nausea and vomiting, which is a rare effect of the drug.

Case 6.—"In one case a lad of twenty-seven years of age swallowed six fluid drachms of the tincture without any permanent injury."—(*Dr. King.*)

ANTIDOTES.—Unless the person is seen immediately after the drug is taken emetics, it is said, are not safe or advisable, on account of the additional prostration they may cause. In fact none but the most stimulating emetic substances would have any effect upon a stomach paralyzed by a large dose of Gelseminum. Probably the best emetic remedy is mustard, a teaspoonful of the ground seed in half a cup of warm water. Ammonia is a valuable antidote to the prostrating effects of the drug, as also are Quinine, Capsicum, and Brandy. Dr. King states that a piece of common coarse salt, about the size of a pea, chewed and swallowed, will produce a restoration in five or ten minutes in many instances. A spoonful of salt and water may be given, if the patient be too weak or insensible to chew it. Electro-Magnetism is a powerful antidote to its paralyzing influence. In bad cases it should be perseveringly used. A strong preparation of Xanthoxylum would prove a reliable stimulating antidote. The Homœopathic antidotes against the primary symptoms of prostration, etc., are Aconite, Verat. viride, Verat. alb., Arsenicum album, Secale, Chloroform, Carbo veg. and China. Against its specific effects on the head and eyes, Opium, Bellad., Stram., Hyos., Agar., and Spig. are indicated in small quantities. The proper antidotes to its secondary symptoms, convulsive, spinal, etc., are Nux vom., Ign., Æsculus g., Cuprum, Agar. and Æthusa. The warm bath, mustard to the extremities, and cool applications to the head and spine would be valuable palliative means.

GENERAL EFFECTS, ON THE NERVOUS SYSTEM—*Nerves of Sensation.*—Gelseminum does not exert the decided and specific effect upon the nerves of sensation that we witness from the effects of Aconite. It causes none of the numbness, tingling, prickling and crawling sensations which mark the action of that poison.

The *pains* which may be caused by Gelseminum are not, in my opinion, caused by a primary affection of the nerves of sensation, but depend upon a certain morbid condition of the nerves of motion. Such pains are caused by cramp-like contractions of muscles and tendons, constricting certain nerves or blood-vessels, or they may arise as in case of Aconite from irritation of the ganglionic nerves, about the blood-vessels—many are probably congestive in their nature, like the pains in the head and eyes. In pure Neuralgia, this remedy can be of but little service; although it may be very useful in removing many consensual symptoms, such as excessive nervous irritation, drawing and twitching of the muscles of the affected parts, etc. Dr. Douglas, however, declares that "A majority of all cases of Neuralgia will be promptly relieved by Gelseminum but it sometimes requires to be given in pretty large doses, repeated every half hour till the pain is relieved." He says: "My experience does not perfectly coincide with your remark upon the action of the Gelseminum upon the nerves of sensation. It does not, certainly, 'cause the numbness, tingling, prickling and crawling sensations' of Aconite, but in my individual experience, it causes the pains. In my own provings, I have frequently experienced a succession of acute, sudden, darting pains evidently running along single nerve branches in almost every part of the body and limbs, sometimes so sudden and acute as to make me start. At one time a quick succession of these acute sudden pains coursed down the outside and front of the tibia for over half an hour, leaving a line of considerable tenderness marking its track. These pains which seemed clearly neuralgic, gave me the palpable indication for its employment in this disease. And it has certainly been successful. But while it has promptly cured some distressing cases of neuralgia, in which Aconite had been fully tried without benefit, there have occurred some other cases in which it has failed and Aconite has succeeded. What is the explanation of this? If we suppose that in some cases of this disease there exists a real inflammatory state of the nerve, and in others a mere excess of sensitiveness, the explanation is easy: Aconite cures the first, and Gelseminum the last." Dr. P. P. Wells, says, "we feel warranted in predicting that the class of fevers to which Gelseminum will be found related, is that based on blood dyscrasia, with a tendency to decomposition of its hæmatine and globules, or to fevers of a miasmatic origin, which Aconite seldom or never is."

Nerves of motion.—Gelseminum, like Nux vomica, Angustura, Æsculus, Ignatia and Strychnia, does primarily affect the nerves of motion, but in an opposite manner. It depresses and paralyses these nerves which they excite and irritate. But while the action of Gelseminum differs from that of Strychnia in this respect; in another it affords a remarkable resemblance. Both cause hyperæmia of the spinal marrow, which may increase to actual engorgement or extravasation. This condition is not brought about as soon by Gelseminum as by Nux vomica, but the condition when obtained has very nearly the same results. But while the active congestion of the spinal marrow caused by Nux vomica, is accompanied by an exalted and tense state of the motor nerves, even to tetanic spasm; the passive congestion of Gelseminum is accompanied by a paralytic or debilitated state of those nerves, or a condition exactly opposite to tetanus. Gelseminum may cause death by prostrating and exhausting primarily the energies and vital power of the nerves of voluntary and involuntary motion.

While Strychnia, Nux vomica, etc., would produce death from the same cause, but the fatal prostration would be secondary; the exhaustion being preceded and caused by the primary irritation and spasmodic action of those nerves. Gelseminum may also cause death by congestion and apoplexy of the brain and spinal marrow. Nux, Ignatia and Strychnia may also cause death by producing such a congested condition of the spinal cord and its membranes as to lead to fatal hemorrhage into those important tissues.

CLINICAL REMARKS.—The primary homœopathicity of Gelseminum to paralysis from loss of motion will be discussed in other places. Its use in very many forms of *Convulsions* may here be alluded to. The other schools of medicine, viewing this drug as a powerful anti-spasmodic, would see it indicated in nearly all forms of convulsions. It has been used in both clonic and tonic spasms; in Epilepsy, Chorea, Hysteria, etc. I gave it in one case of severe Hysterical Epilepsy, a young girl after suppressed menses had attacks every evening, lasting an hour or two, during which time so severe was the spasm of the glottis that asphyxia seemed really impending. The attacks had been every day for two weeks. Five drops of the tincture were given at three and again at six, P. M. At seven, the usual hour, no spasms appeared, and did not return until the next menstrual period, when the remedy had no effect; and Asafœtida, in one grain doses, every four hours was resorted to, which brought on the menses and cured the spasms. I have treated many cases of Hysteria from various causes with Gelseminum, and I know of none more generally useful.

Eclectic writers claim to have cured cases of *Chorea* with Gelseminum. In the three cases treated by me, one recovered, one was benefitted, and one, a case of years continuance, seemed to be aggravated.

In *Tetanus*, it would seem to be one of the most powerful antipathic remedies, yet I cannot find a single recorded case treated with this remedy. After testing the medicines homœopathic to the disease, like Nux Vomica, Ignatia, Aconite, etc., I should resort to the Gelseminum with a good deal of confidence. We know that it produces its peculiar prostrating effects, even to an extreme degree, without causing any local lesion. Now it often happens that no material traces of disease can be discovered either in the brain and spinal marrow of persons who have died of Tetanus. Dr. Gerhard declares that of the twelve cases he examined no lesion whatever could be detected. Some of the secondary symptoms of Gelseminum strongly resemble this disease. Some months after writing the above, we have the following report from Dr. O. G. Strong "I tried the Gel. two weeks since, in a severe case of *Tetanus*. I gave ten drops of the mother tincture, fifteen minutes apart. After the third dose, the spasmodic action entirely ceased, and the patient recovered. It produced the most satisfactory specific action of any remedy I ever tried in such a case."

In *Hydrophobia*, also, no appearances have been found which could account for the fatality of the disease. In this terrible malady,

Gelseminum ought to be found useful if not curative. In material doses, it relaxes all the muscles, calms the fury of nervous excitement, relaxes the glottis and prevents spasms. Why should it not be valuable in Hydrophobia? The spasms in this disease are brief and clonic, similar to the secondary ones of Gelseminum. The circulation is much disturbed (excited). A dog killed with it could not drink while under its influence. Were I to become hydrophobic, I should take Gelseminum and "await the end."

Since writing the above, several of my colleagues have reported to me cures of *spasmodic croup* in children, made with Gelseminum, used according to my suggestion. I have no doubt but it will prove an invaluable remedy in that malady, named by Wood—"*Infantile Spasm of the Glottis*." It is known in medical works under the name of Laryngismus stridulous, Asthma of Millar, etc. The essential nature of the disease is a general morbid excitability of the nervous system, directed especially to the muscles of the glottis, which contract spasmodically. It has been said to arise from irritation or inflammation of the cervical portion of the spinal marrow, (that portion most irritated by Gelseminum) the presence of worms in the intestines, etc. From whatever cause it may arise, the Gelseminum, if not a curative remedy, properly, will be a valuable palliative, used in drop doses of the first dilution or mother tincture, frequently repeated; it must procure relief in the majority of cases, while during the intermediate time, it should be alternated with Bell., Hyos., Ars., or Moschus.

Muscular System.—The most prominent of all the effects of Gelseminum is to induce a profound and intense prostration of the whole muscular system. Its effects are first manifested on the voluntary muscles, afterwards on the involuntary, No remedy so suddenly and surely destroys the tone of muscular structure; but it acts not by causing any disintegration or disorganization, but by impairing the vitality of those nerves which supply it with life. This property of Gelseminum can be made subservient to the physician in many ways.

In cases of obstinate tonic convulsions and cramp-like rigidity, full doses, sufficient to bring the muscular system under its pathogenetic action, will promptly remove such morbid conditions. There is no danger in this method of administering the remedy, for one of the peculiarities of its action is, that there is no permanent injury done to the tonicity of muscular structure, unless its use is long persisted in, and wantonly abused. In this respect it acts wonderfully like chloroform.

Like chloroform, it will be found very useful to the Surgeon, when in cases of dislocation or fracture, reduction is rendered difficult or impossible by a rigidity of the muscles of the part. In such cases the system may be brought under its influence very readily. It does not, however, give that insensibility to pain which is the prominent effect of chloroform.

It is freely used by some obstetricians in cases of rigidity of the *os-uteri*, or external parts. King advises it in all such cases as being much superior to Lobelia, as well as pleasanter, as it does not nauseate nor cause that sense of deathly prostration so peculiar to that drug. I have used it successfully in such cases, as well as for those severe spasmodic pains which sometimes come on in labor. In such instances it must be given in appreciable doses, of five, ten or fifteen drops, repeated if required; a slight dimness of sight is a good indication that the remedy is acting.

Dr. Moore, of Illinois, reports to me, relative to the curative action of Gelsemenum in muscular pain (Myalgia), from great over exertion. He stated that after a day's fatiguing walking, such as usually laid him up with lameness and stiffness for several days, he took thirty drops of a common tincture of Gelseminum. In half an hour the peculiar weakness and pains in the limbs and muscles were ameliorated, and he shortly fell asleep. In the morning, much to his surprise, he awoke feeling as comfortable as though he had not walked so unusually the day before. He had no lameness or soreness, as usual. This case illustrates the specific affinity of Gelseminum for the *motor* nerves and the voluntary muscles under their control. It should prove one of the best remedies for acute *Myalgia* which we possess.

Vascular System—*Heart and Arteries.*—Pulse frequent, soft, weak,—so feeble as to be sometimes imperceptible; fluttering pulse; pulse full 120; pulse slow and full, or slow and soft; sensation as though the blood had ceased to circulate; pulse reduced from 112 to 55 in twelve hours; heart's action slow and feeble; the beats of the heart cannot be felt; the action of the heart and arteries much depressed, with cold hands and feet, chills and pain in the head. —(*Douglas*).

Dr. P. P. Wells (Amer. Hom. Review, Vol. 4 p. 84,) states that from the twelfth dilution he had the following spmptoms: "A peculiar irregular action of the heart which had never been experienced before; this was a sensible motion of the heart as though it had attempted its beat, which it failed fully to accomplish, and the pulse then each time intermitted; this occurred at irregulr intervals, and more frequently when in repose than when in motion, the worst and most frequent attacks being in the evening and worst of all on lying down in bed when retiring for the night, and these attacks aggravated by lying on the left side." These symptoms lasted eight or ten days. Dr. Finke stated to me that he experienced similar symptoms from a higher dilution. In Philadelphia, Dr. Lippe, Henry and others are using the Gelseminum in the thirtieth, two hundredth and one thousandth potencies, with apparent good results; I notice this fact however, that they find these high attenuations curative for the *primary* smptoms of the medicine.

Clinical Remarks.—In diseases of the heart, particularly in those in which the chief indication is to diminish the action of that organ, Gelseminum will be found a valuable remedy. In some forms of functional derangement it will often effect a cure. In material doses it will alleviate those cases of excessive action of the heart from plethora, congestion, neuralgic or rheumatic irritation, or hysteric palpitation.

Like Aconite and Veratrum viride, Gelseminum is not homœopathic or curative in any organic affections of the heart; but like the above named remedies and Digitalis, it is a very valuable auxiliary in the treatment of those maladies.

It is an excellent palliative in those troublesome symptoms which affect the head and eyes during the progress of heart disease. The sensation of fulness, heaviness, giddiness, throbbing, jerking, etc., the dimness of sight, and other amaurotic symptoms, are admirably met by small doses of Gelseminum or its resinoid.

Fever.—Within a few minutes, sometimes within two or three, a marked depression of pulse, which becomes ten, fifteen or twenty beats less in the minute, if quiet, but greatly disturbed by movement; chilliness, especially along the back; pressive pain in the head, most generally of the temples, sometimes in the occiput, at others over the head. The chilliness is soon followed by a glow of heat and prickling of the skin, and quickly succeeded by perspiration, which is sometimes profuse and disposed to be persistent, continuing from twelve to twenty-four hours. As soon as the reaction takes place after the chill the pulse rises as much above the normal standard as it was before depressed below it. With these symptoms is a puffy, swollen look, and feeling of fulness of the eyelids, slimy and disagreeable or bitter taste in the mouth, languid feeling in the back and limbs and sleepiness.—(*Douglas.*) Febrile chilliness, cold extremities, especially the feet, heat of head, and face with headache; pulse uniformly depressed and rendered less frequent with chilliness, cold feet, heat and pain of the head.—(*Hull's Jahr.*) Have felt chilly all day, particularly in the morning. This statement regarding the pulse is erroneous. I have found that in both men and animals, it often increased the rate and frequency of the pulse. Sometimes even the volume of the pulse seemed increased, but generally it is diminished. An explanation of this phenomenon will be found in the paragraph "*Head.*" Derangement of circulation as shown in the fluctuations of the pulse from seventy to 120; chilliness with vertigo; headache and coated tongue; cold extremities; inclination to "hug the fire," with chills following each other in rapid succession from sacrum to base of occiput.—(*Dr. F. L. Vincent.*)

Dr. M. E. Lazarus, a well known painstaking prover, could not get any such prominent symptoms as recorded by Dr. Douglas. He however experienced a languor, with inclination to stretch, some slight chilliness, with feeble flashes of heat. He suggests that perhaps Dr. Douglas is very susceptible to the action of Gelseminum. My impression would be the same, as I have given it to healthy persons, in all manner of doses, yet never heard any one mention such decisive symptoms as those of Dr. Douglas. Still it is undoubtedly primarily homœopathic to the pathological conditions upon which all real chills depend; and secondarily homœopathic to febrile conditions or the reaction which follows those conditions. In this respect it is somewnat similar to Aconite, and others of the same group. But it is only a general, not a particular resemblance.

Dr. J. S. Douglas says:—"You and Dr. Lazarus remark that you have not been able to elicit such marked symptoms in your provings as were experienced by me. The symptoms particularly referred to are the chills, the reactive febrile heat with headache, and sweat. Dr. L. suggests that I am probably very susceptible to the action of this drug. This remark suggest an important fact which has gradually unfolded itself in my successive fragmentary provings on some seventy persons, and on myself. The fact, of which I have at length become clearly convinced, is this: The degree of chill, of febrile reaction, of headache, and of neuralgic pains, bear a very uniform ratio to the nervous sensitiveness of the patient. My temperament is decidedly nervous and sensitive. In all the subjects of a nervous, sensitive temperament, the above symptoms are strongly marked. In those of an opposite, insensitive temperament, while the pulse is depressed, and the extremeties cool or cold, there is no chill, or it is very slight, little or no headache, and slight febrile reaction, and consequently little sweat. In several highly sensitive subjects the chill has been equal to a respectable fit of ague, the reaction and pain of head corresponding, and the sweat profuse. These symptoms have been most strongly developed in some female provers of highly sensitive temperaments, by half-drop doses. Some persons seem almost insensible to its effects. One man who had taken several drugs for proving, without any marked results, took three teaspoonsful in one day of the strong tincture, which I know to be good, and reported the next day no symptoms."

(There is one form of rigors, or "nervous chills," as they are sometimes called, in which, with shivering and chattering of the teeth, there is no sensation of chilliness. It is an irritated condition of the nerves of motion, and is seen in hysterical subjects, or appears during a fright or other mental emotion in healthy persons. It is often seen during parturition, and is said to attend relaxation of sphincter muscles. Now, Gelseminum causes just such rigors by establishing similar conditions as the above, and a small dose of the tincture will control readily such morbid manifestations.)

In *Simple Fever*, without functional disturbance, Dr. Douglas declares it to be specific; given at the onset of any fever of simple, uncomplicated character, it will undoubtedly arrest it very promptly. It seems peculiarly adapted to the fevers of children and sensitive women, while Aconite and Veratrum viride are more applicable to adults of robust and rigid constitutions.

In the so-called *Irritative Fever*, it will be found a valuable remedy. It is more capable of meeting the majority of the symptoms of that malady than any remedy which I have used. It corresponds with the excessive nervous irritation; the tendency to irregular convulsive action; the periods of wakeful debility; and the accessions of feverish stupor. In cases however complicated with hepatic or gastric difficulties, it will have to be aided by Mer., Pod., Ipecac. Tart. emet. Should the lungs be implicated it might answer alone, but Phosph., Bry. or Antimonium crudem will be of service. If the bowels are effected, Pulsatilla, Mercurius or Chamomilla may have to be given although some of the provings seem to indicate that Gelseminum affects the intestinal functions. Wood, with doubtful propriety, classes infantile remittent, as well as worm fever, with irritative fevers. There may be some general affinity, as Gelseminum has proved useful in each. Since I have treated infantile remittents with this remedy, I have conducted them safely through their course with better satisfaction than before.

Dr. Neidhard reports the following case;—A child, aged ten, was cured by Gelseminum first dil. two drops every four hours, of a kind of bilious fever, characterized by the following symptoms: Giddiness, dull, aching pain in the forehead and over the eyes. She cannot concentrate her mind on any one thing; cannot read; is very irritable; very thirsty; and has slight chills, followed by much fever; extreme weakness. Was completely cured within eight days.

Dr. R. Ludlam, in his article on the "Therapeutics of Infantile Remittent Fever," in the N. A. Jour. of Hom., says:—"Excepting the Aconite, there is certainly no remedy with which the profession is at present familiar which promises so much as the *Gelseminum* in the treatment of this variety of the remittents of infancy and childhood."

"From personal observation (and these hints have their origin in this source only) we should be inclined to recommend Gelseminum in those remittents which are primarily characterized by excessive irritability and erethism, either of the general or special nervous systems. There is perhaps no single means which, under the various circumstances which ascompany and give good evidence of the aforesaid pathological condition, promises so much as this. We have sometimes failed with Aconite, with Chamonilla, and with Belladona, to allay the excessive restlessness and disquiet occasioned by what the old nurses style an 'inward fever' in a little juvenile, and at other times have succeeded at once in its relief by a few doses of Gelseminum."

"This remedy appears also to be well adapted to the relief of those attacks of this fever which border closely upon intermittents, examples of which might readily be mistaken for a masked fever of that peculiar type. In such cases, as well as those which toward their close degenerate into ague, in one or another of its protean forms, we may prescribe a low attenuation of the Gelseminum with the confident hope of success. In our hands, indeed it has proved almost a specific for those remittents, the diagnosis of which, from a more definitely paroxysmal form of fever was not readily made out. We have also cured several well marked intermittents with it, but its sphere of usefulness would appear to lie somewhere along the boundary between these and the purely idiopathic remittents of which we have been speaking."

The real value of Gelseminum in intermittents is not yet to a certainty ascertained. Some homœopathic physicians, among them Holcombe, Ludlam and Douglas, assert that it will cure agues. Holcombe with characteristic boldness, gives us the following odd prescription for a homœopathic one: For intermittents with cerebral symptoms, with hyperæsthesia predominating—Sulphate of Quinine, ten grains, Gelsemin, one grain; divide into five parts. Begin six hours before the expected paroxysm, and give one part every hour. "Indications for use; when the paroxysm has been marked by violent pains, referable to the cerebro-spinal, rather than the ganglionic system, and by correspondingly intense burning fever, great nervous restlessness, sensitiveness to light and sound, mental agitation or anxiety, delirium, sleeplessness, curious sensations of falling, swimming from giddiness, partial blindness or deafness, especially applicable to nervous, excitable subjects, and to mild fresh cases, without prominent gastric or hepatic symptoms, in short, before any visceral complication has been engrafted on the nervous phenomenon."

(This last clause, I (Hale) regard as well indicating the sphere of action of Gelseminum in agues, but in the "indications" proper, Holcombe has mixed up the primary with the secondary symptoms of the drug, which rarely appear together. The dose, however that he advises is very nearly of the proper quantity. Of the quinine, I think he prescribes altogether too much. In very similar cases, I have succeeded admirably with one-fifth or one-tenth grain doses of Quinine, alternated with one-tenth or one-twentieth grain of Gelsemin, or two or three drops of the mother tincture. Holcombe's prescription would undoubtedly arrest the paroxysms promptly, but it would be apt to give rise to visceral complications, which smaller doses would avoid, and at the same time be equally as efficacious). Dr. Ludlam writes me—"Perhaps in the whole range of its clinical virtues there is no more satisfactory and really valuable use which can be made of the Gelseminum than in the treatment of those intermittents which might properly be styled post-typhoid. It is to this especial form of intermittents, which succeeding upon an adynamic condition of system, are characterized by a want of distinctness in their several stages, and which are of a masked type and intractable in nature, that the Gelseminum has in our experience seemed to be particularly applicable. We have remarked the evident tendency in patients suffering with enteric fever, and who had but recently removed tothe city [Chicago] from miasmatic districts, to sequelæ of this order. Scarcely any such patient has ecsaped this characteristic convalescence, and in none of those cases in which we have ordered this remedy have we failed to witness the best results from its employment, while in years past, such cases were especially perplexing and tedious, we are free to express our pleasure in and appreciation of a means so entirely successful. These patients were all from the Southern States."

John C. Morgan, M. D., author of a short proving in Dr. Shipman's *Journal of Materia Medica*, writes as follows: "It seems worthy to be called a specific for fresh cases of Intermittents, and will modify even old cases, changing double to single tertian. My dose is one-fourth drop in a teaspoonful of water, usually. I send a few clinical cases."

(*a*) "W. S., a swarthy soldier of large frame, on going into camp, May 11, had no blanket; slept on straw under leaky shed;—the night being cold, awoke early in the morning with a severe chill,—but little shaking; fever ensued. Took at a dose ten drops common tincture Gelseminum; fever augmented with slight delirium. Took five drops—some aggravation. During the afternoon and evening took fractional drop doses; no fever at night. The next day took one-fourth drop every two hours. He had no other paroxysm."

REMARKS.—This may not have been an attack of Intermittent. Such chills, followed by fever, are often the result of exposure, or of getting wet. Still had it not been for the Gelseminum, it might have resulted in some form of protracted fever. (Hale.)

(*b*) "A soldier of sanguine temperament had Diarrhœa and rheumatic pains, with symptoms of Intermittent; took for several days one-fourth drop tincture Gelseminum, and was cured."

Intermittent Fever—Case 1.—"In one case I had used all the usual anti-periodics, as Cornine Salicine, Quinine, etc., without success. Even after producing the constitutional effects of Quinine the chills would sometimes, return every day for awhile, then every other day. Thus the case continued for several weeks, until I despaired of success with the other anti-periodics, so I determined to try the tincture of Gelseminum. Accordingly, I left an ounce of the tincture of the fresh root, directing it to be given in doses of thirty drops every two or three hours, until the eyes were affected; then the medicine was to be suspended until that passed off, then again resumed as before, and so on until the fever was broken. I saw the patient just as the chill was gone off, and commenced the tincture of Gelseminum immediately. The fever did not rise very high, nor continue long, nor did the chill ever return. The patient recovered from the time he commenced the medicine, and was soon up at his usual avocation. Now, what still more astonished me was, that the medicine never affected his eyes in the least, yet it suspended the chills immediately. I had frequently combined the tincture of Gelseminum with the other anti-periodics before and met with very prompt success, yet I attributed it to the other articles; but this time I determined to try the Gelseminum alone."—[Sensible!—Hale.] (Dr. Goss, *Eclectic Medical Journal.*)

Case 2. Nov. 4.—Intermittent Fever (tertian type). Has been affected six months; has pain in the head, and pains over the body, when he has no chill; tongue not much coated; other symptoms common to the disease. Treatment—Alkaline bath once a day; tincture Gelseminum, one-half dram three times a day. Nov. 17, discharged, cured.—*Newton's Clinical Reports.*

The above are the only two published cases of Intermittents cured by this medicine alone. Very many cases are reported of pretended cures by Gelseminum; but, as it was always given so mixed with Quinine, Hydrastin, or other drugs, no reliance can be placed upon the reports.

Dr. Holcombe writes me that the Gelseminum was the basis of several celebrated patent medicines, noted at the South for the cure of remittent and intermittent fevers; that it certainly was the principal ingredient in "Speed's Tonic," which at one time was popularly considered an unrivalled febrifuge, but, failing to cure those cases attended with organic complications, it fell into disfavor, although it is still used by many people in the South. "From large doses I have seen blindness, partial deafness, singular torpor, stupidity of feeling, inability to open the eyelids, and nervous prostration; such symptoms as would follow a state of nervous excitement, or hyperæsthesia. In small doses I have found it valuable in the opposite condition. I class it with Aconite, Bell. and Cham. I have used it in the summer months, for weeks at a time, as I would Aconite. I believe, in addition to its febrifuge power, it has a specific anti-periodic influence."

Dr. Douglas praises the Gelseminum, in drop doses, very highly in simple, uncomplicated Intermittents, when indicated by the symptoms, and speaks of having met with much success in its use. Dr. Ludlam has cured several well-marked cases of Intermittent fever with the low dilutions. Several of my colleagues report cases of Ague, successfully treated with Gelseminum. I have used it frequently in Intermittents, and have succeded in some severe cases in curing the disease, after it had been arrested with Quinine, but showed an obstinate tendency to return. These cases were reported in full in the August number of the North American Journal of Homœopathy for 1861. It can be used both during the apyrexia, and in the paroxysm. In larger doses during the former state, than during the latter. It will be found to control the painful nervous sensations which arise during the fever, better than Aconite, if indicated. An Eclectic physician, engaged in a large practice in the State of Ohio, informed me that except in severe congestive cases, he relied altogether upon Gelseminum to break up the paroxysms of Fever and Ague. He stated, however, that he always gave a sufficient quantity to cause almost complete blindness during the apyrexia. I can hardly doubt the veracity of my informant, but I suggested to him that he might break the patient, as well as the ague. He had no fears of that result, however.

I am not aware that any Homœopathist has advised, or used Gelseminum in *Typhoid fever*. But its pathogenesis and physiological action has many points of resemblance to that form of Typhoid designated as Nervous fever, i. e., when there is no intestinal lesion or any particular local complication. It is specifically indicated in those cases in which the patient, from some great excitement, or over-exertion, suddenly sinks into a low typhoid state, with great prostration of all the vital forces, and when he experiences strange sensations in the head, with morbid condition of the motor nerves, manifested by local paralysis, or continued jactitation of certain muscles. Women are more subject to this variety than men. With the former we have many hysteric symptoms, such as nervous dysphagia, even hysteric spasms, sleeplesness, aberration of sight, etc.

Gelseminum should here be cautiously given in drop doses, or pellets of the 2nd or 3d.

In true enteric fever, I should not place much reliance on Gelseminum. There are other remedies which pathologically correspond, and are consequently more specific; among these are Bapt., Rhus tox., Phosp. acid, Ars., Terebin. and Mur. acid.

In *Yellow Fever*, Gelseminum has not been used by the Homœopathic school, I believe. Drs. Holcombe, or Davis, make no mention of it in their reports to our Homœopathic Journals. They relied upon Aconitum, Belladonna, Arsenicum, Lachesis, and Argentum nitricum. The Eclectic and Allopathic schools have used it to some extent, but the only published report I can find relating to it, is a pamphlet by Drs. White and Ford, of Charleston, S. C. This report was entitled the "Bradycote (whatever that may mean) treatment of Yellow Fever by Gelseminum sempervirens." They prepared a tincture from the fresh root, as follows:—Radix Gelsemini, four ounces; Alcohol (95 per cent.) and Aqua communis, each eight ounces. To adults they gave of this twenty or thirty drops; to children from five to twenty, every hour for the first four hours; then at longer intervals, and with doses half as large. Total number treated with Gelseminum twenty-five; all of which recovered. Of these, fifteen were males and nine, females; adults twelve; children twelve; whites twenty-two; blacks two. Of the whole number treated, two vomited black vomit, five passed black vomit downward. In three cases hemorrhage occurred from the tongue, gums, or nasal passages. One woman was in the sixth month of her pregnancy, and did not abort. Average duration of treatment; about eight days.

No marked prostration was caused by this remedy; the pulse being, however, much less quickly reduced than by Veratrum Viride. In few cases was the heart's action fully lowered in less than twelve hours, and it was well controlled throughout the rest of the disease, in the majority of cases. The concurrent treatment was the same as with Veratrum. Mercurialization was complete in ten cases; incomplete in fourteen cases. In a few instances a marked redness of the tongue was observed, a condition that was not distinctly noticed during the administration of Veratrum. [This symptom has been often noticed in my provings.—*Hale*]. The Gelseminum appeared to produce a general calming influence, even during the early period of its administration, but was not found to possess any marked narcotic properties. It seemed to promote the action of the kidneys, and during its use only, in several cases, an *erythema* of the skin was noticed. This drug appeared to influence the volume of the pulse, before it affected its frequency, and in most cases for the rest of the disease to control both conditions in an equal manner. Emesis was not observed to ensue upon the administration of this medicine; the gastric irritability peculiar to the disease being moreover, to all appearances, favorably influenced. There were treated by *Veratrum viride* 117 cases, of which fifteen died. Of six treated by the ordinary method [without Veratrum or Gelseminum] three died.

In *Scarlet Fever* the Gelseminum bids fair to rank with Belladonna. Besides being indicated in the peculiar, intense fever, with nervous erethism, its well known action on the skin will render it of value in impelling the eruption to the surface. It causes a peculiar erythema, which has some resemblance to the eruption in Scarlatina as well as some forms of Purpura. Its analagous relation to both Belladonna and Aconite, strongly commends it to our favor, and if we are to judge its curative powers from its pathological effects, it will be be found efficient, alone, where the former remedies are indicated. Dr. H. W. White speaks very highly of its effects in *Scarlatina.* He asserts that it will control the pulse, calm the nervous erethism, determine the eruption toward the surface, relieve pain, and lessen the cerebral congestion, in a manner superior to Bell., or Aconite. Cases which seemed quite formidable at their commencement, soon assumed a milder character, and terminated safely. He considers it effectual, alone, to control the majority of cases. Should the disease assume a malignant character, Dr. White alternates it with Amm. carb., Carbo.veg., Mur. acid, or Ars. Its use should be suspended if symptoms of prostration set in.

In *Measles* the Gelseminum appears to be specifically indicated during the forming and inflammatory stage [the eruptive]. Among its pathogenetic symptoms we find prominent catarrhal conditions, as "chilliness, watery discharge from the nose, hoarseness, with feeling of soreness of throat, and in the chest, cough, etc." Among its effects upon the skin we find "a papulous eruption, very much the color of measles, which it closely resembles, but the papulæ are more distant and distinct. It appears most frequently upon the face." Relying upon these fragmentary, yet prominent indications, I have treated several cases of Rubeola with this remedy, and apparently with good results. It seemed to prevent a continuance of the cough beyond its proper limits, and to act as a prophylactic to chronic catarrhal affections, bronchitis, or pneumonia.

Dr. Douglas considers it quite capable of modifying the disease in a marked manner, when given in the first stages, after which Pulsatilla, Euphrasia, and Sulphur will be more useful. Dr. Lodge states that he has used Gelseminum in measles, in some cases to the exclusion of any other remedy, and is satisfied that it is a valuable medicine in this disease.

In the treatment of *Erysipelas*, Gelseminum may be found of unequivocal benefit. It is certainly homœopathic to the febrile symptoms, if not to the peculiar eruption or external manifestations of the disease; yet, Gelseminum causes an erythema, which certainly bears a resemblance to some of the milder forms of Erysipelas. It is also homœopathic to those dangerous, and often fatal congestions, or internal metastases, which often complicate the malady. I gave it one severe case of Facial Erysipelas, in alternation with Rhus. The case progressed very favorably. Dr. Coe advises it as a topical application: "We have found the tincture beneficial as an outward application in erysipelatous affections. Diluted with from four to eight parts of water, we have applied it with excellent results. The parts should be kept covered with cloths wetted in the diluted tincture. It abates the local inflammation, and has a very soothing and pleasant influence."

In *Variola* the Gelseminum may prove as useful as Aconite and Bellad., in allaying the intense and painful fever which accompanies that disease. It has been used advantageously in Varioloid.

In all eruptive fevers, especially in children, there is a strong tendency to convulsions, at or about the time of the appearance of the eruption. I know of no remedy which is so likely to prevent that unpleasant, and often fatal complication, as the one under consideration.

In the treatment of *Rheumatic Fever*, and *Rheumatism* generally, Gelseminum has its advocates in the Homœopathic school of the North-west, or that portion of them which have adopted the use of the remedy.

The Gelseminum is highly praised by some practitioners, in *Hectic fever*, and there are some reasons for supposing it to be peculiarly adapted to that form of fever.

VENOUS SYSTEM.—Dr. Marcy declares Aconite to be "homœopathic to intense or excessive venous congestion, with entire paralysis, or depotentization of all the arterial activities, carried up to the point of actual cyanosis." I [Hale] once supposed Gelseminum to be homœopathic to the same condition, but recent investigations have satisfied me that Holcombe's remark is true, that "Gelseminum holds a position *midway between* Aconite and Belladonna." It is rather difficult to define exactly what this condition is, but it is certainly more homœopathic to arterial congestion than Aconite or Veratrum viride. Still, one of the effects of Gelseminum in moderate doses, is undoubtedly similar to Aconite; for, like it, it "depotentizes the arterial activities."

It needs further trial and investigation to determine the exact relation of Gelseminum, to the venous system. It may be asserted, however, that while Aconite and Veratrum viride are only homœopathic to primary passive *venous* congestion, Gelseminum is primarily homœopathic to that form of *intense passive congestion, of both veins and arteries, in which an irritation of the congested organs sets in*, nearly as severe as though the congestion had been active. This condition may be attended by inflammation or hemorrhage, and *may end* in active arterial congestion, etc. Eclectic writers seem to be aware of the danger of using Gelseminum in some cases. King says, "It is contra-indicated in congestive fever, in cases where there is great muscular and nervous prostration with relaxation, and when there exists a determination to the brain or other important viscus."

LYMPHATIC SYSTEM.—Although Coe, and some other writers, crudely declare Gelseminum to be an "alterative," we have no direct proof of such action. I have never seen any indications of its action on the glandular system, nor can I imagine any such action, unless it be from congestion to certain large and important glands, which it may induce.

LOCAL EFFECTS.

Mind.—Irritable and impatient mood; incapacity to think or fix the attention; confusion of mind; stupid, intoxicated feeling; dulness of all the mental faculties, in one case great mirthfulness; inability to concentrate the mind; depression of spirits; anxiety; incoherency of thought. The sensorial modification consisted of a mistiness within the brain, not much affecting the lucidity of thought, but somewhat confusing perceptions, so that I experienced some difficulty in attending to the physical details connected with my practice. There was at first a cheerful, careless morale, afterwards depression of spirits. Rather dull and stupid for some days, with disinclination to conversation. This was remarked by my friends who knew nothing of my taking the medicine. Aversion to study; melancholy and depending mood. I found it to affect the power of concentration very materially. I could not fix my mind on the contents of a newspaper, although the matter was of an exciting character. I could not pursue one train of thought for any time; ideas would vanish and leave a vacancy of mind which was quite annoying.

Clinical Remarks.—Gelseminum is particularly recommended when there is excessive irritability of body and mind, in mental derangement with vascular excitement. No remedy is more useful in the causeless nervous excitement of hysteric patients; or in those feverish conditions accompanied by great restlessness, tossing about, sleeplessnes and irritable mood. In those conditions, one or two drops of the tincture every hour, will be the most proper mode of administration. It is indicated in those attacks of frenzy, attended with congestion or inflammation of the brain; also in those stupid, comatose conditions attending typhoid fever, and in a low muttering delirium of typhus.' Here we should give drop doses of the second or third dilution.

I have found it homœopathic, or curative, to that state of semi-stupor, with languor and physical prostration, caused by protracted night-watching; also in that mental apathy which follows intoxication from use of ardent spirits.

Hysterical insensibility is much more readily controlled by this medicine than with Opium or Cann. indica. Hysterical catalepsy is a similar malady, and one in which Gelseminum is primarily indicated; also many other hysterical states of body and mind, while Platinum, Asaf., Val., and Scut., are secondarily homœopathic to similar states.

Head.—Pain in the head across the forehead; after breakfast experienced a dull aching pain in the head in region of occiput, which increased in severity as the day advanced; excruciating headache, accompanied by slight nausea; the pain seemed slightly mitigated by shaking the head, but the relief thus obtained was not marked. Headache extending from occiput to os frontis; great heaviness of the head; sensation as if the brain was heavy; heaviness of the head with dulness of mind; dimness of sight and vertigo; pain in the head quite constant, dull, stupifying, and pressive; most frequently in the forehead and temples; bruised pain above and back of the orbits; tightness of the brain; often more or less headache with nausea; giddiness is pretty constant; an intoxicated feeling and tendency to stagger, often with dizziness and imperfection of vision, aggravated by smoking; heaviness, with sense of fulness in the head, which increased to a severe headache relieved on the third day of the proving by copious urination, after which a pleasant languor pervaded the system for some hours; dulness in the head with stupor; dry mouth, coated tongue, bitter taste; pulse full, and 80; intoxication, vertigo unto falling; sort of mistiness within the brain, not much affecting the lucidity of thought, but somewhat confusing perception; staggering like one intoxicated; swimming sensation in the head; head felt very light, with vertigo. He could not hold the head erect. Pain over the whole top of the head, extending back to the occiput; general dizziness, and disagreeable pain in the head; a band-like pain which surrounds the head, with shooting pain in each jaw and parietal bone; pain in left side of head, extending from the prominence of the parietal bone to the mastoid process of the temporal and is periodical in its nature; dull headache in right ride of head; in the morning on rising a dull pain in occiput, and a slight tendency to throbbing in right side of head; headache in the top of the head, in the left occipital region, then changing to the sides and vertex; a settled, dull, dragging headache, mainly in the occiput, mastoid, and upper cervical region, extending to the shoulders; relieved when sitting by reclining the head and shoulders on a high pillow. These last symptoms delineate a form of headache very often met with, and in which Gelseminum is a specific remedy. No remedy has a greater influence over the circulation of the blood in the vessels of the brain. It causes intense hyperæmia of that organ, which stops just short of inflammation. But its paralyzing influence on the great reactive forces of life, prevents that termination by destroying the reactive power of the system. In this respect it differs from Bellad., Stram., and Quinine.

Clinical Remarks.—It is homœopathic to that intense and overwhelming congestion of the brain which often attacks children during the period of dentition. In these cases the nervous energies soon lose their integrity. No reaction comes on, and the patient dies comatose, or in feeble convulsions. Owing to its primary homœopathicity to this condition, Gelseminum should be used in the second or third decimal dilution, repeated every fifteen minutes.

It is also homœopathic to *Coup de soliel*, a condition very similar to the above. In the so-called "brain fever" of children and adults, it will be found beneficial in alternation with Acon., Bry., Bell., or Hyos. In inflammation of the membranes of the brain, it will be found a valuable auxiliary to other well-known and reliable remedies in that affection. It is homœopathic to many varieties of headache, in which it has been successfully used, both by homœopathic and allopathic physicians. In *nervous headaches*, where the pain commences in the cervical portion of the spinal column, and spreads thence over the whole head, it will afford prompt and timely relief. Dr. Pattee says: "Headache of the nervous kind may often be relieved, and I have found no one medicine so useful in this troublesome disease." *Hemicrania* when accompanied by abnormal symptoms of the eyes, such as dimness of sight or double vision, or with great sensitiveness to all sounds, will be promptly relieved by it. The so-called *nervous sick headache*, will generally be arrested by a few doses of a low dilution of Gelseminum, while the true sick-headache, which arises from gastric derangement, will only be palliated by this remedy; a cure can only be effected by proper diet, and the patient use of Puls., Iris vers., Nux vom., Pod. and Sanguinaria.

Those who wish to understand the specific action of thi drug in causing and curing these nervous affections of the head, will find an admirable explanation on page 12 of Peters' Ruckert on Headache. Gelseminum undoubtedly causes a weakened and debilitated state of the great sympathetic nerve; and thence arises the pain, heat, congestion, &c., of the head. It is primarily homœopathic to those headaches which come on suddenly, with dimness of sight, or double vision, with dizziness, followed by great heaviness of the head, semi-stupor, dull, heavy, expression of the face, great muscular relaxation, slow, full pulse, etc. Allopathists claim to cure chronic headaches of long standing with Gelseminum.

In *Coma* and *Apoplexy*: it is homœopathic to these disorders when they arise from intense passive congestion, with nervous exhaustion, and as these are the primary conditions caused by Gelseminum, it must be given in very small doses. If the apoplexy depends on active arterial congestion, in persons of tense fibre, the doses must be larger.

I have found Gelseminum very useful against those distressing pains in the head which often follow fever and ague. These pains are of a crampy, drawing, or tearing character, and are aggravated by study or exertion. They generally occupy the region of the occiput. Also for those sensations and pains which in some persons precede attacks of ague, such as drawing, or shooting, dull pains in the region of the mastoid process.

Eyes.—Great heaviness of the lids; difficulty of opening the eyes or keeping them open; eyes closed in spite of him, on looking steadily at an object; fullness and congestion of the lids; diplopia when inclining the head towards the shoulder, but vision single when holding the head erect; dryness of the eyes; misty or glimmering appearance before the the eyes; pain in the orbits, sometimes excessive; diplopia which I could correct by an effort of the will; distant objects seemed indistinct as I rode or walked, and one evening I could read but with difficulty. These symptoms are characteristic, as my sight is perfectly good, and I never have anything the matter with my eyes. Dilatation of pupils; amaurosis; diplopia; blindness; dimness of sight: Stitch, traversing the eyelids on the right side, vertically; vertiginous sensation, followed by confused vision, especially of distant objects; the sense of sight is tardy in following the movement, things appearing for several seconds to be blurred, and the remaining unfixed in its new direction but no sensation of gauze or film. It is accompanied by a disposition to partially close the eyes as if to steady the balls. Confusion of sight with heavy looking eyes. [Similar to that produced by alcohol.] Pain in both eyes; particularly the left; dimness of sight; drooping of the eyes; indistinct vision; in the evening, eyes felt quite sore, and as if there was some foreign substance irritating the conjunctiva. At night eyes quite sore; not much pain, but merely soreness with sensitiveness to light and lachrymation; Eyes yellow. Eyes much inflamed and weak, with great flow of tears at intervals; great heaviness of eyelids. Pains of a shooting character in the frontal sinus, extending to the eyes and jaws. The pain in the eye is of a pricking character, extending from the bridge of the nose to the eye. Pains deep in the ball of the left eye, extending from above downwards. Pain in the eyes is of a pricking character, extending from the centre to the angle. The pains seem to wind round the right eye. Pain extending from the bridge of the nose to the eye. Deep-seated pain in the eye of the left side, extending from above downwards. Smoky appearance before the eyes, with pain above them. Total blindness ensued in a very short time after taking thirty drops with violent dizziness.

Clinical Remarks.—Gelseminum has a remarkable and peculiar affinity for the organs of vision. No other remedy except Bell., so promptly and so specially affects the eyes. It must become, in time, a valuable homœopathic remedy for many serious internal and external diseases of these organs.

Before its relaxing effects are felt in the general muscular system, its local effects upon the eye-lids become apparent. The lids feel heavy, and are lifted with difficulty. After a time complete paralysis of the lids obtain. This constitutes an affection designated by opthalmic writers as *Ptosis*. It may arise from paralysis of the levator muscle, or from an affection of the third pair of nerves. Gelseminum may cause Ptosis by inducing either of those conditions. But there is some reason to believe that the Ptosis caused by this drug may have a deeper seated origin. Mackenzie (Diseases of the Eye) says:—"The cerebral variety may be either sudden or slow; the sudden, arising after fatiguing exertion, violent mental excitement, exposure to the direct rays of the sun, intoxication, blows on the head, concussion of the body, etc. The slow, from organic changes going on in the brain. The disease often wears an apoplectic aspect." Mackenzie gives several cases, evidently caused by congestion of the brain. It is to such cases of Ptosis that Gelseminum will be found curative. It will probably be found efficient in the Ptosis of drunkards, from exposure to the sun, and the so-called rheumatic variety. It is eminently homœopathic to those cases caused by paralysis of the third pair of nerves.

Diplopia is another prominent and primary effect of Gelseminum. Double vision, according to Mackenzie, may proceed from paralysis of some of the muscles of the eyeballs. Doubtless Gelseminum causes such a form of this disease, and would be found curative to paralytic cases. But diplopia often proceeds from a congested state of the encephalon. I suspect that Gelseminum is homœopathic to such a morbid state, as also to the Diplopia caused by alcohol and chloroform, to which it seems to have a great resemblance in many respects. Gelseminum is homœopathic to *asthenopia* or debility of the eyes; in those cases of weakness of sight caused by exhaustion of the nerve from over-exertion of the eyes, especially when accompanied by dimness of sight; feeling of weight in the head and eyes, with some dryness and double vision. It is not indicated in chronic cases. In these, China, Iron and Nux vomica will be found useful. In one case the prover complained of having *Strabismus*, and a constant inclination to squint. It may be useful in some paralytic cases, but probably not curative in the strabismus which comes on in the course of hydrocephalus.

The *Amaurotic* symptoms caused by Gelseminum are many and distinct. It seems peculiarly indicated in that malady, and if we can ascertain the exact sphere of its action, may prove useful to the oculist in relieving amaurotic patients. It is undoubtedly homœopathic to many forms of amaurosis, viz: to those caused by apoplexy of the retina; congestion of the brain, apoplexy, and even those cases which arise from the presence of worms in the intestines. When administered for the cure of amaurosis it should be given in small doses. The medium or even high potencies will prove efficient. The following case is reported by Dr. Kenyon. It is illustrative of the curative powers of Gelseminum in some forms of *Amaurosis:* "Rev. Mr. ——, aged about 35 years, nervous bilious temperament, previously suffering from intermittent fever, and had taken Quinine, largely, complained of being tormented with a constant floating of spots before the eyes, at times black, and even dazzling—no other symptoms. I gave him Belladonna, and did not see him again in three weeks, when he said the trouble was slightly relieved for a day or two, and then increased; he ceased taking the remedy, thinking it might be an aggravation, but the trouble continued to increase, and after a week he resumed the remedy with no effect. The sight is gradually growing dim, so that he cannot read or write; the words all run together, and he cannot tell a person across the room. There is considerable heat in the eyes, and extending into the forehead; the floating spots are all black ones now; the pupil of the eye slightly contracted; with this exception perfectly healthy in appearance, and there is no indication of former troubles. I then prepared and gave him of the 6th and 30th dilution of Gelseminum—a dose of the 6th each morning, and of the 30th each evening. I did not hear from him again in several weeks, when he wrote me that in two days from the time he commenced the remedy he could see an improvement, when he, according to my directions, omitted the remedy; and in two weeks every trace of the trouble was removed. I saw him months after, and he remained perfectly well." (Seventeenth Annual Report Amer. Inst. of Homœopathy). Dr. D. W. Rogers, of Quincy, Mich., relates a case in the North American Journal, (August, 1861, p. 104) where the Gelseminum was useful in a case presenting symptoms of intense heaviness of head; stupid drowsiness; dimness of vision; also double vision; vertigo; throbbing of the carotids; pulse slow and weak. Other cases could be reported, but sufficient has been presented to direct the attention of physicians to the great value of Gelseminum in this affection.

I have never noticed that it caused anything like photophobia. On the contrary, it frequently causes a *thirst for light*, It might cause photophobia as one of its secondary or remote effects. I judge so from the fact that I once removed permanently a fear of light, more especially candle or lamplight, which had resisted Phosphorus and Conium, and was probably caused by an idiopathic over-sensitive state of the optic nerve, as there was no trace of inflammation. I used drop doses of the tincture, however. Dr. Peters declares Belladonna to be antipathic to photophobia. It must resemble Gelseminum in this particular symptom, and probably many others.

Under the action of Gelseminum the pupils are always dilated. I have never witnessed contraction. Aconite on the contrary, generally causes contraction of the pupils. It will be well to bear this fact in mind, as it is an important diagnostic symptom in many cerebral diseases.

Ears.—Rushing and roaring in the ears; sudden and temporary loss of hearing; the pains which ascend from the back to the occiput often affect the ears; digging in the right ear; stitches; pain behind both ears.

Clinical Remarks.—There are no instances on record of its being used in affections of the ear. One of the symptoms of catarrh in the head, or a common cold, is roaring in the ears, with sudden deafness. In such cases it might prove of benefit. It may be found of service in neuralgic otalgia, also in paralytic deafness. Coe says, "The diluted tincture dropped into the ear will soften the accumulation of hardened cerumen, and relieve the ringing roaring, from diseased secretion."

Nose.—Watery discharge from the nose; sneezing with dull headache; tingling in nose; bloody mucus discharge.

Clinical Remarks.—Dr. Douglas considers it a specific for colds in the head accompanied by a discharge of watery fluid from the nose, hoarseness, cough, soreness in the throat and chest. Dr. D. W. Rogers prized it highly in an epidemic of influenza in which he tested it. It has been a valuable remedy in my practice in mild and severe attacks of influenza, with loss of smell, coryza, headache, etc. Dr. Pattee says, "In coryza, or cold in the head, this is one of the best remedies I have ever used; it cures the severest cases in from twelve to forty-eight hours."

Face.—A papulous eruption on the face, very nearly resembling measles; erythema of the face and neck; heavy, besotted appearance of the face; sensations of stiffness in the muscles of the jaws; the muscles of the face seemed to contract, especially the orbicularis oris, somewhat impeding speech; numbness of the face; pale face; cold face, covered with perspiration. [Toxical effects.] Itching of small points on the face; pimples on the temporal ridge; yellow complexion.

Clinical Remarks.—It has been used successfully by myself, and some other homœopathists, in the treatment of facial *neuralgia*. It cured one case of neuralgia of the infra-orbital nerve, which did not yield to Acon. or Bell. One drop of the tincture was given every hour, and the diluted tincture rubbed on the affected part. Dr. Coe says, "Neuralgia, when arising from functional disturbances of the nervous system, is successfully treated with Gelseminum." It is best indicated, when, in connection with the pain, there are contractions and twitching of the muscles near the portion of the face affected; also in those cases accompanied with extreme general nervousness, and loss of control over the voluntary muscles, giving rise to odd, irregular motions. Dr. Douglas has found it curative in several cases of prosopalgia.

Prof. Ludlam writes me, "In some cases of *orbital neuralgia*, characterized by distinct paroxysms of acute pain, of a quotidian type, located along the superciliary ridge, especially over the left eye, with contractions of the eyelids, and a peculiar expression in the eye of the affected side—the organ appearing to the observer as if the patient were laboring under a maddening delirium, the opposite eye appearing quite normal, meanwhile—we have given the Gelseminum with good effect. In one example, where Quinine had failed at the hand of another physician, the Gelseminum afford- prompt relief. In most cases thus remedied, the relief of suffering has been gradual, the pain tapering off quietly and imperceptibly. We have never employed it locally in this disorder. To speculate upon its *modus operandi* would perhaps be of little service, but that it has the property of interrupting certain nervous disorders, of which the more prominent system is their periodicity, there can be no question. The introduction of the element of time, into the organism, whether viewed in a physiological or pathological light, is one of the most marvelous and entertaining phenomena connected with the history of the species; and any remedy capable of relieving abnormalities of this function—if such we may style it—in any of their protean forms, merits our study and most earnest attention. If it be demonstrated by actual experiment that the Gelseminum is capable of palliating and removing a local hyperæsthesia of the supra-orbital nerves, or indeed of any other nerves, the profession should be made aware of this fact; and it is for this reason that we are led to record our own limited experience in the direction indicated." It may prove useful against *erythema* of the face, also to certain palpulous eruptions of the face, not of a constitutional character. The sensations of tension, stiffness, and contraction of the muscles of the face and jaws, would seem to indicate that it might be useful in some cases of *Trismus.* (Scuttellaria causes similar symptoms.) Acting upon this suggestion I once gave it to a female patient, who, in a hysterical attack of unusual severity, had such rigidity of the muscles surrounding the mouth and jaws, that it resembled an attack of tetanus. The jaws could not be forced open, nor hardly the lips. I succeeded in getting two or three drops between her teeth. In eight or ten minutes the jaws began to gradually relax, and in a short time had assumed their normal condition. In *Erysipelas of the face*, the internal and external use of Gelseminum is sometimes of much benefit as a palliative remedy.

Teeth and Jaws.—Stiffness of the jaws; difficulty of opening the mouth; on the right side, pain extends from the last back tooth up to the temple; pains of a shooting character in the frontal sinus, extending to the eyes and jaw.

Clinical Remarks.—In some cases of *facial neuralgia*, especially in nervous females, when the jaws seem to be spasmodically affected, Gelseminum may be useful in combating that symptom. In

Odontalgia from a cold, or when purely nervous, Gelseminum may be useful. It is said that a bit of cotton wet in the tincture and applied to the tooth, or pushed into a cavity, will relieve the pain.

Mouth and Tongue.—Dryness of the mouth; astringent sensation in the mouth; thickly coated tongue; painful dryness in the fauces; tongue red; tongue red, raw, and painful; sensation as if the tongue was paralyzed, impeding speech; partial paralysis of the glottis and tongue. (Toxical effects.) Tongue coated with light, whitish coat; several times during the day saliva was found colored yellowish, and all the latter part of the day a bad, foul taste and breath; yellowish white fur on tongue; yellow coat on tongue.

Clinical Remarks.—From its effects upon the tongue and glottis, we may find it curative in many cases of irritation, or paralysis of those parts.

Throat.—Dryness; irritation and soreness of the fauces; difficulty of swallowing; paralytic dysphagia; when vomiting, the fluids passed through the nostrils; acute sensation of heat and astringency. (Toxical effects.) Painful sensation of something having lodged in the œsophagus.

I once observed the following symptoms, which occured in a woman, to whom it had been given to arrest daily hysteric convulsions. The patient had never experienced similar symptoms before. The tinc. Gels. was given in doses of ten drops every four hours. The spasms were much relieved, and their periodicity broken up, but on the second day of its administration there appeared dryness and burning of the fauces; red tongue inflamed in the middle; severe burning in the œsophagus, from the mouth to the stomach; spasmodic sensation, and cramplike pains in œsophagus; hawking up of bloody matter. During the spasms, bloody, brown foam would run out of the mouth. The burning sensations at times seemed intolerable; deglutition was painful; food and drinks, warm, aggravating. At this juncture I was called, and for the relief of these symptoms gave Arsenicum 3d, then Carbo vegetabilis 3d, with mucilaginous drinks, but without much benefit. A more careful study of the symptoms determined me to try Phosphorus. Pellets of the second dilution were given with prompt success; relief followed in a few minutes after the first dose, and in a few days the symptoms disappeared. In this case there must have existed Œsophagitis,—a true inflammation of its mucous tissue. As the Gelseminum was taken largely diluted with water, it must have been a specific and not a mere local effect.

Clinical Remarks.—It may be found a valuable remedy in inflammation and irritation of the œsophagus, from acrid secretions of the stomach. Dr. White, of Coldwater, Mich., praises the Gelseminum highly in Tonsilitis, and inflammation of the pharynx, palate, and uvula, He considers it equal to Belladonna in Scarlatinous Angina. I have only used it in slight catarrhal inflammations of the fauces and tonsils, in which it seemed to act favorably. It would seem to be perfectly specific to paralysis of the glottis, and all other portions of the organs of deglutition. In all the above affections, the medium or high dilutions are best indicated, especially if the patient be susceptible to the action of the drug; if not, large doses must be used. Its action on the throat resembles very much the effects of Belladonna. Dr. Douglas advises it in inflammation of the tonsils, and other throat affections. In the spasmodic affections of the throat, so frequent in hysteric females, it is superior to any other drug, but will have to be given in material doses.

Dr. Lodge, reports, that the Gelseminum has proved very useful in cases of paralysis succeeding diphtheria, particularly in paralysis of the organs of deglutition and aphonia. He relates the following case: "A young man of 18 who had been treated for diphtheria by an allopathic physician was found with the following symptoms: great prostration; partial paralysis of the right side; desire for food, but difficulty of swallowing, and vomiting after taking ever so little; cannot speak above a whisper; great difficulty in articulation; cough with expectoration of frothy mucus streaked with blood; severe pain in different parts of the body, immediately after lying down, preventing sleep; pulse 120, and small. He had been kept up by stimulants. *Treatment*—Gelseminum tincture, five dops in half a tumblerful of water; teaspoonful every hour. Commenced the medicine at 3, P.M.; rested better the following night; pains very much less; next day could swallow easier; in four days could swallow well and partook moderately of roast turkey, with relish. The improvement continued under the use of the Gelseminum, all the symptoms disappearing, *except those of bronchial irritation*, which Gel. did not remove. Phosph. and the ordinary remedies were then resorted to, and the cure completed. This youth is now in the enjoyment of good health.

Taste, Appetite, Gastric affections, &c.—Thirst during the sweat; mawkish taste; clammy feverish taste; great hunger; eructations, nausea; hiccough; yellowish-white coating of the tongue, with fœtid breath; alternate increase and loss of appetite, slight nausea; sour eructations; bitter taste; bad, foul, spoiled taste and breath, with frequent need to rinse the mouth, or spit; raising of tasteless, semi-solid matter in the œsophagus, with flatus.

Clinical Remarks.—It is homœopathic to loss of appetite from debility of the stomach, or a paralytic state of the organs of digestion, or increased appetite caused by active hypœremia of the coats of the stomach. It does not seem to be homœopathic to many gastric conditions, as it rarely causes nausea or eructations. It does not induce vomiting, like Verat. viride, Ipecac., or Tart. emet. It only causes vomiting when taken in large quantities; then it irritates by its bulk and acridity only. If useful in any variety of vomiting, it is in that form which arises from atony of the stomach, in which case Nux vom., Iron, and China are better.

Stomach.—Feeling of emptiness and weakness in the stomach and bowels; distension of the stomach with pain and nausea; sensation as of something wanting in the epigastric region; rumbling, and dull pains in the epigastrium, relieved by expulsion of flatus; burning in the stomach extending up to the mouth.

Clinical Remarks.—Sensations of great weakness, emptiness,

"goneness" at the stomach, arises from a debilitated state of the great sympathetic nerve, and may be uncomplicated with any other morbid state, in which case Gelseminum may be useful, in small doses. It may, however, arise from congestion of the portal system, and a torpid state of the liver, in which case Nux vom., Acon., Lept., Pod. or Mer. would be applicable, alternated with Gelsem. It is often caused by uterine congestion, or prolapsus, when Cimicifuga, Helonias, or Sepia must be given. Ignatia, Coffea, or Thea, in cases caused by mere nervous excitement, or sudden emotion. It is primarily homœopathic to accumulation of *flatus* in the stomach, distention, eructations and dull pain, probably caused by want of tone in the muscular fibres of that organ. For such symptoms the 2d or 3d dilutions will suffice. It is secondarily homœopathic to many forms—*gastralgia, cardialgia, cramps in the stomach*, and all spasmodic conditions of that organ. It is homœopathic to *congestion* of the stomach, with hyperæmia of its mucous lining. The symptoms indicating its use are: sensation of a heavy load, with weight, tension, and dull pain; sometimes with empty, faint, sensations in the epigastrium, and a false hunger—a kind of gnawing. Of late, the Gelseminum is much used in all active *hæmorhages*, by the Eclectic and Allopathic schools. They rely upon its sedative power. Many other remedies, however, will prove more useful in these affections. In active hæmorrhages, Hamam., Ipecac., and Erigeron; in the passive variety, Trillium, Terebinthina, and Sulph. acid, will be found efficient remedies.

Abdomen and Stool.—Rumbling and rolling in the abdomen, with emission of flatus above and below; periodical pains in the abdomen, with yellow diarrhœa coming on in the evening; pain in the left iliac region; bowels loose, but great difficulty to discharge anything; there seems to be great strength in the sphincter muscles; dull pain in bowels, which becomes quite severe towards morning; dull aching pain in the umbilical region; palpitation of muscles of the abdomen, which continued about three minutes; slight pain in the transverse colon; gnawing pain in the transverse colon. Seventeen hours after taking the drug, was awakened by severe gripings in the lower abdomen, soon followed by a very natural stool, but followed by no diminution of pain until another large, deeply bilious discharge, followed by instant relief of pain. Evacuation of flatulence both ways; movements of flatus in the lower bowels; slight colicky feeling, as if the bowels would be moved, and constant eructations of wind and bland fluid. At breakfast, dull-ache on the right side of the head; gastric oppression; had to loosen the waistbands; after which colicky sensations to the left of the navel, as if a stool would shortly be passed; slow stool, leaving a sensation of more remaining to be passed, and of abdominal repletion. Pain behind the fifth rib, to the left of the stenum, from flatus relieved by eructation. Stool at first consistent, then papescent, bilious, homogeneous, preceded all the morning by flatulence. Coincident with the intoxicated feeling, gastralgia and colic. Colicky pains below the navel, extending to the testes, and causing flatus; relieved by its expulsion; stool of a deep yellow color and papescent; soft, bilious stool, preceded by threatenings of diarrhœa; Colic; attempted stool, much wind only passed; tea-colored, semi-solid stool; dull pains in the abdomen; sharp pains in the bowels with stools of a light creamy color and pappy consistence; sleep disturbed by lancinating pains in abdomen, relieved by copious discharges of flatus; intoxicated feelings, with painless but slightly diarrhœic stool; tenderness of the abdominal parietes.

Writers of the dominant and eclectic schools have decreed that Gelseminum does not act as an internal irritant, or a purgative; they assert that it is not known to increase any of the intestinal secretions. Homœpathic provings seem to lead us to different conclusions, as many of the above abdominal symptoms demonstrate.

Clinical Remarks.—If Gelseminum be homœopathic to *Colic*, it is to the spasmodic and flatulent. As either of these varieties may run into and induce the other, we will consider them in one paragraph. Flatulence is generally caused by the imperfect digestion of articles of food, some kinds of which, such as raw vegetables, and substances of a fermentable nature, are more prone to have that effect. But in a perfectly healthy state of the digestive organs, all varieties of food may be eaten with impunity. The powers of digestion then, must be morbidly enfeebled before flatulent or spasmodic colic can ensue. Any cause, therefore, which is capable of debilitating digestion, may act as a cause of flatulence. In *Peritonitis*, we cannot expect much specific benefit from Gelseminum except from its power to control the fever, and the nervous erethism from excessive pain. While it might not be as valuable as Aconite, it would be better than Veratrum viride or Tartarus emeticus. An external application of the tincture in peritoneal inflammation might allay the pain somewhat. I have used Aconite for that purpose with the best results. In *Enteritis* it may prove more valuable. As it causes congestion and hyperæmia of the intestines, it may prove homœopathic to the first stages of acute Enteritis. It will probably be useful to restrain the spasmodic action of the bowels, which is often a distressing symptom of this disease. In Neuralgia of the Intestines I have found the tincture, in single drop doses, given every fifteen minutes, to be a successful remedy. The symptoms were acute, lancinating pains in the bowels, with great agitation and restlessness, cold hands and feet, rapid pulse, and a tendency to general spasms. In *Strangulated Hernia*, the Gelseminum in sufficient pathogenetic doses, ought to be a most valuable aid. More relaxing than Chloroform or Lobelia, or Opium, it is surprising that physicians and surgeons of the other schools have not resorted to its use. It would be the first medicine I should resort to, and no remedy holds forth greater promise of usefulness in such dangerous accidents. Its internal administration would be aided much by external application. In *Diarrhœa*, Gelseminum may prove useful when the stools are bilious, papescent, and accompanied by much flatulence; also when there is much nervous prostration—more weakness than the discharge could cause. It *will not* be found useful in diarrhœa with watery, mucous, or profuse discharges; or in looseness from indigestion. Dr. Morgan noticed that while proving the drug, any exciting news would bring on "threatenings of diarrhœa." This fact is suggestive. We know that in certain impressible people, whose nervous system has become enervated, any fright, excitement, or emotion will cause a temporary looseness of the bowels. Now, the effects of Gelseminum on the system are just such as would make it homœopathic to such conditions and its effects. Dr. Lippe, of Philadelphia, reports to me, several cases of diarrhœa, caused by fright, grief, and depressing emotions, treated with the 1000th dilution, a single dose sufficed.

In *Dysentery*, so far as my experience goes, the results attained are very similar to those noticed from the use of Aconite, viz: subsidence of the inflammatory symptoms, disappearance of blood from the stools, less fever, and a mitigation of the tenesmus. I have treated many severe cases with it, in alternation with Merc., Podoph., Ipecac. and Aloes. Besides its internal administration, I adopted the suggestion of Coe and others, and used the tincture in an enema, in the proportion of ten drops to four ounces of warm starch or gum water; injecting all at once, and repeating every few hours. It mitigated the severe tenesmus. In *Constipation*, Gelseminum does not appear to be primarily indicated, in many cases. It may be useful in simple retention of stool from deficiency of tone in the muscular coats of the intestines [in 2d and 3d dilution]. It may be useful, also, in constipation, from spasm of the muscular coats at some point in the intestinal tubes, in drop doses of tincture. In the Southern States it is much used, in infusion, as a domestic remedy for intestinal *worms*, and with alleged success. Dr. Coe advises the Gelseminum in half or one grain doses, two or three times a day, combined with Podophyllin and Santonin, and says it has proved effectual in expelling the ascaris lumbricoides and tricocephalus dispar. I have had unusual success in treating worm affections with the Gelseminum, 2d trituration, alternated with Podophyllin 1st or 2d, and Santonin one-tenth, each in grain doses, two hours apart. After two or three days the worms are either expelled in large numbers, or the verminous symptoms all disappear. A weak dilution of the tincture injected into the rectum, will often bring away large quantities of ascarides.

Liver and Spleen.—The provings of Gelseminum so far do not show any pains or abnormal sensations referred to the hepatic or splenic regions. Its effect upon the alvine evacuations, however, show that it has some effect upon the liver. For instance, we have, "large, deeply bilious discharge; bilious, papescent stool; stool of deep yellow color, and papescent; soft bilious stool;" all denoting increased action of the liver. We have also, "tea-colored stool; stool of a light creamy color, and pappy consistence," indicating a deficient amount of bile in the evacuations.

Clinical Remarks.—Judging from these symptoms, we may consider it primarily homœopathic to some forms of *bilious diarrhœa*, probably from a relaxed condition of the biliary ducts, or the ductus communis choledochus, or it may be hepatic hyperæmia. It is probably primarily homœopathic to passive congestion of the liver denoted by prostration, and a languid circulation; languor, dullness, drowsiness, or depression of spirits; dimness of sight, and dull headache. *Jaundice*, with prostration, clay-colored stool, etc. There are two symptoms above mentioned, viz.: tea-colored, [slate-colored ?] and creamy, papescent stool, which indicate that Gelseminum causes either deficiency or retention of bile. Now, from what we know of the action of the medicine, it is hardly to be supposed that it can cause, primarily, any excessive secretion of bile; but it may cause deficient secretion, from atony of the liver, in which case the yellow coloring matter of the bile would fail to be eliminated from the blood, and its accumulation in the circulation would be a necessary consequence. This, Wood believes to be the most common origin of Jaundice. Gelseminum, 3d dilution, alternated with Merc., Leptandria, Podophyllum, would be most applicable in such conditions.

The Gelseminum seems to have a specific effect upon the nerves and muscles of the rectum. Dr. W. H. White has seen it cause paralysis of the sphincter ani, with tendency to prolapsed rectum.

Urinary Organs.—Urine rather increased in quantity; clear and watery; frequent micturition; frequent emission of clear and limpid urine, with seeming relief to the dullness and heaviness of the head; urine at times clear and limpid, at times milky and turbid. Urine much increased in quantity. [Bird, "Urinary Deposits," p. 210, says that it is characteristic of phosphatic urine to be pale and colorless; also that such urine deposits pale urate of ammonia, nearly white. Phosphatic urine is often fœtid). "The effects of Gelseminum were dissipated within a few hours. As I have remarked an augmented secretion of urine, I suppose my kidneys eliminated the drug rapidly, and so prevented its action on the divers organic spheres." I [Hale] have noticed symptoms similar to the above, whilst under the influence of the drug; and in nearly every instance the profuse emission of watery urine was accompanied by transient chilliness, tremuloussness, and an evident alleviation of the sensations of heaviness of the head, dullness of mind, and dimness of sight. Several persons who made partial provings for me, noticed the same symptoms, with the alleviation. Contrasting the effects of Gelseminum on the urinary organs, with some of the phenomena of disease, and they become interesting and significant. In real *Diabetes*, Gelseminum cannot be of much service. It is probably not pathologically indicated. In *Nephritis*, *Cystitis*, *Urethritis* it may be used as we would use Aconite in similar diseases, viz: to reduce the local hyperæmia. In these affections we must rely entirely upon the secondary action of the drug; using it in larger doses.

In my practice it has benefited some cases of frequent urging to urinate, with scanty emission, attended with tenesmus of the bladder.

In *Enuresis*, Gelseminum ought to prove as valuable a remedy as Belladonna, for like that drug, it induces a paralytic state of all the sphincter muscles. Those cases, then, of involuntary micturition depending on a relaxed or paralytic condition of the sphincter muscles of the neck of the bladder, may be much benefitted, or cured by the use of the dilutions of Gelseminum. Gelseminum will probably prove useful in *spasms of the ureters* from the passage of *Calculi*. In this most painful affection, the object is to produce, in the promptest manner possible, a relaxation of the ureters. This is generally accomplished by the use of hot sitz baths, Chloroform, and Lobelia or Nux vom. Gelseminum, if properly administered, would prove as efficient as either of the above means, and secondarily more homœopathic to the condition. In that most distressing affection, *Spasm of the bladder*, it would certainly prove useful, by promptly relaxing the circular fibres of that organ. This disease is often, in the case of females, confounded with uterine spasm, and in males with spasmodic colic. But in either disease Gelseminum will prove a valuable remedy, aided in some cases by Cauloph., Cimicif.,Colocynth, or Nux vomica.

Case reported by Dr. Neidhard:—"Mr. T. S., one of the most celebrated artists in the United states, upwards of eighty years of age, was afflicted for more than four months with a constant involuntary discharge of urine, every quarter to half hour, day and night. The disease seemed to consist in a relaxed, paralytic condition of the sphincter muscles of the neck of the bladder. It was impossible for him to hold his water. Cantharides, Bromide of Potash, Dulcamara, and some other remedies were prescribed, without the slightest beneficial effect. It was now thought best to omit all remedies for several weeks, but without any improvement. Having lately studied the pathogenetic effects of Gelseminum nitidum, it was resolved to try it in the above case. Five drops of the 2d dil. were administrred three times a day. In a few days its beneficial effects were already perceptible, and in the space of a week the whole disease was conquered, and has not returned now within six months."

Genital Organs.—(1) MEN. Some irritability of the right testis, and afterwards dragging pain in the same, extending to both groins, and the hypogastrium, followed by escape of flatus; irritation of small spots on the mucous surface of the prepuce, with surrounding congestion; painless redness about the orifice of the urethra; agreeable sensation during micturition, throughout the course of the uretha; *involuntary emission of semen, without an erection.* One of the most careful and conscientious provers in our ranks, writes me as follows:—"A seminal weakness, formerly removed by Conium, returned during this proving, and was the chief reason why I discontinued it." This statement throws much light on the action of this remedy upon the male generative system, and accounts for its alleged usefulness in seminal emissions. My own provings of Gelseminum developed the following symptoms: In connection with the general prostration, accompanied by diuresis, there was always much flaccidity *with coldness of the genital organs.*

CLINICAL REMARKS.—Gelseminum is primarily indicated in *impotence* from muscular paralysis and atony; in *seminal emissions* with or without amorous dreams, but caused in all cases by direct debility of the genital organs, or, rather, of the great nerves upon which depends their healthy condition. It is also secondarily homœopathic to seminal emissions from excessive irritation of the organs of generation, either from emotional or local congestive causes, and when accompanied by a condition similar to Satyriasis.

In the former cases, small doses of the dilutions may prove efficient, but in the latter, large quantities will have to be administered—two or three drops of the tincture every two hours. I have used the first trituration of Gelseminum in cases marked by local irritation, and succeeded in effecting a cure, when other remedies had failed. Cases from allopathic authorities. Coe says:—"For spermatorrhœa, in connection with tonics we have found it of exceeding utility. It many cases it is better to administer the Gelseminum alone for several days, or until a remission of the symptoms is induced, and then follow with tonics—Cerasin, Lupulin, or Hydrastin."

Case 1.—From Keith's Journal, in a letter from a physician:—"About four years ago, I was badly afflicted with spermatorrhæa, and had nearly despaired of finding relief, for I had tried every plan of treatment suggested by my medical friends. I acceded to your advice to try Gelseminum and took but four doses [of how much?] before the emissions ceased; and by continuing the medicine my appetite returned, the peculiar cadaverous hue of my face yielded to a more healthy color, and, as subsequent years have proved, I was cured of my disease." In another number we have the following statement: "We believe it to be, in the treatment of spermatorrhœa, as near a specific as any medicine can be. Administer the following powder each night, on retiring:—Gelseminum, one-half grain; Lupulin, three grains; mix. Gradually diminish the dose as the patient shows signs of improvement. We have cured several cases with from six to ten doses." The above prescription could only benefit those cases belonging to the irritative variety, due to some local congestion, or exalted state of the nerves of those organs. The Lupulin alone has a deserved reputation for curing similar cases of the disease.

In *Gonorrhœa* the Gelseminum has been much used, and highly praised by some enthusiastic eclectics. According to Coe, "Gelseminum has gained considerable repute in the treatment of Gonorrhœa. We have employed it for some three years past, in that disease, but have never relied on it exclusively. Our principal object in employing it, is to overcome the urethral inflammation and prevent chordee, and for these purposes we have found it reliable. We usually administer it at bed time, finding that the patient is more apt to enjoy a quiet night's rest thereby. We cannot say with certainty whether the Gelseminum possesses any specific alterative value in the above disease, or not, but we believe it does." He advises it in two grain doses, but small powders of the first decimal trituration, or repeated doses of the first dilution, will probably be found as useful, and less hazardous than the one large dose.

Case.—Dr. J. S. Douglas states that some thirty years ago a patient came into his office with Gonorrhœa, of several months standing, which had been improperly treated. One of his pupils begged him to allow him to treat the case, saying he could cure the most obstinate case in a few days, with the root of Yellow Jessamine, A small handful of the root was put into a common junk bottle of whiskey, and the patient ordered, in a day or two, to take a tablespoonful of the mixture night and morning. He took but a few doses when he became much alarmed with the effect upon his eyes, thinking the medicine had destroyed his vision. Every symptom of gonorrhœa had, however, disappeared, and the cure was permanent. Since that time he has treated many cases with it, and invariably with the same success. Dr. Morgan writes me:—"The Gelseminum is in repute for the cure of *spermatorrhœa;* and an allopath of my acquaintance uses the tincture in the very largest doses in Gonorrhœa with, as he asserts, perfect success, even in old cases.

(2.) Women.—Besides the few pathogenetic symptoms which I have observed, none of the provers of our school give us any symptoms of Gelseminum upon the organs of generation of women. The following symptoms came under my notice: Sensation of heaviness in the uterine region, with increase of the white, leucorrhœal discharge; a feeling of fullness in the hypogastrium [in a girl of 17]; slight uterine pain (to which she had not been subject); aching across the sacrum—a sensation as when the menses are coming on. [These symptoms appeared from taking five drops of the tincture every two hours—in a pregnant female in the ninth week. On examination, the os was slightly open, and somewhat patulous. Notwithstanding the small amount of experience which the profession possess relative to the action of the Gelseminum on the organs of generation of women, there seems to be considerable unanimity of opinion among Eclectic authors, regarding its effects in that direction. We will examine the testimony. Dr. King, who seems to understand its sphere of action very well, and who has had much practical experience in the use of the medicine, says: "In obstetrics it has been efficaciously employed in dysmenorrhœa, gastralgia, cramps, and odontalgia during pregnancy; in rheumatism of the uterus, rigid os uteri, hour-glass contraction, retained placenta, and puerperal fever, puerperal convulsions, etc.

We will examine its merits in the above affections briefly in detail:

In *Dysmenorrhœa* of a neuralgic or spasmodic character, the Gelseminum would undoubtedly prove beneficial in material doses; minute doses would fail to reach the malady, because dysmenorrhœa is not one of the primary effects of the drug. Its neuralgic and spasmodic symptoms are secondary. But in the congestive form the dilutions will be useful. In the inflammatory form, King advises it, in connection with tincture of Aconite, both in large doses. Coe asserts that "for relieving the pain of Dysmenorrhœa we know of no single remedy equal to it." He gives one-half grain of Gelseminum every two hours, and frequently alternates Caulophyllin or Viburnin with it; both of the latter remedies I know to be valuable in this affection. He further says:—"When caused by functional derangement we deem it specific; we have earned the gratitude of many sufferers by its employment." I would advise a candid trial of the remedy in the hands of homœopathists. In

Amenorrhœa, Coe advises it, and says the menses will frequently return under the use of half grain doses of Gelseminum, three times a day. In the congestive variety, induced by a cold, it will undoubtedly prove of service. In *Abortion*, King recommends it on the ground that it will have the same effect as blood-letting in preventing that accident. Coe says: "The opinion has been entertained by some that the Gelseminum is capable of producing abortion, but our experience with it, inclines us to the contrary belief. As before stated, when administered in *small doses, it gently stimulates uterine contraction*, but when given in *large doses, it will arrest the progress of labor with much certainty.* Still, we are unable to say that it will NOT produce abortion under some circumstances, although we have never seen any evidence of its power to do so, and we have administered it to women at all the different stages of utero gestation." Drs. White and Ford thought that when used in Yellow Fever, the Gelseminum rather prevented abortion, as one woman so treated, was in the sixth month of pregnancy, and did not abort. Still, my observations convince me that under some circumstances the medicine may be capable of causing abortion. The pathogenetic symptoms above noticed would go far to substantiate such a belief. Let it be borne in mind that anything which has a severe depressing influence upon the nervous and vascular systems may cause miscarriage. Thus, profuse bleedings, a chill, debility from acute disease, grief, fright or other depressing emotions, will in some constitutions tend to such an accident. Now the effects of this drug on the female organism, are very similar to the above, and may therefore under similar circumstances bring on the same results. Its general action on the uterus will be considered further on. In the *vomiting* and *gastrodynia* of pregnant females, when of a spasmodic character, Gelseminum may prove beneficial. Some writer has called attention to the similarity between this vomiting and sea-sickness. It is a curious fact that the remedies found beneficial in one, are those most useful in the other. Thus Nux vomica, Cocculus, and Chloroform are the remedies for sea-sickness, and I have found them equally reliable in the severe vomitings of pregnancy. As Gelseminum bears a remarkable resemblance to the last mentioned agent, I would advise its use in single drop doses, in cases where the usual medicines had failed to give relief, and where there was present considerable nervous, debile irritability. The troublesome *cramps of pregnancy*, although generally amenable to the usual Verat. alb., Coloc., and Nux vom., may be controlled as readily by the use of Cauloph., Vibur., and Gelseminum. Dr. King in his Obstetrics, speaks of it in *hour-glass contractions*, and *inversion of the uterus*, in order to aid manual operations, but doubts its safety under all circumstances. In those cases it would be expected to have many of the effects of Chloroform, especially *relaxation.* He also strongly advises its use in *puerperal convulsions.*

Cases reported by Dr. J. S. Douglas:

Case 1st.—On the night of the 3d inst., (Nov. 1861) a young married woman, of highly nervous temperament, and seven months pregnant with her first child, was attacked with violent convulsions, frequently repeated, and soon followed with complete unconsciousness, and the wildest delirium.

This state of things continued till the afternoon of the 5th, when she was delivered of a dead fœtus. The convulsions now ceased, but she continued in a state of wild delirium, incessantly talking and without a moment of sleep for three days and nights. During the next half day her delirium was somewhat more subdued, the incessant talk less furious, and she seemed to sleep once or twice for a minute or two. During all this time, the arterial action was inclined to be excessive, as in acute inflammatory disease, though no such state could be detected. This excessive action was successfully controlled by the frequent use of Aconite.

I now resolved to try the effect of Gelseminum. She accordingly took tea spoonful doses of a mixture of three drops, third dilution, in one-half a tumbler of water. During the night, after two or three doses, she had three sleeps of from one to two hours, and in the morning gave the first evidence of consciousness. This, however, was of short duration. A few minutes of mental effort seemed to exhaust the power of the brain and she relapsed into wakeful delirium. But whenever she has become delirious and sleepless, the Gelseminum, in the above doses, has uniformly and promptly procured quietness and sleep. The intelligent nurse has come to rely implicitly upon it whenever needed. The patient has steadily improved from the above date to the present, Nov. 23d, though it has been necessary to give occasional intermediate doses of Aconite, which alone has controlled the excessive arterial activity. She now leaves her room, though her mind is weak, and wanders when too long excited.

In this case it is evident that Gelseminum has uniformly and perfectly succeeded in quieting excessive nervous irritability and delirium, and procuring sleep, where Aconite, Bellad., Cham., Coffea, Hyos., Ign., Puls., Stram., etc., had proved powerless.

Case 2nd.—On the 5th inst. I was called to see a lady eight months pregnant, the mother of four children, the two last of which had been born at about the same period (of eight months). All her labors had been exceedingly tedious, from three to six or seven days, apparently from the great rigidity and unyieldingness of the os uteri. In her last confinement she had violent puerperal convulsions. When I was called on the 5th she had had regular labor pains for three days, but, accustomed to protracted labors, she had not thought it time to send for me till she was seized with a convulsion, which was repeated before my arrival. I found the pains quite active and frequent, but on making an examination not the least result was observable. The os uteri was not in the least developed, but rigid, and perfectly closed.

With the vivid recollection of her last two labors, at the same period of eight months, their extreme tediousness, the violent and alarming convulsions which now bid fair to be continued through a labor of days—perhaps many days; of all the exhaustive appliances formerly employed to subdue the convulsions and to stop or hasten the premature labor, with nearly all my time necessarily occupied with the case above related, no one will marvel at my extreme anxiety and perplexity. On reflection, as all other known means had, on the former occasions, proved so fruitless, I resolved to try the effect of Gelseminum. It might, by its great sedative power, subdue the spasms; it might allay and put a stop to the premature labor pains. If it failed of accomplishing these objects, it might relax the rigidity of the os uteri, and thus facilitate the labor. She was not of a nervous, but a bilious temperament. I gave five drops of the tincture, directing it to be repeated after each spasm, or, if no spasm occurred, every hour unless the pains were abated, or she experienced some of the characteristic symptoms of the drug. After three doses I saw her. No more spasms had occurred. The pains were unchanged. Directed one drop every two hours. Six hours after, the pains were nearly the same, but a very palpable change was effected in the state of the os uteri, which was now soft, relaxed, and sufficiently dilated to admit the finger easily. I had no doubt the labor would now go on, and from the much more rapid relaxation of the os uteri than on former occasions, would be much less tedious. I left to call again in six or eight hours, or to be notified if needed sooner. At my next visit the pains were much less frequent and much lighter. No symptoms from the drug. Continued one drop every four hours. On the following day, the pains had altogether ceased and the patient was feeling entirely comfortable. Three days since she was in her usual good health and attending to her usual duties. She was safely delivered at the proper time, and after an easy labor. Others can draw their own inferences from this case, and I will not comment upon it, except to say, it is obvious that Gelseminum accomplished in it what every hitherto known means had entirely failed to effect, on two precisely similar occasions, with the same patient.

Case reported by Dr. C. A. Williams:—Mrs. S———, a large woman of plethoric habit, about twenty-eight years of age, in her sixth month of pregnancy, was taken, April 25th, 1864, with flowing. It not being very severe, the patient, from some cause, allowed it to continue to the 28th, when, thinking she was about to be confined, sent for me. (I attended her through a case of the same kind the year previous.) On calling I found the above history, with the following condition: considerable flowing, but no pain. On examination, I found the os slightly dilated, and at once proceeded with the usual remedies, to check the hemorrhage, but with no success, and the discharge continued until the eve of the 29th, when the waters were expelled. Immediately previous to the last act, she had had two or three quite severe pains. On examination I found the os uteri rigid, with the orifice about the size of a three cent piece. As she was free from pain I put her on Caul., two grain doses every two hours. I continued this until the 30th, 11 A. M., when, on examination, I found no change. The patient had been comfortable, with the exception of slight nausea; I then gave her Caul., first dec. trit., three grain doses every two hours, until the eve of the same day. Still no change. I then gave her Gelseminum fld. ext., two, drop doses, every hour. The following morning, May 1st, I called again. She had rested well, had flowed but very little, and concluded she was no better. I made an examination and found the os fully dilated, and the head of the fœtus partly expelled. I very soon delivered her, and cut the cord; the child lived nearly an hour. The placenta was retained, and about ten minutes after the child was expelled, the os had contracted, and was rigid as before. I again gave her Caul., in its various potencies, with no success. I then gave Ergot, but got no effect except nausea. This occupied the time from May 1st, until the 3d, Friday, the os still rigid. I gave Gelsem. as before, and with the happiest results, as in a few hours the os uteri was fully dilated, and the placenta expelled. Mark, that during the whole course of this case there were no pains, except the few before the liquor amnii was discharged. The patient progressed finely, and in a few days was convalescent. The discharge was quite light after confinement, and of a pale color.

In the treatment of the form of puerperal convulsions depending on Uræmia, I should place much reliance on the remedial powers of Gelseminum. It will be found of much service in moderating the violence of the fits, as well as to run off by its diuretic effects, some of the urea and carbonate of ammonia upon which the primary morbid condition depends. Of the use of Gelseminum in *rigid os uteri*, Dr. King says: "It has within the last few years, been recommended to overcome this difficulty, and I have administered it in a considerable number of cases with benefit. It possesses an advantage over Lobelia in not causing nausea and vomiting, but as a general rule its influence is not so readily experienced as with that drug, and when once effected is of a more permanent character." (Do not give so much then, Doctor.) Prof. Cleveland, Dr. L. E. Miller, and many other writers eminent in the Eclectic and Allopathic schools speak very highly of the use of Gelseminum in difficult labor, from rigidity of the os or vagina. They consider it much more efficient, and its administration attended with less suffering and danger than Chlorof., Bellad., Lobelia or artificial dilatation. I think that Gelseminum, in rigidity of the os uteri, is superior to any remedy usually recommended in our school. It may be applied locally to the os, in the form of the glycerole of Gelseminum; one or two drams should be rubbed into the rigid *os*, with the finger. Croserio advises the administration of a few pellets of the 30th [!] of Belladonna. Jahr says, "If the neck should remain closed, and a hard rim should be felt all around the orifice, three globules of Belladonna dry upon the tongue will bring about the regular evolution of the progress of labor," or "if the dilatation of the vagina proceed too slowly, or be too painful, a few doses of Coff., Sec., Puls., or Nux vom., will remedy this trouble." This latter prescription is much more scientific than the former for Coff., See. Puls., and Nux vom. undoubtedly cause rigidity of the vagina and os uteri, as a primary effect. But there is not a particle of proof that Bellad. does. On the contrary, the

27

well-known and invariable primary effect of Belladonna is to cause paralysis or relaxation of all the sphincter muscles. Gelseminum has many points of resemblance to Belladonna, but none more similar than its effects on the sphincter and circular muscles, all of which are primarily relaxed, and even paralyzed. It dilates the pupil, paralyzes the glottis, relaxes the sphincter of the bladder and rectum, and those muscles of the os uteri and vagina, upon which their contractile power depends. While, then, it has a similar action to the Belladonna, it can be used with greater safety, for its effects are generally transient, and may be controlled, if excessive, by such a general remedy as common salt; or specific, such as Secale or Caulophyllum. The large doses of Gelseminum advised by Eclectics, are not necessary. From two to five drops of the tincture, or even first dilution, if good, will, in most cases, be found sufficient. There is one other argument for the use of Gelseminum in some difficult labors, which, if made reliable by the test of observation and experience, will bring the medicine into deservedly high repute. I allude to the statement made by several prominent writers, but particularly by Coe, whom I quote, as follows: "Some division of opinion exists in relation to the true action of this remedy upon the uterus. We have had considerable experience in the treatment of female disorders, and have used the preparations of Gelseminum quite extensively. For five years past we have employed it as a parturifacient, and with better satisfaction than any other remedy. We use it for the purpose of relieving cramps, or other spasmodic difficulties, vertigo, nervous irritability, wakefulness and other symptoms accompanying gestation. It seems to prepare the system for the parturient effort, and labor is completed in an unusually short period of time. When administered in small doses, it *gently stimulates uterine contraction*, but when given in large doses it will arrest the progress of labor *with much certainty*." The same writer seeks to account for this and other peculiarities of its action as follows: "Gelseminum is one of those medicines which are peculiarly governed in their action, by the quantity administered. Thus, in small doses it acts as a gentle stimulant and tonic to the nervous system, giving vigor and harmony of action; while in large doses it proves a powerful relaxant, completely prostrating the muscular system, and by over stimulating the brain and nerves, produces irregular and disturbed nervous action." This sentence undoubtedly embodies the real sphere of action of this wonderful remedy, as well as the true rationale of its curative powers in disease. The explanation is worthy the staunchest disciple of Hahnemann, for it indicates as strongly as words can, that it cures according to the law of *Similia*, i. e., *it cures in small doses, that which it causes in large.*

Air Passages.—Paroxysms of hoarseness, with dryness of the throat; voice seems weak; sneezing followed by tingling and fulness in the nose; sneezing with dull headache; tingling in nose; paralysis of the glottis, with difficulty of swallowing; ineffectual efforts to articulate; voice thick, as if the tongue was too large; cough from tickling and dry roughness of the fauces; burning in the larynx and down in the chest, under the sternum; a sensation of soreness in the chest when coughing.

CLINICAL REMARKS.—Dr. Douglas considers it almost a specific for ordinary *catarrhal fever*, with the usual symptoms of sneezing, watery coryza, soreness of the throat, and cough, with rawness in the chest. During the winter of 1860–61 I treated a great many cases of severe *influenza*, then epidemic, in which the symptoms much resembled the above, only more intense, often nearly approaching to acute bronchitis. Gelseminum was the principal remedy relied upon. It seemed to act very favorably in cutting short, or modifying the disease. Only a few cases needed Phos. or Mercur. iod. in alternation. In *Acute Bronchitis* it will doubtless be found as useful as Aconite or Tart. emet. In *Aphonia* from catarrhal paralysis it is fully indicated, in small doses. (See case reported under head of "Throat.")

Thoracic Organs.—Stitching sensations in the region of the heart; constrictive pain around the lower part of the chest; short paroxysmal pain in the superior part of the right lung, on taking a long breath with stitches from above downwards. The pain in the lungs is one of the most prominent symptoms. Periodical pains in the pectoral muscles; offensive breath; slow breathing and slow pulse, (primary), followed by rapid breathing, and quick, weak pulse (secondary). Sudden sensation of suffocation, as in hysteria; respiration almost imperceptible; sighing respiration. (In men) Breathing unnaturally slow; heavy and labored respirations; inspirations, were of a sighing, catching character; slow breathing with rapid pulse (primary). Respiration hurried and seemingly painful; inspirations; long with croupy sound; expirations sudden and forcible.

Pathology.—The following pathological appearances have been observed by Dr. Miller and myself, in animals poisoned by Gelseminum: Active hyperæmia of the lungs; lungs highly congested; heavy, sinking in water, but evidently not inflamed; lungs bluish at the base, crepitating but little, and filled with venous blood.

CLINICAL REMARKS.—But few painful symptoms of the chest have been observed by the provers of Gelseminum. This I presume can be accounted for on the supposition which the pathological appearances seem to uphold, that it does not cause inflammation, or any disturbance of the nerves of sensation of the thoracic organs. In this respect it ranks with Aconite and Veratrum viride. It undoubtedly first attacks the nerves which control the respiratory movements, acting primarily as a sedative, causing more or less paralysis; and secondarily, irritating the same respiratory nerves into irregular and spasmodic action, with concomitant hyperæmia. The venous congestion, I imagine to be the resnlt of an inability of the veins to return the blood to the heart, from paralysis. The secondary symptoms shown by the dogs, were evidently of a spasmodic character, as regards the respiratory efforts, while the primary respiratory symptoms, were as evidently the result of a sedative influence on the nerves.

The therapeutic sphere of Gelseminum in thoracic affections may be briefly summed up: It is primarily indicated in *paralysis* or debility of the lungs, of a nervous origin; and in passive congestion; it is secondarily indicated in all affections of the lungs and pleura, which are marked by erethism, or vascular irritation; or when congestion is to be feared, or is already present; also in all spasmodic affections of the lungs and diaphragm, such as convulsive hiccough, certain forms of asthma, spasms of the air passages, convulsive coughs, etc. In real *Pneumonia and Pleurisy*, it is not truly homœopathic, but may be used with benefit. Dr. J. S. Douglas, says: "A word in regard to the homœopathicity of Gelseminum in inflammations, as pneumonia, etc., etc. In all inflammatory diseases, there is a forming or congestive stage, characterized by chilliness, depressed pulse, etc. According to my view, to this stage, and this only, is Gelseminum homœopathic. When this stage is passed, and congestion gives place to inflammation, the indication for Gelseminum ceases, and that for Aconite begins. This is the clear distinction which I make between these two valuable drugs. I do not, however, mean to exclude Aconite from the congestive stage of inflammatory diseases, but I believe Gelseminum still more strongly indicated."

The remarks of Dr. Marcy, relative to the action of Aconite on the lungs, are perfectly applicable, it appears to me, to Gelseminum:—"It is highly probable, as I have already observed, that many of the pulmonary symptoms, produced by Aconite, are due to its specific action upon the brain, rather than any direct impressions on the lungs. Normal respiration and circulation can only be sustained by an unimpaired condition of the brain. Even when the impression upon this organ is slight, we observe an immediate change in the action of the heart and lungs. The inhalation of Chloroform or Ether, for example, which exercises a specific influence upon the brain, causes an almost immediate acceleration of respiration and circulation—the pulse often rising to 140, and the respirations to 26 or more, in the minute."

I have called attention already to the similarity of Gelseminum to Chloroform. It is probable that as soon as the Gelseminum produces a decided impression upon the brain, the symptoms of pulmonary sedation cease, because counteracted by the cerebral influences, and we have acceleration of the respiration and circulation. Let it be borne in mind too, that in some spinal diseases, various spasmodic affections of the lungs set in. The influence of Gelseminum on the spinal cord may induce similar symptoms. Dr. Douglas, says: "In the first stage of the disease (Pneumonia) as in most other inflammatory diseases, Gelseminum is capable of breaking up the disease in the first twenty-four hours, by producing free perspiration. Repeat it as occasion requires till the fever and pain abate. Gelseminum is more prompt and effectual than Aconite and Bryonia if given at an early stage."

Back and Neck.—Dull, aching pain in back, particularly in lumbar and sacral region; pains in the neck, which confine themselves to the upper part of the sterno-cleido mastoid muscles directly back of the parotid glands; dull pain under scapula of left side; pain in the back as in the cold stage of ague, (in many cases); chilliness and chills running up the back from the loins to the nape of the neck; rheumatic pains in the left side of the neck; contractive sensations in the right side of the neck; a settled, dull, dragging headache, mainly in the occiput, mastoid and upper cervical region, extending to the shoulders, relieved when sitting, and by reclining the head and shoulders on a high pillow; aching in the left anterior part of the trapezius muscle; aching in the sacro iliac and lumbar regions, and the lower part of the left thigh, as when a fever is commencing.

CLINICAL REMARKS.—No remedy so certainly causes *Myalgia* by its seconadary action, than Gelseminum, and no remedy is more certain to relieve *such pains*, temporarily, at least. (See Dr. Moore's case on page 180). It is most useful in the acute variety; when chronic, myalgia must be treated by China, Nux, Helonias, etc. (See Inman's treatise on myalgia.) It is homœopathic and curative, as I have often verified, in many of those aches and pains in the back, shoulders, neck, and occiput, which so often precede or follow attacks of ague or nervous fevers; also when these or similar pains are of a neuralgic nature, arising from some form of spinal irritation; or come on as the result of a cold, having somewhat of a rheumatic character. It will doubtless prove to be homœopathic to many of those anomalous cases of spinal irritation, or chronic myelitis, which resist the usual remedies. In paralytic conditions of the lumbar or sacral muscles, it is especially indicated.

Upper Extremities.—Deep seated, dull aching pains in upper and lower extremities, and joints generally; severe pain in both upper extremities; seemed to be deep-seated in muscles; the pains were most in left arm and fore-arm; severe aching pain in left elbow; rheumatic pain in extremities; sharp shooting in last phalangial joint of right thumb; dull pains in muscles of right arm and shoulder, and some of the time in the left arm; sharp pain in right wrist; weakness and numbness of both arms; coldness of the wrists and hands; itching about the elbows and fore arms; some heat and dryness of the hands; the palms feel hot and dry; drawing-ache about the left elbow. From large doses the arms become powerless, with loss of voluntary motion; sensation remains intact.

In dogs, poisoned with Gelseminum, the fore legs were not paralyzed until some time after the hinder limbs. In attempting to walk—dragging the posterior extremities—the fore legs tottered as if weak, and finally gave way; then clonic contractions seized them.

It would seem to be homœopathic to paralysis of the arms, with loss of motion, but not sensation (the reverse is true of Aconite), also when the paralyzed arms are affected with cramps and contractions. It may be found useful in some forms of rheumatism of the arms, induced by a cold, and not inflammatory, attended with loss of motion.

Lower Extremities.—Dull pain in the left thigh; dull pain in left humeral region, also in lower extremities—these are deep-seated in the muscles; rheumatic pains in bones and joints of extremities, and in the back; deep-seated aching pains in muscles of extremities, relieved by motion; severe pain in calves of both legs; paroxysmal pain in the left lower extremity; shooting pain in calf of right leg; violent shooting pain in the leg, which comes on in paroxysms; every one is more violent; the pain is half way between the knee and ankle; pain in hip of left side, confining itself tothe joint; it at times extends to the outside of the thigh; the pain is of a drawing, sharp character, and much worse on motion; pain in little finger and the one next to it; pains in left foot and ankle, with spasmodic contraction and drawing pains in the toes; excessive drawing, contracting, and crampy pains in the lower limbs, extending from the thighs to the toes—the pains seem to proceed from the bones as well as the muscles; excessive crampy pains in the whole right foot; during and after a walk, the symptoms are much aggravated; it seems as if the limbs could not be made to move another step; when the pains are felt above the knee, they are not felt below, and vice versa; excessive drawing and contracting pains in the gastrocnemius muscle of the left leg; the other pains in the limbs all abate while sitting; this does not; no position seems to relieve it; drawing and aching pains, which seem to come from bones; heaviness and feeling of weight in the limbs; coldness of the extremities, especially the feet, often severe; feet feel as if in cold water, aguish feeling, with pain in the legs; pain in popliteal spaces; aching in the left rectus femoris muscle, and drawing in the right calf; transient crampy pain in the inner part of the thigh when walking: rheumatic pain in the right knee, and left side of the neck—the latter when lying down; the former when walking; while walking, a feeling in the knee joint as if the relation of the bones were deranged, and did not fit, as in partial luxation; pains in the left thigh and knee; sudden catch or twist in the inside of the patella. Paralytic symptoms made themselves manifest throughout the entire muscular system—first experienced in the knee, and then in the inferior tibial region, increased unto falling. Loss of voluntary motion in the lower extremities; fatigue of the lower limbs after slight exercise; soreness in the gastrocnemii muscles as if they had been beaten. The *paralysis* caused by Gelseminum is first manifested in the lower limbs, which become weak and then powerless, but with no loss of sensation, at least not until the near approach of death.

It seems to be homœopathic to rheumatic (myalgic) pains in the legs, accompanied by crampy sensations and weakness of the knees.—(See case reported under heading "Throat.")

Skin.—The Gelseminum produces a very marked eruption in most of the cases. It appears on the face most frequently, but sometimes also upon the back, and between the shoulders. It is papulous, very much the color of measles, which it closely resembles, but the papulæ are more distant and distinct. Though very conspicuous, they are attended with little or no sensation—the patient being unaware of any eruption until he happens to see himself. Persons have frequently been asked what was the matter, or if they had the measles, when they were not aware of the eruption. It generally appears the second or third day of the proving, and continues one or two weeks more. An eruption of vesico-pustules —painless, but having no other analogy with measles—appeared, during proving, on the inside of the thighs.

Intense but transient itching of small points on the face, at the edge of the hair, and on the scalp; pimple, quite sore, having the areola embracing the diameter of a pea, red and inflamed (such an eruption not experienced at any other time). The pimples appeared on the forehead and neck, sore to the touch, and seemed like a small cutaneous induration, or minute furunculi. They finally disappeared without suppuration. During its use in yellow fever a constant *erythema* of the skin was noticed, and a redness of the tongue; neither appearing during the administration of Veratrum viride.

Clinical Remarks.—Its action on the skin is at once specific and peculiar taking into consideration its catarrhal symptoms, we may consider it indicated in measles, as well as some other painless non-suppurating eruptions. Its use in erysipelas and exanthematous fever, has already been alluded to. *Dr. Coe* writes: "We have found the tincture an excellent remedy for poisoning by the Rhus toxicodendron, and Rhus radicans. Dilute the tincture with from four to eight parts of water, and apply as directed for erysipelas, keeping the parts constantly moistened with it. If there be any febrile excitement present, administer the tincture internally at the same time. * * * We have experienced the value of this remedy in our own person, and can recommend it as reliable. Other practitioners have used it with success. * * Many forms of skin diseases [*what?*] may be benefited and cured by the internal and external application of the tincture."

Sleep.—Very restless; during the night was very restless with unpleasant dreams after midnight; but little inclination to sleep; when it does come on, dreams much of business, etc.; disposition to sleep; a sort of stupor; cannot keep the eyes open; is obliged to lie down and sleep. Drowsiness and long sound sleep are very general symptoms. Drowsiness with dimness of vision; kind of drunken stupor; heaviness of the eyes as after night watching; at first it seemed to cause drowsiness; afterwards aggravated the habitual sleeplessness; unusually sound morning sleep, with difficult, weary waking (after taking twenty-five drops the day and evening previous); languor and drowsiness when trying to study; slept an hour in the afternoon, and on being roused felt unwilling at first to move; eyes transiently bloodshot. It cannot be considered a narcotic, ranking with *opium*. Still it has some narcotic traits, in common with Aconite, Chloroform, Alcohol, or Hyoscyamus. Unless taken in large quantities, it rarely induces sleep by its *direct* effects, but it may give sleep by removing nervous erethism. It more resembles the so-called *nervines*, *Scutellaria*, *Cypripedium*, *etc.*

We have the following opinions of writers of other schools: Professor Tully considered it a narcotic, and places it in a group with Spigelia. "It must be borne in mind that *Gelseminum* is *narcotic.* Some division of opinion exists as to whether the *Gelseminum* has a narcotic property. We should think that a very slight experience would be sufficient to decide this question. When the patient is brought fully under its constitutional influence, the symptoms are so marked that we cannot conceive how the remedy should be deemed otherwise. On attempting to move about, the patient appears as if intoxicated; the muscles refuse to obey the mandates of the will, while the head is dizzy and the senses confused. In some respects the symptoms much resemble those produced by Stramonium, and in like manner pass off as soon as the remedy is discontinued; at other times the patient appears as if under the influence of Alcohol, and evinces a decided disinclination to motion, and tendency to sleep, from which he awakes invigorated and refreshed." (*Dr. Coe.*) "Whether it is a narcotic, is not yet satisfactorily established." (*Dr. King.*)

Clinical Remarks.—In those comatose states caused by cerebral congestions, we shall find it a valuable remedy. I have called attention to its usefulness in the stupor attending the fevers of children. [Infantile remittents.] It will be equally useful in the stupor of typhus cerebralis, or any form of typhoid, when coma is a prominent symptom, and the other symptoms correspond. It may also be beneficial in the low delirium of typhoid fever. When used for the above, the low dilutions are advised. In that peculiar stupor, or drowsiness, felt by students and persons of sedentary habits, especially in hot weather, and *not* caused by hepatic torpor, this remedy in small doses, continued for many days, is as capable of affording relief as any drug I have ever used. When depending on hepatic derangements, it is removed by Podoph., Lept., or Nux Vomica. In *Delirium tremens*, or morbid wakefulness of drunkards, large doses (five or ten drops) of the tincture repeated as often as necessary, will be found as useful as opium, in *some* cases, and more efficent in others. No remedy so happily controls the sleeplessness and agitation of teething children, students, persons laboring under mental excitement, or hysteric females. The first dilution will usually suffice.

Case.—Reported by Dr. Lodge. A commercial traveler asked for advice under the following circumstances:—He said that he was engaged during the day taking orders, settling accounts, etc., nerves on the stretch all the time; that at night he would go to bed with a feeling of exhaustion, and great desire for sleep but without obtaining any rest; the transactions of the day would be turned over in his mind again and again—repose coveted but not gained. I gave him a drachm vial of tincture of Gelseminum, with directions to take three or four drops in water when retiring. The prescription was successful. A few months afterwards he reported that it was only necessary to resort to the Gelseminum occasionally, but that when he did use it, it calmed his nervous system, produced slight prespiration and quiet refreshing sleep. In sleeplessness, from nervous irritation, it is invaluable.

General Symptoms.—Weakness and trembling through the entire system; listless and languid; great lassitude; *feeling of lightness in the body;* fear of falling; easily fatigued; general feeling of illness as in fever, so prostrated that he can neither move hand or foot; no power over any muscle; strange, indescribable feeling through the entire system.

Clinical Remarks.—The only symptom in the above which we need to notice in this place is the one in *italics*. It very frequently appears in persons suffering from *spinal exhaustion*, particularly when caused by *onanism*. This fact I have observed in several cases. A very few other remedies in our Materia Medica have this symptom. (Ambra-grisea.)

GOSSIPIUM HERBACEUM.

(*Cotton Plant.*)

The Cotton plant is a native of Asia, but is extensively cultivated in this country.

No proving of the Cotton root has been made, and its medicinal effects are so uncertain and unreliable that it will be mentioned merely to call the attention of the profession to the agent, and stimulate some one to institute provings on the healthy, in order that we may have some reliable data for its use.

Dr. Bouchelle, of New Orleans, I believe, was the first to call attention to its powers as a uterine motor-stimulant. He published his observations in Southern medical journals, and other physicians substantiated his statements. He says:—"The inner bark of the cotton root has a special affinity for the sexual organs, modifying their functions in a remarkable manner; it not only possesses oxytocic properties, invigorating feeble contractions of the uterine fibres, but it *originates* expulsive contraction at any period of gestation, and will induce immediate abortion when taken in the proper quantity, and without any detriment to the health of the female." He asserted that it is "habitually resorted to by slaves in the South as an *ecbolic*, for the criminal purpose of inducing abortion, a fact which I have had named to me a number of times by Southern practitioners." Dr. B. infers, from its influence on women, that the use of it destroys the generative capacity, rendering the person sterile, without impairing the health. Dr. King, in his Eclectic Obstetrics, quotes the above, and says: "Should this eventually prove to be the case, this agent will become a most important article of our Materia Medica, a boon to physicians, and likewise to females with deformed pelves." It is used in strong decoction—four ounces of fresh bark to one quart of water, boiled down to a pint—dose, two fluid ounces every twenty-five or thirty minutes. He adds:—"A tincture of the bark in spirit of nitric ether, and administered in doses of from thirty to sixty drops, several times a day, has produced the most decided and prompt relief in *Amenorrhœa* owing to a torpid condition of the uterus, or a mere derangement of its functions, not connected with disease of other parts. It has likewise proved efficacious in cases of recent dysmenorrhœa. I have successfully used it in a few cases of uterine hemorrhage, in combination with ergot and cinnamon." How mercilessly would Hahnemann have criticized this last statement! How can a sensible physician write such a sentence? Which was the efficient agent? Which had any power over the hemorrhage? Yet, of such loose statements is the ordinary Materia Medica of the opposite schools made up!

Drs. Jones and Scudder place the Cotton root among the Emmenagogues, but at the same time assert that it is "not Abortiva or Parturient in the slightest degree." They say, "It may be emmenagogue; at least, in some cases in our practice, the warm infusion, drank freely, with other auxiliary measures, has reproduced the menstrual discharge. It is hard to determine, however, in such cases, how much to attribute to the agent, as any warm fluid, taken freely, with the use of the warm foot and hip bath, will sometimes be sufficient to reproduce the discharge."

Coe's statements are all loose, and are of no reliable character. He recommends it for all sorts of uterine diseases. (His employers, Keith & Co., manufacture the *Gossipin*, and wish it lauded in the highest terms.) I commenced experimenting with the Gossipium, about eight years ago; I have given it in small and large doses, to the healthy and the diseased, *and have yet to see the first symptom of pathogenetic or curative action arise from its use.* I have ordered it in strong decoction in Amenorrhœa, and also in the third dilution of the tincture; I have prescribed the *Gossipium* in massive and minute doses, in dysmenorrhœa, uterine hemorrhage, etc., but never noticed the slightest effect; nor have I ever seen anything which would lead me to suspect it was an abortivant or parturient. Dr. Holcombe, of New Orleans, and other Southern physicians, inform me that they have no confidence in its alleged virtues. On the contrary, we have the testimony of many Eclectic and Homœopathic physicians, that the Cotton root is a remedy which really does exert an influence over the generative organs of women, and has been found useful in uterine pains, cramps, hemorrhages, atony, amenorrhœa, and as an efficient agent in difficult labor pains.

"Mr. Shaw, of Tennessee, writing to the *Nashville Journal*, says: 'I consider this root one of the very best emmenagogues of the materia medica, and I think it should be so classed. My reasons for considering it such, are grounded upon the different experiments which I have made with it, within the last twelve months. I sometimes use a decoction, and at others an infusion, but most generally a decoction, prepared thus: Cotton root, four ounces; water, two pounds. Boil down to one pint. S.—A wine glass full every hour. This produces the most salutary effect in dysmenorrhœa; it acts as an anodyne in allaying the pain, and as an emmenagogue in aiding or augmenting menstruation; its action is very speedy; after its exhibition, in this case, it produces an effect which, indeed, appears almost natural, that is, almost without pain; the patient, after its exhibition, feels but little inconvenience from pain, which soon subsides, and menstruation is immediately augmented, without acceleration of the pulse or gastric uneasiness. There are few other emmenagogues that can claim this feature.

"'Its action in amenorrhœa I think superior to any other emmenagogue belonging to the materia medica, though it would be proper to pay some attention to the general health of the patient before exhibition. It is superior to anything that I have tried in the way of emmenagogues. I have had cases in which I first tried the usual emmenagogues, with but little effect, or success, when I would determine on trying the decoction of this root, which would far surpass my expectations, by acting with the most marked effect; menstruation being produced on the following day after its exhibition. All of the symptoms disappeared on exhibition of this medicine. I believe this to be the best emmenagogue that we can employ in mere suppressio mensium, where there is no other disturbance in the general health.

"'With the usual emmenagogues, I was unable to produce the catamenia on a young lady, which continued for about twenty-four hours, then suddenly became very sparce and painful; and in a few days after this period had passed, I employed the infusion of the cotton root as a means of exciting this function, which it did on the following day, a plentiful discharge being produced, which continued for five or six days. She has been regular at every period since that time, and has enjoyed good health with the exception of a few simple attacks, which caused no derangement of the menstrual function. For about twelve months previous to the exhibition of this medicine, her health was very much impaired, but she commenced improving, and soon recovered her health. I could detail other cases similar, in which I have tried the decoction with the same effect, but I deem it unnecessary to mention its action in each individual case.

"'As a parturient agent, I think it superior to ergot in one sense of the word, and in another about its equal, its action being about as prompt as that of ergot, and attended with much less danger. I have tried both in parturition, and found the cotton root decoction to act with fully as much efficacy as ergot. In some cases in which I have tried it, the pain was to some extent allayed, and labor promoted with as much speed as when ergot was administered. It appears to be perfectly harmless, from the fact that its action is almost unattended with pain. It causes neither gastric distress, or acceleration of the pulse—if it does, it is not perceptible—both of which are occasioned by ergot to some extent.

"'I have witnessed its action in retained placenta with good effect, which was an expulsion of the mass in about twenty minutes after the exhibition of the first dose. It may be proper to say, that I gave two doses before the placenta was thrown off. I believe it to be safer as a parturient agent, or an emmenagogue, or at least as safe, as any other article of the materia medica.

"'It should have a fair and impartial trial by the profession generally, because it will prove itself worthy of the time and labor spent in its investigation. It is handy to all, and free of expense.

A few trials by the profession will confirm the truth of this short essay. Give it a trial, and it will prove itself in some cases of amenorrhœa, dysmenorrhœa, or probably in some lingering case of labor, which may require the assistance of medicine, to produce contraction of the uterus for the expulsion of the child. I think it worthy of the attention of the profession, in the above cases.

" '*Tincture of Cotton Root as a Tonic.*—There is a condition of the system in which this tincture acts as a valuable restorative. These cases are of a leuoco-phlegmatic temperament of both sexes, but it is to the female sex that I wish to draw the attention of the reader. Where there is general bad health, accompanied with tardy menstruation, I have used it with the happiest effect; in a few cases of emansio mensium, caused by anæmia, where the patient was troubled with pains in the loins and giddiness of the head, with a derangement of the digestive organs, such as anorexia, accompanied with an uneasy, depressed feeling at the scrobiculus cordis, every month, which was promptly relieved by the tincture, but not with the effect of producing the menstrual flux, which was afterwards produced by the decoction, I find it necessary to continue the tincture from two to four weeks. The strength of the tincture that I have been in the habit of using, is prepared thus:—Bark of the root (dry), eight ounces; diluted alcohol, two pounds; digest fourteen days, then filter and give it in one drachm doses, three or four times a day. The tincture which I used was prepared by myself; and as I have seen no account of its use, I claim the first preparation of it, as well as the first experiment with it. My brother, Dr. H. J. Shaw, has since tried it, with the same good effect; in fact, his experience coincides with mine throughout.'

" 'The cotton seed has acquired considerable reputation as an anti-periodic in cases of intermittent fever, the use of which originated with a planter in South Carolina, who says:—'I have never failed to cure a patient, with a single dose of it, even where large doses of quinine have failed.'

" 'It is, however, in the peculiar active properties, of the *root*, that the profession will be chiefly interested. The, oftentimes, great danger in administering ergot, prevents its use, even when its specific effects seem to be called for. If these specific effects can be obtained by the use of the cotton root, and this too, without the liability of injury to the general system (and these have been attributed to it), the profession would do well to give it a thorough and extensive trial."—(*Tilden's Journal*).

I here leave the consideration of this plant for the investigation of my colleagues.

HAMAMELIS VIRGINICA.

(*Witch Hazel.*)

This is an indigenous shrub, sometimes called *Winter-bloom*, *Snapping-hazlenut*, *Spotted Alder*, etc. It consists of several crooked, branching trunks, from the same root, from two to six inches in diameter, ten or twelve feet in height, and covered with a smooth, gray, and *spotted* bark. It is a much larger shrub than the edible hazle-nut, which has a *straight* trunk, *not* spotted, but *brownish*. The Hamamelis vir., grows in almost all sections of the United States, especially in damp woods, flowering from September to November, when the leaves are falling, and maturing the seeds the next summer. The bark and leaves are the parts used in medicine; they have a pleasant, aromatic odor, and a bitter, astringent taste, leaving a sense of pungency and sweetness in the mouth. Water extracts their virtues. The shoots are used as "divining rods" to discover water and metals under ground, by certain adepts in the occult arts. They have been used, also, by certain superstitious quacks, for the cure of old ulcers, etc., by *rubbing* them on the diseased surface. Strange as it may seem, cures are alleged to have been made in this manner. There has always been a large amount of superstition connected with this shrub. The popular preparation known as "Pond's Extract of Hamamelis," is made from the leaves and twigs, by a process of distillation. It is used by all the schools of medicine as an *anodyne* application. It cannot be expected, however, that it will relieve or benefit all the diseases mentioned on the extensive labels of the manufacturer, and the physician who pins his faith thereupon will be disappointed. This remedy, like all others, has its limited sphere of usefulness.

General Application.—Allopathic authors deem it hardly worthy of mention. Wood barely notices it in his Dispensatory, as a mild astringent, and discutient. Eclectics make more mention. King says it is tonic, astringent, and sedative; useful in hæmoptysis, hæmatemesis, and other hæmorrhages; also diarrhœa, dysentery, and excessive mucus discharges:—"It has been employed with advantage in incipient phthisis, in which it is supposed to unite anodyne influences with its others; used as an application to painful tumors, and external inflammations; also, as a wash for sore mouth; an injection in bowel complaints, prolapsus ani and uteri, leucorrhœa, gleet, piles, and ophthalmia." These authors say that the decoction may be taken internally, in any quantity, and applied externally of any strength. No fears are entertained that it will prove injurious. The Hamamelis has been used in homœopathic practice for twelve or fifteen years. Several physicians claim the honor of introducing it to the profession, among whom are Hering, Okie, and Preston. I believe Dr. Okie was the first to write concerning the medicine, although he says Dr. Hering was the first to call his attention to the remedy. Dr. Hering, it seems, became acquainted with its virtues while attending Mr. Pond, the proprietor of the Extract, who informed him what it was. Dr. Okie says:

"Hering proceeded at once, by scientific trials, to discover for himself whether the remedy did, or did not, possess any or all of the virtues attributed to it by its proprietor." Hering informed Dr. Cushing that he had used Pond's Extract in "chronic effects from mechanical injuries," painful and bleeding hæmorrhoids, and "severe pleuritic stitches supervening on tuberculous phthisis." He considers it a "union of Aconite and Arnica." It is a little strange that no regular proving has been made. If Dr. Hering has made any proving the profession has never seen it. Dr. Preston made a fragmentary proving, which was published in the Philad. Jour. of Hom., vol. 1., page 460. We shall have to make use of that, and the pathogenetic and clinical notes scattered through the various journals.

Vascular System—*Arterial System.*—Hamamelis does not seem to affect the heart and arteries *directly*. It does not appear to control arterial inflammation, or congestion, or hæmorrhage; but, according to all observers, its sphere of action is especially upon the *Venous System.* Of the few pathogenetic symptoms we have, not many point unmistakably to an affection of this system. But we have abundant clinical experience to prove that this remedy is one of the most prominent we possess for inflammation of veins, venous congestion, hæmorrhage, etc. In Dr. Preston's proving will be found the pathogenetic symptoms in full, such as "crowding fulness of blood in the head and neck; sense of suffocation, etc.; also "uterine hæmorrhage," "Epistaxis."

Clinical Remarks.—As early as 1851, Dr. Preston writes: "It has been used by many physicians in Rhode Island, in cases of venous congestion, and hæmorrhage, with great success." "*Ex uso in morbis*," I have made many trials of the efficacy of Hamamelis. Have given it successfully in a number of cases of Epistaxis, some of which were of an alarming character, and the cure has been prompt and effectual. One case of active uterine hæmorrhage, caused by a fall, was promptly relieved by it, but its particular sphere seems to be in passive hæmorrhages and venous congestions. I have cured many cases of passive uterine hæmorrhages with it, and have given it with success in a few cases of pulmonary hæmorrhage. But the crowning point of its virtue rests in its peculiar, prompt action in cases of phlegmasia alba dolens, and in varicose veins. In old cases of varicosis I have never seen its equal, and have cured many cases of varicose veins of the leg and foot, which have resisted all other treatment for years." Dr. Preston states that Dr. Henry, then of Selma, Alabama, was the first to recommend the Hamamelis to our use, and thinks he might furnish us with valuable therapeutic and pathogenetic information, but I have not been able to find anything from his pen on the subject. Dr. Okie estimates the Hamamelis highly, in phlegmasia alba dolens, varicose ulcers, and varicoses. He has used it successfully in hæmoptysis, epistaxis *purpura*, bleeding and painful piles, etc. (Phila. Jour. of Hom., vol. 1, p. 536).

Dr. Belcher reports the following cases, which I have somewhat abridged:—

Case 1st.—Vomiting and purging of blood (see "*Intestinal*").

Case 2nd.—A boy, aged fourteen, growing rapidly, with a good appetite, has had Epistaxis at irregular intervals of from four to twenty-four hours, by which he has become pale and much enfeebled. Ham. 3rd, one-eighth of a drop twice a day was given, and since the first dose to the present time, three months, he has had no return.

Case 3rd.—*Melœna* (see "*Intestinal*").

Case 4th.—A case of *Varioloid.* At a certain stage of the disease there came on Epistaxis, which lasted about an hour, ceased, and returned in a few hours, and continued. "The blood was dark, discharging freely in drops; the pulse rapid; breathing hurried; lips and mouth dry; the face and body were covered (besides the papulæ, which seemed to me not to have progressed, but to have shrunken) with a dusky red erythema, with purpural spots, varying from the size of a pin-head to that of a three-cent piece, here and there—but over the abdomen, which I more particularly examined, occupying one-third of the surface. The vessels of the conjunctiva were so congested, as at first sight to appear like chemosis. Gave *Hamamelis*, three drops of the first dilution in a tumbler of water, of which a table-spoonful was given every fifteen minutes. In twenty minutes the hemorrhage had ceased entirely, and returned no more. The medicine was then continued every hour. The next day he had one ejection of a dark, bloody character, but the purpura had not increased, and he had slept some. Gave Rhus. 2, and Ham. 2, alternately every hour. In two days he was out of danger, and convalesced rapidly—(N. A. Jour. vol. 3, page 463.) Dr. Belcher states that "hemorrhage with asthenia or anæmia, or from asthenic tendency, is of itself an indication for the use of Hamamelis." He considers sulphuric acid an analogue of Hamamelis, but its action is not so prompt. Further notice of its action in venous diseases will be mentioned under other heads.

Head.—A crowding fulness of blood in the head and neck. The epistaxis was accompanied with a feeling of tightness of the bridge of the nose, and considerable crowding pressure in the forehead, between the eyes, with a benumbed sensation over the whole os frontis.—(*Preston.*) A painful fulness of the brain, especially at the top, with a desire to hear lofty, sublime conversation, attended with perfect indisposition to talk, myself; feeling as if a bolt was passed from temple to temple through the head, and tightly screwed, accompanied by a feeling as if she ought to be reverenced by all around her.—(*Burrett.*)

Clinical Remarks.—The above symptoms would seem to indicate a condition of passive congestion, or venous stagnation, resulting in hemorrhage from the overloaded vessels. In *headache*, arising from congestion, and resulting in epistaxis, this may prove an excellent remedy. Many cases are only relieved by bleeding from the nose. The Hamamelis acts by removing the *cause*, and in this manner arrests the bleeding, if present, and removes the condition upon which it depends. We have but little clinical testimony as to its value in *Cephalalgia*. It will probably never be found as useful as Belladonna, Aconite, or Geiseminum.

Nose.—*Epistaxis*, with a feeling of tightness of the bridge of the nose, and considerable crowding pressure in the forehead between the eyes. (This was caused by one drop of the 3d, in Dr. Preston, who never before had bleeding from the nose.) *Profuse Epistaxis* (ten hours after taking one drop of the 3d).

Clinical Remarks.—We have found in the various Journals, over one hundred cases of epistaxis, some of them of an alarming character, which were promptly arrested by the use of Hamamelis in some form. A few of these cases have been given under the head of "Venous System," and others, of a notable character, are given briefly below. Dr. Belcher cured a severe case in a boy aged fourteen, with Hamamelis 3d, one-eighth of a drop. The bleeding had not returned several months after. Dr. Preston in an article on venous hemorrhages writes:—"Epistaxis, or bleeding from the nose, forms the most common hemorrhage of childhood, and in a great proportion of cases is simple and perfectly harmless. When it is dependent upon active congestion it is usually arterial, and proves its own remedy; when it is the result of mechanical congestion, or forms one of the developments of the hemorrhagic diathesis, it is passive and probably venous." Dr. P. gives an interesting case, illustrating its treatment with Hamamelis.

"An old gentleman, hemiplegic, who had been subject to occasional attacks of hæmorrhage from the nose, often profuse and very debilitating, and on several occasions requiring Mr. Abernethy's operation of plugging the nostrils, before it could be stopped. He had now been afflicted at intervals of several days with slight oozing of very dark blood from the schneiderian membrane, particularly three times a day and shortly after meals, corresponding to the rhythmical exacerbation of the pulse; after the afternoon meal the bleeding was very profuse. He was able to walk about, but complained of feeling very weak and faint, with occasional vertigo or confusion of ideas; his countenance was pale, and his pulse decidedly hemorrhagic. I ordered him home, and to keep perfectly quiet; to use a strong nourishing diet, with wine at each meal, and gave him China and Hamamelis 3rd, in alternation every two hours. I was sent for to his house in the afternoon and evening, and the bleeding had been almost constant, but, slowly oozing from his nose since he got home; by evening he was too weak and faint to set up, but lay in bed with his head raised; gave China and Hamamelis 1st. The hemorrhage increased however, all the next day, when small pieces of linen were wet with Hamamelis tincture, rolled up in the shape of a funnel, and pushed as far into the nostrils as possible. The next morning the bleeding had been very slight, exhaustion much less, and all other symtoms improving. In three days he was able to go about his business." Dr. Burnet, of N. O., reports "a lady of plethoric habits, had epistaxis twenty-four hours, which all ordinary means had failed to relieve. At a previous attack she came near bleeding to death; I gave her Hamamelis 3rd, and a wash of diluted tincture for her nose. The hemorrhage was arrested in a few moments, but returned, by coughing, the next day. It was again arrested by the same means, and did not return."

Mouth.—Dryness of the mouth; burnt sensation on the tongue.

Clinical Remarks.—I have used the Hamamelis satisfactorily in bleeding from the buccal cavity, bleeding and spongy gums, and hæmorrhage from the cavity after extraction of a tooth. In cases of *burns* of the tongue and lips, from hot drinks, a weak solution of this medicine held in the mouth gives prompt relief.

Eyes.—It has proved curative in painful inflammation of the eyes; excessive congestion of the conjunctiva and bruises of the orbits. It is useful in extravasations under the conjunctiva, and painless sugillations on the eyeball. During pertussis the eyeball sometimes becomes congested, and the minute vessels are ruptured. A wash of Hamamelis quickly dissipates the extravasations.

Throat.—Dry, thirsty feeling of the throat, which water would not relieve, lasting full twenty-four hours.—(*Burritt.*) Fulness in the neck; have to sleep with the neck free of any covering.

Clinical Remarks.—There is a condition of the fauces, and throat, which might not inaptly be designated as *varicosis*, the posterior fauces, uvula, and pharynx are of a blueish hue, caused by distended veins which ramify on the surface; this causes a fulness, with cough, and pain in swallowing, and sometimes hawking of dark colored blood, mixed with mucous. In one case of this character the internal and topical use of Hamamelis proved curative.

Stomach and Bowels.—*Hæmatemesis, Constipation, Hæmorrhoids.*

Clinical Remarks.—The primary effect of Hamamelis in material doses, is to diminish the secretions of the mucous surfaces of the intestinal tract; a form of constipation is the result. In none of the fragmentary provings which we possess is there any symptom relating to congestion, or hæmorrhage from the stomach and bowels, but our clinical experience is rich in cases of such hæmorrhage. Dr. Burnett in *Am. Hom. Review*, vol. 1, page 512, reports: "a lady who had been expected to die for several days, from hæmatemesis. I had none of the Hamamelis by me, and ordered a decoction of the bark—a teaspoonful every three hours. It cured the patient immediately." Writing of hæmorrhage from the bowels, or melæna, Dr. Preston says: "I have given Hamamelis with-success in arresting hæmorrhage, when I knew the bleeding proceeded from carcinomatous ulceration, as well as where it arose, from simple mechanical congestion of the portal circulation. To show that others have had like success with the same remedy, I relate a case of melæna, probably of the latter kind, reported to me by my brother-in-law, Dr. George S. Green, of Hartford, Ct. July, 1855, Mr. M——, aged twenty, light hair, dark eyes, spare figure, etc., came home from his business with a violent headache, and took a dose of Calomel at night, followed by one of Castor Oil in the morning; this he did on his own responsibility, and the consequence was a severe diarrhœa, for which Dr. Schae was called upon to prescribe. Dr. S. attended him ten days, and reports his discharges to have been very profuse and watery, as often as every half hour, accompanied with more or less fever, but no pain. After ten days the Dr. left him convalescent, but quite weak, and, intending to leave for his home in Massachusetts. Two days after, quite early in the morning, he had a very large discharge of dark clotted blood, and within an hour, two more discharges, the three filling a large-sized chamber pot; very offensive but attended by no pain. At this time I first saw him, in consultation with Dr. S. I examined the discharges; found the patient pale and much exhausted, aware of danger but not frightened; pulse 120–130, weak, intermitting, hæmorrhagic; no tenderness on pressure in any part of the abdomen; no enlargement of liver or spleen that could be felt; no pain, nothing but great weakness, and occasional faintness. A week previous to this hæmorrhage he had two discharges from the bowels, that were liquid, and brick colored, with a greasy scum; his appetite had been unusually good, but his countenance pallid and sunken. On the seventh day after this attack, when I was called, he had another discharge from the bowels, of dark, grumous, offensive smelling blood, which continued to pass away from him with a gurgling noise, until three large sheets were saturated. On the next day he passed about a tea-cupful of bright red blood, and the hæmorrhage ceased. He was sick in the house eight weeks; his hair fell off, and he was somewhat anasarcous in the lower extremities, but from the first, had no pain, and, after the hæmorrhage, no fever; his recovery, perfect. The only remedies used were stimulation, China, and Hamamelis virginica. This case was unquestionably one of mechanical congestion of the portal circulation, and the hæmorrhage was probably caused by the action of the powerful cathartics taken in the commencement. It is unnecessary for me to say, that in my opinion, both the diarrhœa and hæmorrhage might have been avoided by judicious treatment in the beginning, because the congestion might have been removed without such violent result; but the symptoms having been caused, the treatment certainly proved successful." We might relate several other cases of melæna, as well as of hæmatemesis, dependant upon other causes besides mechanical congestion, in all of which Hammamelis was of great service in arresting and preventing hæmorrhage, which otherwise would probably have proved fatal. George E. Belcher, M. D., of New York, reports the two following cases: *Case* 1., James (a porter), aged about thirty, a well-built, muscular Irishman, after complaining about three days (as near as I could ascertain) of fullness, and grumbling, aching pains in the abdomen, and irregular febrile flushes, was attacked with vomiting, and purging of blood, which gradually increased. In the morning of the day the hæmorrhage began, his employer sent him Nux v. 3, and *Acon.* 3; to be taken alternately; but, as by evening there was no improvement, I was sent for, and gave *Ipec.* 1, and *Merc.* sol. 2, alternately, every hour. Early on the following morning I received information that the hæmorrhage continued, and that he was faint, cold, and sweating profusely. I found him so, indeed, with a weak, rapid pulse, restless, and complaining of the fullness and grumbling in the abdomen; but, owing to the imperfect domestic arrangements,

I could not ascertain how much blood had been vomited or purged. I gave *Hamamelis*, two drops of the tincture dissolved in half a tumbler of water, of which a dessert-spoonful was given every fifteen or twenty minutes, until improvement took place. This was very apparent, when I called two hours afterwards; a reaction was moderately but firmly established, and the patient *felt* better. He had vomited once only, and but a small quantity of blood; and the melæna from this time diminished, so that it disappeared, nearly, if not entirely, in two or three days. I substituted *Chin.* and *Merc.* for the *Ham.* in about twenty-four hours after improvement had begun, and continued them, on account of the apparent hepatic congestion, to convalescence.

Case 2. W. A. B. A man aged about forty, temperate, of a spare habit, after complaining two or three days of fulness through the hypochondria, and attacked with diarrhœa, on account of which he called at my office, and for which I gave him *Ars.* 3. The next day, not being relieved, I was sent for; found him feeble, with blank, dingy-reddish countenance; thirst; frequent pulse; and having a loose evacuation about every three or four hours, which he described as offensive, and of the color of dark rosewood. Not seeing it, I concluded that it must be melæna, and gave *Ham.* and *Acon.*; a solution of two or three drops of each in tumblers of water, of table spoonful doses, were directed to be given alternately every two hours, until better. The next day I found him feeling decidedly improved, having had but one small discharge since. From this time he rapidly convalesced.

Dr. L. Pratt communicated to the Chicago Hom. Medical Society, 1859, the following case of *Intestinal hemorrhage.* A young man whose health had been injured by ague and quinine, was attacked, during the course of a typhoid fever, with copious bleeding from the bowels. The blood passed by the rectum amounted to at least two quarts before I saw him. He had stools of blood about once in fifteen minutes; it was of a dark grumous nature. Four drops of the mother-tincture of Hamamelis, in a tumbler of water, a desert-spoonful to be taken every ten minutes until the discharges were arrested, for an hour—omit for an hour—then to take one dose more. Afterwards omit until a relapse occurred. The next day ascertained that the bleeding had twice returned, but was at once arrested by a single drop each time. The patient recovered under the use of Arsenicum and China. In this case the bleeding probably originated in ulceration of some portion of the intestines; was of a passive character, and perhaps venous. It would seem from the above cases, that Hamamelis is curative in several forms of hemorrhage from the bowels.

(1) That caused by portal congestion.
(2) From a ruptured vessel.
(3) From ulceration of the bowels.
(4) From a hemorrhoidal vein.

In *Dysentery*, the Hamamelis is indicated when the amount of blood in the stools, is unusual in quantity, and amounts to an actual hemorrhage. The blood in such cases is generally dark, in small clots or patches, scattered through the mucus. Dr. Dunn, of Ill., (Ill. State Hom. Ass., 1858) said he "had not found Mercurius so effectual in the treatment of dysentery, during the past summer, as it had formerly been; but he had been highly successful with Hamamelis, in cases of dysentery, in which the alvine evacuations were largely loaded with blood."

In the so-called *hæmorrhoidal* dysentery, this remedy is almost specific, alone, although it may sometimes have to be alternated with Aloes or Podoph. In my practice benefit has accrued both from the internal and topical application. A few drops of the tincture or lower dilutions, every hour or two, internally; and an enema of one drachm of tincture Hamamelis to four ounces of cold water, or starch water. The decoction of the bark (one oz. to one qt. water) is even better than the above preparation for an enema, both in dysentery and bleeding hemorrhoids.

In *Diarrhœa*, the Hamamelis is said to have been found useful, but the indications for its use are not ascertained. It will require more extended provings and clinical experiments, to establish its applicability to diarrhœa. I would suggest that it may be useful in mucus and serous discharges. It is in *Hemorrhoids*, that the Hamamelis has achieved some of its greatest victories. It seems to have extraordinary power over this disease, not only as externally manifested in the form of hemorrhoidal tumors, but against the primary cause, which is often located in the portal system. It has been used in this affection from the earliest history of the country. The aborigines first imparted a knowledge of its curative virtues to the first settlers. It is mentioned as a remedy for piles, used *externally*, in the works of the early "*Botanic*" physicians. When Pond first sold his Extract, it was recommended particularly for this complaint. Dr. Hering was Pond's family physician, and was induced by him to try its efficacy in some diseases. In 1850 Dr. Hering informed Dr. Cushman, a pupil of Dr. Okie, that he had used it successfully in "painful and bleeding hemorrhoids." Dr. Okie was then induced to test its virtues, and in a letter to Hering, published in 1853, he says: "I next made use of the Hamamelis in a number of cases of *painful* and *bleeding* piles. Those cases in which it has proved most beneficial in my hands, are characterized by burning, soreness, fulness, and, at times, rawness of the anus; in the back a weakness or weariness, or as the patients graphically express it, 'Doctor, my back feels as if it would break off.' The hemorrhage is generally profuse, and I have in several instances seen this latter symptom cured completely, with shrinking of the over-loaded hemorrhoidal vessels, so that the full, pouting look of the anus was changed to its own more natural and demure pucker, while the burning and itching, depending more upon cutaneous irritability, or some herpetic taint, still remained. I have here likewise made a wash of the remedy, applying it externally while giving it internally in the more dilute form. Mr. T., a highly respectable agriculturalist, somewhere in the fifties, had been troubled with painful and bleeding piles for a number of years. On examination I found the anus surrounded with a crop of tumid hemorrhoidal veins, bluish in color, and the whole anus encircled by a red erythemic halo. I found he suffered with 'back-ache,' has a 'pasty mouth,' digestion tolerable, was not much constipated; I gave Hamamelis first dilution six drops night and morning and applied a lotion, one-third of the remedy, two-thirds distilled water. In a fortnight he called again and I found him much relieved. I repeated the prescription, to be taken once a day. Since which time he has remained well."

Dr. Davidson, (*Monthly Hom. Review*, London,) reports a case of "burning, painful hemorrhoids," in a lady, who had been subject to attacks of piles for the last ten years. Her symptoms were "great suffering from weight, and pressure, at the anus; hemorrhoids protruding; great exhaustion from frequent hemorrhage from the rectum; bowels constipated; severe frontal headache; restless nights; mouth parched and dry on awaking. Hamamelis 6, ten drops in six ounces of water; one table spoonful three times a day. The third day after, the hemorrhoidal symptoms were much relieved, but she complained of severe pains in the back. Continued the medicine. Five days after, the hemorrhoids were painful and protruding. A new symptom had also developed itself. My patient wished me to examine her arms, as during the past two days she had suffered severely from a peculiar *pricking pain, from the wrist to the shoulder, which pain is increased on pressure.* On examining the arms, I found that the patient indicated the direction of the pain along the course of the superficial veins. Ordered *Sacch. lactis* to be continued the next three days, when the pricking pain had quite left her arms; but the hemorrhoids were still troublesome. Hamamelis 6—thirty drops in six ounces of water, to be used as a lotion. A pledget of lint, saturated with this, to be applied to the protruding hemorrhoids every night. Six days after she reported herself well. Six months after, the same patient applied again. She was suffering from protruding hemorrhoids, accompanied by severe inflammation. she also had catarrhal symptoms, and was very desponding. Hamamelis 6 was given as above, and the lotion used as before. She took only five doses, because,—'after the fourth dose she became very much alarmed by a *pricking pain* in the region of the heart. The hemorrhoids, however, were much relieved. Ordered *Sacc. Lact.* Two days after, the pricking pain "about the heart" was still very severe; it was also now felt in the courses of the superficial veins of both arms. These pricking pains continued for a period of ten days, increasing in intensity during that time. At length I prescribed Arnica 12, three times a day. Two weeks after the patient states that she feels better than she has done for years; and the piles, to use her own expression, 'have been completely vanquished. I must not forget to record, that while under treatment, this patient had been relieved, by the Hamamelis, of a peculiar tightness of the chest, from which she had suffered from childhood." This case presents some interesting peculiarities, namely: the apparent pathogenetic symptoms caused by the Hamamelis, simulating inflammation of the veins, and even the heart.

The question might arise, would not the same pains, etc., have arisen during the course of an attack of inflammation of the hemorrhoidal veins, had the Hamamelis *not* been administered? However, Hahnemann would undoubtedly have placed these symptoms in the pathogenesis of Hamamelis, and we may do the same; still, we could wish that further experiments would substantiate the reliability of these symptoms as purely belonging to the drug, in which case they would be very important as indicating, unmistakably, its sphere of action.

Urinary Organs.—Scanty, high-colored urine.

CLINICAL REMARKS.—The Hamamelis has been found useful in *hæmaturia.* Several cases presenting the symptom—bloody urine—have been reported, cured by this remedy.

"In Hæmaturia"—writes Dr. Preston—"China and Hamamelis are the principal remedies, unless there be ulceration of the prostate, or neck of the bladder, when these should be alternated with Asterias-rubens. In all hemorrhages dependent upon *Scirrous*, or carcinomatus ulceration, we have used Hamamelis to control the hemorrhage, and Asterias rnbens to arrest the ulcerative process, and we have had more than ordinary success with these remedies in a number of cases. In *urethral* and *renal* hemorrhages, China, Cantharis, Mezereum, and Terebinth, are recommended, but we have had cases of congestion of the tubuli uriniferi, following Scarlatina, and attended with discharges of black blood from the kidneys, when neither of them, nor Dig. Hamamelis, Zinc, and a host of others, had any good effect, that were cured in two or three days by the use of Gallic acid, in three grain doses three times a day."

Dr. Belcher reports the following case, which perhaps can be classed among *renal* effections: "A lady, who, while pregnant, had alburminaria and general anasarca, with occasional vaginal discharges of blood. She was prematurely confined, when about six and a half months advanced, and then had adherent placenta, which, until detached, caused her to flood so profusely as to be faint and fainting for four or five hours. About twelve or fourteen days afterwards she was attacked with dysentery, which lasted four or five days; about ten or twelve days after this, with the ague and fever; after this, flooding again, which last attack was controlled without difficulty by the Hamamelis second, repeated every three or four hours."

Organs of Generation of Women.—Hemorrhage from the uterus, of bright and fresh blood, not coagulable, about midway between the menstrual periods, (from one drop of the third—(Dr. Preston). Active uterine hemorrhage in a young lady. (See Preston's fragmentary provings.)

CLINICAL REMARKS.—Dr. Preston, who reports the pathogenetic symptoms referred to above, remarks that in the first case, that "a *leucorrhœa* which the lady had been troubled with for years, ceased as soon as she began taking the Hamamelis, and has not again appeared." It is a common and popular domestic remedy, in form of a decoction, used as a vaginal enema, and generally with considerable success. Eclectic writers recommend it in leucorrhœa with relaxation of the vaginal walls, but consider its action that of an "astringent." True, the Hamamelis contains *tannin* in quite an appreciable quantity, but even tannin is homœopathic—secondarily—to some forms of leucorrhœa. *Hamamelis*, used internally and topically, is one of the most useful medicines in those varieties of leucorrhœa which similate a hemorrhage, and constitute a drain on the system as severe as a bleeding. In most cases, however, it should be alternated with Pulsatilla, Sepia, Helonias or Senecio gracilis.

Dr. Okie, in his letter to Dr. Hering, says he found it useful in *Ovarian Disease*: "My first use of the remedy was in the case of a colored girl, twenty-two years of age, of plethoric habit, who at the age of eighteen, had received a violent blow over the left ovarian region, and since that time had suffered with violent pains, at times concentrating themselves in the seat of the original injury, and again producing a diffused and agonizing soreness over the whole abdomen; the touch aggravated these sufferings intensely; the left ovarian region was swollen, flat on percussion; the menses were irregular, very painful, with exacerbation of all the sufferings at the catamenial epoch. Examination per vaginum, disclosed exquisite tenderness of the canal, a swollen and tumid os uteri, which was likewise extremely sensitive; passing the finger by the side of the neck of the womb, and pressing upward toward the left ovarian region, likewise caused extreme suffering. This patient was frequently afflicted with retention of urine, and I had been obliged to use the catheter for several days together. I made use of the Hamamelis in this case, both internally and externally. I made use of Pond's extract. After using it she was much relieved; could bear pressure upon the swollen part (the swelling having notably diminished); the diffused soreness was less marked. She bore the vaginal examination with more ease. A gradual return to health set in, from the time the Hamamelis was commenced." Dr. R. Ludlam informs us that he has found this medicine a most important remedy, internally and locally, in all ovarian diseases, accompanied with *swelling* and *tenderness* of those organs. He advises compresses, wet in the dilute tincture, constantly applied to the sensitive locality. It was found very useful by Dr. Burnett, in varices during pregnancy.—"A woman in the fourth month of pregnancy with her seventh child. She was compelled to labor for her livelihood; suffered almost always with varicose veins; at this time she was very lame; suffered much pain and could scarcely move about. I gave twelve globules of Hamamelis third dil., and a wash of diluted tincture. She took four pills at a dose, two doses a day. The first day she felt entire relief from pain, and could exercise with ease. She required no further treatment; I attended her in her confinement and found no trace of her former malady." "A lady pregnant with her fourth child. She complained of a painful stiffness and a sensation of swelling and weakness in her left leg, which continued to some extent during pregnancy; but the Hamamelis gave her prompt relief, and there was no return of it after confinement." "A woman pregnant with her fifth child. During her last three pregnancies she had been troubled severely with varicose veins, which, after the fifth month, had burst above the ankle and bled profusely. When I was called to see her, she was only four months advanced in pregnancy, but the bleeding had commenced, and she was anticipating a serious time. I gave her Hamamelis three times a day, diluted tincture for a wash. She had no more bleeding, and is now well." Dr. F. Burnett, of New Orleans, found the Hamamelis useful in Dysmenorrhœa:—"A colored woman aged thirty-five. Two years previous, at the time the menses should have appeared, she experienced severe pain through the lumbar and hypogastric regions and down the legs; fullness of the bowels and brain, with severe pain through the whole head, resulting in stupor and deep sleep, lasting twelve to thirty-six hours, from which it was impossible to arouse her; after which she gradually returned to her natural state, and so remained till the time for the next menstrual period, when the same suffering was repeated. She was brought to me at the commencement of one of these paroxysms; the pain in the back, pubic region, and head, had already commenced. I gave eight globules of the fifteenth dilution of Hamamelis, to be taken in two doses, four hours apart, which established her menses perfectly without any further medication, and she continued to menstruate regularly afterward." "An Irish girl, aged eighteen, strong, robust make. She had never menstruated, but had suffered instead with hæmatemesis, constant constipation and varices of the legs. I gave her Hamamelis fifteenth, to be taken three times a day. Her menses appeared immediately, her legs got well, and I knew of her perfect health for three years afterwards, during which time she became a mother." This case illustrates its curative virtues in *vicarious menstruation*, when the condition is in correspondence with that caused by Hamamelis. An interesting case of *vicarious menstruation* is reported by Dr. Kenyon (Amer. Hom. Review, Vol. 2, p. 412): "Mary F., aged fourteen, has always enjoyed tolerable health until the last eighteen months, when she menstruated. The first time there was considerable pain in the back and head, for several days preceeding it, with nausea, vertigo, etc. The flow was natural, and recurred two succeeding months quite regularly, and without any of the unpleasant sensations which preceded the first. When the fourth period came round, there was no indication of menstruation, but in place of it, quite free *epistaxis*; this continued for several months, increasing in severity each month. She was emaciated very much; no color in the cheeks or lips; pulse 140, and feeble; action of the heart very labored, but not giving any signs of organic lesion; extremities considerably bloated; stomach very irritable; bowels constipated; urine scanty and clear; some cough, and great dyspnœa. It was the day when the bleeding was to return, and I watched the case; there was over a quart of blood lost; it was thin, forming very slight coagula. I gave her the sixth and thirtieth dil. in alternation, two doses of each in the twenty-four hours, which was all the medicine she got during the month following, except a few doses of Arsenicum for dyspnœa, when it was troublesome. When the next month came round, she menstruated regularly, and had no more bleeding, and from this time she went on rapidly to a perfect recovery, under the use of Hamamelis." In *Uterine Hemorrhage*, it is highly extolled by some physicians. Dr. Preston cured a case of "*active* uterine hemorrhage caused by a fall; it was promptly relieved by it;" but, he thinks, "its particular sphere seems to be in *passive* hemorrhages and venous congestions." He has "cured many cases of passive uterine hemorrhage with Hamamelis." Dr. W. E. Payne states, that he has not used the Hamamelis successfully in uterine hemorrhages, except when the blood flowed *steadily*, was *venous* in its character, and *without* uterine pains. My own experience accords with that of Dr. Payne's; therefore, I would not advise the use of this remedy in hemorrhage after labor, for here we want a remedy like Secale or Erigeron, which causes contraction of the muscular tissue of the uterus, and perhaps of the arteries. *Erigeron* is antipodal to Hamamelis. It is as directly indicated in active, *arterial* hemorrhage, as the latter is in passive *venous* bleedings.

Organs of Generation of Men, etc.—We are not in possession of pathogenetic symptoms relating to these organs, but it has been used in some diseases affecting the veins, testes, and contiguous tissues. Dr. Preston, in an able paper on "Diseases of the veins" (N. A. Jour. of Hom. 1857,) says. "The homœopathic treatment of *Circocele*. (Varicosis of the spermatic veins) is very much the same as for varicose veins in the leg, and in a number of cases under my own observation has been found successful. To illustrate this treatment, I prefer to give the following report of a case, sent me by Dr. Geo. Barrow, of Taunton, Mass.—"A friend of mine, about thirty years of age, a merchant of Chicago, of scrofulous tendencies, was taken some three months since with drawing pain in the left spermatic cord, with swelling heat, redness and pain in the cord and in the left testicle, for which an allopath treated him four or five days with warm fomentations and laudanum applied to the part. The testicle swollen four or five times its usual size; very hard and painful, was closely enveloped with collodion frequently applied (*to support the tumor*?) while seidlitz powders were given to keep the bowels open. As this treatment gave no relief, but the symptoms rather grew worse, my friend was easily pursuaded to abandon it and try the homœopathic plan. In consultation with Dr. Smith, of Chicago, where I happened to be present on a visit, I gave the patient, Bell., Puls., and Clematis, for a week, with very little benefit when I proposed to try Hamamelis. I accordingly obtained a bottle of "Ponds' extract," of which I administered drop doses every two hours, and enveloped the scrotum in a bandage wet with a solution of the same medicine, one part of the tincture to about ten parts of alcohol and water. In twenty-four hours he was free from all pain, the swelling gradually disappeared, and with the help of a silk suspensory bandage, he was able to resume his business in a few days, and now is entirely well." The Hamamelis was at one time highly lauded as an excellent remedy in the treatment of *Gonorrhœa*. It was advised to administer the remedy internally, and use the diluted tincture (or Ponds' ext.) as an injection. Dr.

Small informs me that in the first stage of this disease it has appeared to be of benefit, in allaying pain and inflammation. It may be useful in all stages, but cannot be looked upon as a specific remedy. I have advised it in long standing cases of *Gleet*, with apparent benefit. In *Orchitis*, it is highly praised by Dr. Ludlam. He states that under its *external* use the tumefaction and pain rapidly subsides. He considers it to have some specific power over inflammatory affections of the testes and ovaries.

Thoracic Organs.—Return of inflammation of the diaphragm with the following symptoms:—labored respiration; opressive tightness of the lower part of the thorax, inability to make a deep and full inspiration; when attempting to assume the recumbent posture breathing became almost impossible; a crowding fullness in the neck and head, and a sense of suffocation so as to prevent his lying down; unable to make a deep inspiration when standing up. (*Preston.*) Pricking pain in the region of the heart; felt also in the superficial veins of both arms. The pricking pains in the heart continued for ten days, increasing in intensity all the time. (Arnica twelfth was then given, and the pains disappeared.)—*Davison.*

Clinical Remarks.—Hamamelis has cured cough, and hæmoptysis, with taste of sulphur in the mouth, and dull frontal headache." Also "tickling cough, with taste of blood on waking." In *Hæmoptysis*, it is considered by some as a remedy *par excellence*, applicable to nearly all cases; but this is going too far. It can never take the place of Aconite. Dr. Preston (Diseases of Veins) says:—"In general we look upon Hamamelis as a specific for passive venous hemorrhages, and we have seen it successful in arresting this particular form of bleeding from the pulmonary mucous membrane; but we speak from only a few years experience, and that a few observers, and therefore we must be impartial enough to mention a few of those remedies which other practitioners have recommended as useful in the cure of some forms of hæmoptysis:—Aconite, Ipecac., Ferr., acet., Arnica, Millefol, etc. Dr. E. M. Payne (U. S. Jour. of Hom. Vol., I. p. 730) reports the following case:—A young lady aged sixteen, was seized while at school, and without any premonitory symptoms, with blood-spitting. The patient was of slender build, light hair, blue eyes, fair complexion, lax fibre, and phthisical diathesis; menses regular and normal. The blood-spitting commenced with a slight hack, and continued, with scarcely a moment's intermission up to the time of my visit, a period of nearly an hour. I found her lying upon a sofa, calm, with a napkin in hand nearly saturated with apparently pure venous blood, and spitting about the amount of a tea-spoonful at intervals of one or two minutes. The blood came into the mouth without any effort. She described it as issuing about ten inches below the right clavicle, in a warm current, making apparently a tortuous course, and at the same time there was a sensation in that region, as from the pressure of a hard body. Pulse somewhat accelerated, eighty-five. Ferrum aceticum was given but caused no improvement in three hours, Millefolium, Acon., Ipecac, and Belladonna caused no amelioration. Hamamelis, four drops of the tincture to half a tumbler of water. A spoonful was given. The bleeding immediately ceased, and did not afterwards return. I have never used the Hamamelis successfully, in cases of blood-spitting when the blood was of light fluid red, frothy in appearance, and raised by much cough." Dr. Okie reported an interesting case in which hæmoptysis was present, in a complicated lung affection. Hamamelis controlled the bleeding, but was powerless to *cure* the patient. A girl, aged, nine, was said to be in a dying state. She was sitting upright, supported by pillows, her breath greatly oppressed. She had been ill about two years, dating her first loss of health to a cough, which was said to have resulted from swallowing a small piece of straw; since that period, she had been tormented with incessant cough. She bled from the lungs pints at a time. She had raised large quantities of offensive matter; at one time "nearly a tumblerful." Examination elicited general anasarca, great swelling of the lower extremities; the abdomen swollen from the areolar infiltration; face much puffed, closing the eyelids; a number of spots resembling *purpura were found* upon the lower extremities; she had been troubled with profuse epistaxis. Auscultatory examination elicited the presence of a very long cavity, extending from the mammary region to near the base of the right side. The respiration in the left lung was puerile, with a mingling of rhonci and mucous rales. The urinary secretion was almost null, the urine itself of a deep brandy color, depositing a heavy lateritious sediment. I feared a fatal result, and speedily. The scant urinary secretions and pleuritic pains, the hydropic tendency, and the state of the thoracic organs, led me to fear the superventon of anæmia and serous effusion into the pleural sac. *Iodine* was given; for about a fortnight she improved; the urine was much increased; the dropsy lessened; the respiration easier; petechiæ did not appear; cough about as usual. At this time she was seized with *Epistaxis and Hœmoptysis* pulse full, etc. *Hamamelis* checked the hamorrhage promptly, and there was no recurrence. The strength, appetite, and general health of the patient improved, so that she was up, and about her usual avocations. She lived about eighteen months, but finally died from pulmonary abscess.—*Philal. Jour. Vol.* 1. *p.* 538.

Back.—Tearing pain across the small of the back, with fulness of the joints of the legs.—(*Burritt.*)

Clinical Remarks.—It has been found useful as an external application to lumbago, "crick in the back," myalgia, bed-sores, and petechia.

Upper and Lower Extremities.—*Pricking* pain in the superficial veins of both arms, extending from the wrists to the shoulder. (*Davison.*) Painful fulness of the joints of the legs, as if they would burst, which soon extends to all the joints of the body; after the fulness of the joints disappear, then there was a dread of moving the limbs, as if it would cause suffering, with a weary, stiff, full feeling.

Clinical Remarks.—The greatest triumph of Hamamelis, has been in the treatment of *varicoses* of the limbs. Dr. Preston, writing of *varicoses* remarks:—"Homœopathy has, as in many other cases, directed us to a specific remedy, which in my practice, as well as in that of a number of my colleagues in this section of the country, has been attended with uniform success in the treatment of this annoying disease. "Since 1851 (six years) I have prescribed Hamamelis in upwards of fifty cases of varicose veins of the lower limbs, and in no single instance has it failed to make a decided curative impression; but in the great majority of cases, it has, thus far at least, proved a radical cure. My plan is, first, to bandage the limb tightly from the arch of the foot to a little above the knee, or to the hips, if the varices are above the knee, and the best bandage, in my opinion, is an elastic silk stocking, manufactured for the purpose. Under this, compresses of linen are laid over the dilated veins, and kept wet with Hamamelis tincture, or Pond's extract. I give the 3d dil. internally, two or three times a day. Some few cases, with large, indolent ulcers on the tibia or malleolus, have been under treatment a year, but most of them have been cured, or at least have disappeared, in less than half that time. The crowning point of its (Hamamelis) virtues, rests in its peculiarly prompt action in cases of phlegmasia alba dolens, and in varicose veins. In old cases of varicosis, I have never seen its equal; and have cured many cases of varicose veins of the leg and foot, which had resisted all other treatment for years." Dr. Belcher reports several cases of varices in pregnant women, cured by Hamamelis. (See cases under "Organs of Generation of Women." Dr. Barrows found this medicine a valuable auxiliary in the treatment of a child, with the following symptoms:—"Inflammation of the femoral vein, with the erysipelatous spot near the groin, and over the vein, spreading over nearly one half of the thigh, with flexion of the leg; swelling of the entire leg and foot, with tension; heat and pale appearance of the limbs; scanty urine, stiffening the linen (albuminous); tympanitis; œdema of the whole body, limbs, and face. Calc., Hepar and other remedies, were used. (See case in full, in N. A. Journal, vol. 6, page 317.) Dr. R. Ludlam informs me that he considers the Hamamelis of the greatest advantage in all cases of articular rheumatism, with swollen and painful joints; as a *local application* it seems to possess decided anodyne properties. He advises that cloths, or cotton wool, wet in the dilute tincture, be applied constantly to the painful parts.

NOTE.—Just as this paper was ready for the printer, I received the "Hom. Review," for April, 1864, which contains a case of Phlebitis, reported by Dr. H. Robinson, Jr., cured by Hamamelis. The symptoms were: "Great pain in right leg, from the knee to the hip; leg much swollen, and quite sensitive to the touch. The cutaneous veins were hard, knotty, swollen, and painful. The skin erysipelatous; pulse small and wiry; much thirst; no appetite; bowels costive; urine red and scanty; veins of abdomen, hard, like cords, red and painful. Gave Hamamelis 1., five drops in half a goblet of water." Cured in ten days.

HELONIAS DIOICA.

(*False Unicorn Root.*)

This plant is known by the names of Drooping Starwort, Devil's Bit, etc. It is indigenous to the United States, growing in woodlands, meadows and moist situations. It is found in Canada, and as far south as Georgia and Louisiana. "The plant is sometimes mistaken for the Aletris Farinosa, but may be identified by the leaves of the *Aletris* being sharply pointed, with a straight, slender spike of scattered flowers, while the *Helonias* is not so sharply lance-shaped in its leaves, and has a thick plumose dioical spike. The *root* is the officinal part; it is tapering, fibrous, about an inch and a quarter in length, and from two to six-eighths of an inch in diameter, very hard, transversely wrinkled, and abrupt or præmorse at the end, appearing as though it had been cut or bitten off. There has been, and still exists, much difficulty among druggists, in determining the difference between the roots of the Aletris farinosa and Helonias dioica. It has often been the case that these roots have been indiscriminately bought and sold."—(*King.*) King, in his Dispensatory, gives a very minute description of the root of the Helonias, which I would advise our pharmaceutists to examine, for it is highly important that the preparations used by our school, should be genuine. It is quite probable that much of the fluid extract and active principle, Helonin, made in this country, is prepared from both plants mixed.

General Properties.—"The Helonias is *tonic*, diuretic, and vermifuge; in large doses, emetic; and when fresh, sialagogue. The plant is said to kill cattle feeding on it, and the decoction to kill insects. In doses of ten or fifteen grains of the powdered root, repeated three or four times a day, it has been found very beneficial in dyspepsia, loss of appetite, and for the removal of worms. It is reported beneficial in colic, and atony of the generative organs, etc."—*King.* "It is tonic, stomachic, diaphoretic, and pectoral; it is adapted to atonic states of the system; it has been recommended in cases of chronic rheumatism, jaundice, strangury, etc., also in colds, and coughs; it has been used as a remedy in low grades of fever, as a stimulant, with success, etc."—*Jones and Scudder.* "It is alterative, tonic, diuretic, vermifuge and emmenagogue, used in prolapsus uteri, amenorhœa, dymenorhœa, leucorrhœa, to prevent miscarriage, dyspepsia, worms, etc."—*Coe.* We can glean but little information as to the general sphere of action of this medicine, from the above farrago; that it has been used with benefit in the above mentioned diseases and conditions, I do not doubt, but we are still at a loss for any *special* indications; those which can only be obtained from a thorough proving.

The great majority of medical men of other schools do not realize the value of physiological experiments. They rely more upon uncertain empirical data, judging of the curative virtues of a medicine by its effects upon the sick. That this method has its value, we do not dispute; indeed, we may always feel confident that, a medicine which will *cure* a given group of symptoms, will cause similar ones, in healthy persons. We, therefore, look upon curative effects, as indication of pathogenetic effects. We have but a meagre proving of Helonias, and that only on the male. This I regret very much, for its action on the organism of women is notable and peculiar. I shall be able to present to the profession, however, some suggestive clinical facts, which will throw some light upon its remedial action. The following symptoms are obtained from a fragmentary proving sent me by Dr. C. H. Burr, of Portland, Maine. The proving in its original form, appears at the end of this article.

General Symptoms.—An unnatural degree of languor and a feeling of weariness and weight in the region of the kidneys; general weariness. (Burr.) "Decided increase in *muscular power* which continued as long as the remedy was taken" (in large doses).—*Dr. Close.*

Clinical Remarks.—This medicine is a peculiar and powerful "tonic," or, as Headland would have it "restorative." It is considered, particularly indicated when the disease has proceeded, (1) from disease of the *generative organs*, (2) or from functional disorders of the *stomach;* hence it is considered valuable in anæmia and chlorosis, in alternation with Ferrum; and in dyspepsia, in alternation with Nux vom., if indicated. It does not belong to the China group, because it has no anti-periodic powers; nor does it cause a hyper-stimulation of the nervous and vascular systems like that powerful drug. Neither does it have much more affinity for the Nux vomica group, for it does not excite or irritate the spinal system. It is more nearly allied to Ferrum than any other article of the Materia Medica, while, at the same time, it has some points of resemblance to the members of both groups above referred to. China and Nux vomica, together with their analogues, cause a condition, which may be described as increased tonicity of muscular fibre. China brings about this condition, through its influence upon the processes by which the blood is formed; it probably tends to augment the quantity of that fluid, and to render it richer. Thus, by its own operation upon the nutrition of the heart, and through the agency of the enriched blood, it gives greater energy to the contractions of that organ; and hence the fuller and stronger pulse, not unfrequently resulting from its moderate and continued use. But in cases of anæmia, chlorosis, and some other conditions of the system, China will not improve, apparently, the condition of the blood, or at least, the tissues do not respond to the stimulus of the improved blood. Then it is that Ferrum, or Nux vomica, given alternately with it, will place the diseased tissues in a condition to be benefitted by the circulating fluid, and a cure is soon effected. Nux vomica increases the tonicity of tissues, mainly through its influence upon the spinal system. It is a spinal stimulant, and nearly all its therapeutic effects arise from this action. In a great many cases of atony of any organ, or tissue of the body, this medicine will, alone, effect prompt and permanent cures; but, like China, it will sometimes fail, unless superseded or assisted by the action of China or Ferrum. There are also other instances wherein China, Ferrum and Nux will fail to improve the abnormal conditions for which they seem indicated, and the Helonias will here come in play, and be found very useful. Helonias enriches the blood, through its influences upon the nutritive processes; not as iron does, for iron is a metallic substance, and a vegetable substance cannot act in the same manner. But Helonias does not act like China or Quinine, for the latter stimulates by its direct primary action, while the former does not.

Mental Symptoms.—Mind dull and inactive. The previous cheerful state was followed by dullness, and gloominess; irritable; could not endure the least contradiction, or receive any suggestions in relation to any subject; all conversation was unpleasant; desire to be left alone; he desires to find fault with every one around him. (This state of mind lasted several days—see proving.)

Clinical Remarks.—One cannot help being struck by the similarity of the above symptoms, to those mental states common to diseases of the *genital organs* in both *sexes*, particularly in women. Such symptoms are quite common to uterine disorders, and to unhealthy pregnancies. In disorders of *digestion* we also meet with a similar group of symptoms. I consider such symptoms to be an excellent guide, in default of other pathogenetic ones, to the selection of Helonias in uterine disorders, etc.

Cerebral Symptoms.—Slight pain through the temples, with a feeling of fulness in the head, and vertigo; a feeling of pressure from within upward to the vertex, aggravated by looking steadily at any fixed point; pain in the occiput, with pulsative pain in the vertex—increased by stooping, attended with vertigo; pain in the forehead as if a band about an inch wide was drawn across from temple to temple. (Iod., Merc., Stann., Nit. ac.)

Gastric, etc.—Wakes every morning at 5 o'clock (an unusual hour) with the lips, tongue and fauces dry, and a bitter taste in the mouth; appetite not as good as usual. Soon after taking each dose sensations of pain, tightness, and pressure felt in the stomach, which was partially relieved by the eructation of tasteless gas; *cramp-like* pain in the stomach; motion and rumbling in the intestines, as if diarrhœa would come on. "In Ohio, and many of the Western States, it is in very general use as a common *emetic*, operating with great certainty, but with more activity than Ipecac. or Eupatorium."—*Lee.*

Clinical Remarks.—Dr. Coe says the "*Helonin* will be tolerated by the stomach when other tonics are rejected. It invigorates the appetite, promotes digestion and depuration, and so improves the quality and increases the quantity of the blood. In this way the foundation for a cure is laid, by improving the tone of the entire system." A thorough proving would doubtless show that this medicine produces a long train of gastric symptoms, beginning with *hyper*-stimulation, and ending in *atony*. I have found it very useful both in idiopathic functional diseases of the stomach, and especially in those sympathetic gastric disorders, which accompany diseases of the uterus. Loss of appetite, eructations fulness, cramp, and painful congestion, with lowness of spirits, are the chief indications for its employment. Dr. Close (Tilden's Jour. of Mat. Med., vol. 2, p. 297) reports the case of a woman with general dropsy: "Her stomach was in a very irritable condition, rejecting her food and medicines. After giving Helonias (fl. ext.) I remained and watched with no little solicitude its effects, expecting it would be likewise rejected; but instead, I had the satisfaction of seeing it retained, and in a little time she became less restless, the moaning noise which she had been accustomed to make almost constantly, ceased, and at the end of half an hour after it was given she fell asleep; the pulse became decidedly softer, and slower, than it had been for a long time. When she awoke there was a decided increase of muscular power." (Dose of fl. ext. one to three drachms, according to Tilden. Dr. C. probably gave as much.)

In Dyspepsia, etc., I have generally used the lower dilutions and triturations.

Urinary Organs.—Kidneys somewhat stimulated, and a larger amount than usual, of clear, light colored urine has been voided.

Clinical Remarks.—It is deemed to be a *diuretic* by medical writers: "In the treatment of the various forms of dropsy, the Helonin has proved of remarkable utility. It operates in a general manner, and is, seemingly, a powerful resolvent. The only manner in which it proves evacuant, is, in some cases, as a diuretic—except when given in over-doses, when it is emetic."—*Coe.*

There are few forms of dropsy which are not due to an asthenic state of the system, or which do not bring on this condition during their course. Therefore, not only do we need to use in dropsy such remedies as Apis, Apocynum, Colchicum, which act specifically upon the kidneys, but possess no "tonic" power; but we are obliged to resort to such medicines as China, Arsenicum, Phosphoric acid, etc. Indeed, these latter medicines have, alone, cured many cases of general dropsy by their influence over the general system. The *Helonias* will be found valuable to the homœopathist in that class of cases, when there is anasarca, with general debility, and an atonic condition of the generative organs, such as chlorosis, amenorrhœa, dropsy from uterine hemorrhage, etc.

Generative Organs.—Pain in lower part of the back, through to the uterus, like inflammation, piercing, drawing; *breasts* swollen, very tender, and will not bear the pressure of even an ordinary dress; *nipples* very sensitive and painful; great uterine hemorrhage came during the proving, and continued until the medicine was discontinued. [The above pathogenetic symptoms were noticed by Dr. E. Clark, of Portland, Me. He states he has noticed the same train of symptoms in six or eight cases. The medicine was given at the first trituration (Helonin). These symptoms were received after the following was written.]

Clinical Remarks.—The Helonias is one of those indigenous medicines, which from the earliest days of medicine in this country, has had a peculiar reputation—first with the Aborgines, then with the early white settlers, and finally with the medical profession in the country—as being a remedy, even *the* remedy, for those disorders generally termed "uterine," and which depended upon an *atonic* condition of the organs of reproduction. I regret exceedingly that I cannot present the profession with a proving upon the organism of women. I have given it to healthy women, but never observed any notable symptoms. Primarily, it always increases the tone and physilogical activity of the generative organs. I therefore consider it *secondarily* homœopathic to those diseases or conditions for which it has been used so successfully. Were it not so, it never could have been used successfully in the doses usually administered by the opposite school of practice. It would have produced *aggravations*, and been by them considered *contra-indicated.* Before giving the clinical experience of our own school, I will quote the opinions and clinical remarks concerning this remedy, which I find in the records of allopathic literature.

Prof. C. A. Lee writes (Tilden's Journal of Mat. Med. II., p. 123):—"Numerous trials have satisfied us that it has a specific action on the uterine organs,—an alleviative, regulating influence over their functions. Hence, in *Amenorrhœa* marked by general atony, and an anæmic and torpid condition of the system this, plant proves of great service; giving tone to the digestive organs, favoring nutrition and sanguification, and promoting the secretions generally. So, in *Leucorrhœa*, associated with similar conditions of the general system, it will be found equally serviceable. Its influence as an uterine tonic is also well marked in cases of atonic or passive *Menorrhagia.* Here, by imparting tonicity to the muscular fibres of the uterus, and by a stimulating power over the plexuses of organic nerves, which supply the pelvic viscera, the exudation of blood is checked, and he predisposing, as well as the proximate cause of the disease, removed. If it has the power of obviating sterility and impotence, as is alleged by some writers, it must be by a similar mode of operation. It may be slightly aphrodisiac, but there are no well-attested facts bearing on that point. It is very probable, however, that it may, in common with Senecio and other uterine tonics, produce such effects; but if it does, I have no proof of the fact, except what may by drawn from analogy. It is very probable, also, that in cases of *dysmenorrhœa* and liability to *abortion* from atony of the reproductive organs, it may prove highly advantageous by a similar mode of action, just as we find in the case of Iron, and other tonics which improve the general health. But, in addition to this, it would seem to be endowed, to a considerable extent, with specific properties and powers. Dr. Coe (Conc. Org. Med.) is very enthusiastic, he says:—"No agent of the Materia Medica better deserves the name of *uterine tonic.* The remarkable success attending its administration in the diseases peculiar to females, has rendered it an indispensible remedy to those acquainted with its peculiar virtues. Like the Senecin, it is alike appropriate in the treatment of diseases apparently calling for dissimilar properties, as, for instance, amenorrhœa and menorrhagia. Its alterative and tonic influence will account, in a measure, for its utility in those complaints. In the *treatment of amenorrhœa*, it will be found most beneficial in those cases arising from, or accompanied with, a disordered condition of the digestive apparatus, and an anæmic habit. It has an especial influence on the organs of generation, independent of its general constitutional influence. For this reason it has proved of eminent value in the cure of *prolapsus uteri*, tendency to miscarriage, and atony of the generative organs; *sterility* and *impotence* have also been relieved and cured by this remedy. Certain writers have classed it as an aphrodisiac, and stated that its continued use induces an abnormal desire for sexual indulgence. Such a statement could only have been made in the absence of actual knowledge, and as the legitimate fruit of a prurient imagination. We have probably used the Helonin quite as extensively as any other practitioner, and we must confess to a want of sufficient penetration to discover any such results from its employment. The only aphrodisiac we recognize, is the natural proclivity of a sensual mind. That the Helonine is a special tonic to the organs of reproduction we are well aware, but only to a normal and healthy extent. Did its action extend further than this, it would be a disease-producing, and not a disease-curing remedy. When a medicine so acts upon a diseased organ as to restore it to a physiological condition, we very naturally conclude that said organ will manifest the fact of its restoration by the resumption of its functional activity. This is precisely the case when the Helonin is employed. If administered for the cure of indigestion, the appetite improves, the food is digested, absorbed, and assimulated, and thus the curative action of the remedy manifested. If, on the other hand, the case be one of amenorrhœa, sterilty, menorrhagia, or impotency, secretion is restored, tone imparted, and the healthful flow of returning stimulus is manifested by the usual physical signs. The sexual appetite is sequent, and not the antecedent of the restoration of the ability of the organs to perform the functions assigned them by nature."

A portion of Dr. Coe's remarks, namely, that which relates to the effects of *curative* doses of medicines, is in the main correct. But his general statement contains one great, fundamental error, which has ever been the glaring fault of allopathic therapeutics. He states that Helonin is a special tonic to the organs of reproduction, but *only to a normal extent;* did it extend *beyond* this, he remarks, it would be a disease-creating remedy. The old school of medicine, has always been wilfully blind to the truth, that all medicines may be disease-producing. That a medicine is a "special tonic" to any particular organ, is the strongest proof that it is capable, if long continued, even in small doses, of causing disease in that organ. If, then, Helonias be given for uterine atony, and acts curatively, when that organ has regained its tone, if the remedy be continued, it will urge or *elevate* the physiological functions of that organ, and induce an abnormal condition, the result of hyper-stimulation. If Helonias *is* a special tonic to the organs of reproduction, we do not doubt, that if given to a healthy individual, it would cause an *excess* of sexual desire, congestion of the uterus, ovaries, etc., and even amenorrhœa, or menorrhagia, dependent on active congestion; then, after a time the *irritability* of these organs would be worn out and according to a well-known physiological law, we shall have an exhausted or atonic condition of the tissues previously over-stimulated. The conditions and diseases enumerated by Dr. Coe, as within the curative range of Helonias, are those which it would cause by its *secondary* action. It is capable of causing an almost equal number by its *primary* action. My theory of *Dose*, accounts for the curative operation of the material doses used by the allopathic schools. The curative action of Helonias in the lower attenuations, is chiefly directed towards those atonic states which it causes secondarily. But if given for its *primary* effects, it must be given in the middle or higher attenuations, else, we should get up injurious medicinal aggravations.

Resume.—The Helonias is *primarily* homœopathic to the following diseases, when occurring in persons of plethoric habit, strong digestion, and great muscular power:—Active congestion of the uterus, causing, besides the usual symptoms of that condition, *suppression* of the menses, (congestive amenorrhœa); *menorrhagia*, from active congestion; prolapsus or retroversion from congestion; abortion from undue afflux of blood to the uterus. The special *symptoms* which would indicate in these diseases, can only be obtained by a thorough proving. Helonias is *secondarily* indicated, and has proved eminently curative to diseases of the reproductive organs, occurring in persons of a lax, or anæmic habit, and in which there is a loss of normal tone. As diseases of the same name may be caused by opposite states, so the primary amenorrhœa of Helonias may be due to congestion, while the secondary amenorrhœa is due to lack of blood and normal activity of the uterus, etc.

The clinical experience of our school with this remedy is not large, but quite successful. Dr. C. H. Burr, of Portland, Me., says:—"I have given it in similar cases of *prolapsus uteri* with very satisfactory results; also in cases of frequent and profuse menstruation, when the patients lose more blood than is manufactured in the inter-menstrual period, with pain in the back, and frequent palpitation of the heart; in such cases it will seldom disappoint those who are disposed to use it."

Dr. Geo. S. Foster, of Meadville, Pa., reports to me the following cases:—"Mrs. ——, aged thirty-two, had prolapsus uteri and ulceration, for nine years, up to the summer of 1862, with all the symptoms incident thereto. All the physicians in town during that time had been trying to cure her; the usual pessaries and cauterization, and all they could do, with no success. When I took the case in hand in September, 1862, I gave her but little encouragement, as you may suppose. I examined her; found ulceration of neck of womb, constant dark, bad smelling discharge; great irritation of vagina, so much that a soft sponge pessary could not be retained; she had lost her "reckoning," the discharge being constant, with flooding on lifting a bucket of water, or anything of weight; countenance sallow, and such an expression as one would have from the suffering she had endured; could with difficulty, walk up the stairs, or across the room; the least exertion would bring on flooding. I did not keep an account of my prescriptions, but prescribed remedies for symptoms present—the principal, Nux., Bell., Secale., Sabina, etc. I repeatedly replaced the womb; the treatment was very discouraging to myself; but symptoms would give way to the action of the remedies readily. About seven months ago, I procured the Vaginal Syringe, and had her use it with water and Tannin. About six months ago I replaced the womb for the last time, and did not prescribe again for four or five months, when she called on me, informing me that it had not been down since my last services, then five months; but still she looked rather badly, and still a dark, ugly discharge, pain in the small of back, etc.

"December 19.—Helonin seond dec.; three a day, for two days.

"December 21.—Improving; twelve powders, about one grain, three a day.

"December 25.—Reports marked improvement in general health the discharge had changed to a bright red—more like the menstrual.

"December 30.—No discharge for five days; she could dance, run up and down stairs; her cheeks have the bloom of health, and in spirits she equals the youngest. So you may see what a few doses of the Helonine has done; finished up the case in grand style, very much to my own and her gratification.

"*Case* 2.—A young woman who has hadtwo abortions at four months; she was in her fourth month again, with all symptoms of again aborting. Left Secale; saw her again in a day or two; it was then time for her courses, and I was fearful that would augment her trouble; she was suffering the usual pain as in such cases. I left her Helonine second dec., and saw her in town yesterday; she had walked in; has had no trouble since taking the last prescription. You may be able to glean but little from the foregoing; but it still points to the remedy as sure to be the foremost in the rank of uterine remedies."

The following cases came under my own treatment, and I have since used the Helonin in similar cases with good results:

Case 1.—A woman, aged 25, the mother of two children, and enciente with a third. The usual symptoms of pregnancy were not present, but in their stead, a peculiar prostration of the nervous and muscular system obtained. She was anæmic—pulse small and feeble; skin sallow and pale; digestion bad; no desire for any kind of food, and all kinds of food caused distress and epigastric oppression. She became emaciated, debilitated, and very low spirited. There was also present constipation, and almost constant uterine distress and pain, of a pressing down character; also leucorrhœa. China, Sepia, Pulsatilla, Ferrum, Nux, and Ignatia were given, with but slight benefit. Upon purely empirical data, I prescribed Helonias, five drops of the mother tincture, one hour before each meal. The effect was surprising. In a few days her appetite increased; all dyspeptic symptoms disappeared; strength returned rapidly. The blood improved in richness, as was manifest by the returning color, and healthy complexion. The uterine disturbance ceased, and a normal pregnancy resulted.

Case 2.—A lady, aged 45, at the climacteric period suffered much from frequent and repeated floodings, profuse serous leucorrhœa, and dropsy. She had also much uterine and ovarian pain. Her complexion was very sallow, unhealthy looking, earthly, and pale. She had taken muriated tincture of iron from an allopath, for some months, but grew worse under its use. A report of the treatment of the whole case would be of interest, but want of space prevents its narration. The floodings subsided under the use of Trillin one-tenth; the dropsy and ovarian pain was removed by Apis. 2; the uterine pain was palliated by Sepia and Macrotin. But she still remained weak, emaciated, and the complexion did not improve. Leptandrin 2nd improved it somewhat; the icterus had disappeared. Helonias 2nd dec. trit., two grs. every four hours was then prescribed. Under its use the nutritive functions rapidly recovered their tone; strength and increased vitality returned, and in a few weeks she felt quite well.

Back, etc.—A feeling of weariness and weight in the region of the kidneys; sharp, spasmodic pain in the back, running to the crest of the left ileum; severe rheumatic (?) pain in the right hip joint, worse during motion; pain, and a feeling of lameness, in the whole back; pain in lumbar region, about the upper portion of the sacrum, and pelvis; the pains in the back are more troublesome during the night. (See generative organs.)

Clinical Remarks.—Pains in the back, also lameness, stiffness, etc., located in the sacra-lumbar region—a common symptom in all uterine disorders, and even in diseases of the male organs of generation. Helonias seems to cause these pains in quite a notable degree; they often simulate *rheumatic* pains, and may be mistaken for them.

PROVING OF HELONIN, BY DR. C. H. BURR, OF PORTLAND, ME.

The preparation used in this proving was a solution of thirty grs of Helonin in one ounce of alcohol, diluted with half an ounce of water. It was thought best to commence with small doses, and increase hourly, until decided symptoms were produced, and Oct. 15th, in accordance with this idea, two drops were taken at 10, A. M., four gtt., at 11; eight gtt. at 12 M. Soon after taking each dose, sensations of pain, tightness, and pressure were felt in the stomach, which was partially relieved by the eructation of tasteless gas. At 1 P. M., twelve gtt. were taken; at 2, sixteen gtt.; at 3, twenty gtt.; motion and rumbling in the intestines as if diarrhœa would come on. At 4, thirty gtt. were taken; at 5, forty gtt.; at 8, fifty gtt. Slight pain was now felt through the temples, together with a feeling of fullness in the head, and vertigo. At 10, P. M., took fifty gtt.

October 16th.—The symptoms produced yesterday were not of a decided character. Took at 7, A. M., forty gutta; at 9, fifty gtt.; at 11, sixty gtt.; at 12, sixty gtt. Still, but little effect is produced, and I should be unconscious of being under the influence of any remedy were it not for an unnatural degree of languor, and a feeling of weariness, and weight, in the region of the kidneys. At

2, P. M., sixty gtt.; at 3, sixty gtt. At this stage of the proving, the alcoholic preparation was put aside, and an aqueous one substituted; Helonin twenty grains, water one ounce; of this, forty gtt. were taken at 4, P. M.; at 7, fifty gtt. The symptoms mentioned as occurring in the head, are more decided; the sense of fulness increases, and there is a feeling of pressure from within, up to the vertex; the latter feeling is aggravated by looking steadily at any fixed point; the kidneys have been somewhat stimulated and a larger amount than usual of clear, light-colored urine has been voided during the last twelve hours; the pulse ranges at eighty-four, full, and a little irregular. At 9, P. M., took sixty gtt.; no new symptoms.

October 18th.—No medicine was taken during the 17th, until evening, when at 7, half a drachm was taken; at 9, half a drachm; at 12, half a drachm. In the afternoon and evening, there was a great deal of weariness, and feeling of weight in the region of the kidneys, and with much more general fatigue than usual; mind dull and inactive.

October 19th.—Took at 8, A. M., half a drachm; at 12, half a drachm; pain in the vertex; the pain in the head is increased by stooping, and attended with increased vertigo; sharp, spasmodic pain in the back, running to the crest of the left ilium. At 5 P. M., took half a drachm. Have awoke every morning since the proving was commenced, at 5 o'clock, an unusual hour, with tongue and fauces dry, and a bitter, disagreeable taste in the mouth. The symptoms during the day have been more marked, and principally confined to the head and back; the appetite has not been as usual.

October. 21st.—Took at 12, M., one drachm. Soon after taking this dose felt a cramp-like pain in the stomach. At 8, P. M., took one drachm; severe, rheumatic pains in the right hip joint, worse during motion; pain in the forehead, as if a band about an inch wide was drawn across from temple to temple; pain and feeling of lameness in the whole back, and dryness, and bitter taste in the mouth.

Oct. 22nd.—Took at 9, A. M., one drachm; at 12, M., one drachm. Last evening was engaged in singing until 8 o'clock, at which time I took one drachm. Previous to taking the remedy, I never felt better, more cheerful, or in better spirits. Ssoon after taking it, there was an entire change in surrounding circumstances; I very soon became dull, gloomy, and irritable; could not endure the least contradiction, or receive any suggestions in relation to any subject; all conversation was unpleasant, and what I most desired was, to be left alone, reserving to myself the privilege of finding fault with every one around me. I consider that this moral condition was not accidental, but purely a pathological state, produced, and kept up by the action of the medicine. Previous to the 22nd, this state assumed an intermittent form, but after that date, it was unchanged for several days, and was one of the most constant and marked effects.

October 26th.—No medicine has been taken since the 22d. Pain in the lumbar region, about the upper part of the sacrum and pelvis. These pains during the last twenty-four hours have been more constant and severe than at any other time; the pain in the back seems more troublesome at night than during the day."

HYDRASTIS CANADENSIS.

(*Golden Seal.*)

This well-known plant is indigenous. It has a perennial root, which is the officinal portion. It consists of a tortuous, knotty caudex, with numerous long fibers, and is of a bright yellow color internally. The plant is found growing in shady woods, in rich soil, and in damp meadows, in different parts of the United States, but is more abundant west of the Alleghanies. It flowers in May and June. The *root* in its fresh state is juicy, and when dried looses much of its weight. Its odor is strong and somewhat narcotic, with a very bitter taste. Its virtues are imparted to water and alcohol. A peculiar nitrogenous, crystallizable substance called *Hydrastin*, is considered the active principle of this plant. In homœopathic practice we use *five* different preparations of this agent.

(1.) A tincture and dilution of the fresh root. This should be made with diluted alcohol.

(2.) A trituration of the pulverized root.

(3.) A trituration of the *Hydrastin.*

(4.) A glycerole made with the tincture.

(5.) A cerate.

The Hydrastin is not considered to possess all the virtues of the root. It stands in the same relation to it, as Quinine does to Peruvian Bark (China). It possesses all the *tonic* properties of the root, but not all the peculiar specific action on the mucous tissues, which is possessed by the preparations of the root. We ought to have a good proving of both preparations.

General Effects.—There is no medicine in use in eclectic practice about which there is such a general unanimity of opinion as to its therapeutical effects. The unequivocal testimony is that it is.

(1.) A mild, certain, and permanent *tonic*;

(2.) An *alterative* to all the *mucous surfaces*, and indeed to all tissues with which it is brought in contact. When we come to speak of special indications, its various applications in disease will be fully considered. I hope to be able to show that this agent, so truly valuable even in empirical practice, is realy homœopathic to nearly every condition for which it has been used successfully by eclectic physicians. The allopaths seem to know or care but little about this remedy. *Wood* thus mentions it in his Dispensatory. "It probably possesses the ordinary virtues of the vegetable bitters, and is said to be employed as a tonic in some parts of the country. In the form of infusion, it has been used in the Western States as a topical application in ophthalmia, and the Indians are said to employ it in the same manner, in old ulcers of the legs. The notion of its efficacy in cancers, originating in a report which reached the late Professor Barton, that it was used in the cases of this complaint by the Cherokees, is probably altogether groundless." In his "Therapeutics" and "Practice" Wood does not mention it. In homœopathic practice it has been used for a few years, but only upon empirical data.

General Symptoms.—The universal testimony of those who have had experience in the use of Hydrastis, is, that it increases in a marked manner the physical strength, and elevates the functions of the stomach, as regards digestion, assimilation, etc. It probably increases the appetite, and acts in many ways as *China* does when given during convalescence from disease, or in diseased states characterized by debility.

This is to the Eclectic, what Quinine is to the Allopath, and China is to our own school. The first-named school look with surprise upon the indifference with which this, their favorite *tonic*, is treated by their rival school. I have known eclectics in large practice, rely upon it almost to the exclusion of Quinine or Salicine, in intermittents and other malarious fevers. They usually prescribe one drachm of the tincture or fluid extract, or one or two grains (even as high as six grains) of Hydrastin, every one, two, or four hours, as the case seems to demand, and assert that it always acts as a pure *tonic*, and that its effects are not attended with any stimulation of the circulation, or congestion of the brain, as is the case with Quinine. Yet, curiously enough, English homœopathists assert that a "few drops of the mother tincture will cause a sensation of physical prostration." It could not do this by its *primary* action, like china—its scondary effect may be prostration. Drs. McLimont and Marston state that "one of us has for upwards of a month at a time, endeavored by experiment, to ascertain its pathogenesis; but we have been unable to elicit any very decided symptoms, except upon the sensorium and heart, which were affected for a very short time, by doses of half an ounce and upwards, smaller quantities appearing to pass off without any effect at all." The tincture used by the gentlemen must have been of a very poor quality, or half an ounce would have shown its effects in quite a decided manner. They state, however, that they "know of no medicine which has caused so great an improvement in the general health of our cancer patients as has this, an improvement which, in most cases, has become visible in the bettered expression of the countenance, to all who had previously known the patients."

It is appropriate in this place, that I should give some account of the use of Hydrastis in cancers by our English colleagues. In the October No., 1863, of the *British Journal of Homœopathy*, we find an article entitled, "Cancer; its Pathology, etc.," by Drs. McLimont and Marston. After mentioning other remedies, as Arsenicum, Aurum, Hyoscyamus, Conium, and Carbo. veg., they proceed to notice the Golden Seal. They say: "We are not sure who it was that first adopted and recommended the use of Hydrastis c., but have reason to believe that this application of the root was first made in America." We have looked through the various works published in this country, in which this plant has been noticed, but do not recollect that it is once mentioned as having been used in cancerous affections. King, Jones and Scudder, Kost, and others, mention that it possesses a marked action upon mucous surfaces, and is curative in ulceration, chronic inflammation, etc., of those surfaces; also old ulcers on the extremities, etc. In domestic practice it is used somewhat as we use Arnica, as an application to bruises, abrasions, and sprains. The first mention of the use of Hydrastis in cancer is found in the earlier numbers of the *British Journal.* Dr. Bayes and Dr. Pattison both reported cases cured with an external application of the drug. But Dr. P. published his cases in a pamphlet, much as the cancer doctors of this country publish their wonderful cures, and there was much room left for doubt, as to the genuineness of the statements. Drs. McLimont and Marston do not, however, rely entirely upon the use of Hydrastis alone, but consider it necessary to "enucleate" the tumor. This process of enucleation is described in full (see page 628). Hydrastis was applied to the tumor, after it had been incised. But it will seem strange to American homœopathists, who have always loked upon their English brethren with something akin to reverence, when they learn the manner of its application. "A piece of lint is applied to the surface, spread with equal parts of a paste composed of a strong decoction of Hydrastis root, *chloride of zinc, and flour, and stramonium ointment.*" Shade of Hahnemann, have mercy upon English homœopathists! Is this Homœopathy? What, in the name of common sense, can a mild, non-caustic medicine like Golden Seal do, mixed up with such caustics and narcotics as chloride of zinc and stramonium? Is the *British Journal* so badly in want of original articles, as to be obliged to publish such absurdity under the name of homœopathy? It is equally ridiculous with old school practice. If the Hydrastis was to be tested, why not do it in a proper manner, by applying it in a concentrated form to the diseased part? In some of the cases reported, a "lotion" of Golden Seal was applied with apparent good effect. Of the constitutional treatment they say: "This"—the Hydrastis—"is the medicine upon which we chiefly rely in our treatment of cancer, usually putting our patients under a course of it for a month or so, before commencing the enucleation of the mass. Our doses vary from one or two drops of the sixth dil., to drop doses of the mother tincture; the lower forms being used chiefly in those cases in which the cachectic condition is fully marked; and we must confess that we know of no medicine which has caused so great an improvement in the general health of our patients as has this. We continue the medicine during the whole of the treatment, and for some weeks after. "In some cases, however, the ulceration has extended into such parts as to prevent much treatment by the application of the paste, and here we have obtained much good from the Hydrastis *lotion*, combined with its internal administration; the pain decreases, the fœtor diminishes, the discharge is lessened, and the ulceration progresses less rapidly. * * Our experience, on the whole seems to lead to the conclusion, that for the most part the health (as connected with the disease) improves more rapidly under Arsenicum than under Hydrastis, while on the other hand, the local condition participates more decidedly in this amendment when Hydrastis is taken." Several example cases are given to illustrate the curative effects, a few of which we condense:

Case 1.—A lady had observed for some years a hard substance in her right breast, which, for a few months before coming under treatment had rapidly increased in size, and had become so painful as to prevent all rest by night. On examination, a tumor of strong hardness, and about the size of a duck's egg, was discovered in the upper portion of the left breast. It was non-adherent, but the skin was slightly puckered, and the nipple retracted. Another physician had called the tumor a malignant one. Hydrastis sixth was administered in drop doses. The pain was at once relieved. The enucleation of the tumor, however, was decided upon. The wound speedily cicatrized, and the patient remains perfectly free from disease.

Case 2.—"A lady had suffered for six months from a swelling in the left breast. The pain—which was compared to knives thrust into the part—had become almost unbearable, and the patient was already beginning to assume that worn appearance so characteristic of the cancerous diathesis. The tumor, which attained a considerable size, was hard, heavy, and adherent to the skin, which was dark, mottled, and very much puckered, the nipple also being much retracted. The patient was at once advised to come to town for the enucleation of the tumor. This, however, her circumstances prevented, and without any expectation of affording much relief, a lotion of Hydrastis was ordered, with the internal use of the same medicine. The pain almost immediately ceased, and the tumor so speedily decreased in size that at the end of two months it had altogether disappeared, leaving but the puckered skin, which had otherwise regained its natural appearance. When we last heard of this patient she continued perfectly well. It is needful to state that her health rapidly improved under the treatment, and that her countenance regained the aspect of health." This is a notable case, and if the Hydrastis will always act as well, it will prove a great boon to humanity.

Ten cases are given, in which the Hydrastis was used. In most cases it relieved the pain, and in some it checked the progress of the disease. The writers claim that it failed to give relief in no case. They predict great advantage from the use of this medicine. But we protest against its combination with powerful caustics and anodynes, if we are to have all the good effects of the "paste" attributed to the Hydrastis. I would suggest that American homœopathists test the pure paste of Hydrastis (pulv. root) applied to the "incised" tumor, or the lotion, or even a strong cerate, giving at the same time the remedy internally. The Hydrastis is also recommended for Lupus. Three cases, says Drs. McL. and M., have been treated successfully with it.

I have been treating a case of scirrous of the breast by the use of Hydrastis. The lady had a scirrous tumor extirpated from the right breast six years previously. Three months before I was consulted she noticed a small induration, or tumor, near the site of the one which had been extirpated. It gradually increased in size and became very painful. The pain was lancinating, and extended up to the shoulder and down the arms. I applied a lotion of Hydrastis, one-tenth in water, and ordered her to take five drops of the one-tenth three times a day. It is now one month since she commenced its use. The pain ceased the first week, and the tumor has decreased rapidly in size. Dr. H. M. Saxton, of St. Joseph, Mich., writes me that he has had considerable experience in the use of Hydrastis as an external application; and gives the following cases illustrating its use:

Case 1.—A girl seven or eight years of age fell, and lacerated the scalp above the left temple. The wound was several inches in length, in the form of a crescent. It suppurated, and became a troublesome sore. After cleansing the surface, the Hydrastis, in fine powder, was applied. It checked the suppuration, allayed the inflammation, and under its use, the ulcer healed in a few days.

Case 2.—Was an ulcer from a burn, on the back of a child's hand. It was much inflamed, very painful; she could hardly move her wrist. The powdered Hydrastis was applied lightly. Although the child irritated it a good deal, it soon healed, and left the cuticle smooth, and without a cicatrix.

Case 3.—*Infantile Intertrigo.* "Excoriation in the folds of the neck." The dry powder was applied, and it healed in three days.

As a wash, one part of the tincture to ten of water I have found more useful in obstinate excoriation of the skin, in children, than Arnica. Glycerine is a better vehicle than water. The Glycerole of Hydrastis is used with great advantage in cases of intertrigo, sore nipples, and ulcerated surfaces. While Arnica seems specific for contusions, with extravasations, and Calendula for incised and lacerated wounds, even when unhealthy suppuration ensues, the Hydrastis seems the best remedy for chronic ulcers, arising from either of the above causes, or from burns, scalds, or some diseases of the skin.

Skin.—Enough has been said above to indicate the conditions of the skin, etc., for which Hydrastis is indicated. It is probably not specific against any idiopathic diseases of the skin, but only for some of the effects of such diseases. It has been found useful against *lupus*, psoriasis, rhagades, and excoriations. It may be employed as a simple lotion, a glycerole, or in the form of a cerate. If the general condition of the system is *cachectic* its internal use will be found beneficial.

Sleep.—Awakened several times during the night by severe pains in the small of the back, and hypogastric region, with dull pain in the umbilicus.

Fever.—Chilly sensation all night, notwithstanding abundance of covering; chilliness, with aching in the back and limbs.

CLINICAL REMARKS.—Its use in Intermittent fevers has already been alluded to. It is most serviceable in *quotidians*, when there is considerable gastric disturbance, jaundice, and a general cachectic condition. Also in cases where mercury and quinine have been used injuriously. In the debility which follows gastric, bilious, and typhoid fever, it will be found very useful.

Mind.—Feel very sad and gloomy.

Head.—Dull, heavy frontal headache; constant dull headache, with pain in the hypogastrium and small of the back of a dull aching character; *dull* frontal headache present most of the time.

CLINICAL REMARKS.—I have found it useful in headache from gastric difficulties, those arising from dyspepsia, and in those frontal headaches which occur in chronic catarrh. It has been found curative in headache from habitual constipation.

Eyes.—Mucous membrane of the eyelids much congested; discharge of large quantities of thick white mucus; profuse secretion of tears; eyelids agglutinated together; mucous membrane of lids congested; smarting of the eyes; burning of the eyes and lids.

CLINICAL REMARKS.—We find here distinctly manifested, the specific action of Hydrastis. It affects all mucous membranes, that of the eyes seems to be prominently affected by the pathogenetic influence of the drug. We also find that this remedy has been used very successfully by eclectic practitioners, in diseases of the eyes. In catarrhal conjunctivitis, after the acute stage has passed, it has been used as a collyrium with unequivocal benefit. *King* advises it in *opacity of the cornea.* Jones and Scudder assert that, "A decoction of it is very useful as a detergent and antiphlogistic application to the eyes, either in acute or chronic inflammation; in acute ophthalmia we have obtained much advantage from applying a poultice of equal parts of Hydrastis and ulmus fulva, wet with cold water; it relieves the pain and burning, and in many mild cases will effect a cure without any other application. In the chronic form of the disease we employ it without the ulmus fulva, directing a large poultice to be applied to the affected eye upon going to bed, and retained on through the night, wetting it occasionally with water if it becomes dry." Were it not for the senseless combinations which they use, some valuable clinical experience might be gleaned from the works of writers on eclectic medicine. From the above testimony as to the use of Hydrastis in Ophthalmia, we may deduce some practical suggestions. The "eye symptoms" noticed by the provers show that Hydrastis is an analogue of Pulsatilla, Euphrasia, Hepar sulphur and Sepia. The two former correspond more particularly to acute catarrhal inflammation, while the latter, and Hydrastis are more appropriate to the chronic condition. (Æthusa effects the eyes similarly to Euphrasia.) Pulsatilla is but indicated when the discharge is thick, mucus, or even muco-purulent, and there may be superficial ulceration of the conjunctiva. But the discharge for which Hydrastis is indicated, proceeds from a more obstinate catarrhal inflammation, in which ulceration is a prominent symptom. It is a little strange that the above mentioned writers do not mention or advise the use of this remedy internally in Ophthalmic diseases. It may be remarked, however, that the older allopathic writers do not mention the internal use of Pulsatilla or Euphrasia, although they used them as topical agents, in the same diseases for which we use them.

Dose, etc.—In *acute* conjunctivitis give the third dilution, and apply about the same attenuation, (in distilled water), to the eyes. In the chronic, attended with ulceration, use the one-tenth or one-hundredth internally and as a collyrium.

Nose.—Very much stuffed up; *constant discharge of thick white mucus from the nose;* constant coryza with profuse secretion of tears; obstruction of the nasal passages with frequent coryza; constant coryza with frontal headache; (B) "excessive secretion from the mucous membrane of the nose, so much so that the secretions were removed in long tenacious shreds or pieces."—(*King.*)

Clinical Remarks.—This last symptom, which I find in King's Disp., shows very clearly the sphere of action of the drug; also that the mucous membrane of the nose is specifically affected; this symptom was caused by *internal* administration. For several years I have been in the habit of treating chronic nasal catarrhs, ozæna, and diptheritic affections of the nose, with Hydrastis. In simple catarrh, the second dil. may be given internally and used as an injection into the nostrils, two or three times a day. When there is ulceration the first dec. trituration will afford more satisfactory results. In Ozæna, it may be used still stronger, and in alternation with injections of Baptisia, giving at the same time internally, Iodide of Arsenic, or Nitric ac. In acute coryza, with copious secretion of white mucus and tears, nightly chilliness, despondency, etc., I would suggest the use of the high potencies. Its internal and topical application may prove of benefit in nasal polypi. If its asserted power of discussing scirrous and other tumors be but substantiated, it may prove useful in cancer of the nose.

Mouth.—Large apthous sore on the mucous membrane of the under lip; flat taste in the mouth; "excessive secretion of tenacious mucus from the buccal mucous membrane, so profuse that it may be removed in long tenacious shreds."—(*King.*)

Clinical Remarks.—We have here the same blenorrhagic symptoms noticed under "*Nose.*" Hydrastis has always been a favorite domestic remedy in "sore mouth." Many physicians use it in all forms of stomatitis with alleged success. It has been found useful in common apthous stomatitis of children; in simple ulceration of the buccal mucous membrane; in mercurial sore mouth; and in stomatitis materna. I have witnessed the most obstinate varieties of these affections, yield to the local application of Hydrastis in decoction or powder, after the mineral acids, astringents, nitrate of silver of the old school, and even homœopathic remedies had been tried in vain. The best method of application is to put one drachm of the tincture into half a pint of water, use this as a wash every four hours; enough will be swallowed or absorbed, to exert its specific constitutional action.

In Dr. Ludlam's report on "stomatitis materna. (Trans. Ill. Hom. Society) mention is made of the use of this remedy in that disease. Dr. Murch has been very successful in many cases, using it as a wash, and the dry powder applied to ulcers in the mouth.

Fauces, Throat, etc.—Tingling and smarting in the throat; hawking up of tenacious, yellow or white mucus, with rawness of the fauces; some pain on swallowing, as from excoriation.

Clinical Remarks.—It is a favorite remedy with many homœopathic physicians in the West, as a gargle in cases of simple ulcerated sore throat; also in *Angina* with ulceration, when accompanying scarlatina; it does not, like Baptisia, remove the fœtor in a direct manner, but its curative effect over the ulceration tends to remove any putrefactive condition. I consider it as useful in *Diphtheria*, as any remedy we are acquainted with. (Use as directed under "Mouth.") The pathogenetic symptoms are quite similar to those for which Dr. Gray, of New York, so highly recommendsMerc. Iodatus; and the pathological condition, namely, inflammation and engorgement, with profuse secretion of mucus from the mucous follicles of the throat, very much resemble the condition which Mercurius causes. In some varieties of *Chronic* Angina, we find the mucous membrane of the fauces studded with round, protuberant spots, of a red color, as if injected with blood, and the patients complains of an aggravation from the least exposure to cold. For this state of the throat Hepar sulphur is generally prescribed, but its permanent curative effect is much aided by the internal and local use of Hydrastis. *Syphilitic Angina*, has been benefited by the use of this medicine; indeed, in its action on the glands of the mucous membrane, Hydrastis is an analogue of the mercurials. There is a kind of sore throat, which often attends dyspepsia; it is sometimes known as "bilious sore throat," although the name is inappropriate; it is a sympathetic disorder, arising from irritation of the stomach and lower portions of œsophagus; for this troublesome affection, the Hydrastis internally is an excellent remedy.

Gastric Symptoms.—Eructations of sour fluid; faint feeling at the stomach; dull *aching* pain in the stomach, which causes a very weak, faintish feeling; burning pain in the umbilical region, with a faintish "goneness" in the epigastric region; *cutting* pain in the stomach.

Clinical Remarks.—This remedy seems likely to prove as prominent a remedy for those conditions which are known under the name of dyspepsia, as Nux vomica, Sulphur, or Pulsatilla. We will glance at the testimony of eclectic physicians on this subject: "It is successfully administered in dyspepsia and chronic affections of the mucous coats of the stomach; in chronic inflammation of the stomach it is very valuable; it will be found of especial advantage in the treatment of persons who are intemperate, gradually removing the abnormal condition of the stomach, and in many instances destroying the appetite for liquor.—(*King.*) "In anorexia, indigestion, and general debility, arising from a languid, or atonic state of the stomach, it is unsurpassed, restoring tone to the stomach, promoting the appetite, and acting as a general restorative. It may also be employed in those cases of chronic gastritis and chronic irritation of the stomach with altered secretion, which constitute the worst and most persistent forms of dyspepsia. In *acid* indigestion the Hydrastis, associated with calcined magnesia or prepared charcoal, will be found truly valuable, especially when attended with a torpid condition of the bowels. In those sympathetic diseases of the digestive organs, arising from uterine disease, we have obtained more benefit from this than from any other agent.—(*Jones & Scudder Mat. Med.*) "The cases in which we have known this plant used with most success, were atonic dyspepsia, attended with torpidity of the liver; languid circulation, and constipated bowels." (*Professor Lee*, Allopath.) The few pathogenetic symptoms which we have, point to its use in dyspepsia with *acidity*, and dyspepsia from *atony*. The *faint* feeling, is quite suggestive of congestion of the portal system; but we should be guided, perhaps, more by the general action of Hydrastis upon mucous membranes. We know that it causes (1) *blenorrhagia*; (2) excoriation and ulceration (*superficial?*); and a condition simulating chronic inflammation. I have used this medicine in gastric disorders, for several years, and my experience, together with a knowledge of its general effects, lead me to consider it homœopathic to the following conditions; I use the nomenclature of Dr. Chambers—(see Disorders of Digestion):

(1) Mucous Flux (chronic.)
(2.) Excess of epithelium (chronic).
(3.) The Anæmic state.
(4.) Chronic Inflammation, (mucous).
(5.) Ulcer of the stomach.
(6.) Deficiency of gastric juice.

It may prove of value in cancer, or scirrous of the stomach, if the experience of our English colleagues should be verified; it palliates those symptoms of flatulence, distention, and painful digestion, so common to dyspeptics.

Stomach and Bowels.—Slight pain in the umbilical region, with a hot sensation in the same parts; severe cutting pain in the hypogastric region, extending into the testicle, where it is of a dull aching character, occurring after stool and accompanied by a very faint feeling; constant distress in the umbilical region, with loud rumbling in the bowels; dull pain in the hypogastrium and small of the back; dull pain in the umbilicus, aggravated by moving, and accompanied by great rumbling in the bowels; severe pains in the hypogastrium with very faint feeling following stool; constant dull pain in the right side of umbilical region; constant dull aching pain in the stomach that produces a gone, or faint feeling; constant pain in the cardiac portion of the stomach, that produces a very weak, faint feeling; severe cutting pains in the stomach and umbilical region; at intervals sharp pain in the region of the spleen, with constant dull pains in the stomach and bowels, accompanied by a hot burning sensation; the aching pain in the umbilicus prevents my sleeping; great deal of pain in the umbilical and cœcal regions, continuing all night, with pain in the whole bowels all the following day; sharp pains in the region of the cœcum.

Clinical Remarks.—It will be well here, to inquire into the general action of Hydrastis upon the intestinal tube. It is not considered as a *cathartic*, yet I have known large doses of the powdered root to act as a purgative. This, however, may have been in part owing to the irritating effects of the woody fibre in the powder, as the tincture does not, in quite large quantities, have that effect. *King* says that in some instances "it proves laxative, but without any astringency, and seems to act in therapeutical action between Rhubarb and bloodroot." Prof. Lee says it "proves laxative to the bowels." Dr. Burt, who made a portion of this proving, writes me that he did not have any very loose stools during the experiment; that he did not notice any mucus in the evacuations; the burning pain in the bowels was quite troublesome; but his proving was not continued a sufficient length of time to develope its peculiar blenorrhagic effects upon the intestinal mucous membranes. We feel safe in asserting that Hydrastis is not primarily or directly homœopathic to *diarrhœa*, unless in the catarrhal, in which it should be used highly potentized; but it is decidedly homœopathic to the following conditions:

(1) Chronic mucous flux of the intestines. (This condition has been treated under the name of intestinal catarrh, blenorrhœa of the bowels.) It seems to be a near analogue of Ammonicum muriaticum in its effects upon mucous surfaces.

(2.) Erosion, chronic ulceration, etc., with "defective absorption;" it is also homœopathic to flatulent colic; and pain in the bowels when accompanied by faintness.

Stool.—Soft stool, followed by severe cutting pain in the hypogastrium, with dull aching in the testicles, accompanied by a very faint feeling; soft, mushy stool, with great rumbling in the bowels. (Burt). Obstinate relaxation of the bowels; griping pains in the bowels; tenesmus.

Clinical Remarks.—Prof. Lee (allopath), says this medicine has been used with most success in atonic dyspepsia, attended with languid circulation, torpidity of the liver, and *constipated bowels*. If it really proved curative in material doses, in constipation, it must be *secondarily* homœopathic to that condition. The reports of our English colleagues seem to support this theory by actual cases. Dr. Hastings, Surgeon (British Hom. Journal, Vol. XVIII, page 317,) writes: "My assistant, Mr. Clifford, uses it extensively in very chronic and obstinate cases of constipation, and says, that a drop of the mother tincture, in water, first thing every evening, has been most effectual in these cases." The following cases, illustrating the use of Hydrastis can. in constipation, were reported by Dr. Rogerson in the British Journal, Vol. XVIII., page 526:—

Case 1.—"Margaret Shaw, aged thirty-eight, came to the dispensary, with the following symptoms:—for the last eight years, she had been troubled with constipation, during which time her bowels had never been moved more than once or twice a week, and then only by the aid of opening medicine. Castor oil and pills generally had been taken, consequently she complained of constant headache, more especially in the morning; bad taste in the mouth; foul tongue; pain in the back and shoulders; a sense of constriction in the hypogastric region, which was only relieved by opening medicine; rather bilious; yellow complexion; skin smooth and dry; great pain after each stool, which was of a hard nodulated consistence, and of a brown or gray color. I now ordered her to take *Hyd. c.*, every morning and evening, and to leave off taking all opening or purgative medicines; after four days had elapsed, her headache, pain in the back and shoulders, were much better; the bowels having moved. Four days afterward, the headache had entirely disappeared; free from pain; stool quite easy and healthy; yellow hue disappearing from the face; the appetite much better, and at the end of four weeks she reported herself quite well."

Case 2. "Sarah Howarth, aged twenty-nine, complaining of sore neck and throat, the latter much relaxed and inflamed, more especially the posterior part; headache, cough and spit; pain in side while stooping and rising from a recumbent position; breath bad; tongue foul and coated with a thick white fur; appetite bad; and bowels for some seven or eight weeks very much confined; had been obliged to resort to opening medicines every Saturday evening; they were generally moved three or four times every Sunday, and not again until the medicine was repeated on the following Saturday. She was ordered Hydrastis c. every morning and evening; one week afterward, she felt rather better; breath not so bad; tongue moist and more healthy; appetite increasing; bowels moved every day since she commenced taking the medicine; continued the Hydrastis; one week later she feels nearly well, excepting a slight pain while swallowing any food; bowels free from all uneasy sensation, and move every day; appetite greatly increased and gaining strength every day; continued the medicine, which resulted in a perfect cure at the end of two weeks longer."

Case 3.—Thomas Oscar, aged forty-six. Has been for several months troubled with general anasarca—difficulty in making water, which was of a high color, depositing a cloudy sediment while standing; and having been in active service during the Crimean campaign was accustomed to sleeping out in the open air, and being so exposed for a series of weeks and months, suffered from an acute attack of rheumatic fever, which laid the foundation of his present illness; his bowels for the last two months having been very much confined, so much so, that he was necessitated to resort to opening medicine once or twice a week. On my first visiting him, however, on the twenty-first of April, I prescribed Hydrastis every morning and evening.

April 29th.—Has, since taking the medicine, had his bowels moved two or three times every day; he also makes much more water—more freely and of a better color; continue Hydrastis.

May 4th.—His bowels have been moved every day, with the

exception of yesterday; his water increases; tongue better; sleeps very well, and feels in every respect great relief from his former sufferings; continue Hydrastis every morning.

May 26. Bowels more quiet, regular; swelling much diminished; water freer, clear and copious; feels now nearly well; continue Hydrastis every other morning."

"The above cases are only a few of the many in which I have tried it with great success; it seems to act most beneficially on those who have undergone, or constantly resort to a course of opening medicine; it also seems to act best on those who have spent an active life, but have become of sedentary habit." It is to be regretted that Dr. Rogerson did not give the *doses* he used. Hydrastis is indicated in some forms of dysentery; in mucous enteritis when of a catarrhal character, and the inflammation sub-acute, the Hydrastis at the third dilution will prove curative. In chronic enteritis, when the discharges are tenacious, slimy, and accompanied with tenesmus; or when the fæces are in the form of hard balls, coated over with yellowish, tough mucus; this medicine will be of service in the first and second potency. The topical application of the remedy must not be forgotten in these cases. Enemas of Hydrastis will be found useful, and will bring about a cure unaided, or at any rate materially aid its internal action; when the disease is located in the *rectum,* this form of application will be found particularly beneficial.

In *Ulceration of the rectum*, occurring after bad cases of dysentery, the local application of Hydrastis will effect prompt cures; also, in *fissure* of anus. (The cerate will be the best preparation in these cases).

In *Hæmorrhoids*, this plant has some reputation. Reliable practitioners have assured me that they have cured the most obstinate cases by the alternate use of Hydrastis and Podophyllum, using enemas of Hydrastis every night.

In *Excoriations of the anus*, as it occurs in little children, or even adults, in diarrhœa and dysentery, no better remedy can be advised; it should be used in the form of *glycerole.*

Liver.—Our provings do not point to any particular symptoms, relating to the liver, but it is considered valuable in hepatic disorders, by the Eclectic school.

Coe says:—"Upon the liver it acts with certainty and efficacy; as a chologogue and deobstruent it has few equals; it is of inestimable value in the treatment of chronic derangements of the liver and portal circulation; it seems to exercise an especial influence over the portal vein, and hepatic structure, generally; resolving biliary deposits; removing obstructions; promoting secretion, and giving tone to the various functions. It may be relied upon with confidence for the relief of hepatic torpor. In intermittent fever, we have found it most reliable in those cases in which the prolongation of the disease depended upon a disordered condition of the functions of the liver." *King* does not mention its applicability to hepatic diseases. Other writers, however, recommend it in affections of that organ. If the liver eliminates the principle of the

Hydrastis, we may safely assert that it will disorder its functions. I have quoted the above, to draw the attention of our school to its alleged uses. There is one condition of the liver, however, in which I consider the Hydrastis homœopathically indicated; I allude to to "catarrhal inflammation of the mucous membranes lining the gall bladder, biliary ducts, etc.

Urinary Organs.—Dull, aching sensation in the region of the kidneys; dull, heavy weight in the lumbar region; urine increased from twenty-eight to sixty ounces per day, and changed from an acid reaction to neutral." (B).

CLINICAL REMARKS.—No mention has been made of the *diuretic* action of Hydrastis, yet it would seem to have such effect; it needs confirmation, however, and further provings may clear up the matter. From analogy, it is more than probable, this medicine has the same effect upon the mucous membranes of the urinary organs, that it has upon the mouth, nose, and fauces, above alluded to. The resinoid principle of the drug, may be eliminated through the kidneys, the same as Turpentine, Copaiva and others; if so, it would undoubtedly cause those blenorrhagic conditions of the bladder, urethra, etc., for which it is considered almost a specific. *King*, and every other Eclectic writer on therapeutics, assert its "great value in gleet, chronic gonorrhœa, *incipient stricture*, *spermatorrhœa* and *inflammation* and *ulceration of the internal coat of the bladder*." "Many cases of ulceration of the internal coat of the bladder have been cured by the decoction of Hydrastis alone. It must be injected into the bladder, and held there as long as the patient can conveniently retain it—to be repeated three or four times a day, immediately after emptying the bladder." It may be prepared as follows: Tincture Hydrastis, c., one drachm; hot water, one pint; inject about blood-heat. Its internal use alone would undoubtedly cure the disease, but it would require a longer time. (I have cured cystic blenorrhœa with Copaiva, Chimaphila, and Uva-ursi internally.)

In *Gleet*, it is beneficial, used in the same manner as above recommended. Dr. Hastings, U. S. Marine Hospital, San Francisco, California, reports in the *Pacific Journal*, his treatment for Gonorrhœa. Patients in the acute stage are freely purged; kept quiet; placed on half rations for three days; after which they are allowed full diet. The urethra from the time of the reception, is injected night and morning with a saturated infusion of fresh Hydrastis. He is first directed to urinate, and after the injection, to lie on his back for an hour or so to retain it. After the first purgation, no medicine is given internally. This treatment allays the chordee and ardor urinæ immediately, and in the course of a few days the disease is removed. Dr. H. says that, having used all kinds of treatment, he finds this produces a quicker cure, with less pain to the patient, than any other. Dr. Hastings has also employed the Hydrastis as an injection into the bladder in *Cystitis*. For this purpose, the temperature should be brought to blood-heat, and about four ounces thrown in daily. The pain on micturition is remarkably relieved." From this crude treatment, we may draw some practical suggestions. We can use the Hydrastis in minute quantities, with just as good effects as are gained from massive doses. *Dr. Coe*, says, it should be given *internally* in small and repeated doses in chronic inflammation of the blader. In congestion of the ureters, chronic suppression of urine, and gravelly affections, also in incontinence of urine, and diabetes, it will be found highly useful." This may be taken *cum grano salis*.

Generative Organs of Men.—It is homœopathic to chronic gonorrhœa, gleet, balanitis, balanorrhœa, etc. For the debility after spermatorrhœa it is an admirable remedy. (See urinary organs.)

Generative Organs of Women.—We regret that we have no provings of Iris v. upon women. But the clinical experience relating to use in some disordered states of the reproductive organs, is quite extensive. From its peculiar, specific action on other mucous tisues, we should consider it homœopathic to conditions marked by abnormal secretions, such as uterine and vaginal catarrh, or *mucus leucorrhœa* (which according to Tyler Smith is a hyper-secretion of the glandular portion of the cervix uteri). In this form of leucorrhœa the discharge is tenacious, sometimes hanging from the os, in a long viscid string. It should also be useful in *epithelial abrasion of the os and cervix uteri, and vagina*, especially when *superficial ulceration* is present. When these conditions are accompanied with considerable debility, and disorder of the digestive functions, I have found the Hydrastis one of the best of medicines. It should be given internally, in the lower attenuations, and used as an injection, of about the strength of one drachm of the tincture to one pint or quart of water. The enema should be retained five minutes, repeated twice or three times a day.

The following Eclectic testimony may not be inappropriate in this place:—"It is of singular efficacy in leucorrhœa when the complaint is complicated with hepatic aberration."—(*Dr. Coe.*)

"In those sympathetic affections of the digestive organs, arising from *uterine* diseases, we have obtained more benefit from it than from any other agent. Not only does it exercise a tonic influence upon the digestive organs, but if there is one agent more than another that deserves the name of *uterine tonic*, we believe that this is the agent. As a vaginal injecion in leucorrhœa, or inflammation, (J. & S. Met. Med.,) of the cervix uteri, it has no superior."

Dr. H. M. Saxton, of St. Joseph, writes me that he has used it very successfully in various forms of leucorrhœa. Very many other practitioners of our school consider it indicated in this class of affections, not from any special affinity for the generative organs, but by its general sphere of action, both as a restorative, and from its power to influence the conditions of mucous membranes.

Catarrhal Symptoms, etc.—Dull, frontal headache, with frequent coryza and constant secretion of tears; nose very much stuffed up; constant tickling of the larynx, with a dry harsh cough; chilliness; itching of the back and limbs; eyes smart and burn; scraping sensation in the larynx; constant rough, hacking cough.

Clinical Remarks.—Although our eclectic colleagues recommend it in "all *chronic*, and even acute inflammations of mucous membranes," yet they make no mention of its use in catarrh of the air passages. The above pathogenetic symptoms point directly to its effects on the respiratory tract. It causes many notable catarrhal symptoms. I would reccommend it, theoretically, in acute catarrhs-nasal, laryngeal and bronchial (in the sixth dil.), also in chronic catarrhs of those passages. It is homœopathic when the discharge is thick, yellowish, very tenacious, "stringy," and profuse. In these cases the low attenuations should be used, aided when practicable by the topical application in the form of injection. In the bronchial catarrh of old people, with debility, loss of appetite cachectic conditions, it should prove very useful.

Back and Upper Extremities.—Aching in the lower region; weariness in the arms.

Clinical Remarks.—I once treated a lady, during her climacteric period, whose chief complaint was an intense *aching* pain in the small of the back. This pain sometimes changed to a burning. The profuse menses, were lessened with Platina; the nervous symptoms by Lachesis and Pulsatilla, but neither these nor Sepia relieved the pain in her back. Upon the recommendation of a nurse she drank a decoction of Hydrastis, with the effect of removing the back-ache in a few days. The cure seemed permanent.

Lower Extremities.—Legs feel very weak, and ache; pain in the small of the back; severe pain in the right knee, lasting all day, and much aggravated by walking; dull aching in the loins.

Clinical Remarks.—In *irritable* ulcers on the legs, this medicine may be used in the form of a very weak wash, also internally. In *indolent* ulcers, a stronger preparation, even the pure tincture would be more useful.

DR. BURT'S PROVING OF HYDRASTIS.

Nov. 9th.—Feeling well, bowels regular once a day; urine natural; took ten grains 3. P. M., all day constant, slight pain in the umbilical region, with a hot sensation in the same parts, 7. P. M., soft stool, followed by severe cutting pains in the hypogastric region and dull aching pains in the testicles, accompanied with a very faint feeling; eructations of sour fluid; dull-heavy weight in the lumbar region.

Nov. 10th.—Feeling well, 9. A. M., took twenty grains 12 M.; dull, heavy, frontal headache; constant distress in the umbilical region, with loud rumbling in the bowels; dull aching sensation in the region of the kidneys; took fifteen grains 5. P. M., dull headache; slight constant, pain in the umbilical region; dull pain in the region of the kidneys; took forty grains; constant dull headache, with great deal of dull pain in the hypogastric region and small of the back; slight stool, with a faint feeling afterwards; legs feeling very weak, and ache; urinated twenty-eight oz. acid.

Nov. 11th.—Awoke several times in the night, with severe pain in the small of the back and hypogastric region, and dull pain in the umbilical region, aggravated by motion, with great rumbling in the bowels; stool at 6. A. M., soft, papescent, followed by a very faint feeling and severe pains in the hypogastric region; dull headache; eyes secreted large quantities of thick white mucus; mucous membrane of the eyelids good deal congested; nose very much stuffed up; slight hacking cough, with a scraping sensation in the larynx; took fifty grains at 10. A. M. 5. P. M., constant dull frontal headache; nose secreting constantly a thick white mucus; constant rough hacking cough; soft mushy stool at 2.P.M. with great rumbling in the bowels; constant coryza; my right knee has pained me very severely all day—walking aggravates it very much; took sixty grs. 9. P. M., there has been constant dull headache; frequent coryza with profuse secretion of tears; nose running constantly a thick white mucus; constant, slight, hacking cough; constant dull pain in the umbilical region; soft mushy stool; urinated forty-two oz. acid—heat has no effect upon it.

Nov. 12th.—Slept well; eyelids agglutinated together; mucous membrane of the lids congested; obstruction of the nose with thick mucus; frequent coryza; slight, hacking, rough cough; constant dull pain in the right side of the umbilical region; soft mushy stool; dull aching in the loins; apthæ-like sore on the mucous membrane of the under lip; took seventy grains at 10. A. M., 12. M,. there is a constant, dull, aching pain in the stomach, that produces a gone or faintish feeling; dull, frontal, headache 5. P. M., there has been constant pain in the cardiac portion of the stomach, that produces a very weak, faintish feeling; soft mushy stool; feeling very sad and gloomy; took eighty grains; constant pain in the stomach and umbilical region all the evening; dull heavy back-ache; urinated thirty-six oz., acid.

Nov. 13th.—Awoke a number of times with severe cutting pains in the stomach and umbilical region; nose stuffed up; apthæ is better; soft papescent stool; 10. A. M., took 100 grains; 12. M., constant dull pain in the umbilical region by spells quite sharp pains in the region of the spleen; feeling very gloomy; all the afternoon, dull pains in the stomach and bowels, with sharp pains in the region of the spleen, accompanied with a hot sensation; 4.P. M., took seventy drops of the tincture; constant dull burning pains all the evening, cramps in the umbilical region, with smarting of the eyes; urinated forty-one oz., slightly acid.

Nov. 14th.—The dull, heavy aching pains in the umbilical region prevented me from sleeping, most of the night; dull heavy headache; eye-lids agglutinated together; mucous membrane congested; nose stuffed up; soft mushy stool; 9. A. M., took fifty drops of Tildens fluid extract; 12. M., there has been constant, dull, burning pain in the umbilical region, accompanied with a faintish goneness in the epigastric region; dull frontal headache; burning in the eyes; took seventy-five drops; same symptoms were present all day; urinated sixty-one oz., slightly acid.

Nov. 15th.—Was very chilly all night, notwithstanding I had an abundance of clothes over me; great deal of pain in the umbilical and cœcum region all night; pain all day in the whole of the bowels; soft, mushy stool; urinated fifty oz.

Nov. 16th.—Feeling quite well.

IRIS VERSICOLOR.

(*Blue Flag.*)

DESCRIPTION.—This indigenous species of Iris has a perennial, horizontal, fibrous root, and a stem two or three feet high, round on one side, acute on the other, and frequently branching. The leaves are sheathing at the base, sword-shaped, and striated. The flowers are from two to six in number, and are usually blue, or purple, though varying much in color. The capsule has three valves, is divided into three cells, and when mature, is oblong, three-sided, with obtuse angles, and contains numerous flat seeds. The Blue Flag is found in all parts of the United States and Canada, flourishing in low wet places, and flowers in June. The root is the medicinal portion and yields its virtues to water, but more especially to alcohol.

MEDICAL HISTORY.—It is probable that its employment as a remedial agent, was first suggested to the profession by the Indians, who, it is said, value it as one of their most powerful medicines. Indeed, so important a place does it hold in their estimation, that a traveler among the tribes in Georgia and Florida, mentions having seen an artificial pond in almost every village, covered with a luxuriant growth of the *Iris*, and which was constructed especially for its cultivation. In times of prevailing sickness, they would partake freely of a decoction of the root, which, together with prayer and fasting, they considered an efficient guard against an attack of the epidemic. In allopathic practice it has been considered useful in dropsical affections, on account of its power as a diuretic, but it is more especially mentioned in the books as a cathartic and emetic, and is highly spoken of by some physicians for the promptness and certainty of its action in the direction its classification indicates. Dr. Bigelow states that he has found it efficacious as a purgative, though inconvenient from the distressing nausea and prostration which it is apt to occasion.

DR. WM. H. BURT'S PROVING WITH IRIS.

May 15th.—Took three grains of the green root at 3 P. M.; the acrid property was strongly marked; back part of the mouth and fauces felt on fire all the afternoon, with profuse flow of saliva; 8, P. M., took three more grains; slept well, but had a discharge of semen with amorous dreams, something I am not accustomed to.

May 16th.—Mouth and tongue feel as though they had been scalded, natural stools; anus feels sore, or as if sharp points were sticking in the parts; 8 A. M.; took ten grains; so acrid it was with difficulty that I could get my breath; constant discharge of ropy saliva dropped from my mouth during conversation; constant distress in the anus, feeling as if it was prolapsed. 1 P. M.; took twenty grains of the dried root; no acridness to it, great distress in the stomach half an hour after taking it; lasted two hours; no other symptoms.

May 17th.—Took thirty drops of a poor tincture; no symptoms, except that the next morning I awoke feeling very irritable.

May 18th.—Took forty grains of the green root; fifteen minutes after, profuse flow of saliva and tears; mouth and stomach feel on fire; almost impossible to breathe, it is so acrid; one half hour of great pain and distress in the stomach; it is awful to bear; continued all the afternoon and evening; it is not a sharp pain, but an awful, burning distress; appears to be deep in the region of the pancreas, cold water does not touch it; profuse flow of saliva all day; constant eructations of tasteless gas; sleep; very restless all night, with bad dreams.

May 19th.—Awoke at 4 A. M., with great rumbling and distress in the umbilical and hypogastric regions, and with great desire for stool, followed immediately by a copious, thin, watery stool, which could not be retained a moment without much pain; mouth feels as if it had been scalded, tongue thick and rough. 8 A. M., another thin, watery stool, with great rumbling in the bowels; no appetite; loss of taste. 11 A. M., took forty grains; acridness not felt so much. 1 P. M., in great distress in the epigastric region; the distress is horrible to endure; profuse flow of saliva. 2.30 P. M., the distress in the epigastric region is still increasing; very restless; cannot be still one moment; think I cannot live; very much frightened; copious discharge of thin water from the bowels, but no abatement of the awful agony in the epigastric region; inhaled chloroform, which gave a little relief. 3.15, P. M., another large stool of water, tinged with bile; the water ran from the bowels in a continuous stream; nearly two quarts of water passed; there was great rumbling in the bowels, but no pain; this gave great relief; felt quite well at bed-time; sleep, very restless; amorous dreams, with discharges of semen.

May 20th.—Very irritable through the day; otherwise quite well. I had constant eructations of tasteless gas during the whole period.

June 9th.—Took fifty grains of the green root, chewed it, and swallowed the juice, at 11.30 A. M.; immediately a great burning distress in the epigastric region, but not much in the mouth; profuse flow of saliva; the burning in the stomach is awful; cold water does not seem to reach it. 2.30 P. M., large, yellow, papescent stool; with great rumbling, but no pain; five minutes more, another large watery stool; the burning in the pancreas is fearful to endure; constant rumbling in the bowels, but no sharp pains. 2.45, P. M., another watery stool with colicky pains in the epigastric region; flow of saliva abating. 5.30, P. M., there has been severe colic in the epigastric and umbilical region for the last two hours; every few moments copious watery stool, with great rumbling in the bowels. 6 P. M., great pain and distress in the bowels, followed by a large watery stool; still the pain continues; begin to feel very faint and exhausted; knees weak and tremble. 6.30, P. M., another watery stool; anus feels on fire. 7, P. M., another watery stool, with disposition to strain and bear down; great burning in the anus; food rises very sour. 9, P. M., another watery stool with straining; anus feels on fire; becoming very much exhausted I was compelled to retire. At 4 A. M., great rumbling in the bowels, with desire for stool; had a profuse one of a watery nature; followed by great straining, with the passage of a little mucus. 5 A. M., another watery stool, followed by great straining, with the passage of blood and mucus. 5.30 A. M., another stool of mucus, streaked with blood, with great tenesmus. 7 A. M., stool of water and mucus with great straining; mouth tastes flat; tongue feels thick. 9 A. M., another copious stool of water and undigested food, with great straining; have become very much exhausted; eyes much sunken in; teeth feel too long, and are very sore; dull, heavy headache; very hoarse; urine very scanty—deep reddish color; stomach very sour; bowels very tender on pressure; loss of appetite. 10.30 A. M., another stool of mucus and water, with great tenesmus, and rumbling in the bowels; dull heavy headache in the forehead; calves of the legs pain very much when walking, especially the right; thick flat taste in the mouth. 12.45, P. M., small stool of mucus, with great tenesmus; constant rumbling in the bowels; almost impossible to walk, my limbs are so weak and painful; for the last six hours the mucous membrane of the anus has been prolapsed with great smarting pains. 3 P. M., another small stool of mucus, with severe tenesmus; urine very scanty, and burning when voided; constant eructations of sour gas; flying pains all through the bowels.

June 10th.—Dull, heavy headache in the frontal region; flat, thick taste in the mouth; quite hoarse; urine very scanty, red and burning the whole length of the urethra for half an hour after voiding it; inflammation of the glans penis; it is very much swollen and red; severe back-ache; teeth all feel sore and elongated.

June 11th.—Feel quite well; little hoarse; inflammation in glans penis about gone.

June 13th.—At 4 P. M., natural stools, urine about natural.

June 15th.—Very hard lumpy stool; anus feels prolapsed; pained all day.

June 16th.—Very severe back-ache, but otherwise well; for two weeks occasionally, severe, shooting pains would pass through my temples several times a day. I was surprised that no constipation followed such a long course of diarrhœa.

DR. BURT'S PROVING WITH IRISIN.

May 26th.—At 11 A. M., took four grains of the first decimal trituration. 12 M., dull, heavy headache in the forehead; by spells sharp pains in the temples; tight constrictive feeling of the scalp; 3.15, P. M., food rises very sour; 4.30 P. M., took eight grains; 10 P. M., soft papescent stool without pain, but rumbling in the bowels; dull headache in the frontal region; very restless night; dreams of fighting, etc.

May 27th.—Great deal of rumbling in the umbilical and hypogastric regions, with desire for stool; had a soft, papescent stool, without pain; flat taste in the mouth; teeth feel elongated and sore; back, upper, and lower molars—dull, heavy, aching pain in them for three hours; pain in the forehead and left temple; pain in the

34

temple very sharp by spells; passed water but twice during the day—very red color; restless night; discharge of semen, with amorous dreams.

May 28th.—At 9 A. M., took ten grains; frequent eructations of tasteless gas; rumbling all the afternoon in the umbilical region; pain in the right kidney—lasted three hours; teeth still feel elongated and sore; great desire to sleep in the day time; fell asleep while reading; dreamed of dissecting a woman hanging up by the heels in my office; awoke very much frightened; made several attempts to get up to shut the door, but could not; it was a regular night mare. 4.30, P. M., took fourteen grains; soft papescent stool at 9 P. M.; hands hot and dry all day; dreamed of snakes, and every thing bad; discharge of semen; restless night; teeth still sore.

May 29th.—Took twenty grains at 9 A. M.; hands hot and dry all day; cannot fix my mind on my studies; constant eructations of tasteless gas; great diminution of the secretion of urine; made a very little water morning and night, followed by great burning in the urethra for half an hour after voiding it; dull heavy headache in the forehead and temples; by spells the pains in the temples are very sharp and shooting; dull heavy pain in the lumbar region all day; soft papescent stool at 2 P. M. At 5 P. M. took thirty grains; restless night; horrid dreams; great rumbling in the bowels all the time; discharge of semen, with amorous dreams.

May 30th.—Mouth tastes flat; tongue coated white; dull heavy headache in the forehead and temples; at times the pain in the temples is very sharp; constant pain in the lumbar region, aggravated by motion; urine very scanty and high colored; very soft, yellow stool, with great rumbling in the bowels but no pain.

May 31st.—Took forty grains at 8 A. M.; dull, heavy headache all day; great pain in the lumbar and sacral regions; almost impossible to walk. 12 M., took eighteen grains; soft, mushy stool at evening, with great rumbling, but no pain; restless night; bad dreams.

June 1st.—Dull, heavy headache; back pains me very severely; very much worse by walking. 8 A. M., soft, papescent stool with great rumbling in the bowels; constant eructation of gas.

June 2d.—Took five grains of the pure Irisin; good deal of pain in the forehead and temples. 5 P. M., severe colic in the umbilical region; pains come on every few minutes; lasted two hours; great rumbling in the bowels; soft, papescent stool in the evening; restless night; dreampt of digging up dead people, and finally fell into the grave which awoke me, feeling very much frightened.

June 3d.—Top of the head has twenty-six pustules on it, some of them as large as a three-cent piece; the pustule is situated upon an inflamed base of a rose color; with red streaks running from one to the other; they contain yellow matter; very tender to the touch; gradually disappeared in four days. Took ten grains at 4 P. M.; dull heavy pain in the forehead and temples; great rumbling in the bowels; very restless night; dreampt of the dead, as usual; discharge of semen.

June 4th.—Flat taste in the mouth; teeth sore; natural stool; took twenty grains at 9 A. M.; dull heavy pain in the forehead and temples; the pain in the temples is very sharp at times; very restless night; awful dreams of the dead; discharge of semen.

June 5th.—Flat taste in the mouth; headache is very troublesome to-day; dull, heavy pain in the lumbar region all day. 5 P. M. soft, papescent stool with pain in the umbilical region; restless night with bad dreams; discharge of semen.

June 6th.—Dull, heavy headache; back pains me very much; had the soft, painless stools, with great rumbling in the bowels; great increase of urine; urinated eleven times profusely.

June 7th.—Natural stool; backache all gone, but voided urine in large quantities.

June 8th.—Feel well, but pass urine in large quantities; stool natural.

I would advise Allopaths to use Irisin for constipation, if they must use cathartics to cure it. In the last number of Braithwaite's Retrospect is a short notice of Irisin. It states that "the effects of Irisin are very similar to those occasioned by a combination of blue pill, rhubarb, and aloes. It seldom fails to produce a mild catharsis with bilious evacuations, and appears to possess the advantages (1) of not requiring the addition of murcurial, (2) not irritating the rectum as aloes is apt to do, (the green root does irritate the rectum very much); and (3) it has no astringency and therefore does not produce subsequent constipation, like rhubarb when given alone. (This last statement is correct, constipation does not follow the use of Iris.) In a sluggish state of the bowels, arising from torpidity of the liver, or when the stools are pale, particularly as we find them in the intervals of overt attacks in gouty persons, we have found the Irisin one of the best aperients, much gentler than Podophyllin, and more reliable when a slight cholagogue action is required, to be maintained for a lengthened period." (*Lancet*, Aug. 30, 1862, p. 239.)

PROVINGS BY J. G. ROWLAND, M. D.

The following provings, with one or two exceptions, were made from the *tincture* prepared in the customary manner. The attenuations used were made on the decimal plan. No. 1 used the third and first dilutions, and the mother tincture; No. 2 and No. 3, same; and No. 4, the first trituration.

No. 1.—About fifteen minutes after taking the third dilution, an uneasy feeling was experienced in the scorbiculis cordis, together with rumbling in the lower part of the abdomen; these symptoms increased until the lower part of the sternum seemed protruding; nausea and eructations of wind; dull pain in the right parietal protuberance, which increases steadily until it becomes a hammering pain, and so much aggravated by motion, that for the moment it appears unbearable, but by continuing movement it gradually abates, returning again when at rest; rheumatic pain in the right shoulder, worse on motion, especially by raising the arm; a disposition to feel displeased with everything and everybody, which gives place to a feeling of liveliness and activity, immediately after taking the first dilution; sneezing; nausea and slight vomiting of watery and extremely sour fluid; about two hours after, stitch in inferior part of occiput, more on the right than the left side; severe rheumatic pain in the whole right arm and right knee joint, worse on motion, and continuing when at rest; acute and extremely severe boring pain in right parietal protuberance, causing him to bend down his head; pain in the left side, as though the ribs were were pressing hard upon the lower portion of the lung; unable to take a long breath, for the pain in the left lung, which was of a sticking and cutting character; a short dry cough, excited by tickling in the larynx; slight toothache in a warm room; headache, much aggravated by coughing; rumbling and uneasiness in the stomach, accompanied by diarrhœa, with little pain; stools lumpy, brown, and very offensive; sweat over the whole body, particularly in the groin; dry cracked lips; a sharp cutting pain in the urethra, when commencing to urinate; after taking medicine five days, several small vesicles appeared on the right wrist, which gradually formed into pustules, having a depression in the centre; these dried up in the night, leaving crusts, which remained nine days before disappearing. (The prover thinks it proper to state he had been attending a severe case of small pox.) Half an hour after taking nearly half an ounce of the mother tincture, a feeling of rawness in the throat; general languor; ill-humor; inability to fix the mind on any subject; when writing, mind will wander to other things; diarrhœa, with colic; nausea, and vomiting of a thin watery fluid, of an exceedingly sour taste; constant nausea for more than an hour, and vomiting several times; diarrhœa, with rumbling and cutting in the lower part of the abdomen; heat over the whole body, then chilliness, with cold hands and feet; head feels very heavy, the eyes dull, with pain directly over the left superciliary ridge; severe burning pain in the internal canthus of the right eye; the eye filling with tears; sensation of fulness of the head; head feels hot, and face flushed; whenever attempting to laugh a sensation as though a band were drawn tightly around the forehead; the day after taking mother tincture, feeling of sleepiness, with great chilliness, only at all comfortable when near a hot fire, and even then, cold, chilly sensations are felt down the back; violent tearing pain in the right hip-joint, knee and shoulders, very severe, indeed; the most severe only lasting about three minutes; vomiting of the sour matter before mentioned; and great chilliness over the whole body the whole night, although abundantly covered; weakness; despondency; thinks he is going to be very sick, then a disposition to laugh at his fears, which, however, soon return; dreams of suffocation and fire; cutting and sticking in the urethra when making water, with coldness and itching over the genitals, the itching being worse on scratching; six dysenteric stools during the night, with pain and rumbling in the lower part of the abdomen; also great lassitude; after these symptoms have abated, there remains a sore-throat and slight headache.

No. 2. Feeling of weakness and weariness in the lower part

of the back; pain of a dull, aching character, in right hypochondria when walking; pains in the right, then in the left knee when walking; feeling of weariness in the back for several days; sharp pain near outer side of left arm, when moving it; swelling of gums on the inner surface of left side of lower jaw, under the molar teeth; pain in left hip joint, when walking; redness of the conjunctiva, as if from cold; for a day or two much fetid flatulence; pain in abdomen, which is relieved by discharge of flatus; sharp pain in first joint of great toe of right foot, when walking, renewed frequently during the day; pain in last joint of middle finger of left hand; a number of shooting, shifting, and momentary pains in the phalangeal and metacarpo-phalangeal articulations, all of these pains coming on more during the evening, and being worse on motion; boils on back, face and hands; pain along posterior part of cristi ilium of the right side; urine more copious; the pain in first joint of great toe occurs, during walking, for a number of days; pain in left thigh; pulse accelerated; after increasing doses more frequently renewed, empty eructations, and pain in the stomach; unusual restlessness during the night; sleep disturbed by startings; aching pain in the stomach before breakfast; *pains tensive and sticking in right shoulder during motion, particularly on raising the arm.* (This symptom set in soon after commencing the proving, continued six weeks after discontinuing the medicine.) Pains in the metacarpal joints of both hands, muscles of right arm, and pectoralis-major, mostly during motion, and in the evening; woke two hours earlier than usual, with no disposition to renew sleep; pain in the bowels, going off by discharge of flatus; feeling of a greasy coating over mouth and tongue, early in the morning; aching pain in the stomach after drinking cold water; pains through the day in most all the limbs; urine increased in quantity, *tensive, momentary, and constantly recurring pains* in all the joints, but mostly the *smaller;* which *shift rapidly about,* mostly in the evening, that is, from supper to bed-time; pain in abdomen above the crest of the ilium, both sides; after breakfast a diarrhœaic stool, with subsequent pain in the epigastrium; in writing, pains in phalanges of right hand, and in the end of index finger of same hand. (Observed several weeks after proving.) Pain in left thigh; shooting, sticking pain in the right foot; continuous sharp pain along the left side of first phalanx of middle fingers of right hand; sharp pains in the middle fingers of left hand succeeded instantly by a similar pain in the axillæ of same side. (Occurring frequently during about five minutes.) Sudden diarrhœaic stool after supper; sharp, cutting pain, frequent in the metacarpo-phalangeal articulation of thumb of right hand; vexed, irritable mood, disposed to find fault. (Proving No. 2 was made by the same individual, at three different periods.)

No. 3.—Pulse somewhat accelerated; headache for two days; the third day he was seized with a peculiar headache; the pain shot, as he describes it, like an electric shock, from the right temple to the left part of occiput, and continued about half an hour; headache with great depression of spirits and general debility;

crampy pains in right lumbar region in the evening, continuing several hours, and causing a sweat to break out; woke up unusually early, with dry mouth and general depression; headache occurring irregularly during several days; observed a pimple on middle finger of left hand; the next day the inflammation was extended over the hand; the day after it became more violent, and occasioned great pain, and was afterwards opened to obtain relief; no pus was found, but it was subsequently formed, and discharged through the opening, which penetrated as far as the bone; a fungous growth meanwhile had taken place around the edges; pain extended from this hand up the arm; there was much swelling and pains* in the part affected, which had much the appearance of a malignant boil; there was a disposition to a similar formation on the index finger but the inflammation subsided after a time, and finally disappeared; during the proving the urine was very copious, and had a strong disagreeable odor; restlessness for five nights in succession; headache with pain in the bowels; sickness of stomach in the evening, obliging him to lie down; pain in left side of chest.

No. 4.—Colicky pains during the evening and night, obliging him to bend forward for relief, and attended with loss of appetite and great restlessness during the night; this colic continued the next day, but was immediately removed by a dose of Nux vomica; no appetite the next day; restless at night, with troubled dreams; several pimples on lower extremities and other parts of the body, like mosquito bites; constipation several days; languid and feverish in the afternoon; no disposition to mental or physical exercise; next day flushed face, fever, drowsiness and loss of appetite; weakness and languor, with rumbling in the bowels; the morning after, a thin watery diarrhœa, continuing through the day; debility and loss of appetite; diarrhœaic stools the next day, succeeded by pain in the umbilical region; colic in the afternoon, ceasing at night.

CHARACTERISTIC PECULIARITIES.—The symptoms appear mostly in the evening and at night. (In myself the symptoms appeared mostly in the day time.) *Pain aggravated by motion*; right side most effected.

EFFECTS UPON ANIMALS. EXPERIMENTS OF DR. BURT.

June 5th.—Gave a young female cat, weight three and one-fourth pounds, a decoction of Iris ver.; at 2 P. M., five minutes nausea and vomiting of frothy mucus; stares at it as if frightened; ten minutes after, constant nausea, nothing but mucus vomited. Quarter after 2, lies on the lounge and appears quite natural; gave half an ounce of tincture (wasted a little); six minutes after, very restless, crying fearfully; nausea and vomiting. Twenty minutes after 4, nausea and retching; mewing; eyes half closed; respiration very rapid; restless. Half past 4, mewing and efforts to vomit; lies still thirty-six minutes; running across the floor with efforts to vomit; mews; saliva runs from mouth constantly. Forty-three minutes after, desperate efforts to vomit but cannot. Ten

* The pain in the finger was accompanied by perspiration, although the weather was cold.

minutes to 5, nausea and mewing; saliva running profusely. 5, retching; throws her head up and mews fearfully; respiration seventy-two; mouth wide open. Ten minutes after, nausea and moaning. Quarter-past 5, retching and sneezing; head hangs to the floor. Half-past 5, nausea and vomiting; very restless; mewing; respiration fifty-six; does not notice anything; mouth wide open; saliva running profusely; mews and appears in great distress. 6, the nausea continues, with great efforts to vomit; saliva runs from the mouth constantly; groaning and appears in great distress; nose rests on the floor; mouth wide open. 7, still sick at the stomach; saliva runs in great quantities; respiration forty-six; gave half an ounce more; died in five minutes without a struggle.

Post-mortem one hour after death: pupils dilated; the brain was not examined; lungs very much congested; the upper lobes filled with dark venous blood; heart filled with black blood; stomach natural color, but very much distended with gas, with a quantity of meat undigested; pyloric extremity covered with bile; also the duodenum and jejunum was covered with bile and watery mucus; liver is very much congested, of a black color, bleeds profusely when cut into; gall bladder half full of bile; the pancreas is very pale; all other organs natural.

June 23d.—Gave a female kitten, four months old, at 2 P. M., forty grains of Irisin; wasted a good deal. Half-past 2, profuse flow of saliva; mouth wide open; wants to lie down all the time; respiration very rapid; mews constantly. 3 P. M., mews most fearfully; appears to be in great pain; rolls from one side to the other; mouth wide open; great difficulty in breathing; appears to be dying; secretion of saliva is very limited. Quarter-past 3, still lying in the same position, mewing at every breath; mouth filled with froth; walked two feet, staggered very much; dropped on its side; respiration forty-eight. Half-past 3, tries to walk but falls; mews at every breath. 4 P. M., cannot stand; lies on its side; respiration thirty-six; mouth open, filled with froth. Quarter-past 4, respiration forty-eight. 5 P. M., gasping for breath; respiration twenty-four; if spoken to mews fearfully, but cannot get up; in ten minutes crawled two feet; went into a spasm, lasted one minute; the spasms were in its fore legs and back; respiration eighteen; pupils dilated. 7 P. M., on its side gasping for breath; respirations eighteen; cannot stand when lifted up; ears and legs cold; mews fearfully by spells, as if suffering great pains; kicks and scratches at a fearful rate. Half-past 8, appears in great pain; mews every breath. Half-past 9, went into spasms, the forelegs and spine; had a watery passage from the bowels and died.

Autopsy ten hours after death.—Upper lobes of the lungs very much congested; heart, auricles and ventricles all filled with dark venous blood; liver very much congested, especially the left lobe; gall bladder half filled with gall; stomach almost ready to burst with gas; part of the medicine in it; color natural; little food in it; *pancreas red with blood; more congested than any other organ;* the whole of the intestines are filled with mucus, water, and gas; no bile to be seen; all the other organs natural.

General Symptoms.—Nervous; irritable, with prostration of the whole system; weakness, so that he can hardly stand; nearly all the symptoms are aggravatd by motion.

Clinical Remarks.—Nearly all the conditions for which Iris is applicable, are characterized by unusual lassitude, prostration and lowness of spirits; it is most useful in persons of bilious temperament, subject to gastric and bilious disorders.

Skin.—Several vesicles on the right wrist, gradually forming into pustules, which dried up in one night, leaving crusts which remained nine days; malignant sore resembling a boil, on middle finger of left hand, forming a cavity reaching to the bone; pimples resembling mosquito bites, on body and extremities; small boils on the back, face and hands.—(*Rowland*). Twenty-six pustules on the scalp, (vertex) some as large as a three-cent piece; the pustules are situated upon a rose-colored, inflamed base, with red streaks running from one to the other; they were painful on pressure, and filled with yellow pus.—(*Burt*).

Clinical Remarks.—It has been highly recommended for scrofulous affections, and skin-diseases; it would seem homœopathic to certain pustular eruptions.

Case.—Reported by Dr. Burt, treated since he made the proving. "A child aged eight months; the vertex and sides of the head covered with a thick crust from the exudation of lymph; under the scab it looks red, and bleeds if the incrustation is disturbed. There are also scabs at the back of both ears, which look red and bloody. Gave Iris versicoler, ten drops of the mother tincture in a tumbler full of water, one teaspoonfull three times a day; a cerate of the same remedy to be applied twice a day; the head to be washed once a day with castile soap. The one prescription cured it in two weeks. It is now nine weeks, and there is no return of the eruption."

Sleep.—Feeling of drowsiness; sleepiness with chills; unusual restlessness during the night; waking much earlier than usual; startings during sleep; restless every night; dreams of suffocation and fire.—(*Rowland.*) Very restless at night; bad dreams during the whole proving; dreams of the dead every night; amorous dreams, with nocturnal emissions, (from Iris v). Dreams of snakes, of the dead; of dissecting a body; awoke very much frightened; tried to get up and shut the door, but could not. (This attack resembled nightmare). Dreams of fighting; amorous dreams (from Irisin).—*Burt.*

Mind.—Desponding; low spirits; easily vexed, and put out of humor; afraid he is going to be very sick, and afterwards laughs at his fears, which soon return, succeeded by blindness and activity. (*Rowland.*)—*Very irritable;* confusion of the mind; dullness of the mental faculties; cannot fix the mind on his studies; fear of death; waking with fright.—(*Burt*).

Clinical Remarks.—The above symptoms of mind and sleep are probably not due to any direct irritation of the brain, but rather to the disturbing action which the Iris exercises upon the liver and gastric mucous membrane. The lowness of spirits is an indication for its use in hepatic disorders, and perhaps in spermatorrhœa; it would seem particularly applicable to the night cries and "terrors" of children, from intestinal irritation.

Fever, etc.—Sweat, from violent pain in the finger; sweat over the whole body, but particularly in the groin; heat over the whole body, followed by chill, with cold hands and feet; desire to be close to the fire, and even then, chills along the back; chills over the whole body at night, although abundantly covered; feverish, during pains in abdomen; pulse accelerated.—(*Rowland*). Dry, hot skin; hands hot and dry; pulse slightly accelerated (during the whole proving).—(*Burt*).

Clinical Remaks.—It is used by eclectic physicians in bilious fevers, much as the allopath uses calomel; it is considered a sort of "vegetable mercury," causing copious bilious evacuations, salivation, etc. Dr. Kitchen, (North Amer. Jour. of Hom. Nov. 1851), recommended the Iris v. very highly in *typhoid fever*. He reports several cases:

Case 1.—"A boy, twelve years of age, had typhoid fever. I had given a number of remedies without effect; he had fever; muttering delirium; yellow, watery, fœtid diarrhœa; involuntary passage of water and fæces; coated tongue, dry, brown, crusty; edges red; sordes on the gums and teeth; foul breath, and all the marked symptoms of this disease. I gave the Iris, third dilution. It certainly produced a very marked change, showing its effect, first on the tongue and bowels, and thence extending its beneficial action to other parts. It was on the tenth day of the disease when I gave it, and in five days he was convalescent, although I had no idea he could possibly recover; the tongue became moist; diarrhœa eased off, fever subsided; delirium ceased; and he soon became rational, slept well, and had a rapid convalescence."

Case 2.—"An old lady aged eighty-three, had fever; stupor; black, stinking, *involuntary* diarrhœa; tongue dry and brown; fœtid breath. Cured (?) in 48 hours."

Case 3.—"A middle aged woman. Fever; intense headache; pain in small of the back; black dysenteric passages; nausea and efforts to vomit; cured in four days. (After she took a few doses she lost all power over her lower extremities; had cramps of the legs, nausea, and some retching.)"

Case 4.—"A young man, aged fourteen, with an attack of bilious pneumonia; could not retain even a mouthful of water on his stomach; continued easy through the subsequent course of the disease."

The provings here given show Iris to be homœopathic to all the above symptoms in each case.

Head.—Dull, heavy headache in the forehead, accompanied by weakness, nausea, and even vomiting (from Iris); heavy headache in the forehead and temples—at times sharp, *shooting* pains in the temples, (this pain occurred as often as every half hour during the whole proving); pain in the forehead and *right* temple; constrictive feeling in the scalp (from Irisin); dull pain in the right parietal protuberance; (*Burt*), becoming a hammering pain, aggravated by motion, which if continued relieves it—but it soon returns when at rest (see Rhus); severe stitch in the lower part of the occiput, more on the right side; extremely severe boring pain in the right parietal protuberance, causing him to bend the head down; headache aggravated by coughing; sensation of fullness in the head; head and face feel hot; when attempting to laugh, sensation of constriction around the forehead; head feels heavy; lancinating pain under outer extremity of right eyebrow; pain shooting from the temple to left occiput, compared to an electric shock.—(*Rowland.*)

Clinical Remarks.—The Iris-headache occupies generally the forehead and *right* side of the head; *aggravated* by rest, and on first moving the head, but relieved by continued motion: accompanied by lowness of spirits, nausea, and even vomiting. Dr. Kitchen, who published the first clinical experience with this remedy, says of its use in "sick-headache:"—"It is the most prompt and effectual remedy I have ever given in this truly annoying malady. The first dose will arrest the trouble, in some patients. I have experienced this effect in several cases. I have made comparative trials with it and other remedies, telling my patients to observe, and let me know which number would relieve them the most speedily; they have invariably, on the attack, sent for the number attached to Iris; this I consider conclusive respecting this complaint, so that I need not comment on it further than to recommend it very highly, so far as my experience goes. Let it be tested by others."

The Iris has been tested by many homœopathic physicians, in sick-headache, and the testimony is generally in its favor; from our knowledge of the sphere of action of the medicine, it would seem most likely to be indicated in those "sick-headaches" of a *gastric* or *hepatic* origin; in the purely "*nervous* sick-headache" or that variety arising from *congestion*, other remedies may prove more useful. This matter, however, can only be decided by careful observation.

In *Neuralgia* of the head, eyes, etc., Dr. Kitchen recommends the Iris: "A lady afflicted at intervals with this most distressing complaint, and who had swallowed the whole allopathic and homœopathic Mat. Med., with only partial benefit, has been more relieved by the Iris, than by any remedy I have yet administered to her. It is usually in the head, temples, eyes, etc., and attended with most distressing vomitings, of a sweetish mucus; and occasionally, when with much straining, with a trace of bile. It is the only medicine which has much control over the stomach, arresting the vomiting in the few trials I have made with it, very soon, and allaying in some degree, the violent pain of the head, so that I have been asked by her whether I had not given her morphine. I have been asked the same question by patients in bowel affections, they frequently going to sleep after its administration; this is easily accounted for by the cessation of pain, which is almost invariably followed by sleep."

Eyes.—Redness of the conjunctiva, as if from a cold; the eyes feel dull, with pain over left superciliary ridge; severe burning pain in internal canthus, with effusion of tears.—(*Rowland.*) Eyes sunken, with blueness around the eyes.—(*Burt.*)

Clinical Remarks.—Dr. Kitchen relates that while giving the Iris to a child for summer complaint, the mother said to him:—"Doctor, you have not only relieved the diarrhœa, but you have cured my child of *inflamed eyelids*, which it has been troubled with for some time." He states that he has tried it in several cases of that affection, and with success. The cases in which it seemed to be of benefit, were those of simple palpebral inflammation, apparently arising from a cold—nothing that I could perceive of a scrofulous taint—they did not adhere in the morning, at least very slightly.

Ears.—Singing and buzzing in the ears (in a lady—after two grains of Irisin second, given for bilious diarrhœa, which it cured after Chamomilla, Pulsatilla and Ipecac had failed).—(*Burt*).

Mouth, Fauces, etc.—Greasy feeling over tongue and gums on rising in the morning; feeling of rawness in the mouth; slight soreness of throat; dry mouth; slight toothache in a warm room; dry, cracked lips; swelling and soreness of gums, inner part below molar teeth of left side.—(*Rowland.*) Back part of mouth and fauces feel on fire (constant symptom); tongue feels as though it had been scalded; flat taste in the mouth; constant discharge of saliva—it dropped from the mouth during conversation; tongue coated white; diminution of taste; teeth feel sore and elongated; ulcers on the mucous membrane of the cheeks [Iris]; dull, heavy, aching pains in all the teeth; teeth feel very sore and elongated; severe pain in the back upper and lower molars, lasting three hours, [Irisin].—(*Burt.*)

Clinical Remarks.—The Eclectics class this plant among the "sialagogues," Dr. Burt, who proved the fresh root in large doses, does not doubt that it would produce sloughing and deep ulceration, if continued for a long time. There is a rather curious and remarkable similarity between the action of the Iris and that of Mercury; this is all the more singular when we consider that the former is a vegetable remedy; not only does this Iris affect the mouth in a similar manner to Mercury, but this similarity of action extends throughout the whole glandular and mucous systems, and perhaps, all the tissues except the *osseous*. I have taken patients from off the hands of Eclectic physicians, who were so completely salivated by the Iris, that were it not for the absence of the peculiar *fœtor*, I should have taken it for a mercurial salivation. Even the sympathetic fever which the Iris causes, has considerable resemblance to that of Mercury. *Dr. Coe* (Conc. Org. Med.), thus speaks of the *Irisin*:—"Irisin is justly esteemed as one of our most valuable alteratives. It is eminently resolvent, and exercises a marked influence over the entire glandular system. It increases the salivary flow, and has the reputation of producing ptyalism. But a careful distinction must be made between the effects produced by vegetable agencies upon the mucous and salivary glands, and mercurial salivation; the former are nothing more nor less than manifestations of a quickened physiological activity—evidence of special therapeutic stimulus, constituting oftentimes a critical conservative effort—No loosening of the teeth; no sponginess of the gums; no putrefactive odor; no sloughing of the soft parts; *increased*, but not disordered secretion. On the other hand, Mercury induces a pathological condition of the vital constituents of the blood and fluids, and favors the formation of vitiated products; altering from good to bad, and from bad to worse; giving rise to congestions, lesions, putrefactive conversions, and disorganizations of the organic structures. In the former case we have the evidence of a direct therapeutic stimulus, operating upon the vital impressibility of the secretive apparatus, promoting increased activity of the functions for the purpose of eliminating legitimate products. In the latter instance we have an augmented flow of morbid material, resulting from the destructive conversions of the vital constituents by the remedy itself, and which are not the legitimate products of organic metamorphoses. In the former case, the remedy itself is the motor-stimulus, while in the latter instance the mercurial corruptions constitute the stimuli of excitement."

To the superficial student of medicine, the above *reads* very well, but to the physiologist it becomes simply absurd. Only one conclusion can be drawn, namely, that Dr. Coe is *ignorant* or *dishonest*. Nothing but the gravest ignorance of the elementary facts of physiology and pathology, could lead to such special pleading. He must be aware that any *departure from a normal physiological state, constitutes a pathological condition.* Given to a person in perfect health, the Iris causes abnormal activity of the glandular and mucous systems: Mercury does as much. The main difference between the actions of the two medicines is in *degree*. The poisonous effects of Mercury are more pervading and more malignant than the pathogenetic effects of the Iris. Both cause actual pathological conditions, having their peculiarities and characteristic symptoms. When given in disease, if homœopathically indicated, and administered in proper doses, they both restore the tissues, for which they have an affinity, to a healthy condition.

If Dr. Coe was dishonest in his statements with the intention to prejudice the reader against Mercury his conduct degenerates into downright meanness. Mercury, when administered according to the law of similia, is a benificent, and valuable curative agent. When given in this manner, it never causes any pathogenetic symptoms, gives rise to no morbid products, and disorganizes no tissues or secretions. On the contrary it tends to prevent the very calamities which Dr. Coe so much dreads, and which he could cause, *to a certain degree*, by the abuse and prolonged use of even the Iris. I would here make an observation relative to the action of Iris, namely: it is *not* owing to the acridity of the fresh root acting topically, that the pseudo-mercurial symptoms are due, but to a specfic dynamic action of the drug on the constitution. It is true that the Iris *does* contain an acrid principle, but from the fact that the dried root, and even the alkaloid, causes the above-named condition when taken into the stomach, is proof that those effects belong to the whole drug. If this was not sufficent proof, we could refer the physician to the fact that this peculiar action may be caused by the *dilutions* of the remedy, up to the third, and perhaps higher.

THERAPEUTIC DEDUCTIONS.—It is a strange comment on the practice of the opposite school, that they should recommend the Iris highly in *mercurial cachexy*, *syphilis*, *etc.*! No drug is more thoroughly homœopathic to diseases of the mouth, similar to those caused by Mercury, and in the few cases in which I have used it, it has acted well. Even in mercurial salivation it has been found useful, but it cannot be relied on with as much confidence as the Chlorate of Potash. In *Stomatitis*, with or without ulceration (canker), when there is painful *burning* in the mouth and fauces, Iris is strongly indicated. In these cases I would advise the tincture of the green root, administered in the third or sixth attenuation.

Gastric Symptoms.—Loss of appetite; nausea and empty eructations; nausea, and vomiting of a watery and extremely sour fluid; constant nausea and vomiting for an hour; aching in the stomach before breakfast, and on drinking cold water; sickness of stomach obliged him to lie down.—(*Rowland.*)

Eructations of tasteless gas; rising of water, very sour; *great burning distress in the epigastric region*; it could not be allayed by drinking cold water; colicky pains every few minutes in the epigastric region; *Intense burning in the region of the pancreas* (this was a constant symptom during the whole proving.—(*Burt.*) Severe and profuse vomiting; vomiting with much pain in the stomach; distressing nausea and vomiting; vomiting and purging; vomiting with diarrhœa, accompanied with great prostration; burning in the mouth, fauces, and œsophagus.

CLINICAL REMARKS.—The Iris has probably an irritant action upon the gastric mucous membrane, as seen upon the mouth, fauces and œsophagus. By refering to Dr. Burt's heroic provings, this action will be seen portrayed in strong colors. I know of no one of the new remedies which promises to be more useful in gastric disorders, than the Iris versicolor. Even now we have some valuable clinical observations.

Dr. Kitchen in his paper on Iris, says it is useful in *vomiting*: "Effectual in almost all kinds—simple sour, bilious, of food, with or without pain. In every case of vomiting or sick stomach in which I have yet given it, it has been successful, and, in severe cases, on the administration of a few tea-spoonfuls. Such has been my experience. I have recomended it in some cases in which the other usual remedies had failed, and in no case in which I have given it, have I been obliged to abandon it, and resort to other remedies. Such, I again say, has been my experience thus far, but I would not be understood as saying that this will always be the case in future. No doubt it, like all other remedies, has its appropriate sphere, which it will take time and opportunity to make out and define correctly. I merely state what I have discovered up to the present, with the limited opportunities I have had of testing it in different forms of disease. I have for some years attended a little girl, now about nine years of age, who has periodical vomiting spells, coming on once every month or six weeks, sometimes not for three or four months, but certainly three or four times in the course of a year. I have tried in various attacks, all the different remedies usually successful in such cases, but not with much benefit; the attack would last two or three days, and would seem to wear itself out. A single tea-spoonful of the *Iris* arrests it at once. It comes on with vomiting of the ingesta, then sour fluid, and at last, bile, yellow and green, with great heat of the head, some general fever, and great prostration; the perspiration is warm, caused by the efforts of straining and vomiting."—(*N. A. Jou. of Hom.*)

The Iris is eminently homœopathic to some varieties of *gastritis* (mucous), *œsophagitis*, *duodenitis*, and many of those disorders of digestion which go under the general name of *dyspepsia.* In many points it resembles Pulsatilla, especially the tendency to "acidity of the stomach," and "rising of ingesta;" also the sympathetic disturbances having a gastric origin. The peculiar and severe symptoms elicited by Dr. Burt, and referred by him to the pancreas (see proving,) and which, in all probability, were really in the gland, point to its applicability to *inflammation*, and other disorders of that important organ. In that disease known as "Pancreatic salivation" it ought to prove specific. A thorough knowledge of the physiology of the pancreas will lead us to define pretty clearly the derangements likely to be caused by the Iris. The pancreas is usually regarded as belonging to the group of salivary glands. "The pancreatic juice is analagous to saliva. It acts upon starch even more energetically than saliva, transmuting it into sugar and lactic acid; and upon fats, by forming them into an emulsion so that they are readily absorbed. —(*Draper.*) It is generally conceded that a normal pancreatic juice (as regards quality and quantity), is necessary for the digestion of fatty food. Many of the derangements of digestion, are undoubtedly due to deficiency, and unhealthy conditions of this juice. There can be no rational doubt of the action of Iris upon this gland. Even had we not Dr. Burt's suggestive provings, we could judge of its effects upon that gland from analogy. A remedy which irritates and stimulates the salivary glands, must have a similar action on the pancreas—a similar tissue, possessing similar functions.—(Puls., Merc., Iodine, Podoph.)

Prof. Lee (Allopathist) says:—"It acts as a stimulant to the liver and *pancreas*." Our list of pancreatic remedies are five in number, and the symptoms they possess, directly referring to that gland are quite *indefinite*. The *Iris* promises to prove very valuable for the removal of morbid states, induced, directly or indirectly, by functional diseases of that organ. *Dr. Burt* succeded in killing several cats with the tincture of Iris versicolor. One of the most noted morbid appearances noticed on examination was a highly *congested condition of the pancreas*. A portion of one pancreas was sent, through me, to Dr. Ludlam of this city, who subjected it to a critical examination, which proved the presence of intense congestion of the minute vessels, and even a rupture, and extravasation of blood into the tissues of the gland.

Dr. Kitchen says he "cured a case of gastrodynia characterized by violent pains in the epigastric region, coming on at intervals" with Iris. The Iris relieved him at once, and he had no return. He has also relieved and cured, "vomiting of food an hour after meals," with Iris.

Liver, Hypochondria, etc.—Pain in the right hypochondria—worse on motion; pain above the cristi ilii on both sides, first on the right; crampy pains in the right lumbar reigon.—(*Rowland.*) Cutting pains in the region of the liver.—(*Kitchen.*)

Clinical Remarks.—Prof. Lee (allopathic) says, the Iris "*stimulates the liver.*"

A writer in the London Lancet, asserts the *Irisin* to be a powerful and efficient *cholagogue.*

King intimates that it acts upon the liver in a manner similar to the mecurial preparations; not as active as Podophyllin but more lasting. The opposite school believe it stimulates the liver, increasing the secretion and excretion of bile, by virtue of its general stimulative action on the glandular system. Dr. Kitchen (homœopathic) says:—"May it not be administered beneficially in some *affections of the liver?* It undoubtedly acts on this organ. I have had full evidence of that in several cases, producing a manifest secretion of healthy bile."

Abdomen, Stool, etc.—Uneasy feeling in the scrobiculis cordis; rumbling in lower part of abdomen; lower part of sternum seems protruded; cutting pain in the lower part of the abdomen, relieved by discharge of flatus; colic, obliging him to bend forward for relief; fœtid flatulence; diarrhœa with slight pain, accompanied by rumbling and uneasiness in the stomach; stools lumpy, brown, and very offensive; diarrhœa with colicky pains; diarrhœa with rumbling and cutting in the lower part of the abdomen; six *dysenteric stools at night,* with rumbling and pain in abdomen, and great lassitude; sudden liquid evacuation after supper; constipation for some time, succeeded by thin watery diarrhœa.—(Rowland). Colicky pains every few minutes in the epigastric and umbilical regions, with desire for stool (during the whole proving); four yellow, papescent stools, with rumbling in the bowels; fourteen thin watery stools, followed by two stools consisting of water and mucus, *with tenesmus;* watery stool; copious running from the bowels in a continuous stream; stool tinged with green; stool of undigested food; stool of blood and mucus, with great tenesmus, and a sensation as if the anus was on fire; anus feels as if sharp points were sticking in it; mucus membrane of the rectum prolapsed; great smarting and burning of anus after every stool.—(*Dr. Burt, from Iris.*) Swelling of the stomach and abdomen.—(*Kitchen.*) [The Irisin produced severe, intermittent colic in umbilical region, with soft mushy stool; also soft, papescent stools, with rumbling, but *no* pain.]

Clinical Remarks.—The Iris is esteemed by the opposite schools as a powerful cathartic, but one which, they assert, does not leave constipation after its cathartic action. Dr. Burt sustains this assertion by the results of his own proving of massive doses. Prof. Lee says:—"As a cathartic it is said to act on all parts of the canal, but more particularly on the upper portion. It has been rejected by some as unsafe and dangerous; but it was probably administered in over doses." Iris undoubtedly causes bilious discharges from the bowels. Dr. Burt thinks he has seen evacuations of *pure bile* follow its use. The burning and smarting, however, at the anus and rectum, noticed in the proving, is rather the result of its *acridity*, than the effect of bilious fluids; the sensations in the rectum are probably due to the same cause as the burning in the mouth and fauces. Regarding its therapeutic action, we cannot do better than quote Dr. Kitchen's experience:

Colic.—"Some cases I have relieved. The colic of infants is benefited by it. There is a peculiar condition of the abdominal region of the adult also, which may come under this head, and which may be termed a grumbling bellyache. It is most prevalent at the changes of the seasons, Spring and Autumn, and appears to be owing to a vitiated secretion of the liver, and mucous membrane of the bowels, and consists in an almost constant uneasiness and grinding in the bowels; a kind of sub-colic; a mushy passage once or twice a day, in some cases, but in the generality of cases, a very fœtid discharge of wind, of a coppery smell, attended occasionally with an involuntary escape of fluid, soiling the shirt, and sometimes a passage of scybalous matter, together with fluid, mucoid fœces of an offensive, putrid, and coppery odor. It was a case of this kind which first led me to a use of this remedy. I had tried several medicines without the least relief, for nearly a week, and administered the Iris at random, never having given it in any disease. To my surprise the patient was shortly relieved, and had no return; his bowels soon became healthy and regular, and he praised the good effects of the remedy very highly. The sphere of the Iris appears to be chiefly the stomach and abdominal contents."

Diarrhœa.—"I have not yet been able to obtain with any degree of accuracy, the symptoms of those cases in which it proves to be the most appropriate. I think, however, that *burning* in the rectum and anus, after a passage, is one state which it arrests almost immediately. It also seems to be appropriate to cases in which there are pains, and *green* discharges, relieving the pains very frequently in a short time, and changing the green passages after some doses have been given. There is one very curious feature which I have frequently observed, which is, that when the diarrhœa is not arrested after a few doses, it seems, after the administration of it for twenty-four or forty-eight hours, to produce an aggravation; there is an increase of pain and several free fœtid passages, and then the diarrhœa ceases. This generally has taken place about two or three o'clock in the morning. Whether I have given it in too low dilutions, generally from second to sixth, I cannot tell, but such a feature I have frequently observed, and have administered it with perfect success in a few cases of *periodical night diarrhœa*, attended with pain, and two or three free discharges towards morning. I have also cured *all* my cases of *cholera infantum* with it this summer, and some of them in a few days. I look upon it as a very valuable addition to our remedial measures in this complaint.

"In *Cholera morbus*, I have succeeded in every case in which I have yet administered it, even the most violent. A single teaspoonful, of a few drops in a half tumbler of water, has in many very severe cases, put immediate stop to the vomiting. I consider it a specific in this form of disease, and I would earnestly request physicians to try it in the first cases of Cholera Asiatica, which may fall under their notice, and give the result to the profession. In cholera morbus, it arrests the pain which is so violent in many cases at the pit of the stomach, or around the navel, or, in some cases, still lower down in the abdominal region, at or before every fit of vomiting or purging. In fact, it seems, as far as I have as yet been able to judge, the more appropriate the more violent the pain, and in some cases, acting, as the patients and bystanders express themselves, 'like a charm.'

Dysentery.—"Some mild cases I have cured with Iris, but it is not *the* remedy in this disease. The cases which seemed to be benefited were of the nature of *dysenteric* diarrhœa, attended with green discharges, or slimy mucus, without blood, or much straining. (Dr. Burt's proving elicited these very symptoms, however, and quite severely.) In one case it evidently acted favorably on the secretion of the liver, producing a free flow of healthy bile, and an immediate abatement of the unhealthy passages. In those cases in which there was bloody flux, I did not rely on it, not knowing sufficient of its curative powers." The pathogenesis of Iris points directly to its sphere of usefulness in some varieties of dysentery, probably in bilious-dysentery; yet there can be no doubt of the power of Iris to cause *acute mucous enteritis*, but the inflammation *may* be located higher in the intestinal canal, than in ordinary cases of dysentery. (Here it appears the opposite of aloes and podophyllum, which affect the lower portion of the canal, rectum, etc.") It will be seen by the proving, however, that it has many symptoms analogous to Podoph.—the prolapsus of rectal mucous membrane," "pricking in anus," etc. Dr. Kitchen's successful use of Iris in abdominal typhus, proves its applicability in some quite severe forms of intestinal inflammation, and perhaps in organic lesions of that canal. (*See Ferri*). I would simply add, by way of testimony that many homœopathists, with myself, have found the Iris a valuable remedy in nearly every disease of the bowels for which Dr. K. recommends it. I would also suggest its use in *hæmorrhoids*, *bilious colic*, fisure of the anus, fistula in ano, etc.

Urinary and Genital Organs.—A sharp cutting pain in urethra when beginning to urinate; urine copious; strong, disagreeable smell to the urine; cutting and sticking in urethra when urinating; coldness and itching of the genitals.—(*Rowland.*) Dark red urine, with burning in the urethra for half an hour; increase in the quantity of urine; *nocturnal emissions with amorous dreams* (from Iris): profuse urination—eleven times a day—for three days; nocturnal emissions, with amorous dreams for seven consecutive nights; glans penis much swollen and red, (from Irisin).—(*Burt.*)

Clinical Remarks.—The Iris seems to have a special affinity for the genito-urinary organs, causing not only irritation, with increased secretion, but symptoms of inflammation even. Eclectic physicians have elevated this plant to a high position, as a remedy for affections of these organs. *King* says it is a *diuretic.* He recommends it in *dropsy*, but advises it to be given until its hydrogogue effects are obtained. Although such a course will often run off the dropsical effusion, yet it is unnecessary and injurious. As with the Apoc. cann., the Iris, if appropriate, will eliminate the serous fluid through the kidneys, without any action on the bowels. The dropsies in which Iris will be found curative, will probably be found to be *hepatic* in their origin, generally.

Syphilis.—Not only King, Jones, and other eclectics, but Coe and Prof. Lee, positively attest that "In *Syphilis*, either primary or secondary, it acts as a powerful and efficacious agent. In eradicating the syphilitic virus, and correcting the diathesis of the system, it is not only powerful, but positive, and certain. In the secondary or tertiary forms of syphilis, after mercury in all its forms of administration had proven abortive, this agent has restored patients to perfect health. A gentleman who had studied medicine, but abandoned the practice for the ministry, informed us that he had used, and heard of others prescribing it with entire success in a large number of syphilitic cases, after the disease had passed into the secondary or tertiary stages, and often after mercury had been liberally used for a long time. The dose in which he employed it was one or two fluid drachms of the tincture, six or eight times daily."—(*Jones and Scudder's Mat. Med.*) If these recommendations of Iris, in that terrible malady, are reliable—and we have no reason to doubt the veracity of the above named authors—this remedy would be far preferable to its metallic analogue, Mercury. The general sphere of action of the Iris, as developed by our provings, would certainly point us to its use in Syphilis and Gonorrhœa, even if we had no previous intimation of its use in those diseases. Some homœopathic author remarks that in no proving of Silicia, Calcarea, etc., do we get those ulcers, abscesses, etc., for which those remedies are so specific. So it is with Iris. It would be carrying the provings of this medicine beyond proper bounds to produce the ulcers, and other characteristic symptoms of Syphilis, even if it were possible so to do. Dr. Headland's theory of *eliminative* action may explain why Iris, and some other medicines cure Syphilis, namely: by eliminating the virus through the proper glands, thus ridding the system of the poison—*not antidoting it in the system.* Neither my colleagues—so for as I can learn—nor myself, have had any experience in the use of Iris in syphilitic affections.

In *Gonorrhœa* it would appear by its pathogenesis to be indicated. I used it in one case, with apparent good results. It was given at the first dilution, five drops four time a day.

In *Seminal Emissions*, when accompanied by *amorous dreams*, it is very appropriate. When consulted in a case of spermatorrhœa, the first question to be asked is, "Do you have amorous dreams, with emissions?" If the answer is in the affirmative, I consider the case one of *irritation*, and treat it with Phos., Canth., Cann., Puls. and Iris. If a negative answer is received, the case is classed with those arising from want of tone, and lack of vitality and which call for such remedies as Kali brom., Conium, Phos. acid, Agnus castus and Caladium. This method of ascertaining the pathology of this affection, was first laid down by the astute Lallemand, whose researches in this direction have been so valuable. No proving of this medicine upon the female organism has been made. Judging from its effects upon the male organs, we can safely consider it capable of deranging the female organs of generation. Eclectic physicians claim to find it useful in the treatment of "leucorrhœa, congestions of the cervix, ulceration, and other disorders of the uterine system." Coe thinks it "particularly indicated in uterine leucorrhœa, in which affection it seems to be of almost specific value." As this variety of leucorrhœa is the result of a hyper-secretion of the glandular follicles of the cervix, it is quite probable the Iris may act curatively, as its primary effect is to cause a similar condition in glandular tissues. "A physician who had used this article extensively, and had had ample opportunities of testing its virtues, informs us that he had found it more effectual in hemorrhages, particularly *menorrhagia*, than any other agent he had ever tried."—(*Jones and Scudder Mat. Med.*) If the Iris should prove a true homœopathic remedy for syphilitic affections, it will be found useful in many diseases of the vagina, uterus, and ovaries, caused by that pervading poison.

Larynx and Chest.—Short, dry cough; excited by a tickling in the larynx; pain in the left side, as though the ribs were pressing against the lungs; unable to take a long breath for the pain in the left chest, which was of a cutting and sticking character; pain in the left chest.—(*Rowland.*) Hoarseness and ringing in the ears; soreness and rawness of the fauces.—(*Burt.*) Taken in connection with the above symptoms, the experiments of Dr. Burt on animals, are quite suggestive.

Back.—Constant pain, aggravated by motion, in the lumbar and sacral region, was a constant symptom when proving Irisin. —(*Burt.*)

Upper Extremities.—A sharp, tensive pain in right shoulder; worse on motion, especially by raising the arm, and continuing a long time; this pain occurs most in the evening; severe pains; shooting, momentary, and shifting about rapidly, in the phalangeal and meta-carpal-phalangeal articulations; and also in the sides and ends of the fingers, of both hands—these pains more in the evening; sharp pain in the end of middle fingers of left hand, succeeded instantly by a similar pain in axilla of left side; pains in phalanges when writing.—(*Rowland.*) Hands hot and dry all the time.—(*Burt.*) Dr. Rowland advises the Iris in rheumatism of the shoulders, wrists, and hands.

Lower Extremities.—Pain in the right knee joint, worse on motion; violent tearing pain in right hip and knee joints; sharp pain similar to those in the hands, in right hip, right and left knee joints, and in right foot, especially in the first joint of great toe—all worse on motion.—(*Rowland.*) Trembling and weakness of the knees; calves very painful, when walking, especially the right.—(*Burt.*) "After she took a few doses, she lost all power over her lower extremities, but regained it during convalescence. (This can hardly be considered a pathogenetic symptom, as it occurred in a patient with typhoid fever.) Pain in lower extremities and cramps in calves of legs, with nausea and retchings".—(*See Dr. Kitchen's notice of Iris.*) The Iris appears homœopathic to rheumatalgia of the lower as well as upper extremities. Dr. Burt says it caused paralysis of the hinder extremities, and spasm, of the fore-legs, in cats. Its action on the spinal cord may be more intense than we are now aware of. In many of its symptoms, especially the pains in the chest and extremities, the Iris strongly resembles Bryonia alba. I close my notice of this undoubted polychrest, with the hope that from the materials here given, the profession may reap some important benefit.

LEPTANDRIA VIRGINICA.

(*Black root.—Culver's Physic.*)

This is the Veronica virginica of Linnæus. It is an indigenous, perennial plant, with a simple, straight, smooth, herbaceous stem, from two to five feet in height. (For Botanical description see King's Dispensatory.) This plant grows throughout the United States, in limestone countries, in rich moist places, woods, thickets and barrens, and flowers in July and August. The root, which is the officinal portion, is about the thickness of the finger, six or seven inches in length, of a blackish color externally, and brown internally. The powder is dark brown, with a faint odor, and a bitter, nauseous taste. Its virtues are impaired by age. Alcohol and water extract its medicinal properties. The root should be gathered in the fall of the *second* year. There has been no accurate analysis of this plant. King says it contains "an essential oil, bitter extractive, tannin, gum, a *resin*, and woody fibre." To the *resin* the name of *Leptandrin* has been given, but there are other medicinal principles, as the Leptandrin does not contain all the therapeutic properties of the root.

It will be seen by the following proving and remarks, that there are three forms in which this plant may be used. Each preparation will have different medicinal effects, i. e., one preparation will possess qualities which the others do not:

(1).—The tincture of the *fresh* root, which will contain *all* the medicinal virtues of the plant.

(2).—The tincture, or triturtion, of the *dried* root which will contain only a portion of its virtues, as the *narcotic* and *acrid* principles are probably volatile.

(3).—The *Leptandrin*, which possesses about the same properties as the dried root, with perhaps less of its *irritating* qualities.

General Effects.—*King* thinks the *fresh* root is too drastic and uncertain for medicinal use, as it produces vomiting, bloody stools, dizziness, vertigo, and in pregnant females, abortion, unless used with much care. (He should give it in minute doses.) The *dried* root is decreed to be "laxative, tonic, cholagogue, and alterative. * * It exerts a powerful influence over the absorbent system, * * It is thought to possess narcotic properties. Leptandria is by the same author said to be a "powerful cholagogue, with but slight laxative influence." Prof. Hill, when an Eclectic, thought it to be "aperient, alterative, and tonic." Dr. Coe regards it as "alterative, deobstruent, cholagogue, laxative, and tonic." No remedy is held in higher estimation by the Eclectic school than this; and they use it profusely, in all diseases, with the same disregard for special indications, that the Allopaths use mercury. The following proving, and clinical experience, though meagre, may do something toward showing the real pathogenetic and curative power of this agent:

Mucous Membranes.—"No remedy with which we are acquainted, is more to be relied upon in chronic affections of the mucous surfaces."—(*Coe.*) The *fresh* root, especially, seems to have a peculiar irritating effect upon mucous surfaces. This may proceed to inflammation. It may cause pseudo-membranous inflammation in the intestines, as occurs in acute enteritis. Coe says Leptandria is curative in this condition when it occurs in chronic diarrhœa and dysentery. It causes an increased secretion and discharge of mucus from the intestinal surfaces (the mucous follicles), and in higher grades of its toxical action, the secretion is so much increased that the discharges are profuse and watery. It may even cause ulceration, sloughing, and gangrene. (See Intestines, Stools, etc.)

Serous Membranes.—It seems to have some action on these membranes, but probably only indirectly.

Nerves of Motion and Sensation.—Its action upon the nervous system is probably not direct or notable.

Glandular System.—"The glandular system, including the skin, partakes of its healthful impress."—(*Coe.*) Gatchell says it causes pain in the sub-maxillary glands. In Dr. Burt's proving it seemed to cause pain in the inguinal glands. Its action upon the liver seems to be well attested. It arouses its secretory and excretory functions. It probably irritates the whole intestinal glandular apparatus, when given in large doses. In small doses, used homœopathically, it restores these glands to a healthy action.

General Symptoms—Languid, tired feeling; *feel very weak and faint;* very weak and languid, can hardly walk; faintness from the severe nausea at night; general relaxation of the system; great prostration; great lassitude, with disinclination to talk; talking is very laborious; physical and mental depression, with vertigo and drowsiness.

Clinical Remarks.—Notwithstanding the assertion of Eclectic physicians, Leptandria in large doses, depresses the general strength of the system. It is only when it is used in proper medicinal (i. e. homœopathic) doses, that this medicine acts as a *tonic.* It is a tonic in the same manner as Arsenic, Nitric acid or Mercury, by removing abnormal conditions. Dr. Gatchell says "a characteristic indication for its exhibition is *excessive debility.*" Dr. Coe declares that "one great advantage possessed by the Leptandria is its tonic power. It never debilitates, but, on the contrary, invigorates while it deterges." Yet he admits that its operation is frequenty attended with considerable prostration. I have witnessed cases in which a decoction of the fresh root had been administered, where the prostration was excessive, and resembled that caused by mercury.

Fever.—Pulse diminished in frequency; feet and legs from knees down feel cold and numb; pulse full, but reduced from sixty to forty; great lassitude; languor of the whole system; disinclination to talk, which is very laborious; chilly sensation at the shoulders and down the back; tendency to shiver; sore and lame feeling in the small of the back.—(*Gatchell.*) Skin hot and dry; pain in the bowels with chilliness along the spine.—(*Burt.*) Universal chilliness.

Clinical Remarks.—Coe remarks that when the Leptandria is given in disease, and the patient is fairly brought under its constitutional influence, "the skin, which was before hot, dry, and constricted, becomes soft, moist, and flexible; expectoration becomes easy, the *arterial excitement is lessened*, and the patient, before restless, wakeful, and delirious, becomes calm, rational, and inclined to sleep." He considers it a valuable remedy in typhoid fevers, and in this opinion King, Jones, Morrow, and others concur. Some homœopathic practitioners, as Hill, Gatchell, and many of my correspondents, place the same high estimate upon its curative powers in typhoid states, when there is present, *great prostration, stupor, heat and dryness of the skin, calor mordax, or coldness of the extremities; dark, fœtid, tarry or watery stools, mixed with bloody mucus, and an icterode condition.*

In *Intermittent Fever* it is a favorite and much-used medicine by nearly all Western physicians, of both schools, who combine it with Quinine. They assert that it renders the action of Quinine more certain, and prevents the liability to a return of the disease, at least for the season, and is useful in periodic diseases generally, of an obstinate character, in which Quinine alone produces little or no result. In my experience, which was at one time very large, in diseases of the character referred to, the Leptandria did really act in a very beneficial manner. My method was to use it in alternation with Quinine, China, Nux vom., or any other medicine indicated, and always in acordance with what I always considered to be its homœopathic applicability. I do not consider that it has any real anti-periodic power, as some drugs undoubtedly have, but it removes conditions of the liver which often tend to keep up a continuance of intermittent maladies. I usually gave it for the following symptoms: considerable prostration; loss of appetite; heavily coated brown tongue; bitter taste in the mouth; constipation, or diarrhœa, with dark fœtid stools; jaundice; yellow, saturated urine.

In *Bilious fevers*, I have given it for nearly the same symptoms, using Leptand*rin* second or third dec. trit.

In *Infantile remittent*, I have had some excellent results from its use, administering the second or third dilution of the tincture, or the third and fourth trit., as seemed most proper.

Mind, Sleep.—Gloomy; desponding; sleep disturbed by the pains in the head and bowels, sleep more disturbed after midnight; very gloomy and irritable all day; drowsiness; a kind of stupor of of the mental faculties.

CLINICAL REMARKS.—It causes symptoms of the mind, similar to those occurring during disordered conditions of the liver, such as hepatic torpor, congestions, and the like. Some writers consider the fresh root to possess narcotic properties. It seems homœopathic to the drowsiness attending hepatic torpor, or that occurring in typhoids.

Skin.—Skin hot and dry, with frequent pains in the bowels.

CLINICAL REMARKS.—It is probably not homœopathic to any of the various affections of the skin. But may be found useful when they are aggravated by the retention of bile. In the intolerable itching of the skin, occurring in jaundice, in will prove useful. (See Liver.)

Head.—*Constant, dull, frontal headache*, worse in the temples; slight frontal headache, with a dull aching sensation in the umbilicus; dull frontal headache, apparently deep seated in the cerebrum; slight frontal headache, with neuralgic pains in the right temple; *very severe frontal headache*, made nearly unbearable by walking; very dizzy while walkiing; feeling as if the hair was being pulled at; vertigo.

CLINICAL REMARKS.—With the knowledge we now possess of the action of this medicine, especially on the liver, we can very properly decide the above-described headache to be the so-called "bilious headache." It somewhat resembles the cephalalgia caused by Nux and Bryonia. A "bilious headache" is usually accompanied by constipation, furred tongue, bitter taste, indigestion, yellow urine, languor, and depression of spirits. A free discharge from the bowels, of dark-brown, or greenish, feculent matter, usually dissipates the pain. Such headaches are relieved, and even cured, by the use of Leptandria, second or third trituration.

Eyes.—Eyes smart and ache very much (this symptom was present during the whole of the proving); eyelids agglutinated; profuse secretion of tears; eyes smarting constantly, with dull, aching pains in the eyeballs; painful sensation in left eyelid; lids and balls feel constricted.—(*Dr. Gatchell.*)

Mouth, Throat, etc.—Tongue coated, yellow along the centre; pain in sub-maxillary glands.

Gastric Symptoms.—Tongue coated yellow along the centre; flat, pappy taste in the mouth; nausea, with deathly faintness upon rising in the night; painful distress in the stomach, with rising of food, very sour; canine hunger; nausea, with faintness; nausea followed by vomiting; severe vomiting, accompanied by diarrhœa.

Clinical Remarks.—Among the Eclectics, it is considered a "valuable remedy for *dyspepsia.*" This phrase is continually used in reference to Leptandria. But "dyspepsia" may be caused by many various morbid states, both of the stomach and liver, thus: it may depend upon an excess or a deficiency of bile; on gastric catarrh, and degeneration of the gastric glands; atony of the stomach; deficiency of gastric juice, etc., etc. My experience with Leptandria inclines me to the opinion that it is chiefly homœopathic to those varieties of dyspepsia which depend upon disordered states of the liver, and atony of the stomach. I have found it very useful, used in alternation with Nux vomica, in men, and Pulsatilla in women. If there is present constipation, headache, jaundice, and bitter taste in the mouth, I prefer the first decimal trit. If there is diarrhœa, rising of sour ingesta, nausea, pain in the bowels and debility, the third or sixth trituration.

Stomach.—*Constant distress in the lower part of the epigastrium and upper portions of umbilical regions; sharp, cutting pains at intervals in the same parts;* constant aching distress in the stomach and umbilical regions; constant aching, burning sensation in the stomach and liver, aggravated by drinking cold water; severe aching pain in the stomach immediately after rising, and continuing all the forenoon; dull, aching pain in the cardiac portion of the stomach; great distress in the stomach and small intestines, with great desire for stool, that could not be retained one moment; weak, sinking sensation at the pit of the stomach.

Clinical Remarks.—It would seem homœopathic to some forms of gastralgia, cardialgia, pyrosis, and some of the various pains and distressing sensations which accompany indigestion. The "sinking sensation at the pit of the stomach," caused by Leptandria, is probably due to portal congestion, for which condition it is one of the most valuable remedies. It should be administered at the 2d or 3d dec. trit.

Liver.—Dull aching pain in the lower part of the right hypochondriac region, near the *gall-bladder*, with dull aching pain in the umbilicus, and rumbling in the bowels; dull aching in the whole of the liver—the pain extends to the spine, but is worst near the gall-bladder; constant dull, burning distress in the epigastric and hypochondriac regions; dull, aching burning distress in the region of the gall-bladder, with frequent chilliness along the spine; profuse, black, undigested stool, followed by great distress in the region of the liver, extending to the spine; the pain is of a hot, aching character, with chilliness along the spine; sharp, cutting pains near the gall-bladder; great burning distress in the back part of liver, and in the spine; pain in left shoulder and arm.

CLINICAL REMARKS.—The eclectic school of medicine, and even the allopathic, claim for Leptandria, that it possesses a specific affinity for the *liver;* that it profoundly modifies its functions in various ways. *King* says of Leptandria: "It is a cholagogue. It causes the liver to act with great energy, and without active catharsis, and is employed with success in all hepatic affections * * It is indicated by an inactive state of the liver, and all functional diseases of that organ." And of Leptandrin he says: "It is the only known medicine that efficiently stimulates and corrects the hepatic secretions, and removes functional derangement of the liver, without debilitating the system by copious alvine evacuations." Other writers of that school reiterate the same statements, and all eclectic practitioners use it with unhesitating confidence. It is to that school what "blue mass" is to the allopathic, while the Podophyllin is considered to take the place of calomel. But the wide recommendation of Leptandria in "*all* functional derangements of the liver," is too sweeping, and resembles the assertions of the allopaths, that Mercury is the only remedy in "all hepatic derangements." We are aware that the researches of Inman and Thudichum seem to render it doubtful if Mercury acts directly upon the liver; but the great mass of the allopathic school still use it, and probably will, for the next ten generations. Dr. Burt's admirable proving of Leptandria, which we herewith present the profession, establishes the fact beyond all controversy, that this medicine does exercise an influence of no doubtful power over the liver and its secretions. The hepatic symptoms are well marked, both the subjective and objective, and the whole experiment goes to prove what I have so often asserted in my writings: that all the remedies *successfully* used by the allopathic schools, are used strictly in accordance with the homœopathic law of cure; and being administered under that law, *do* effect cures, notstanding the large doses in which they are given—doses which very often produce needless and painful, and sometimes injurious medicinal aggravations. In regard to the real action of Leptandria on the liver, and its secretions, I do not propose to hazard any decided opinion, inasmuch as the action of Mercury even, upon that organ, is involved in considerable mystery. The same may be said of such analagous medicines as Iris versicolor and Podophyllum. But I may throw out a few suggestions, which can be taken for what they are worth: "Calomel," says Draper, "increases the fluid, but diminishes the solid constituents of the bile." It is my impression that Podophyllum and Iris versicolor act in a similar manner. Leptandria, on the contrary, *seems* to increase the solid, and decrease the fluid constituents of that secretion; or, in other words, Leptandria may have the power of facilitating the elimination of the proper excrementitious portions of the bile, or an excess of the non-excrementitious portions. It is at present believed that the retention of cholesterine in the blood is very injurious. That substance acts somewhat after the manner of *Urea*, namely: *as a direct poison to the nervous centres.* Its non-elimination causes headache, vertigo, languor, depression of spirits, painful sensations in various portions of the body, etc. Now, it is highly probable that Leptandria increases, directly, the elimination of this substance, for under its action, when given in proper medicinal doses, the symptoms enumerated above, are rapidly dissipated. The retention of other excrementitious constituents of the bile cause various morbid conditions, and the Leptandria, by its peculiar action, seems to be the remedy most likely to be of benefit when we wish to eliminate such substances through the liver. As it does not appear to increase the fluid constituents of the bile, as does Podophyllum and Iris v., its apparent *tonic* effect, even in material doses, may thus be accounted for. Mercury, however, seems to have in some instances, a similar action with Leptandria. In minute doses, in certain states of the system, it acts as a tonic, *i. e.*, it removes the morbid state by its homœopathic action, and the vital powers resume their normal sway. Some further suggestions relating to the action of Leptandria may not be amiss. Its *primary* pathogenetic action seems to be that of a stimulant, or *irritant of the hepatic cells. Chambers* states that "Mercury, Nitro-Muriatic Acid, and Manganese, cause an increase of yellow matter in the cells of the liver." Podophyllum may have the same effect; so also Leptandria. As a consequence of this primary stimulation or irritation, we have the increased elimination before mentioned, and sometimes acute congestion and inflammation. Leptandria therefore is primarily homœopathic to an irritable condition of the liver, in which the discharges are of the peculiar character described under "Stool," and the pains and abnormal sensations are similar to those under "Liver." The *secondary* effect of Leptandria is *over*-stimulation, or a condition of *exhausted irritability*, in which the hepatic cells refuse to perform their office (particularly that of eliminating the excrementitious substances from the blood?). In such cases we have the following conditions, namely: Jaundice from retention of biliary matters in the blood; so-called "bilious symptoms;" congestion of the liver, and even chronic inflammation of that organ, with its complications of enlargement, abscess, and various other structural changes. Leptandria is therefore secondarily homœopathic to the last-named pathological states. The size of the dose, let me remind the reader, will depend on its primary or secondary homœopathicity.

Abdomen.—*Constant, dull, aching distress in the umbilical region with ocasional, sharp, cutting pains in the same region*: pain and distress in the bowels, preventing sleep; dull pain in the lower part of right hypocondriac region and near the gall-bladder, with dull, aching distress in the umbilical region, and rumbling in the bowels; great distress in the whole of the bowels; sharp, cutting pains, with rumbling and desire for stool; stool followed by very weak feeling in the bowels and rectum; constant, dull, aching distress in the umbilical and hypogastric regions, with sharp pains every few minutes—the pains make me feel very faint; constant, dull, aching pains in the right inguinal region, passing down to the testicle; dull aching in the lumbar region; great rumbling and distress in the hypogastric region, with a profuse, black, fetid stool, followed by slight pains in the bowels; great distress in the hypogastric region, with great desire for stool—the pain is aggravated by drinking cold water; a good deal of distress in the stomach and bowels, with a burning sensation; stool followed by very severe, cutting pains in the small intestines; distension of abdomen; sense of vermicular motion in the colon; sense of coolness in the alimentary canal; pain in the left iliac region; rumbling in the intestines; flatulence.

Clinical Remarks.—The Leptandria is homœopathic to a variety of chronic enteritis, especally that form which is so common in camps, and among the lower class of our population in cities. It should be useful in bilious enteralgia, and the colics from flatulence, etc.

During the course of cases of typhus abdominalis, symptoms will often arise, which call for its administration. Every practitioner has met with cases in which the icteric symptoms, the prostration, and frequently the abdominal pain, and the character of the intestinal discharges, resemble very closely these found in the provings of Leptandria. It is not suitable for conditions of such intensity as call for the use of Arsenicum, but for those cases where the derangement is still functional, and there is yet no real decomposition of the fluids and solids, no ulcerations, etc., such as Arsenicum causes. I have used the second dec. trit., in a few cases of typhus abdominalis, with unequivocal benefit.

Stool.—Hard, black, and lumpy; afterwards soft and mushy stool; stool soft and mushy, and followed by a very weak feeling in the bowels and rectum; great rumbling and distress in the hypogastrium, with a profuse, black, and very fetid papescent stool, followed by slight pain in the bowels; great desire for stool; very profuse black stool, of the consistence of cream, and partially digested, followed by great relief; profuse, black, fetid stool, preceded by severe pain in the umbilical and hypogastric regions; inability to retain the stool, which is followed by great relief; great distress in small intestines and desire for stool, followed by a soft very fetid and black stool; watery stool, followed by *severe cutting* pains in the small intestines; inability to retain the stool, which is very profuse, fetid, and watery, with large quantities of mucus, and followed by very severe pain in the hypogastrium; desire for stool with great rumbling in the bowels, followed by profuse stool of watery mucus intermingled with a yellow matter—the evacuation was followed by very severe pain in the umbilicus; profuse, thin stool, with large quantities of mucus, followed by sharp, cutting pains, and great distress iu the umbilical region.

Clinical Remarks.—It is a stereotyped phrase of eclectic writers that the Leptandria causes "copious, dark, tar-like dejections from the bowels." They teach that when this symptom occurs, after the administration of Leptandria in disease, it is a very favorable symptom, and recovery is confidently predicted. This assumption is based upon the well-known fact, that similar evacuations do often occur during the course of bilious and other fevers hepatic diseases, etc., and seem to be of a "critical" character, *i.e.*, they relieve the system of certain morbid matters, which had caused the malady. I have treated many malarious fevers of a pernicious character, when these tar-like discharges ocurred under the homœopathic use of Arsenicum and Rhus, and when the peculiar evacuations were not due to the medicine, but to the *vis medicatrix naturæ.* I have known them to occur during an attack of supposed portal congestion, when no medicine had been taken. But this pathognesis of *Leptandria* proves that those peculiar dark discharges, are not always the result of natural disease—in other words, that this medicine is not alone an *eliminative* of such morbid matters, but actually cures such evacuations, when given to healthy persons. Eclectic writers erroneously teach that when the Leptandria causes black evacuations, it shows that the system was being poisoned with "vitiated bile," or some other morbid matters. It is this belief that has led them to the indiscriminate routine, and injurious use of this remedy in many diseases. They did not stop to ask themselves the question, whether the tar-like discharges, might not be due to the poisonous action of the drug? I have known patients under eclectic treatment to be kept under the action of Leptandria day after day, until the third stage of poisoning—namely, that state when watery mucus and bloody stools occur; because the physician supposed he must continue the administration of the medicine until the black discharges ceased. When they did cease, then the disease was said to "run into dysentery;" but it was the *dysentery of Leptandria.* So much for the blind adherence to pervading opinion, which is the curse of all medical schools. There are some interesting peculiarities in relation to the symptomatology of the evacuations caused by Leptandria. The *catharsis* caused by it may be divided into *four* stages:

(1) Discharge of black, *thick*, tar-like, fœtid substances.

(2) Thinner, brownish, often fœtid evacuations.

(3) Stool of mixed mucus, flocculent, and watery matters, with yellow bile, or blood.

(4) Mucus, bloody stool, mixed with shred-like substance—often pure blood is discharged.

Now, to prescribe a drug successfully, we should know the different stages of its pathogenetic action. This is just as important as to know the stages of disease. The *catharsis* of Podophyllin differs materially from that of Leptandria, and although it causes *some* of the varieties of stool, they occur in a different *order.* If we are called upon to prescribe for a diarrhœa, we should investigate its history; if that history corresponds in *order* and *nature*, with the Leptandria-disease, then that drug is the specific remedy. In the treatment of a dysentery the same rule holds good; dysentery occurs in the fourth stage of Leptandria-poisoning, while it occurs in the *second* stage of podophyllum-intestinal-irritation. With some drugs, scanty, bloody, and mucus stools, occur, as a primary symptom, as in cases where the *rectum* is the seat of inflammation.

Teste was the first to call attention to the importance of selecting remedies upon this data, and the practitioner will find the rule a valuable one.

Dr. P. P. Wells, of New York has lately called the attention of the profession to the importance of the *characteristic* symptoms of drugs; those symptoms which make it differ from all other drugs. Thus, there are many remedies for "*black stools*," but not all will remove that condition; the *collateral* symptoms must correspond. This subject will be noticed in another place. In the subject of the proving of Leptandria, it should not escape the notice of the physician, that the evacuations *per anum* are accompanied by some peculiar symptoms: The pains in the intestines usually occur *after stool*; in the podophlyllum diarrhœa they occur *before*, while the diarrhœa of mercury, and many others, the *pain* is severe *during* the stool. It will also be noticed that the evacuations are not followed by *tenesmus*. The proving here given does not mention it, nor do I find it mentioned in any article refering to its action. In practice I have not found it useful when there was marked tenesmus attending the disease. Such remedies as Podophyllum, Aloes, and Mercurius are more applicable.

I am inclined to believe that Leptandria does not have any *direct* specific effect on the *rectum*. Its action on the liver and portal system, undoubtedly causes it to effect the rectum and hemorrhoidal vessels but this action is *indirect*. If we carefully study the symptoms of Leptandria, after the method proposed by Dr. P. P. Wells, we shall find it a drug possessing a distinct itdividuality, as much as any other drug in our Materia Medica.

In *Acute Diarrhœa*, we shall find this medicine often indicated, and it will prove a valuable specific when administered for the pathological conditions in which it is indicated—those, and the *symptoms*, are well shown by the proving.

In *Chronic Diarrhœa*, this drug is even more reliable for the general condition, which is shown by the following extracts from my lecture on Leptandria, delivered before the class of Hahneman Medical College, in the winter of 1864:—

"The three principal varieties of chronic diarrhœa, in which Leptandria will be found useful, are:

"(*a*) From chronic inflammation or irritation of the mucous membrane.

"(*b*) Dependent on hepatic derangement.

"(*c*) Diarrhœa of debility.

"Some of the indications for Leptandria in the first-named variety, I have already given. But I will here call your attention to one form of this affection, which bears the common name of "Camp Diarrhœa." This disease is usually contracted in camp, where the soldiers are illy protected from atmospheric changes, and are exposed to cold, dampness, and fœtid exhalations, from refuse matter, decaying vegetation, etc. These, together with improperly cooked food, and bad water, are the principal causes of this malady. Its onset is sometimes gradual, lasting for days and weeks before the surgeon's attention is called to it by the patient; but it often attacks its victims suddenly, and assumes the character of a cholera morbus, or acute enteritis. It is one of the most intractable diseases with which our army has to contend. Under allopathic treatment it is almost incurable, and sometimes resists all medication, so long as the man remains in camp or barracks, exposed to the same influence which caused it, and obliged to subsist upon the usual hospital diet. In the acute stages, the following treatment will be found most applicable: If it is evidently caused by a cold, or exposure to dampness, Dulcamara, Aconite, or Pulsatilla will be found most efficacious. When caused by bad diet, and improper food or water, Pulsatilla, or Podophyllum will be most useful. If hepatic derangement is evidently present, Mercurius, Podophyllum, Leptandria, or Iris versicolor will be indicated. If the attack is choleraic in its character, Arsenicum, Veratrum alb, or Euphorbia cor., and perhaps Aconite, should be selected. But when it assumes a chronic character, and persists in spite of altered diet, change of location, etc., then Leptandria or Leptandrin will be found an invaluable remedy. In many cases its persevering use will alone effect a cure, although there are cases in which we may be obliged to resort to the auxiliary aid of Phosphoric acid, Nitric acid, Arsenicum, Sulphur, or Mercurius corrosivus.

"It is in most cases absolutely necessary that the patient (the subject of Camp Diarrhœa) should be removed from camp, or barracks, as soon as possible, and transferred to some healthy locality. For obvious reasons, a return to the patient's home is to be preferred. Here his military dress should be changed for his former civilian's apparel and his diet should consist of plain, nutritious, easily-assimilable substances. My experience has been that patients do the best upon a milk diet; plain bread and milk being the best form of its use. In addition, he should have a certain limited amount of good fresh beef, mutton, or game, every day. Taking the hint from the practice of an eminent Russian military surgeon, who successfully adopted the treatment in the great military hospitals, I have advised the use of raw, or nearly raw, beef, and in most instances, with the most satisfactory results. Tender, lean steak should be selected, and chopped very fine, a very small quantity of salt may be added if the patient insists. Of this an adult may eat one or two ounces, three times a day, with his bowl of bread and milk. Potatoes, salted meats, warm bread, raw fruit, pastry, coffee, preserves, and liquors, should be prohibited. Moderate exercise will be of advantage; too much, injurious. If the chronic diarrhœa depends for its continuance on debility, and resembles the colliquative diarrhœa of phthisis, accompanied by hectic fever and colliquative sweats, the Leptandria is still useful, but should be given in alternation with Phosphorus, Arsenicum, China, or Ferrum. The two latter are especially indicated if a lientery is developed, and the food passes the bowels unchanged, or in a state of putrefactive fermentation.

"In some cases such is the debility and relaxation of the mucous membrane, that the serous and even fibrinous parts of the blood escape, attended sometimes with more or less of the red coloring matter. An increased degree of the same affection constitutes passive hemorrhage. It is not unfrequently associated with a watery state of the blood, which becomes incapable of sustaining a due energy in the extreme vessels. In such conditions, Leptandria is still useful, but should be aided by those remedies which are capable of bringing back the blood to a normal condition. First in importance stands Iron. The preparation I prefer is the Phosphate, given in the form of syrup of super-phosphate of Iron, thirty drops after each meal, or a few grains of the first decimal trituration of the Pyro-phosphate. Next in value are Hydrastin, Helonin, Muriatic acid, and sometimes Nux vomica. The Citrate of Iron and Strychnine is often one of the most efficient remedies for chronic diarrhœa when we have two conditions; namely, an impoverished state of the blood, and an atonic state of the muscular tissues of the intestines. When these states obtain, we usually find alternate constipation and diarrhœa, deficient digestion, accumulations of flatulence and hæmorrhoids.

Dr. Small is very successful in the treatment of Chronic Diarrhœa: he relies upon Nitric Acid and Arsenicum.

"Chronic ulceration of the intestines often occurs during the course of a chronic diarrhœa. Dr. Chambers says: 'There is no disorder in which emaciation is so marked a feature throughout its whole course, as chronic ulceration of the small intestines. Ulcerations of the cœcum and colon, tubercular or not, produce as much, nay, often more diarrhœa; but they are not, by any means, so distinguished in their power of reducing the patient. In this lesion of the ilia, even the parts which are not the actual seat of disease, seem incapacitated from absorbing nutriment, and the victuals pass through the alimentary canal in the same state as when they left the stomach, except being made putrid by chemical decomposition. All the stages of digestion are equally suspended.'

"These lesions are more common during infantile life, and thousands of children are yearly carried off by this malady in every large city. In this affection Arsenicum, Merc. cor., Sulphur, Nitric acid, and Phytolacca are indicated. The Leptandria has also been of use in my hands, when, with the usual symptoms, there was present a jaundiced hue of the skin, sallow complexion, pain in the region of the liver, lack of bile in the evacuations, and great debility. In such a condition I would advise you to use, for adults, the first decimal trituration; for children, the third trituration.

"When the ulceration is tubercular, you will have to resort to a different class of remedies, prominent among which I would advise the hypophosphate of lime (calcis hypophosphis), which has all the curative properties of calc. carb., together with the recuperative qualities of phosphorus. The second or third dec. trit. will prove the most satisfactory. Leptandria may be called for, even in this disease, if we find disorder of the liver complicating the case. I believe it increases the absorbent action of the intestinal mucous membrane, and thus prevents the excessive emaciation. In respect of the action of Leptandria on the mucous membranes of the intestines Dr. Coe, gives a case which is quite interesting. He says: 'No remedy with which we are acquainted, is more to be relied upon in chronic affections of the mucous surfaces. Its value in this respect is peculiarly apparent in chronic dysentery and diarrhœa, and other diseases of the bowels. When false membranous formations have occurred in the smaller intestines produced by the gradual exudation of plastic lymph., the Leptandria may be relied upon for their removal, with great confidence. * * * We have also used it with great success, in the cure of constipation and piles. We recently treated a case of the latter complaint, accompanied with frequent hemorrhage from the rectum, of twelve years standing. A short time after commencing its use, the patient discharged considerable quantities of false membrane, in shreds and patches, and a number of pieces several inches in length, forming complete tubes. The evacuation of this matter was attended with an amelioration of all the symptoms, and at the present time the patient declares himself well. The bowels are regular, appetite good, the hemorrhage has ceased, and the distressing pain, so long experienced beneath the sacrum, entirely gone.'

This is quite an important clinical fact, and although the cases were treated with massive doses two to four grs. twice or thrice a day, we cannot doubt that the remedy was homœopathic to the disease mentioned.

In Woods' Practice, article "Chronic Enteritis," we find that "occasionally portions of false membrane are discharged, and in some rare instances, tubes of considerable length, obviously the result of a plastic inflammation, throwing out coagulable lymph upon the surface of the mucous membrane."

Dr. Cumming of Edinburg has given an account of a peculiar variety of pseudo-membranous inflammation of the bowels (quoted by Wood). In this variety, Dr. Simpson used Arsenic, a remedy homœopathic to the disease, and Dr. Cumming used tar and electro "galvanism," successfully.

Believing, as I do, that all medicinal remedies cure only under the law of *similia*, it seems highly probable to me that Leptandria, in the case given by Dr. Coe, caused the expulsion of the membrane and effected the cure, by virtue of its power to cause a similar pathological state.

Chronic Dysentery is often associated with chronic enteritis, and it is not always easy to determine, how far the two portions of the bowels are severally involved in the inflammation, nor is the decision a matter of much importance. Chronic Diarrhœa and Dysentery are very nearly allied in their anatomical character, and we often find cases where the symptoms of both maladies are intimately blended. But chronic dysentery, when not thus combined, is distinguished from chronic diarrhœa by the frequency and comparatively small quantities of the evacuations, their character, and the tenesmus with which they are attended. The greater number of the stools consist chiefly of mucus, sometimes mixed with pus-like matter or blood. Occasionally, however, feculent or bilious matter is mixed with the proper dysenteric discharge. When the disease occupies the rectum and lower portions of the colon, the feculent discharge is often consistent, and instead of being uniformly mixed with mucus, is either irregularly pervaded by it in layers or streaks, or enveloped in a thick coating of it, derived from the surface of the bowel with which the fœces lay in contact. There is usually more or less tormina, and tenderness on pressure; the pulse, skin, and appetite are affected as in chronic diarrhœa, and there is nearly the same emaciation. Chronic Dysentery is seldom an original disease, but when it occurs, is almost always in consequence of an acute attack. It is very often a result of acute attacks of "camp dysentery," and even "camp diarrhœa" may run into a chronic dysentery. In this disease we have in Leptandria a valuable and efficient remedy, but it is more applicable to those cases in which a chronic enteritis complicates the disorder.

In *Cholera Infantum* it has proved a very useful remedy. Dr. King (Eclectic), says:—"In cholera infantum, a disease which sometimes sets at defiance all the skill of the physician, I have met with excellent success by the following combination: Leptandria six grs., Quinia three grs., Camphor one and a half grs., Ipecacuanha three-fourths grs., mixed and divided in twelve powders, of which one may be given every two or three hours, and its use continued thus for several days. Its action at first is to increase the alvine passages, and apparently augment the disease, but in a few days the character of the evacuations change, become more and more normal, as well as more regular in their appearance; after which, one or two powders per day for a week will render the cure permanent."

I have quoted the above, to show that this mixture, absurd as it is, really cured the disease homœopathically.

Leptandria, the main ingredient, is eminently homœopathic to the disease in most cases, as the proving shows conclusively.

Quinia, for which we substitute *China*, is indicated by the general condition (prostration from loss of fluids), and by the special symptoms (copious, dark, or light, watery stool, etc).

Ipecac. is one of our best remedies, when there occurs *vomiting* with the diarrhœa, and *Camphor*, as shown by Hahnemann is quite homœopathic to choleraic symptoms, with considerable prostration. By the use of Leptandria third trit., China second dil., and Ipecac., first or second, with Camphor tenth, as an intercurrent remedy, the homœopathist, can cure his patients, without the danger of doing injury to the organism, especially in cases of children, that is apt to occur from such massive doses as is advised by King, who admits that the disease is apt to be aggravated at first by the medicines.

Dr. B. L. Hill, when an Eclectic, wrote as follows concerning the action of Leptandria, in dysentery.

"In the epidemic dysentery which has prevailed for the last two seasons (1854,55,) in many parts of our country, this article has been of great service. It was usually given with the best success, after evacuating the bowels freely, with a combination of Podophyllin and Leptandria, or Rhubarb. For this purpose give from one-half of a grain to a grain every hour, gradually lengthening the intervals as the discharge becomes darker. Though it may not be applicable in all cases of dysentery, it is doubtless one of the most useful articles in this dangerous disease."

The epidemic referred to was of an adynamic character, quickly prostrating the patient, and often ran into a typhoid condition. For the same epidemic, Dr. Hill would now advise and use with as good results, minute doses of Leptandria, Podophyllum, Arsenicum, and Baptisia. It may be remarked here that Podophyllum is indicated for a much higher grade of inflammation and irritation of the bowels, than Leptandria. The following was Dr. Hill's estimate of the action of Leptandria:—"It is not strictly cathartic. It is aperient, alterative and tonic. In cases of children affected with summer complaint, where there is evidently a lack of the proper biliary secretions, but when owing to the already irritated condition of the bowels, the ordinary remedies for arousing the liver are inadmissible, this article seems to be the very thing needed. While it acts freely upon the liver, instead of purging, it seems to change the discharge from the light, and watery, or slimy condition, to a darkened and apparently bilious state rendering them more and more consistent, until they become perfectly natural, without having been arrested entirely, or at any time aggravated. It at the same time seems to act as a tonic, restoring the tone of the stomach, and increasing the strength and activity of digestion."

Dr. Hill the homœopathic, values the Leptandria as highly as did Dr. Hill the eclectic, but he accounts for its action in a more rational manner. As the latter he gave one-fourth to one grain every hour or two, in acute cases, or one to two grains three times a day in chronic cases; as the former he finds one-tenth or one-hundreth of a grain equally servicable. In those severe cases of disease which clearly resemble the primary symptoms of poisoning with the fresh root of Leptandria, the thirtieth, if prepared from a good tincture, would doubtless act curatively.

Urine.—Urine at first slightly acid, then neutral and rather scanty; urine very red, and does not affect litmus paper; dull, aching pain in the lumbar region.

Clinical Remarks.—King says "it exerts a powerful influence upon the absorbent system, and in combination with cream of tartar, has been successfully used in obstinate cases of dropsy."

If Leptandria is homœopathic to any variety of dropsy, it is probably that dependent on *disease of the liver.* In order to test its value in dropsy, or, indeed, any disease, it should be given alone. To combine medicines is to lose all data concerning the real action of any single agent.

It is doubtful if Leptandria exercises any specific action on the functions of the kidneys, yet a medicine may be useful in dropsy without being a diuretic. It may act curatively by a certain general restorative power. Thus *China*, *Iron*, Helonias, etc., may remove dropsies by bringing the organism up to a normal condition. Any cause which obstructs the circulation in the portal system of veins, will induce dropsy. Chronic tumefaction of the liver, and organic diseases of that organ; also inflammation of the portal vein, are the principle causes of the varieties of hepatic dropsy.

Thorax.—Soreness in left side of the thorax, especially about the cardiac region.

Clinical Remarks.—In affections of the liver, we may have sympathetic disturbances of the heart's action; so also from dyspepsia.

Indirectly the Leptandria may prove useful in some derangements of the functions of the heart.

Back.—Sore and lame feeling in the small of the back.

Upper Extremities.—Both wrists are very lame, and ache severely, lasting some hours; pain in left shoulder and arm; chilly sensation at the shoulders and down the arm.

Clinical Remarks.—Pain in the left shoulder is a symptom of disease of the posterior portion of the liver.

Lower Extremities.—Feet and legs, from the knees downward, feel cold and numb.

DR. BURT'S PROVING OF LEPTANDRIA.

January 29th, 1864.—Am perfectly well; good appetite; bowels regular, once a day; urine acid. My temperament is sanguine-nervous, with a little of the bilious. Took one grain of Leptandrin, at 10 A. M.; 10.15, natural stool; 12 M., constant, dull, frontal headache, worse in the temples; constant distress in the lower part of the epigastric region, and umbilicus—by spells there are sharp, cutting pains, in the same parts. Took two grains, 3 P. M.; slight, frontal headache, with a dull, aching sensation in the umbilicus. Took three grains, 5 P. M.; constant, dull, frontal headache, very severe, deep in the regions of causality; constant, dull, aching distress in the umbilicus—at times there are very sharp pains in the same region. Took four grains, 9 P. M.; the frontal headache has been very severe; eyes smart, and ache very much; constant, aching distress in the umbilicus, with sharp pains at times; feeling very gloomy. Took 5 grains.

January 30th.—Feeling very tired; slept middling well; awoke several times, and found that I had a severe frontal headache. Took six grains at 7 A. M.; 10 A. M., slight, dull headache, with slight distress in the bowels. Took eight grains, 12 M.; constant, dull headache, very much worse in the regions of causality; eyes sore, and smart severely; constant, aching distress in the stomach; with great distress in the umbilical region. Took ten grains 2 P. M., had to ride ten miles on horseback, did not notice any particular symptoms. At 6 P. M. took fifteen grains; 9 P. M., slight, frontal headache; eyes ache, and smart severely; constant, aching distress in the epigastric and umbilical regions, with sharp, cutting pains, by spells; urine slightly acid; no stool to-day.

January 31st.—Had a restless night after midnight; the pains and distress in the bowels prevented me from sleeping; feeling very languid; dull pain in the lower part of the right hypochondriac region; tongue coated yellow along the center. Took twenty grains at 8 A.M.; stool, first part hard, black, and lumpy, afterwards soft and mushy; 12 M., slight, frontal headache; eyes smart very much; frequent, dull, aching pains in the lower right hypochondriac region, near the gall bladder, with dull, aching distress in the umbilical region, and rumbling in the bowels. Took twenty-five grains, 2 P. M.; dull, aching distress in the whole of the liver that extends to the spine; the most distress is in the region of the gall-bladder; great distress in the whole of the bowels, with sharp, cutting pains, rumbling, and desire for stool; stool, soft and mushy, followed by a very weak feeling in the bowels and rectum; 5 P. M., frontal headache; eyes smart a great deal; constant, burning, aching distress in the region of the stomach and liver; dull, aching distress in the umbilical and hypogastric regions. Took twenty-five grains, 9 P. M.; dull, frontal headache that is very deep in the cerebrum; eyes smart very much; burning distress in the whole epigastric and hypochondriac regions; constant, dull, aching distress in the umbilical and hypogastric regions, with very sharp pains every few minutes; makes me feel very weak and faint; constant, dull, aching pain in the right inguinal region, that passes down to the right testicle; it is very hard to endure the pain in the testicle; dull aching in the lumbar region; urine rather scanty, and does not affect blue litmus paper.

February 1st.—Had a restless night after midnight; skin was very hot and dry, with frequent pain in the bowels; eyelids agglutinated; unpleasant; flat taste in mouth; tongue coated yellow, along the centre; great rumbling and distress in the hypogastric region, with a profuse, black, very fœtid, soft, papescent stool, with slight pain in the bowels afterwards; feeling very languid. At 6 A. M., took thirty grains; 11 A. M., frequent, dull, aching distress in the umbilical and hypogastric regions. Took forty grains, 2 P. M.; for the last two hours I have been in awful pain and distress in the epigastric, umbilical, and hypogastric regions; drinking cold water aggravates the pain and distress very much; dull, aching, burning distress in the region of the gall-bladder, with frequent chilliness along the spine; great distress in the hypogastric region, with *great desire* for stool; very profuse, black stool, about the consistence of cream, with undigested potatoes in it. This gave great relief, but was followed by great distress in the region of the liver, extending to the spine; it is of a hot, aching character, with chilliness along the spine; 5 P. M., slight, frontal headache; there has been constant distress with very sharp pains by spells, in the lumbar region; 10 P. M., slight frontal headache, with sharp pains in the temples; there has been constant distress, with pains in the whole of the abdomen, since 5 P. M., but, for the last half hour, the pains in the umbilical and *hypogastric* regions have *been awful* to endure, with rumbling and great desire for stool; a very profuse, black, fœtid stool, that ran a stream from my bowels, and could not be retained a moment; this gave great relief, but, did not stop the pain altogether; urine very red, does not affect blue litmus paper.

February 2nd.—Slept soundly; feeling very languid; both wrists are very lame and ache quite severely the left one aches the most, pain lasted until noon; tongue coated, yellow along the centre; flat taste in the mouth. Immediately after getting up, a very severe, aching distress came on in the epigastric region. At 10 A. M., the distress in the stomach is constantly getting worse; I cannot sit or stand still, it is so severe; food rises very sour; 12 M., the painful distress in the stomach has been unendurable all the forenoon; it is a hard, aching, burning sensation, and appears to be in the stomach; 9 P. M., the painful distress in the stomach has not been so hard, but have had severe pains in the umbilical region all the afternoon; urine neutral; no stool to-day.

February 3rd.—Slept soundly; awoke at 5 A. M., feeling very hungry, with great distress in the epigastric region, and continued until I had breakfast; frequent pains in the epigastric region all day.

February 4th.—Slept well; feeling quite well; great desire for food; stool, first part natural, last part soft and mushy.

February 5th.—Awoke at 2 A. M., feeling very hungry; have a great appetite; 11 A. M., took twenty drops of the fluid extract of Leptandria; 12 M., dull, frontal headache; profuse secretion of tears; dull, aching distress in the stomach and umbilical region; 3 P. M., slight headache; constant, aching distress in the umbilicus with sharp pains by spells; sharp, cutting pains near the gall-bladder. Took thirty drops, 4 P. M., dull, frontal headache, with a sensation as if the hair were pulled at; good deal of distress in the stomach and bowels, with a burning sensation; 6 P. M., dull, aching distress in the umbilicus. Took forty drops; 10 P. M., there has been a great deal of distress in the umbilicus, with a great burning distress in the back part of the liver and in the spine; soft, mushy stool; took fifty drops.

February 6th.—Slept well; arose once in the night; immediately I became sick at my stomach, with a deathly faintness; tongue coated yellow; flat taste in my mouth; 7 A. M., took six drops; 10 A. M., slight headache; great distress in the small intestines, and desire for stool; stool soft, very fœtid, and black. Took seventy drops; noon, dull, aching distress in the umbilical region, with very sharp pains by spells. Took eighty drops; 3 P. M., slight frontal headache; eyes smart a good deal; constant, dull, aching pain in the cardiac portion of the stomach; great distress in the umbilicus. Took one hundred drops; 10 P. M., slight frontal headache, with neuralgic pains in the right temple; eyes smarting constantly, with dull pains in the eyeballs; have had very severe pains in the stomach and small intestines, with great distress and desire for stool; stool soft, very fœtid, and mushy; have been very gloomy and very irritable all day. Took one hundred and twenty drops.

February 7th.—Up all night with a very sick patient; had frequently severe pains in the umbilical and hypogastric regions; stool, 3 A. M., that run a stream from my bowels, followed by very *severe cutting* pains in the small intestines; 8 A. M., very severe frontal headache, walking makes it almost intolerable; great distress in the stomach and all of the small intestines, with great desire for stool, that could not be retained one moment; run a stream from my bowels, very fœtid, with large quantities of mucus in it, followed by severe pain in the hypogastric region; Took one hundred and sixty drops. 10 A. M., there has been constant and very violent frontal headache; great distress in the stomach and small intestines, with frequent pains in the umbilicus that make me feel very faint and weak; great rumbling in the bowels; stool that could not be retained, consisting of water and large quantities of mucus and a little yellow matter, followed by very hard pains in the umbilicus; very dizzy while walking; quite weak and languid, can hardly walk; 12 M., severe frontal headache; constant, dull, aching, burning distress in the whole of the bowels, with frequent pain and rumbling, and great desire for stool; stool of water and mucus, followed by very hard pain in the hypogastric and umbilical region; 2 P. M., another very profuse, thin stool, with large quantities of mucus; great frontal headache; very weak and languid, compelled to go to bed; 4 P. M., slept two hours, awoke with great distress in the whole of the bowels, and great desire for stool; profuse, watery stool mixed with mucus that could not be retained; 5 P. M., another stool of mucus and water, with part natural fæces, very fœtid; 6 P. M., another stool, with large quantities of mucus in it, followed by sharp, cutting pains, and great distress in the umbilical region; feeling very weak and faint; 9 P. M., another profuse stool that could not be retained, followed by severe pains in the bowels; very severe frontal headache.

February 8th.—Slept soundly, feeling very languid; tongue coated yellow along the centre; dull, aching distress in the bowels; during the night have had frequent pains in the umbilicus, with much rumbling all day; no stool; great appetite.

February 9th.—Lost my sleep last night, and am feeling very bad to-day; have had frequent pains in my bowels all day, with severe headache; no stool.

February 10th.—Slept well; feeling very well, excepting frequent pains in the umbilical region; soft, yellow, papescent stool, preceded by pain in the umbilical region.

NUPHAR LUTEA.

(*Small flowered, yellow Pond-Lily.*)

This well-known plant is found all over the United States, growing in ponds and stagnant waters, is of a similar habit to the white pond-lily—the leaves always floating in deep water, and are erect in shallow. The petioles are semi-cylindrical; color of the root and flower, deep yellow. Dr. Marcy says the species used by Dr. Petit, the prover, was the *small*, and flowered, yellow pond-lily, *n. lutea*, not the *large*-flowered, common yellow lily—from which, however, it is said to be sometimes difficult to distinguish it.'

This proving was made with the fourth, sixth, seventh and eighth dilutions, by Dr. Petit, and translated from the *Jour. de la Societe Gallicane*, and may be found in the North Amer. Jour., Vol. 3, p. 250. I have arranged the pathogenesis according to the general plan herein adopted.

General Symptoms.—Weakness; restlessness; diminution of the strength; and flush, healthy complexion.

Emotive Sphere.—Excessive moral sensibility, giving one great pain on witnessing the suffering of animals; great impatience at the slightest contradiction.

Skin.—Toward the end of ten or twelve days which followed the commencement of the proving (first), there appeared, on different parts of the body, a number of red blotches, tolerably regular in outline, oval or circular, prominent, and covered with little scales, of a silvery white; in short, resembling *psoriasis*. There were a few on the posterior surface of the arms, but they were most abundant on the anterior surface of the legs; they itched violently, especially in the evening. Friction removed the little scales, which were rapidly reproduced; remained a few days, then fell off again from the scratching induced by the itching. This eruption lasted a month and a half. As it disappeared, and the scales ceased to be reproduced, the skin at the place of each blotch became pale, red or yellowish. It would be impossible to mistake the character of psoriasis in these symptoms. Were they pathogenetic or unconnected with the remedy."—(*Petit.*) Aggravation of a moderate *ptyriasis* capitis, of several years standing; morning and evening, especially, the itching is intolerable, and the comb brings away a great quantity of hair (second proving). (Dr. P. doubts whether this was a drug symptom, as the pityriasis was constitutional with him.) Sensation like flea-bites in different parts for several days; a red, slightly prominent patch, covered with little white scales, and itching violently, on the interior surface of the right arm, near the axilla; a red, oval, prominent patch, as large as a five-cent piece, on the internal surface of the left arm, exactly like a patch of psoriasis, covered with silvery scales, falling off, and renewed again every few days, itching violently especially in the evening.

With very commendable frankness Dr. Petit offers the following:

Remarks.—"We have seen during my first proving, an eruption like psoriasis appeared on my lower limbs. Although of an eminently psoric constitution, manifested in childhood by temporary enlargements of the cervical lymphatics, chilblains, catarrhal inflammation of the eyelids, etc., and in adult life by symptoms resembling, at one time, the commencement of tubercular consumption, and which only yielded to homœopathic treatment, it was nevertheless the *first* occasion in which I had been affected with an eruption of this nature. It continued for a month and a half. In the second proving, subsequently instituted a few months after, there was no eruption. But in the *third*, five months afterwards, two patches appeared on the internal surface of each arm. Four *years* afterwards, while an *interne* at the *Hospice de la Salpêtrière*, and brought every morning in contact with some hundred patients affected with itch, I was seized with a general psoriasis, which lasted more than a month, without being in the least affected by any medicament, and only yielded, at the end of three or four weeks, to the alternate use of *manganum* and *nitric acid.* Every year since has been marked by the appearance of two or three patches of psoriasis. Quite recently I again proved the *Nuphar l.*, and in less than a fortnight the patches of psoriasis appeared on all sides. * * * What conclusion shall we draw from these facts? Did the *Nuphar* act three times in succession to produce the eruption? Or did it simply act by awaking the pathological susceptibilities of the economy, and depressing the vital functions, and thus favor the appearance of the disease? Or is the whole thing a mere coincidence? I shall willingly adopt the latter conclusion as the wiser one, until further provings, and an extended clinical experience shall have thrown more light upon the subject."

This conclusion does honor to his judgment. Let further provings on *healthy* persons be made.

Head.—Pressive headache in the forehead and temples, ceasing in the open air; boring pain in transitory attacks in the left anterior part of the forehead, in the evening; dull, or teasing pains, sometimes in the forehead, at others in the whole upper part of the head; heaviness in the whole head, in the middle of the day; dull, deep lancinations behind the left frontal eminence; dull pain in the left anterior central lobe; very painful, bruising, shaking in the brain at every step when walking; dull pain and sensation of painful weight in the orbit all day, in the right anterior cerebral lobe, and right side of the occiput; painful heaviness in the orbit, at the base of the brain—a very frequent symptom since the beginning of the proving; lancinations in the left anterior part of the brain; weight in the temples in the morning.

Clinical Remarks.—The pains about the orbital regions are peculiar. Dr. P. is of the opinion that its action is deep, direct and primary on the nervous centers.

Eyes.—Dull pain, and sensation of weight in the orbit; discolored eyes, (*around the eyes? H.*) (For other symptoms of the *orbit, see Head.*)

Face.—Face pale; discolored eyes; though otherwise as well as usual.

Gastric and Intestinal Symptoms.—Sweetish taste several times a day; sense of weakness; slightly painful over the whole anterior surface of the stomach; soft stool, preceded by some colic, for several days; diarrhœaic stools, morning and evening, preceded by violent colic pains in the rectum; six stools from 8 P. M., to 6 A. M.; diarrhœaic stool during the day, after breakfast and another after dinner; yellow diarrhœa, especially in the morning, for three days, five or six stools a day, without colic or epigastric trouble, except at times a sense of weakness in the epigastric region; the stools are always more numerous toward five or six o'clock, A. M.;

emission of flatulence in evening, with wind colic; smarting, and burning pain at the anus, after every stool; stitches, as from needles, in the rectum.

Clinical Remarks.—"In the chronological order of the symptoms, those which are seated in the digestive organs do not commence until a number of days after the disturbance has been manifested in the nervous functions. Their seat, so far as can now be judged, is in the lower part of the digestive canal. Thus the pains which accompany or precede the stools, are principally seated in the *rectum.* The appetite is not at all disturbed, still the strength is not renewed, nutrition languishes, the face becomes pale, the eyes dark colored. The stools are sometimes soft, generally languid, yellow, most frequent between four and six o'clock, A. M. It is indicated in acute or chronic cases of entero-colitis., when the aggravation takes place, in the early morning, and generally in cases where there is depression of the virile functions."—(*Dr. Petit.*)

Case 1.—"M. B., *æt.* twenty-eight, had had a morning diarrhœa for three months. He had to rise every morning towards five o'clock, several times for this purpose of going to stool—never any colic. Bryonia and Sepia, did no good in a fortnight; the diarrhœa continued of the same character, and the slightest error in diet aggravated it. *Nuphar* cured it rapidly.—(*Ib.*)

Case 2.—"M. Louis B., *æt.* twenty-one, Professor of Literature, had scarce returned from the country, towards the end of last autumn, when he was taken with a morning diarrhœa, with colic. Between four and six, A. M., he had two or three stools, and commonly one in the evening. This state had lasted eight days. After first dose of Nuphar, taken at night, the diarrhœa ceased."

Case 3.—"M. L., *æt.* forty-three, musician, had suffered three years from entero-colitis, contracted by excesses at the table, and venery, and domestic troubles. He had exhausted the resources of the old school, and of quackery, without benefit; and when he consulted me, towards the end of last November, he presented the following case:—Appetite good, sometimes excessive; frequent regurgitations of an acrid and corrosive taste; digestion slow; colic and rumbling every night, awakened several times from five to seven, every morning, to go to stool, which was liquid or soft, yellowish, and either sour or fœtid; the least excess, of any kind, produced an aggravation of this state, and generally obliged him to remain in bed for a day or two—ordinarily he was enabled to attend to his affairs; his sleep was agitated; heat in the palms of his hands; frequent pulse; at times a dull pain in the left renal region, which was sensitive to the touch. From the first doses of *Nuphar* he derived more benefit than he had previously experienced from any treatment, and in two months he was well."—(*Ib.*)

Case 4.—"M. D., a jeweler, *æt.* thirty-three, had had a diarrhœa for a fortnight, which obliged him to get up several times for stool, towards five or six, A. M. He had no colic, but experienced burning at the anus, together with general depression. The diarrhœa ceased from the second day."—(*Ib.*)

Case 5.—"M. B., *æt.* thirty-seven, wood carver, consulted me on the 26th of May. He had been sick for three months. His tongue was white, mouth pasty, and his stomach the seat of a painful sensation of weariness; digestion slow. He had wind colic, principally early in the morning, with liquid or soft, sour-smelling stool. For several years the virile functions had been badly performed; he had tolerable frequent pollutions during sleep; constant itching of the scrotum and perineum; small desire for coitus; infrequent and feeble erections; the diarrhœa, colic, digestive troubles, and general weariness, were aggravated on the day succeeding sexual connection. I prescribed *Nuphar*, and eight days after the first consultation, the patient not coming to visit me, one of his friends told me he was better."—(*Ib.*)

This remedy has much resemblance to Iris v., in the character of the intestinal symptoms, and also the seminal emissions, but is not so active and intense in its action.

Urine.—The urine deposits a copious, reddish sand, which adheres to the vessel.

Generative Organs of Men.—Diminution of lascivious thoughts and the sexual inclination for ten days; opposite effects during the succeeding days; complete absence of sexual desire; penis contracted; scrotum relaxed; entire absence of erections and sexual desires; the voluptuous ideas which fill the imagination, do not cause erection; lancinations in the right testicle; dull, transitory pain in the right testicle for several days in succession; a similar pain at the extremity of penis, right side; severe lancinations in left testicle, with pains in extremity of penis, left side; an *interne en pharmacie*, of the hospitals of Paris, took for several days a quantity of tincture of this drug, and remained for two months without perceiving either propensity or power of performing the generative act.

Clinical Remarks, etc.—Nuphar possesses a remarkable power of modifying the vital forces, particularly in the matter of the generative functions, as was already known to the ancients. (*Dioscorides*, *Pliny*, *etc.*) This action is exhibited in depressed phenomena, more and more marked, and lasting sometimes as long as thirty days. The reaction then commences, and proceeds, but with considerable slowness.

Case 1.—Having administered a dose of Nuphar 6th dil., for several evenings in succession, to a patient convalescing from typhoid fever, whose feeble state was aggravated by nocturnal emissions, these latter diminished in number from the first day, and gradually disappeared.

Case 2.—Gave the drug to a man who, for nine years, had had involuntary seminal losses, during sleep, at stool, and when urinating, with complete absence of erections. He was pale and languid, and had been treated in vain, for several months, by Opium, Quinine, etc. The first evening he had violent headache, accompanied by vertigo, as if from intoxication, extending into a part of the night; with soreness, nausea, epigastric pains, and bitter mouth; the next morning general bruised feeling, as if it had been beaten with a club. (There is a connection between these pains, and the bruised pains produced by *Nuphar* in the brain and thorax, which are sensibly aggravated by the shock of every step. (P.) During the following evenings, the patient, who was taking the remedy twice a day, experienced heaviness in the head, vertigo, as if from intoxication (similar, he declared, to those he had felt while taking opium), and bitterness in the mouth. For a month he took the *Nuphar*, at two different times. His paleness diminished, his general weakness disappeared by degrees, and his digestive functions took a new start. At the same time the pollutions ceased, erections came on, accompanied by a decided propensity for the generative act, and before the thirtieth day of the treatment he was able to satisfy it with success, and without fatigue."—(*P.*)

Thorax.—Painful sensation behind the sternum when running, as though the subjacent organs were violently shaken.

Back and Extremities.—Deep, dull pain at the lowest part of the left lumbar region, and in the posterior superior part of the external iliac fossa; it coincides with a similar, but not constant pain in the internal iliac fossa of the same side; weakness of the limbs in the evening.

PHYTOLACCA DECANDRA.

(*Poke.*)

This plant is indigenous, growing in nearly all parts of the United States, in fence corners, and cleared land not under cultivation. The root is collected in November, cut in slices and dried in the sun; the leaves are gathered just before the berries ripen, and the berries when fully ripe. An active principle termed *Phytolaccin* has been obtained from the root, and is much used in place of the tincture, or pulverized root. The tincture should be made with purified alcohol, *from the green root*—the dried root tincture is comparatively inert. Phytolacca is asserted to be emetic, cathartic, alterative and discutient. It acts as an emeto-cathartic, and exhibits some acro-narcotic powers, such as impaired vision, vertigo and drowsiness. In over doses it is said to cause excessive vomiting and purging, with great prostration, and occasionally convulsions. "While the most prominent effects of Phytolacca appear to be produced on the stomach and bowels, the skin, the nervous system, and the urinary and genital organs of both sexes share largely in its influence. When given to animals in large doses it produces vomiting, purging, bloody stools, perspiration, drowsiness or stupor, cough, tremors, convulsive motions, increased urination, and distention of the abdomen. The flesh of wild pigeons and other birds which eat the berries, acquire a highly red color, a disagreeable flavor, and is *destitute of adipose substance;* and in some instances whole families have been excessively purged by eating game which has fed upon these berries, although children frequently eat the berries without any bad consequences. Phytolacca has been successfully used in veterinary practice, for discussing tumors, fistulous ulcers, and in a disease called 'yellow water.'"—(*Trans. Amer. Ins. Hom.*) The Phytolacca is an analogue of Mercury, Iodide of Potash, Iris versicolor, Podophyllum, Arsenicum, and other drugs. It is a little strange that a vegetable remedy should be so analogous in its action to the Iodide of Potash; one symptom is quite notable—the loss of *adipose tissue* in birds which have eaten of the berries. Kali hyd. has this power of causing absorption of adipose in a great degree; so also both are useful in periodical, mercurial, and so-called syphilitic rheumatism.

Two provings are here given, (one found in the Trans. Amer. Inst. of Hom. Vol. II.; the other lately made by Dr. W. H. Burt):

General Symptoms.—Many of the symptoms, especially those about the head and throat, are better after breakfast, while the heat, and many of the abdominal symptoms are worse in the afternoon; dryness of the fauces, most in the morning; some of the abdominal symptoms disappear in the night; the symptoms of the chest are worse after midnight, better in the afternoon, and most of them on the right side; the pains in the head are chiefly in the forehead, and worse after dinner; dullness, giddiness and vertigo; the prominent feeling in the eyes is that of smarting; the symptoms of the eyes and eyelids are worse in the morning, but the vision is worse in the evening; increased sense of hearing, the right ear is most affected; sensation of a lump in the throat; the symptoms of the stomach, throat, and mouth are worse in the morning. The *first* appearance of the pain in the right hypochondrium was in the afternoon, but afterwards it was always worse before daylight in the morning; griping pains without diarrhœa; pain in the left iliac region; the symptoms of the lower extremities are worse in the afternoon; the pains are sometimes followed by itching and burning; the pains shoot inwards and upwards; transitory pains. Many of the symptoms are attended with heat; neuralgia in the perinæum in the middle of the night; the cough is worse towards morning; sudden translation of internal pains to the extremities. During one of the provings, the symptoms of the eyes became so severe, that Sulphur was taken as an antidote, and all the subsequent symptoms appeared on the left side.—(*Trans. Amer. Ins. Hom.*) Great prostration accompanying the vomiting and purging; much debility.—(*Dr. Burt.*)

Mucous Membranes.—This medicine appears to act as virulently upon mucous tissues as Mercury, and the preparations of Potash. Like them it appears to cause something like false membranes (throat), and severe ulceration and inflammation in the intestines, stomach, etc.)

Muscular Tissue.—It seems to exercise a marked influence over this tissue. It causes muscular pains (myalgia) and rheumatic symptoms, and has been found very useful in the latter disease. No remedy is more popular in domestic use, for chronic rheumatism, than a rude tincture of the ripe berries in whisky. I have observed several marked cures of obstinate cases from its use. "The extract of the root is an excellent remedy for the removal of those severe pains attending mercurio-syphilitic affections (ostea-copus), in which it is more beneficial than Opium."—(*King.*) This would seem to indicate that it affected the *periosteum.*

Nervous Tissue.—The Phytolacca has been known to cause convulsions in men and children. Dr. Burt's experiments on animals elicited many convulsive symptoms. According to Dr. King, it causes "a tingling and prickling sensation over the whole surface." In its pathogenesis we found many *neuralgic* pains, which are clearly distinguished from the *myalgic.* No post-mortem examinations have been made of men or animals—poisoned with this plant—with sufficient accuracy to point out the peculiar pathological conditions it causes.

Vascular System.—*Heart, Fever, etc.*—Neither of our provings, contain any mention of the effects of Phytolacca upon the vascular system. I find no "fever symptoms," and but one "heart symptom." "Occasional shocks of pain in the region of the heart; as soon as the pain in the heart ceases, a similar pain appears in the right arm." This is quite a valuable symptom, as it appears in some rheumatic affections, and may indicate grave cardiac disease. I find no mention of its use in any form of *fever*; it is quite probable, however, that a remedy of such power will be found useful in some febrile diseases. (Enteric gastric, etc.)

Glandular System.—It is esteemed very highly in glandular affections. In our pathogenesis we find the following symptoms:—"A very peculiar tension and pressure in the parotids; hardness of a gland on the right side of the neck; suppuration of a tumor behind the right ear, with a discharge of matter and blood." Dr. Burt found the Phytolaccin to cause swelling and inflammation of the tonsils. Several homœopathic physicians, with myself, have found it useful in swelling and induration of glands; it seems to have a specific affinity for the mammary glands (see "Generative Organs of Women".) According to King, "the root excites the whole glandular system, and has been highly extolled in syphilitic, scrofulous, and cutaneous diseases. It is said to hasten the suppurative process; it has been used with alleged success in bronchocele.

Cancer, Scirrous, Ulcers, etc.—King says: "An inspissated juice of the *leaves* has been recommended in indolent *ulcers*, and as a remedy in cancer." According to Coe: "Phytolaccin has been much employed in the treatment of carcinomitous affections. It is undoubtedly as efficient an alterative as can be safely employed in that disease; its beneficial effects are most apparent in cases of open cancer. The patient's system should be freely brought under its constitutional influence, and the dry Phytolaccin applied to the ulcer. The Phytolaccin applied either in the form of a paste with water, or in strong alcoholic tincture, has been found quite effectual in that species of cancer known as *lupus*, when used in the early stages." Other eclectic physicians advise the Phytolacca in old, indolent, and fistulous ulcers, both as an external and internal remedy. I have found it fully equal to our best anti-psorics, in the treatment of old ulcers, even when of a syphilitic nature; in this respect it is a congener of Silicia, Lachesis, Arsenicum, Kali hyd. Kali bichrom, and Sulphur.

Skin.—A small boil behind the right ear; suppuration of painless tumors; drawing in cicatrices; pustule behind right ear; a painful boil on the right side of the back; eruption of spots on the chest, of the size of lentils, elevated, with great itching.—(*Trans. Amer. Hom. Ins.*)

We have a large amount of testimony from various sources, in relation to the curative action of Phytolacca in cutaneous diseases. *King* asserts its usefulness, and advises an ointment of the pulverized root or leaves in psora, tinea capitis, etc., in connection with its internal administration. Scudder says:—"In ringworm, scabies, shingles, etc., it may be regarded, almost in the light of a specific. At all events it has but few equals." *Coe* states that "Salt-rheum, itch, and other cutaneous eruptions have been cured with Phytolaccin; it is to be employed not only internally but externally." With the country people it has considerable reputation for the cure of obstinate cutaneous diseases. It seems most successful in itch, psoriasis, and certain *scaly* diseases of the skin. An ointment is usually made by stewing the bruised root in lard; this is applied several times a day. I have known this to cure an obstinate and disgusting disease of the scalp, resembling tinea. When the ointment or concentrated alcoholic tincture is applied to the healthy skin, it produces "burning and smarting pains," and may even cause inflammation, vesication, and ulceration. It would seem to act homœopathically even when applied locally, like other escharotics. Many homœopathic physicians value this medicine highly in the treatment of chronic skin diseases. It is to be regretted that we have no exhaustive proving with small and diffusible doses. I predict that it will prove a valuable anti-psoric as well as polychrest.

Sleep.—Yawning; frequent gaping in the daytime; drowsiness; sleepiness; very wakeful at night; restless sleep at night; he lies on the stomach; nausea on being woke out of sleep at night; great inclination to sleep; sleep is very sound; restless at night from pain in the bowels; awoke crying from a very sad dream. It is said to be *narcotic* (acro-narcotic); it will be indicated in the stupor which accompanies some diseases of the bowels, brain or typhoid fever.

Sensorium.—Sensation of soreness in the interior of the head, deep in the brain; dullness of the head; stupefaction; transient giddiness; vertigo with dimness of vision; head feels very light and *hollow*.

Head.—Pains throughout the head; aching; dull feeling in the head; dullness, with the sensation of weight in the forehead; dull pain in the forehead; slight pain in the fore part of the head, with increased sense of hearing; dull, steady, aching pain, principally in the forehead; heavy aching pain about the forehead, after dinner;

aching pain along the lower half of the right orbit; slight pain in the tuberosities of the forehead; headache, with sickness of the stomach from walking; one-sided pain just above the eyebrows, with sickness of the stomach; the pain is increased by looking down and by stooping; headache; slight fullness of forehead with constant gaping; heaviness in the head and especially in the temples; pain in the region of time and mirthfulness, on the right side in the top of the head, and a sensation as if the brain were bruised, when stepping from a high step to the ground; pain in the left temple, followed by burning in the skin in the left region of time; in the left region of combativeness; cold in the head; pressure in the temples and over the eyes; in the temples; in the forehead, after dinner, in the glabella; on forehead and upper part of both eyes, painful; on the temples and constrictive feeling at the præcordia, like the feeling that precedes sea-sickness; slight pain across the forehead, with gaping; sore pain over the head, worse on the right side and in damp weather, as if an attack of sick headache were approaching; slight constriction across the forehead; drawing sensation above the root of the nose; drawing pain in the right temple; moving transitory pains in various parts of the head, almost constantly, generally on one side at a time, but more frequently and most severe on the right side; shooting pain from the left eye to the top of the head, which passes off and returns at short intervals; heat in the head.—(*Trans. Amer. Ins. Hom., Vol. II.*) Dull, heavy headache in the forehead—a constant symptom; sharp, shooting pains in right temple.—(*Dr. Burt.*)

Clinical Remarks.—Phytolacca promises to prove useful in some varieties of rheumatic, catarrhal, and nervous headache. It will probably be found useful in those terrible cephalalgias to which syphilitic patients are liable.

Eyes.—Shooting pain from the left eye to the top of the head; pressure in the eyes; pressure around the eyes in the afternoon, as if the eyes were too large; pressure over the eyes; some painful pressure on the upper parts of both eyes and forehead; burning and smarting sensation in the left eye with great flow of tears; sensation in the eyes like that caused by horse-radish; smarting in the left eye; sandy feeling in the eyes; itching at internal canthi of the eyes, very severe, which caused the application of the finger to rub the eye—the ball became very painful from the slightest pressure; sensation as if a grain of sand were lodged under the left eyelid, causing a secretion and flow of tears from that eye; smarting in the internal canthi of both eyes, but worse in the left one, and very much aggravated by gas-light in the evening; feeling in the eyes and nose as if a cold would come on; soreness on closing the eyelids; reddish-blue swelling of the eyelids, worse on the left side and in the morning; cannot close the eye without pain all the forenoon, better in the afternoon; agglutination of the eyelids during the night; flow of tears all the time from the eyes, relieved in the open air; photophobia in the morning; dimness of sight; long-sightedness.—(*Trans. Amer. Ins. Vol. II.*)

Great smarting in the eyes and lids—(constant symptom); *dull, heavy*, aching pains in the eyeballs, aggravated by motion, light, and especially by reading; sensation as if there was a feather over the sight; eyes agglutinated every morning.

CLINICAL REMARKS.—The Phytolacca has a large number of symptoms of a prominent and suggestive character, relating to the eye, and affecting its various tissues; it is eminently indicated in rheumatic, catarrhal, scrofulous, mercurial and even syphilitic opththalmia. I have used it with success in one case of rheumatic pain in and about the eye, and another of chronic conjunctivitis with granulation. In the "Chicago Medical Examiner" is found the following mention of the curative virtues of Phytolacca in *Granular Conjunctivitis.* Although from allopathic sources, the testimony is worthy our consideration. In this case as in all others, the pathogenesis of the medicine proves its homœopathicity to the disease:

Dr. C. S. Fenner, of Memphis, Tenn., in the N. A. Med. Chirurg. Review, January, 1857, highly extols the efficacy of the Phytolacca in preventing relapses of inflammation in granular lids. "Regarding," he says, "these exacerbations, accompanied with circumorbital pain, soreness in the periosteum and scalp, as of rheumatic origin, about two years ago, I was induced to try the poke, from its well-known efficacy in rheumatic inflammations, and the result has far exceeded my most sanguine expectations. With the aid of this remedy, I have been enabled to effectually cure cases of granular conjuctiva, that, without it, would have resisted all my efforts; indeed, with me it has almost proved a specific for the exacerbations attending this complaint. Patients fully under the influence of the Phytolacca, often expose themselves, and take a severe cold, without affecting the eyes in the least. I use the root in the form of a strong decoction or tincture, and give it in large enough doses to produce fulness of the temples and head; I have not yet seen a severe recurrence of acute inflammation in this disease, where the patient was kept fully under the influence of the Phytolacca."

An allopathic physician claims to have effected several cures of *fistula lacrymalis*, with Phytolacca. I cannot find the paper which makes mention of it in such cases, and therefore the manner in which it was used, is not known to me. But, as in granular conjunctivitis, it was probably used topically and internally.

Ears.—Shooting pain in the right ear, very quick; pain in both ears, worse in the right one; irritation in one of the eustachian tubes; a sensation of obstruction in the left eustachian tube, with a rushing sound in the ear of the same side, and a feeling as if the hearing were dull, while at the same time it is sensitive to the most minute sounds; increased sense of hearing with pain in the forehead.—(*Trans. Amer. Inst. Hom., Vol. II.*)

Nose.—Drawing sensation above the root of the nose; feeling in the nose and eyes as if a cold would come on; cold in the head; stoppage of the right nostril; coryza; flow of mucus from one nostril while the other is stopped; discharge of mucus from one nostril at a time, sometimes one and sometimes the other; total obstruction of the nose when riding, so that one is forced to breathe altogether through the mouth, and cannot relieve himself by blowing the nose.—(*Trans. Amer. Inst. Hom., Vol. II.*)

CLINICAL REMARKS.—Persons engaged in pounding or grinding the root are generally affected with symptoms like severe coryza. Even those engaged in making the second and third triturations of Phytolaccin are similarly affected. It is a powerful irritant to the nasal mucous membrane; it is indicated in acute and chronic nasal catarrhs; in ozæna, and syphilitic ulceration of the nose. It has cured a small cancer on the alæ of the nose.

Face.—Palenesss of the face; heat in the face after dinner; heat on the left side of the face in the afternoon; heat with redness of the face, and a sensation of fullness about the head, and coldness of the feet; eruption on the upper lip, left side; aching pain along the lower half of the right orbit.—(*Trans. Amer. Inst. of Hom.*)

CLINICAL REMARKS.—The inspissated juice of the berries, applied to cancerous or scirrous tumors, and ulcers of the face and lips, has effected cures of such ulcers, etc. It has been found useful in prosopalgia and rheumatic pains in the bones (periosteum) of the face.

Mouth, Teeth, and Tongue.—Small ulcers on the inside of the right cheek, like those caused by mercury; tenderness and heat in the roof of the mouth and on the tongue; flow of saliva into the mouth; mouth fills with water; the saliva is yellowish, and has a metallic taste; dryness of the palate in the morning; swelling of the soft palate; slight feeling of smarting and coldness towards the tip of tongue. Shooting pains in the molar teeth of the upper and lower jaws of the right side; disposition to bite the teeth together; irresistible inclination to bite the teeth together. —(*Trans. Amer Ins. of Hom.*) Tongue feels rough, with *blisters* on both sides, and a very *red* tip; great pain in the root of the tongue when swallowing; teeth all ache, and are very sore, and feel elongatod (the same symptoms were caused by *Phytolaccin*;) metallic taste in the mouth.—(*Dr. Burt.*)

CLINICAL REMARKS.—Some of the symptoms of the medicine strongly resemble those of Mercury, even to the metallic taste, and soreness of tho teeth; it has been used with benefit in mercurial ptyalisim, and mercurial pains of the teeth; it is indicated in inflammation (rheumatic) of the gums, and buccal cavity; rheumatic odontalgia, ulceration of the buccal cavity, and various forms of sore mouth are amenable to its action.

Pharynx and Œsophagus.—Sensation in the pharynx like that caused by eating choke-pears; pressing pain in the right side of the throat; sore throat, and swelling of the soft palate in the morning, with a thick, white, and yellow mucus about the fauces, after the removal of which the throat feels better, and still better after breakfast; soreness of the throat, and a feeling when swallowing saliva as if a lump had formed there; the same sensation is felt on turning the head to the left side; the throat feels very dry and sore, especially on swallowing in the afternoon; general soreness of the posterior fauces, and apparent extension of the irritation into one of the eustachian tubes; roughness in the pharynx; unpleasant sensation of dryness in the pharynx towards morning, which makes him cough; great dryness of the throat; dryness of the throat on going to bed; dryness in the throat, worse in the morning; sensation of dryness of a spot in the fauces on the left side in the morning, continuing until after breakfast.—(*Trans. Amer. Ins. of Hom.*) Great dryness of the throat; roughness in the pharynx (constantly); sensation as of a lump in the throat that causes a constant inclination to swallow; sensation as if an apple core had lodged in the throat; great congestion and swelling of the soft palate and tonsils; the right tonsil is half as large again as the left; both are of a very dark red; feeling as if a ball of red hot iron had lodged in the fauces, and whole length of the œsophagus, when swallowing; the pain was so great that I could eat nothing but fluids for two days, constant choking sensation; roughness and rawness of the throat; tonsils and palate congested, and of a dark purple color; great pain in root of tongue, fauces, etc., from Phytolacca and Phytolaccin; (*Dr. Burt.*)

Clinical Remarks.—One of the most prominent symptoms observed in all cases of poisoning with Phytolacca, is "inflammation of the fauces;" it seems to have a decided affinity for these tissues. Dr. Burt wrote me during the time he was proving the drug, that it would certainly prove a valuable remedy in *diphtheria*, and his prediction has been verified. A few weeks after his provings Dr. Burt had an opportunity of testing the virtues of Phytolacca in that disease. He reports the following cases for the "*Investigator*, *Vol. I*, *p.* 30 *:*

"Miss. B., æt twenty. November 8th had a severe chill at night, with great pain in the back of the head, back and limbs, followed with fever and sore throat. 10th, was called to see her; found her suffering very much, with great headache; worse in the back part; back and limbs aching fearfully; both tonsils very much swollen, and covered with a grayish pseudo-membrane; tongue very red at the tip, coated white; great prostration; cannot stand; if she raises up in bed, she immediately faints away. Prognosis unfavorable. Gave Phytolacca, four drops at a dose every hour, and a gargle of the same between. Morning, decided change for the better. Continued the same treatment for three days, when the false membrane came off, and the fifth day discharged her cured. She took a large spoonful of beef tea every two hours. She had no other remedy. It was remarkable to see how quickly the fever abated under its influence.

"Mrs. B., æt. thirty-one. November 16th.—Throat commenced to feel sore in the morning, followed by high fever all day; right tonsil very much swollen; at noon commenced to see white substance forming on the tonsil. I was called 10 P. M.; found the right tonsil covered completely with a white pseudo-membrane; fauces and soft-palate very much inflamed; deglutition almost impossible; loss of appetite; great frontal headache; bowels moved every two hours, with severe pain in the umbilical region; great prostration; vertigo is so great that she cannot walk. Pulse 127, soft. Gave

Phytolacca, four drops every hour, and a gargle of the same every hour, consisting of fifty drops in a tumbler of water. 18th.—Very much better; pulse 100; throat does not feel near as sore; false membrane beginning to come off; back and limbs ache but slightly; headache nearly gone; continued same treatment three days. Discharged her cured. The diarrhœa stopped the second day.

"Miss. H. æt., twenty-five. December 3d.—Had a severe chill in the night followed by high fever and sore throat. Took Aconite and Belladonna all day, but continued to get worse. Midnight I discovered patches of pseudo-membrane on the tonsils; she complained most bitterly of the back of her head and neck; back and limbs aching. Pulse 120; bowels costive; loss of appetite. Gave Phytolacca, three drops every hour, with a gargle of the same between. 4th, noon.—Feeling better; continued the same treatment. 5th.—No fever; feeling quite well, but thinks her throat is more sore; both tonsils are swollen and covered in patches with false membrane; continued the same treatment, giving six drops at a dose. 6th,—Feeling a great deal better; pseudo-membrane is off of the tonsils; continued same remedy every two hours for two days, when I discharged her, cured.

"A. Snyder, æt. thirty-nine. November 10th.—Throat commenced to feel sore, with severe headache; back and limbs aching severely. 11th.—Was called to attend him, and found the following symptoms: Throat very sore; both tonsils covered with a grayish pseudo-membrane, soft and swollen; palate and fauces violently inflamed; deglutition impossible; severe frontal headache; back and limbs aching severely; high fever; pulse 128; delirious at times; bowels costive; has not slept through the night. Ordered fat salt pork to be put around his neck; beef tea every two hours, and gave Phytolacca every half hour; four drops at a dose, with a gargle of the same. 13th.—Decided change for the better; pulse ninety-eight; head, back and limbs do not ache so hard as they did yesterday; throat feeling very sore, but the false membrane does not seem to be spreading; continued the Phytolacca every hour. 13th.—Feeling much better; pseudo-membrane commencing to fall off, leaving great holes in the tonsils, that bleed a little; continued same treatment. 14th.—Pseudo-membrane all off; tonsils are very much swollen, and look very red and ragged; continued the Phytolacca for three days, once in two hours, when I discharged him cured. I have given the Phytolacca in two cases of children, and two in adults, where the pseudo-membrane was well formed (but there was not so much fever), with the same gratifying result. These are all the cases I have had this fall, and Phytolacca has cured every one of them. I believe there is no medicine in the Materia Medica to be compared to it in diphtheria, if the respiratory organs are not involved. I had no cases where the air passages were involved, to know its effects."

Other cases reported by Dr. Burt to the "*American Homœopathic Observer*."

"Mr. F. æt. twenty-six, Jan. 4th. 9 P.M.—Slight pain in the left tonsil when swallowing; rested well until 2 A.M.; awoke with a severe frontal headache; back and legs aching very hard, with high fever and sore throat; could not sleep any more; 8 A. M., pulse 120 and very soft; head, back and legs are aching violently; throat very sore; left tonsil very much swollen and covered with a grayish false membrane; right tonsil has patches of the pseudo-membrane on it; delgutition is almost impossible; great prostration; can stand up only a few moments at a time, it makes him so faint and dizzy. Gave Phytolacca, four doses every hour, with a gargle of the same, consisting of fifty drops in a tumbler of water. 5th.—Feeling very much better; fever nearly gone; head, back and legs do not ache half as much as they did yesterday; pulse 100; throat is feeling very sore; left tonsil is very much swollen and still covered with the pseudo-membrane; the right one looks very red with small patches of membrane on it; deglutition almost impossible; continued treatment. 6th.—Feeling much better; pseudo-membrane is off from both tonsils; they look very red, and the left one is still swollen; no fever; slight appetite; continued treatment. 7th—Feeling quite well, but throat pains him when swallowing; discharged cured.

"Mrs. G. æt. twenty-one, nursing a babe. Jan. 11th—Throat commenced to feel sore; had a very restless night. 12th.—Slight headache with, a severe pain in her back and legs; very chilly all the time; throat very sore; both tonsils very much swollen, and covered in patches with a dark-colored pseudo membrane; deglutition very difficult; face very much flushed; great prostration; cannot sit up any, she is so faint and weak; bowels regular. Gave Phytolacca, four drops every half hour, with a gargle of the same. 13th.—Feeling very much better; fever all gone; back and legs do not ache any; throat is feeling very sore; tonsils very red and swollen, and covered in patches with the pseudo-membrane; deglutition is very painful. Continued same treatment once an hour. 14th.—Feeling quite well; pseudo-membrane is off from both tonsils; there are large holes eaten into the tonsils; can swallow quite well. Continued same treatment every two hours; discharged her cured the next day. The babe nursed her all the while, and did not take the disease. I attended a lady once before who nursed her babe through the disease, and it did not take it.

"Miss. K. æt. 9. December 12th.—For the last two days has had a fever, with chills all the while; throat has been very sore, and is getting worse all the time; head, back and legs are aching constantly; pulse 130; very weak and soft; soft palate, and tonsils are violently inflamed and swollen; both tonsils are covered with grayish pseudo-membrane; cannot swallow anything; very weak; cannot sit up; has not eaten anything for two days, neither can she be pursuaded to take any kind of nourishment. Gave Phytolacca two drops every hour; morning feeling a little better; pseudo-membrane looks about the same; continued treatment; morning feeling quite well; false membrane is all off, but the throat is feeling very sore; continued same treatment one day more, and then discharged her cured.

"Little Henry. æt. 4. For two days has had a little fever and sore throat; says he is cold all the time; refuses to take food; both tonsils are as large again as they ought to be, and covered in patches with a whitish false membrane; pulse 118; very weak; he lies on the lounge all the time. Gave Phytolacca, ten drops in a tumbler one-half full of water; cured in two days."

A young lad was taken with diphtheria, and treated by an old school physician, and died. His sister, twenty-eight years of age, was taken with it, three days after, and treated by an eclectic, and died the fourth day. A young lady who waited on them was taken down with it four days after the death of the sister. I was sent for, found her with a very sore throat, and the tonsils and soft palate covered with the false-membrane, of a greenish color; both tonsils were twice as large as they ought to be; neck was very stiff; pulse 128. She was very much frightened, was sure she would die; hands and limbs trembled constantly. I tried to quiet her, and gave Bellad. and Iodide of Mercury, every hour, in alternation. Morning found her very much worse; left tonsil was swollen so much that she could not swallow; fever the same; and still trembling. I gave one dose of Aconite, and then a gargle of a tincture from the green root of Phytolacca, every half hour, and gave internally about six drops of the same every hour. Remained with her through the day, and all night; morning, she was not so nervous, and the disease had not made any progress; continued the same treatment; next day about the same; continued same treatment, but made it a little stronger. Morning, decidedly better, the pseudo-membrane looks as if it would soon drop off; continued same treatment. Morning, feeling quite free from fever, and about a quarter of the membrane has come off; she has a fine, scarlet eruption all over the body and limbs, but more on the legs than there is on the body; urine is albuminous; continued the same treatment every two hours. Morning, one tonsil (the right) is free from the membrane, but looks very raw, and burns a good deal; continued the same. Next morning, false-membrane all gone; swelling has disappeared excepting the left tonsil; continued Phytolacca. This case was cured in a few days. Dr. Burt says he has succeeded with Phytolacca in thirty-two out of thirty-four cases of Diphtheria treated.

Case of Scarlatina, with Diphtheritic complications reported, by Dr. Geo. F. Foster; "I had an opportunity last week of trying the *Phytolacca dec.*, in a case of diphthera, with better success as to time of curing patient than with *Bell. Iod. Merc. etc.*

The patient, in the room with a scarlatina patient, was taken sick; high fever, headache etc., not complaining of throat for two days, when the child's mother told me she complained of her throat. I examined it and, sure enough, there was the trouble; both sides covered with the membrane, with rash on the body. I stopped Acon. and Bell., and gave the *Phyto. dec.* (tinct. root), fifteen drops in one-third glass of water two teas-poonsfull at a dose every hour, with gargle of same, three drops to a glass of water. It was the quickest cure of the disease I ever made.

Dr. G. C. Brown says: "I have been experimenting a

little with Phytolacca in enlarged tonsils, and so far have found it very beneficial. In two cases they were so much enlarged as to materialy interfere with deglutition, and had surface ulcers. Were speedily reduced by the use of Phytolacca. a few drops of the tincture in a tumbler of water; a tea-spoonful every two hours."

Dr. C. W. Boyce reports that he has found the Phytolacca universally beneficial in diphtheritic sore throats.

Dr. Stearns, uses the thirtieth attenuation, of Phyto., in diphtheria, with striking curative results.

Appetite and Taste.—Taste like nuts in the mouth—bitter at first, but leaving a slight feeling of smarting and coldness toward the tip of the tongue; raging appetite; hungry soon after eating; diminished appetite; the usual appetite remains, notwithstanding the nausea of the stomach. (*Trans. A. Inst. Hom.*)

Gastric Smptoms.—Eructations; eructations with spitting of water; eructation, with flatus; violent pressure in the stomach on walking in the morning, with accumulation in the mouth—disappears after rising; constrictive feeling at the præcordia, with pressure in the temples; sickly feeling in the stomach; nausea on being awoke out of sleep in the night; feeling of sickness, as if he would vomit; sickness of stomach accompanying the headache; vomiting, with but little distress in the stomach. (*Trans. A. Inst. Hom.*)

Stomach.—Cutting in the pit of the stomach, and in the abdomen; tenderness to the touch of the pit of the stomach; pain in the region of the pylorus (*Trans. A. I. H.*); eructations of air; eructations of sour fluid; great distress in the stomach and bowels; pains in the cardiac portion of the stomach, aggravated by a full inspiration and by walking; nausea with a very faint feeling; nausea with severe pain in the umbilical region; slight nausea with profuse vomiting, without much pain attending it, but good deal of distress in the stomach; nausea and violent vomiting (in dogs). (*Burt.*)

Clinical Remarks.—The vomiting caused by Phytolacca comes on slowly, preceded by nausea, much prostration, and sometimes fainting and convulsions. When the vomiting does set in it is intense, thorough, and composed of bile, mucus, ingesta, worms, and even blood. This medicine ought to prove useful in a variety of gastric affections, and disorders of digestion.

Liver, Hypochondria.—Digging pain in the right hypochondrium, in the upper and lower portion of the liver, preventing motion; first felt at two o'clock in the afternoon, then every morning before daylight; some soreness remaining through the afternoon and evening; pain in the region of the pylorus; cannot lie on the right side after midnight, on account of penetrating pain in the right hypochondrium; violent dull, pressing pain in the left hypochondrium, in the evening, so that he cannot remain in the sitting posture, he lies on the painful side all night and the pain is gone the next morning; *soreness and pain in the right hypochondrium during pregnancy. (*Trans. A. Inst. Hom.*)

Clinical Remarks.—The Phytolacca is recommended in chronic hepatic disorders, also in diseases of the spleen. It undoubtedly has some influence over these organs, by virtue of its tendency to irritate all glandular structures. It has cured "soreness and pain in the hypochondrium during pregnancy.

Abdomen.—Boring pain to the left and a little above the umbilicus, continuing but a few minutes; deep-seated, but not severe pain, in the left iliac region; neuralgic pain in the left groin; cutting in the abdomen; griping pain, as before a diarrhœa; griping all day long, followed by the passage of offensive flatus; the griping disappears in the night; sensation in the bowels, as if a diarrhœa would follow; rumbling noise in the bowels; frequent passage of wind downward. (*Trans. A. Inst. Hom.*)

Stool and Anus.—*Constipation of long standing; hard stools; three stools during the day; the first one is hard, and preceded by griping, and the others with pains moving about in the abdomen; continual inclination to go to stool; mushy stool; diarrhœa attentended with a sickly feeling in the bowels, but no tormina or tenesmus; copious discharges of bile from the bowels; in the middle of the night, neuralgic pain shooting from the anus and the lower part of the rectum along the perinæum, to the middle of the penis, followed in a few minutes by a neuralgic pain in the right big toe. (*Trans. A. I. H.*) Constant dull pain in the umbilical region, worse by motion; severe, colicky pains in the umbilical region; rumbling in the bowels, sometimes with desire for stool; burning distress in the umbilical region; bowels very tender on pressure, and pain severely when walking; stool natural; stool soft and mushy, with undigested food in it, sometimes with straining; stool of mucus, with straining; dark, lumpy stool; soft papescent stool, followed by a very faint feeling; wind passes the bowels constantly, of a very fetid nature; emissions of flatus relieves the pain in the bowels; loss of appetite; canine hunger; vomiting of worms (in animals); pain in the left hypochondriac region when walking; loss of appetite; hiccough with great inclination to vomit, but no nausea; nausea and violent vomiting (in a dog); great rumbling in the bowels, with pain in the umbilical region; great pain in præcordial region, very much worse by walking; great distress in the umbilical and hypogastric regions; stool soft and mushy; dark, papescent stools with undigested food if them; pain in the umbilical region with desire for stool. (*Burt.*) *Toxicological effects*, trachea and lungs filled with mucus; stomach highly congested at the base; colon and rectum appear congested; liver highly congested; kidneys appear very much congested.

Clinical Remarks.—The Phytolacca is an emeto-cathartic. It causes many of the symptoms of a severe attack of cholera morbus. It is homœopathic to some forms of cholera, diarrhœa, dysentery, and hemorrhoids. In piles it has been found curative (by eclectics) in many cases, applied locally, and given internally. It is also homœopathic to enteritis and colic. It has cured a case of "constipation of long standing."

Urinary Organs.—*Urgent desire to pass water; copious nocturnal urination; weakness, dull pain and soreness in the region of the kidneys, most on the right side, and connected with heat;

uneasiness down the ureters; a chalk-like sediment in the urine; a gurgling sensation in the prostrate gland, repeatedly in the afternoon; *pain in the region of the bladder, before and during urination; *dark-red urine which stains the chamber of a mahogany color, and which is hard to get off.—*Trans. Am. Inst. Hom.*

The urinary secretion was at first diminished, afterwards increased. The urine remained *acid* and became decidedly *albuminous*. The *specific gravity* became greatly increased. The bottle used to measure the urine became completely covered with a *white deposit*, about one-sixteenth of an inch thick.—*Dr. Burt.*

Clinical Remarks.—The urinary symptoms in the original proving were quite notable, but those elicited by Dr. Burt, are really of great importance. The urine, under the usual tests, was decidedly albumninous. When we consider how important albuminaria becomes, in Scarlatina and Diphtheria, we can easily realize the full value of Phytolacca in those maladies. It is indicated in many renal and cystic disorders.

Generative Organs of Men.—Complete loss of all sexual desire for two months; no erections during the whole proving; sexual organs unusually relaxed.

Clinical Remarks.—It would seem quite homœopathic to *Impotence*. It seems likely to prove a valuable remedy in Syphilis, although our provings do not bring out any objective symptoms. "The Cherokee Indians, is is said, used to dress the venereal sores with the powder of the dried root; and some physicians aver that it will cure syphilis *without the aid of mercury*." If we are to credit the testimony of eclectic physicians, it has not only been found curative in *primary* syphilis, (chancre, etc.) but in *secondary* and *tertiary* syphilis, (ulcers, eruptions, throat and nasal diseases, bone pains, etc.) "For the cure of syphilis, and mercurio-syphilitic disorders, the Phytolaccin is quite equal to any other organic remedy. * * The severe pains attending tertiary-syphilis and mercurio-syphilitic complications are more effectually relieved by the use of this medicine, than by any other remedy."—(*Coe.*) It is said to be particularly useful in cases of chronic and obstinate gonorrhœa and gleet. Dr. Small thinks highly of it in some forms of syphilitic rheumatism, and I have found it promptly curative in many of the conditions mentioned above. It has cured *Orchitis*.

Generative Organs of Women.—**Metrorrhagia*; *menstruation too copious and too frequent; painful menstruation; violent pains in the abdomen during menstruation, in a barren female; *leucorrhœa; *inflammation swelling and suppuration of the mammæ.—(*Trans. Amer. Inst. Hom.*)

Clinical Remarks.—All the above symptoms are marked with the asterisk, in the original proving. I have no means of ascertaining whether they were originally pure pathogenetic symptoms. The asterisk implies they *were;* but had been substantiated by curative effects. The proving in Symptomen codex, is not accompanied by the name of any prover, or those physicians who contributed clinical notes. In the clinical observations I find the following: "Being given in a case of chlorosis, when the leucorrhœa had been cured by Pulsatilla, it brought the leucorrhœa back again." (Possibly?) It always appeared surprising that eclectic writers should say so little about the Phytolacca in diseases of women. I find no mention of its use in that class of diseases, in King, Scudder, and others, yet the extensive range of action of the medicine precludes the idea that it will not be found useful.

In my estimation the sphere of action of Phytolacca is principally upon (a) the glandular system, (b) the serous and fibrous tissues, and (c) the mucous membrane.

Phytolacca has a specific effect upon the thyroid and mammary, also parotid, and other glands of the throat, and by analogy ought to act powerfully upon the ovaries, and glands of the uterus (also the testes). Accordingly it ought to prove curative in ovaritis, and other affections of the glands, such as neuralgia, etc.; in uterine leucorrhœa, or that variety which proceeds from the glandular portion of the cervix. Its powerful influence over ulceration should make it curative in ulcerated os-uteri, whether of a non-specific, or specific character. Finally, it should cure rheumatic affections of the uterus. The metrorrhagia and frequent menstruation mentioned above, may have proceeded from ulceration of the os; the dysmenorrhœa from rheumatic irritation, and the leucorrhœa may have had a glandular origin. In organic affections of the uterus, as tumors, cancer, scirrous, ulceration, I would strongly advise the Phytolacca, internally and locally applied, and its use persevered in for some time. The action of Phytolacca on the mammary glands is specific and decisive. In No. 84, page 201, of the British Journal of Homœopathy, will be found an article from my pen, which covers this subject as much as the present state of our knowledge will permit. I would urge upon physicians to test its virtues in the various diseases of the mammæ. Since the article was published, I have used it successfully in many cases of mammitis as well as tumors and nodosities in these glands:

"It is the intention of the writer to call attention to only one particular use of this remedy; viz., *in certain diseases of the mammary glands.*

"The various writers on Materia Medica of the dominant and other schools *not* homœopathic, while they recognize its value in diseases of the glands, do not mention this particular sphere of its action. In the homœopathic proving above referred to we find the following:—

"'*Inflammation, swelling, and suppuration of the mammæ.*' But I am not aware that this symptom has ever been put to practical test by homœopathists, with the exception of Dr. Hill, who recommends it in some diseases of the breast. (See *Hill and Hunt's Surgery.*) My experience with the drug dates back nearly fifteen years, before I had seen the proving referred to, or indeed any published statement of its value as a medicine.

"When I was a student of medicine in my father's office (he was then an allopath), a neighbor had a valuable cow, which, after a clandestine confinement, was brought home from the woods with a most enormously swollen udder. It was as hard as a stone, intensely hot, painful, and sensitive, and not a particle of milk could be drawn. In his anxiety the owner came into his office, and asked my father to suggest something to discuss the swelling and engorgement. A dose of Epsom salts was administered, but after twenty-four hours the cow was worse than before. At this juncture an old woman of the neighborhood brought in a piece of a large, white, succulent looking root, which she called *scoke*, and ordered the farmer to cut a portion of it up finely and give the animal in some "bran mash." Another, the larger portion, was made into a decoction, and the cow's udder washed with it frequently. The effect was magical! In less than twelve hours the milk could be drawn, the gland softened, and in a few days the morbid condition was removed.

"This incident was nearly forgotten until a few years after, when I was engaged in practice, and was having trouble with mastitis and abscess of the breast in the persons of my patients. I found the remedies laid down in our books notoriously and obstinately inefficient. In spite of Aconite and Belladonna in high and low attenuations, the inflammatory engorgement would run on to suppuration. I then tried larger doses and other remedies, among which the *Kali hyd.* was most valuable; also topical application of Belladonna, Arnica, Iodine, etc., after the manner of the dominant school, and will give them the credit of preventing much suffering and deformity. But I determined on making a trial of the virtues of the Phytolacca, and before I commenced its use, made inquiry among the farmer's of my acquaintances, and found to my gratification that it was considered a specific in all cases of inflammation and engorgement, "caking" of the udder of cows, and even mares.

"The next case of engorgement of the mammæ which came under my care was an aggravated one. The woman, the mother of several children, had had "broken breasts" with every confinement, and the cicatrices in the glands bore testimony to the truth of her assertion. About four days after delivery she had a severe chill followed by some fever, and in a few hours both mammæ were hard, swollen, and painful. The child made ineffectual efforts at nursing, the nipples became very sensitive, and she was in much distress for fear of the inevitable sufferings apparently in store for her. Here was a case wherein to test the efficacy of the Phytolacca. Ten drops of the first decimal dilution were administered every hour, and a lotion was prepared by adding one-half oz. of the tincture to one-half pint of warm water. This was applied constantly by means of folds of cotton cloth laid upon the breasts. In the course of the next twenty-four hours I had the satisfaction of finding some signs of resolution. The heat, pain, and swelling became less, and in a few days, with the aid of low diet, and careful extraction of the milk, the woman recovered with only a small abscess at the site of an old cicatrix, instead of extensive suppuration, as usual. Since that time I have used it in very many cases, with the same excellent results, and it is only in the severer forms, accompanied with erysipelatous inflammation, that I have had to resort to Belladonna internally and externally.

"But this Phytolacca is not only useful in simple and inflammatory engorgement, causing rapid resolutions, but it is valuable in those cases where suppuration has already commenced. Here it reduces the inflammation, increases the activity of the absorbents, and will often condense an apparently large abscess into the smallest dimensions.

"It is often the case that neglected or ill-treated mammary abscess degenerates into ill-conditioned, fistulous ulcers. In such cases I have seen the best effects follow the judicious use of this remedy.

"*Case* 1.—A young woman, a *primipara*, very corpulent, with very large mammary glands, was taken with chills and fever a few days after confinement. The family were poor, and lived a long distance in the country; no physician was called, and nothing was properly done, but very improperly the breast was poulticed for nearly two weeks, when several large abscesses opened spontaneously and discharged enormous quantities of unhealthy pus. Six weeks afterwards she came to me for advice. The breast affected was a most loathsome sight, long, pendulous, distorted, the seat of several large fistulous ulcers, discharging a watery, fœtid, ichorous pus; the gland was full of hard, painful nodosities, of the size of a walnut and larger. I suspended the breast by the application of long strips of adhesive plaster, placed in various directions across and around the gland, and prescribed ten drops of Phytolacca first, four times a day; also a preparation of one-half oz. of the tincture to eight oz. of distilled water, to be thrown into the fistulous canals with a small glass syringe; this treatment, together with a better diet and a little wine, so much improved the case in a week, that but one small ulcer remained open; and in a fortnight the treatment was suspended. The gland will never return to its normal condition, but will probably retain its irregular shape and knotty feel.

"*Case* 2.—A woman, aged 40, applied to me to be treated for what had been declared an "open cancer" of the breast. It originated one year previously after the birth of her seventh child, and was the result of a neglected abscess. The ulcer was an inch in diameter, gaping, angry, filled with unhealthy granulations; a probe passed obliquely downwards until it reached a hard sensitive tumor about the size of a hen's egg; the discharge was offensive and sanious. The case was treated by suspension and compression, and the use of Phytolacca as above. Cured in two weeks.

"Many similar cases might be cited, but these will suffice, as they are good examples of the many cures made with this remedy.

"It may here be mentioned, that the local application of this remedy is useful in cracked and excoriated nipples. It should be given at the same time internally. If the fissures are syphilitic in their origin, this remedy is still useful. I once treated a case of irritable tumor of the breast as described by Sir Astley Cooper.

It had been present several years, and was very sensitive and painful, most especially at the menstrual periods; the pain extended down the arm of the affected side, and at times causing a sympathetic enlargement of a gland in the axilla. I administered Belladonna, Conium, Phosphorus, and Iodine, but without any good result, and the patient left me. A few months after, I learned to my intense mortification, that an old woman had cured it with a plaster of the inspissated juice of the berries of the Phytolacca. Since that occurrence I have treated several cases successfully with the Phytolacca internally, giving the lowest dilutions, and sometimes the mother tincture. In one case I permitted the patient to use a "salve" of the juice of the berries mixed with mutton tallow. This she applied constantly over the site of the tumor. Whether it hastened the cure or not I cannot say, at least its application did no harm, although it seemed capable of causing some vesications of the skin.

"The same old lady above mentioned had quite a reputation for curing "cancers," and with no other application, as I was assured, than the extract of Phytolacca. I have known the finely powdered root, when applied to fungous growths, have the effect of changing such abnormal into normal or healthy ulcers which soon healed.

"I have found it useful in encysted tumors; in recent indurations; and even in scirrous of the breast; nor should I be surprised if further trials should show it to be useful in cancer of the mammæ.

"In those cases of irritable mammæ where there is no swelling, induration, or tumor, only a painfulness at the menstrual period, I have found it specific in a few cases. The menses became more natural, and the pain in the mammæ ceased. The question here arises: Why will it not prove valuable in certain diseases of the testicles or the ovaries? When we consider the physiological relation of the ovaries to the mammæ, we should incline to predict it will found useful in many ovarian diseases."

To the above article I would add, that the root is in general use among dairymen in this country, to regulate *any* abnormality in the milk of cows. If the milk be scanty, thick, watery, curdy (flocculent), or contains blood or pus, or becomes in any way unnatural, they give the green root, or a decoction in small quantities, and the effect upon the milk is generally favorable. This should suggest its use in abnormal conditions of the milk in women, giving it in the lower dilutions. The higher might be tried in some peculiar cases.

Larynx and Cough.—Tickling in the left side of the larynx, with hacking cough, and aching in the right side of the breast and great dryness of the throat; sensation of roughness in the bronchia; cough towards morning, from dryness of the pharynx; dry bronchial cough, with the sensation of roughness and slight increase of heat in the trachea and bronchia; hacking cough.—(*Trans. A. I. H.*)

Clinical Remarks.—It seems to be Dr. Burt's opinion that when the diphtheria membrane invades the air passages, the Phytolacca is of less value, or none at all, but this remains to be proven. If it is specific to the disease, it may be curative of it, let it be located where it will. It is said to have been used in asthma, and chronic coughs, with benefit.

Chest and Respiration.—Shortness of breath; aching pain in the right side of the breast; pain in the right side of the chest about the region of the nipple, passing through to the back, felt on taking a long breath, and on bending the shoulder backwards, better in the afternoon; pain in the right side of the chest, so bad after midnight as to prevent sleep, aggravated by lying on the right side, disappears after getting up in the morning; tenderness of the muscles of the chest, as if they were bruised; occasional shocks of pain in the region of the heart, and as soon as the pain in the heart ceases, a similar pain appears in the right arm.—(*Trans. A. I. H.*)

Clinical Remarks.—Some eclectic writers suggest its use in pulmonary turberculosis, and analogy might suggest its use in ulcerative diseases involving the lungs and bronchia, but we have no clinical records of its successful use in such cases. I found it beneficial in one case of intercostal rheumatism of several years' standing. It ought to prove curative, as the symptoms indicate in some rheumatic and neuralgic affections of the thorax and heart.

Back.—Pain in the left lumbar region, followed immediately by severe itching; a lasting pain in the left shoulder-blade, as if from a blow; an occasional sensation as if a small piece of cold iron were pressed on the painful shoulder-blade; sensation of weight and pressure on both shoulder-blades, as after carrying a heavy load; stiffness in the right side of the neck, worse in bed, after midnight; a very peculiar pressure and tension in the parotids; hardness of the gland on the right side of the neck; suppuration of a tumor behind the right ear, with a discharge of matter and blood; severe pain between the scapulas, when walking; constant dull, heavy pain in the lumbar and sacral regions, aggravated by motion; the back is very stiff every morning.—(*Dr. Burt.*)

Clinical Remarks.—It is indicated by the symptoms, and has proved curative in cases of "stiff neck," *lumbago*, and even *spinal irritation.*

Upper Extremities.—Dull aching pain and tenderness along the top of the right shoulder, along the superior edge of the trapezius muscle, increased by pressing upon the part and by contracting the muscle; pain throughout the muscles of the left shoulder; pain in the humeral insertion of the left deltoid muscle; slight drawing pains in the right upper arm; pain appears in the right arm after a similar pain ceases in the heart; tenderness in the outside of the left arm just above the elbow, when pressing upon it, and when extending the arm; dull aching pain and excessive tenderness, as if from a bruise in the muscles of the outside of the right upper arm, most severe for about two inches above the elbow, felt particularly when the part is pressed upon and touched, and when extending the arm; twitching and fluttering of the muscles of the right upper arm, while it is resting on a table; weakness and aching in the bone of the right arm above the elbow, aggravated by motion and extension; rheumatic drawing in the right forearm; rheumatic drawing in the left forearm along the ulna, and the same sensation in the right leg; rheumatic pains in the hands and feet, sometimes in the arms and legs; drawing pain in the right hand, now and then, by shocks upwards to the elbow; rheumatic feeling in the little finger of the right hand, very annoying when writing; rheumatic pain, first in the left hand, and afterwards in the right one; shooting, like needles, in the left thumb; violent shooting pain in the fleshy part of the left thumb, lasting about half a minute; lancinating pain in the little and ring-fingers of the right hand; neuralgic pains in the palm of the right hand; occasionally frequent sudden pricking in the points of the fingers, as if from eclectic sparks; shooting in the finger-points, sometimes in one hand and sometimes in the other.—(*Trans. A. I. H.*) Arms ache; ends of the fingers all throb and ache, as if they were going to suppurate, (this symptom lasted three days).—(*Dr. Burt.*)

Clinical Remarks.—Dr. Burt recommends the Phytolacca in whitlow, *felon*, etc., because of the remarkable similarity of the symptoms. It is a popular domestic remedy in those troublesome affections (the green root is applied raw or boiled). Indicated in rheumatic affections of arms and hands. Dr. Burt has cured warts on the hands with the tincture locally applied.

Lower Extremities.—Sciatica; neuralgic pain on the outer side of the left thigh; neuralgic pain in the external part of the right thigh; neuralgic pain in the external part of the left thigh; neuralgic pain in the left groin; heaviness in the knee joints, tired from a little walk; heaviness in the lower extremities, as if they were asleep, in the afternoon; rheumatic pain in the right knee, in the afternoon, increasing in the open air, and especially on a damp day; rheumatic drawing in the right leg and in the left forearm along the ulna; rheumatic feeling in the left knee, with the sensation of shortening the tendons behind the knee when walking; rheumatic pains below the knees and in the arms; pain on the dorsum of the right foot at four o'clock in the morning; coldness of the feet with increase of the capillary circulation about the face and head; free sweating of the feet, most under the toes; neuralgic pain in the right big toe, in the middle of the night; pains at a spot on the ball of the right foot, which had been frost-bitten years before, and in a corn never painful before.—(*Trans. A. I. H.*) Legs ache, and feel very stiff about the knees, aggravated by walking; weakness; could walk with difficulty.—(*Dr. Burt.*)

Clinical Remarks.—It is stated that from the application of the juice of the root to corns "the whole toe became inflamed and turned black, like gangrene." It seems almost incredible that this should have been a direct result of the Phytolacca. It has been used successfully in chronic rheumatism of the lower extremities; for chronic inflammation of the knee joint, with or without effusion, and in sciatica and nightly pains in the limbs. Syphilitic and mercurial rheumatism (periostitis) generally selects the *tibia*, as the chief point of its operations. I have used it successfully in nightly pains in tibia, with nodes, and even irritable ulcers on the legs. It will be found useful in nearly all those cases in which Iodide of Potash is so freely used in allopathic practice, and strangely enough is quite as successful as that salt.

Characteristic Peculiarities.—The pains all partake of the nature of neuralgia; they are pressing and shooting, sometimes sore, drawing and aching; the pains are all made worse by motion and by pressure; the pains in the extremities are always in the outer portions of the limbs; the secretion of tears, saliva, bile, urine and the menses is increased; irresistible inclination to bite the teeth together; vomiting attended with but little distress in the stomach; the diarrhœa appears to be kept up by the increased action of the liver, and consequent redundancy of bile, with but little tormina and tenesmus; with the increase of the secretion of bile, there is a dry, irritative cough, and almost constantly recurring transitory pains in different parts of the head. We find the symptoms predominating in the right side of the head and neck, the right upper extremity, the right side of the chest, and the right lower extremity; when enumerating the symptoms of the eyes only, we find the left one most frequently mentioned; in the above extract there are forty symptoms located on the right side, and thirty-one on the left. In several instances, the symptoms appeared on the left side first, and either passed over to the right, or the next symptom occurred on the right side.—(*Trans. Am. Inst. Hom.*)

PODOPHYLLUM PELTATUM.

(*Mandrake.*)

This plant is also known by the common name of *May-Apple.* It is so well-known that no description is here necessary. It is found in great abundance in all parts of the United States. The fruit is eaten and much liked by some persons, but extremely disagreeable to others. It is slightly aperient, and popularly supposed to cause an eruption of *boils.* The pulp only should be eaten. The fleshy portion contains much medicinal power, but inferior to the *root*, which is the officinal portion. It was well known to the Indians before the whites settled the country, and was one of their most active purgatives. It should be collected soon after the ripening of the fruit; its active principles are readily taken up by alcohol; it contains a resinous principle, called *Podophyllin.* The preparations used in homœopathic practice should be the tincture from the fresh root, a trituration from the dried root, and from Podophyllin; and dilutions made in the usual manner from the third trituration of the last-named preparation, or the tincture.

Toxical Effects.—The entire plant in its recent state is an irritant poison, producing vomiting, hypercatharsis, tormina, stupor, and bloating of the body; the root recently dried, operates as a drastic cathartic and emetic, when given in large doses, but the violence of its action is materially modified by age. Several cases of poisoning by the fruit, in children who had eaten the rind, have been brought under my observation, but in no instance was a fatal result induced.

The following narrative of cases by Dr. D. C. Owen, which I take from the "Chicago Medical Examiner," are of interest, as showing the principal toxical effect of the medicine:—"On the 4th of August, 1860, I was called upon to visit two children of H. C., who, the messenger said, were vomiting themselves to death. I inquired what the children had been eating or taking; he replied, that the parents thought the vomiting was caused by May-apples, which the children had eaten in the morning. I drove briskly on, and arrived at the place in, perhaps, half an hour, where I found two very pretty little girls, aged respectively, six and eight years, stretched upon their beds; bathed in cold perspiration; their faces pale as corpses; eyes sunken in their orbits; noses pinched; pulse very weak, and scarcely perceptible at the wrist; great thirst; and the stomach contracting so hard and rapidly, in efforts to vomit, that the wrenching pain would cause them to utter sharp screams, one after another, for five minutes at a time. I was told that the vomiting had been going on for the last four hours, almost without intermission, it being now 12 M. On examining the matters thrown from the stomach, I found them to consist, for the most part, of seeds, pulp, and membraneous covering of the ripe May-apple, having the peculiar odor of that fruit. I asked them if they had eaten the rinds of the apples. They said, no; but they had used their teeth to rupture the rinds. I informed the parents that the recovery of the oldest child was not to be expected, owing to the prostration already produced; but that the chances for the younger were much better. I gave the oldest, one gr. sulp. morphine, covered the epigastrium and entire abdomen, which was tympanitic and very tender, with a blister; invited the blood to the extremities with hot flannels and sinapisms; gave carbonic acid water, in small quantities, to allay thirst; and, as the bowels had not been moved since the vomiting begun, ordered an enema of castor oil and molasses in warm water. To the younger I gave, perhaps two-thirds gr. morphine, and ordered the same course as for the other, except that for the blister I substituted mustard. They were now kept as quiet as possible for, perhaps, an hour and a-half, when the younger child was sufficiently under the influence of the narcotic to fall into a quiet sleep. The oldest now vomited again bilious matter mixed with blood—the bile dark green and very thick, the blood dark and coagulated. She complained frequently of burning sensation in the throat. Finding that the injections had failed to move the bowels, I gave Hydrargyri sub. mur, gr. xij., Morphine sulph., gr. j. They were now both getting warm extremities, the youngest still sleeping. I left powders of morphine and camphor, one of which was to be given after each act of vomiting, should it commence again, or after each stool, should the bowels act too freely. I directed the parents to do everything in their power to maintain the proper amount of heat in the extremities; and, if the means they were then using were not sufficient to keep up the warmth of the body, to use brandy by enema. For the youngest, I left similar powders and directions, should she require them.

"Called August 5th, at 7 A. M.—Found the oldest past all hope—the eyes glazed and motionless, the death-rattle in her throat, the abdomen swelled almost to bursting, and the under jaw fallen. At half-past eight o'clock she expired. I learned that she had continued to vomit thick bile, with more or less blood mixed with it, about every hour through the night. The youngest child was considerably better, although there was considerable tenderness over the stomach, to remove which I applied a blister; gave Dover's powder to keep her quiet, slippery-elm water for drink, kept the bowels solvent with sulphate of magnesia; and, by the morning of the 8th, she was convalescent. I have endeavored to give a simple statement of the facts in the above cases, as they occurred; and I will decline making comments, more than to say, that, after seeing the deleterious effects of the May-apple in these cases, I would not recommend them as being the healthiest article of diet that we can procure; and I have also kept an eye single on the action of podophylline." In the hands of incautious or ignorant physicians, the Podophyllum and its active principle have been productive of an immense amount of injury to the people of the West. I have treated many painful, severe, and incurable diseases of the stomach and intestines, uterus, and urinary organs, which could be dated distinctly to over dosing with this potent drug. Next to Mercury, it is capable of inflicting more injury to the human organism, when abused, than almost any other drug in common use; yet eclectics denounce Mercury in all its forms, while pouring this poison down their patients. The original and only proving which has yet appeared, was made by Dr. Williamson, of Philadelphia, and published in the "Trans. Amer. Inst. of Hom. Vol. I." I shall make that the basis of this article, and add thereto the pathogenetic and clinical symptoms which have been collected since that publication. It has been used more extensively, perhaps, than any of the new remedies, and is already looked upon by our school as a valuable polychrest. I am indebted to Dr. E. J. Frazer, of Chicago, for the peculiar arrangement of the symptoms of this medicine. Under my directions he has placed the *primary* and secondary symptoms in their proper order, as nearly as our knowledge of the action of the drug will permit. This should be done with every medicine, in order to facilitate the study of its effects, and guide us in the selection of the proper dose. Eclectic physicians, and of late many of the allopathic school, have come to look upon the Mandrake as a sort of panacea for nearly all acute diseases, and useful in almost all chronic affections. With its enthusiastic admirers it ranks with Calomel. Medical adjectives have been exhausted in describing its powers and virtues. It is said to be cathartic, emetic, alterative, anthelmintic hydragogue, sialogogue, deobstruent, febrifuge, anti-periodic, diuretic, etc., etc., etc. It is a fact, that like Mercury it penetrates every nook and cranny of the organism, and there is scarce an organ or tissue of the body but feels its malign influence, when it is introduced into the system in toxical doses. It has been used in nearly every disease in the nomenclature, and is said to have proved curative in those of the most opposite character. I shall try to show in my clinical remarks the causes of its great popularity, and attempt to define its real sphere of action. I will here remark that I shall use the statements relative to the Podophyll*um* and Podophyll*in*, indiscriminately—as I believe both to act in a similar (perhaps identical) manner upon the system. The latter may not have as wide range of action as the former, because it does not contain all the medicinal constituents of the plant. To meet the requirements of an exact science, such as homœopathy aspires to be, there should be a proving of both preparations, but until we reach that desideratum we must do the best we can. In the clinical remarks I shall designate as far as possible which preparation was prescribed, in order that the physician may use the same in similar cases. (I shall, for the sake of brevity, adopt the abreviation "*Pm.*" for the one, and "*Pn.*" for the other preparation.)

GENERAL EFFECTS.—**Nervous System.**—Podophyllum does not act specifically upon the nerves, as does Aconite or Nux vomica. In this respect it ranks with Bryonia, Aloes, and other medicines of the same class. The pains induced by the Mandrake are probably *myalgic* in their character. In idiopathic neuralgia, or indeed neuralgia in any form, it is of doubtful utility.

Muscular System.—We have not sufficient proof, nor do we find anything in the pathogenesis, which would lead us to suppose that Podophyllum acted directly upon the muscular fibre, as does Bryonia, Mercurius, or Helonias. To fully understand the action of Mandrake, and other similarly acting and depressing drugs, one should read that instructive book, "Inman on Myalgia." I would suggest that Podophyllum causes pains, cramps and other sensations and affections of muscular tissue by (a) its irritating action upon mucous membranes, and (b) by its depressing action upon the vital power. According to Inman, all drastic purgatives may cause myalgia, and even cramps, and wasting of muscle. Viewing the action of this medicine as I do, I cannot consider it indicated in rheumatism affecting muscles or tendons. If it has been found beneficial in that disease, it has been from some indirect action, and not from any specific effect. I have known it to cause severe myalgic pains and soreness, and have found it curative in similar conditions, but never in true rheumatism. The Podophyllin has the power to cause other pains besides those referred to the bowels, stomach and other portions of the digestive tract. I have known it to cause pains in various parts of the system, but I believe them to be generally *myalgic*. Dr. Coe, whose testimony is sometimes valuable, says: "Podophyllin is sometimes very tardy in its operation, not acting under eighteen or twenty hours, and frequently it will operate more freely during the second twenty-four hours, than during the first. In cases of chronic disorders of the liver, spleen, and other viscera, *considerable pain* will frequently be experienced in the diseased organs during the operation of the medicine. Sometimes the pain will be in the liver, at others in the spleen, again in the kidneys, (medicinal aggravation), also in the back of the neck and head, in the pleura, intercostal muscles, etc., (myalgic), but these symptoms will subside with the operation of the medicine." He thinks these are favorable indications, "showing that the remedy is at work arousing the dormant energies of the system." It is not necessary, however, to cause these pains, etc.

Mucous Tissues.—In its action on mucous membranes it ranks with Mercurius, Iris v., Veratrum album., and other drastic cathartics. It is powerfully *irritant* to the tissues, especially those of the digestive tract. It is not directly specific in its action upon the mucous membrane of the respiratory and urinary passages. It will however irritate and inflame any mucous surface when brought in contact with it, sometimes acting as a powerful escharotic. Of its power to cause inflammation of any and all portions of the mucous membrane from the mouth to the anus, there can be no doubt. Such effects have been too often observed in practice, by all physicians who have had opportunity to notice its action when adminministered in material doses. It even causes ulceration of this tissue, and may be said to act as Dr. Freligh asserts of mercury—"*as a solvent of the living solids*," but not to the extent of the former poison. Mandrake is homœopathic to enteritis, gastritis, etc., and even to bronchitis and urethritis, under certain circumstances, which will be noticed under appropriate headings.

Serous Tissues.—It is said to affect, by its "alterative action," the serous membranes of the body, and prove curative in pleuritis, peritonitis, synovitis, and even meningitis; but its action in this direction, is not, in my opinion, specific or direct, as is the case with Bryonia.

Glandular System.—It is here that mandrake is a close analogue of Mercury, Iodine, Iris versicolor, etc. When taken up into the circulation, it is eliminated by the glands, and is thus rendered capable of causing irritation, inflammation, and even suppuration of almost any glandular organ or structure. To those who would thoroughly understand the action of that class of medicines termed "Eliminants," I would advise a careful perusal of that masterly work, "Headland on the Action of Medicines." According to King and others, "It produces a powerful and lasting impression upon the glandular system and secretory organs, unequalled by any other article." It is highly recommended and habitually used in scrofula, induration, and swelling; also inflammation and suppuration of glands. It would be useless to waste our space in recording all the laudations of eclectic physicians in relation to its curative action upon the system. Like the praises the allopathist bestows upon mercury, they are too often based upon an unsubstantial foundation.

Vascular System, Fever.—Chilliness while moving about during fever, and in the act of lying down, with perspiration immediately afterwards; chilliness when first lying down in the evening, followed by fever and sleep, which is disturbed with talking and imperfect wakings; fever attended with constipation; fever with incoherent talking (W); slow pulse, scarcely perceptible pulse; pulselessness and collapse. The primary action of toxical doses is to depress the vital energies of the whole system, and therefore lower the action (tone) of the heart and arteries, in a manner similar to Verat. alb. and its analogues. This will be seen by reference to the case of poisoning recorded on a previous page. Dr. Coe makes a suggestive remark on page 245 of his work (Conc. Org. Med): "Podophyllin exercises a remarkable control over the sanguiferous system, removing capillary obstructions, and equalizing the circulation. *Its exhibition is frequently followed by a decided increase of temperature* on the part of the skin, and patients sometimes imagine that the medicine is *going to induce a fever.* Many who have been troubled with unequal circulation and coldness of the extremities for months, are permanently relieved by a single dose." The symptoms I have put in italics, would seem to show that the Mandrake, like mercury, had the power to cause a fever peculiar to itself, a real *irritative fever.* This fever sometimes resembles the mercurial fever, as it is often accompanied by *perspiration*, and pains all over the system. Taking the *ensemble* of the symptoms, we have in the coldness, chilliness, heat, pain, sweat, etc., a very good picture of a febrile attack.

Clinical Remarks.—Eclectics and other admirers of Podophyllum in the "regular" school, make the sweeping assertion that it is useful in the treatment of *all* fevers, and place in the same list those of the highest and lowest grade, the sthenic and asthenic. This is so manifestly absurd, that it were useless to spend time to show its absurdity, but the opposite schools of medicine are so prone to deal in generalities that we can expect nothing better of them. Podophyllum is indicated and has been found useful in the following varieties of fever.

Intermittent Fever.—When the following symptoms are present: "Chilliness when lying down—or in the evening; chill in the morning a 7 o'clock, with pressing pains in both hypochondria, and dull, aching pains in the knees and ankles, elbows and wrists; back-ache before the chill; the shaking and sensation of coldness continues for some time after the heat commences; some thirst during the chill, but more through the heat; the patient is conscious during the chill, but cannot talk, because he forgets the words he wishes to employ; delirium and loquacity during the hot stage, with forgetfulness afterwards of all that passed; violent pain in the head, with excessive thirst during the fever; sleep during the perspiration; loss of appetite during the apyrexia." The above symptoms are given by Dr. Williamson, who does not inform us whether they are purely curative symptoms, or pathogenetic and curative. He further says Podophyllum is indicated in quotidian *tertian* and quartan organs, and for "periodical diseases" generally. The practitioner, however, must not expect too much of this remedy in Intermittents. It cannot be ranked with Nux., China, Quinia, Cornus flo., or any of the "anti-periodic" group of medicines which act curatively by virtue of that power, but rather with

Mercurius, Leptandria, Iris, etc., which act as curative agents in Intermittent fevers, by another power, namely, of correcting the condition of particular organs, as the *liver*, and thus removing the obstacles to a recovery. In my practice, which was at one time extensive, in a district cursed with ague, I had ample opportunity to observe the action of Podophyllum in this disease. I never found it of benefit unless the hepatic, intestinal, and gastric symptoms corresponded with those of the fever; when given for the symptoms of the fever *alone*, enumerated above, it was not curative. In fact it would remove all the *other* symptoms, and the *paroxysms* of fever would still occur in a modified form. But if alternated with Ipecac., China, Cornus, or Nux vomica (in quotidian), Arsenicum, Cedron, or Quinia (in tertian), the cure would be prompt and *permanent*. Those who are opposed to alternation of remedies can use the Podophyllum first, and the appropriate remedy afterwards. As the testimony of eclectic physicians may be interesting on this point, I will quote: "In bilious fevers, either remittent or *intermittent*, it not unfrequently arrests the diseases, at the first prescription, if given in the proper manner, or it so far modifies the attack that the case becomes mild and manageable." (King). Dr. Morrow makes the same statement, but says it is only indicated when there is evident hepatic torpor or congestion. "During the early stages of most febrile diseases, particularly *intermittent* and bilious remittent fevers, podophylline is an agent of superior efficacy. A single dose often arrests the severest attacks of fever." (Jones and Scudder). "In the treatment of fever and ague, we almost invariably precede the employment of the other remedies by the free exhibition of Podophylline. By so doing, in this climate, we cut the disease short at once, and oftentimes have no occasion for further medication. We have known many cases of intermittent fever yield to a single dose of the Podophylline, and, we have no doubt, but the credit of the cure is frequently due to this agent, where it is attributed to other means." (Dr. Coe.) The above embodies the general estimate of the eclectic school, as regards the value of this medicine in agues. No writer pretends that it has any actual anti-periodic power. It has been noticed in many of our provings, that certain *febrile* and even *painful* symptoms were decidedly aggravated, or had a tendency to recur at certain hours in the day, or on alternate days. This peculiarity renders a drug an "anti-periodic." In the proving of Podophyllum, we find that certain febrile and other symptoms, tend to occur in the *morning*, but this I consider rather an indication of its *remittent* action. Future experiments will decide. In *Bilious Fevers*, this medicine is an excellent homœopathic remedy. No other drug so often corresponds with the symptoms, particularly when there is much intestinal irritation. It is admirably indicated in the various forms of *remittent fever*; which in the west are generally considered "bilious" in character. The *febrile* symptoms are quite strongly marked, and may afford some data for the selection of this drug, but we should be guided principally by the general symptoms. As above stated, eclectic physicians, and of late many allopathic, are enthusiastic believers in the power of Podophyllum, when given at the onset of nearly all fevers, in cathartic doses, of arresting or "breaking up" such attacks. But I need not acquaint the homœopathic physician that such practice is sometimes fraught with the most deplorable consequences. When the patient is strong and robust, the vitality of the organism may rally from its depressing action, or medicinal aggravation of the malady; but if such reaction does not take place the *fever*, which may have been mild in its character, is changed to a serious and intractable one. The intestinal irritation which the Podophyllin sets up, will go on and withstand all the rude means of the eclectic to arrest. In this way I have known simple remittents changed into enteric or typhoid fever. In *irritative fever*, and *infantile remittent*, no remedy will give better satisfaction, not even Mercurius. But it should be used with caution in *all* fevers accompanied or caused by intestinal orgastic irritation. In these cases it is primarily homœopathic, and should be used in the fourth and sixth dec. dil., should the symptoms denote inactivity of the liver and glandular system of the intestines, and constipation, with jaundice exist, then the second or third dil. may be used safely. In *Typhoid and Typhus fevers*, (enteric) the Podophyllum is often indicated. It is quite as homœopathic to the irritation, inflammation, and even ulceration of Peyer's glands, as Mercurius and Arsenicum, but it is not so well indicated by the general symptoms; namely, the condition of the blood, etc., as Baptisia, Phosphoric and Muriatic acids, or even Leptandria or Iris. Dr. Hill, (Epitome) says Podophyllin is the *best* remedy for the diarrhœa of typhoids, but homœopathists can accept no such whoselale assertion. If the diarrhœa, in a case of typhoid, corresponds to the Podophyllum-diarrhœa then, and only then is it a specific remedy. The best writers in the eclectic school are aware of the danger of giving large doses of Podophyllin in typhoid and other low fevers, and *all* are particular to warn the physician not to use it when there is much prostration or intestinal irritation existing. Notwithstanding this, the physicians of that and the old school, are generally so ignorant of disease, and so reckless of consequences, as to give this powerful drug in typhoid fever. The consequences are that but few patients, under that treatment, have vitality to resist the toxical effects of the drug and the disease. If Podophyllin is prescribed in true enteric (or typhoid) fever, it should be only the middle and higher potencies—the tenth and upwards. The Podophyllum may be used lower, in the third or sixth. These general remarks, I deem sufficient to point out the applicability of the remedy in the various forms of fever. They will serve to guide the practitioner in the selection of the drug by the special symptoms. Even the *exanthematous fevers* form no exception.

Sleep.—Sleepiness in the day time, especially in the forenoon;

sleepiness early in the evening; restlessness the fore part of the night; distress after the first sleep in the evening; rising up in the bed, during sleep without waking; moaning in sleep with eyelids half closed; *restless sleep of children, with whining at night; unrefreshed by sleep on waking in the morning; too heavy sleep at night; drowsy and difficult to wake in the morning, *a feeling of fatigue on waking in the morning.

CLINICAL REMARKS.—Stupor and even coma occur in cases of poisoning with Podophyllum. The above symptoms form a group very often met with in persons who are supposed to be "bilious," or have "liver complaint." In other words, they are common to "hepatic torper, and are premonitory to many kinds of fever. The symptoms marked *, are said by Dr. Williamson to have been cured by this medicine.

Skin.—*Sallowness of the skin in children; *moistness of the skin with preter-natural warmth.

CLINICAL REMARKS.—The two symptoms above, are the only ones recorded as skin symptoms, and those appear to be curative. I have never noticed any irritation or eruption of the skin appear from its internal use. It is probably not homœopathic to any cutaneous disease. Its topical application, by virtue of its escharotic power, results in redness, vesication and even pustulation and ulcers. It forms an ingredient of the "irritating plaster" of the eclectics. In this manner of application it may prove locally homœopathic, as does Argentum nit., etc. I have known its abuse and prolonged use to cause jaundice, but that symptom more properly belongs to another paragraph. Like mercury, it causes a peculiar irritative fever, characterized by heat of the skin *with* moisture (fever with sweat). This symptom may be of value, in aiding us in the selection of the medicine. Coe says the resinoid "possesses a degree of escharotic power, and when applied to fungous growths will dissolve them down. It produces a rapid pustulaton, which appears first in the form of minute vesicles filled with a serous fluid which speedily changes to a whitish or yellowish hue. This superficial inflammation is at the same time quite severe. The pustules are slow in healing.

Mental Symptoms.—Depression of spirits; imagines he is going to die, or will be very ill.

CLINICAL REMARKS.—According to Dr. Williamson it has been found curative in the delirium of fevers. Beyond this we know but little of its homœopathic use in mental or emotional disorders. It is evidently indicated, judging from its sphere of action, and has been found useful, in depression of spirits, and hypochondriac state of mind arising from hepatic disorder.

Head.—Giddiness and dizziness, with the sensation of fullness over the eyes; momentary darts of pain in the forehead, obliging one to shut the eyes; dullness and headache with sleepiness in the morning; *morning headache with flushed face; pain on the top of the head when rising in the morning; morning headache with heat in the vertex; pressing pain in the temples in the forenoon, with drawing in the eyes as if strabismus would follow; stunning headache through the temples relieved by pressure; sudden pain in the forehead with soreness of the throat in the evening; heavy dull pain in the forehead, with soreness over the seat of pain; headache alternating with diarrhœa; vertigo while standing in the open air; pain in the left frontal protuberance aggravated in the afternoon; vertigo with inclination to fall forwards; *perspiration of the head during sleep, with coldness of the flesh while teething; face pale as a corpse's with pinched nose and a cold perspiration.

Clinical Remarks.—Dr. Williamson found the Podophyllum curative in "rolling of the head during difficult dentition in children;" also the two symptoms marked with the asterisk. The head symptoms are quite notable, particularly the "morning headache" so common in bilious affections; also the "headache alternating with diarrhœa"—one of the most frequent symptoms is hepatic difficulties. We have no proof that this drug will cause inflammation or congestion of the brain or its meninges, but the symptom recorded above as cured by Dr. Williamson "rolling of the head," etc., together with another—wrongly placed under the head of teeth; namely, "grinding of the teeth at night, especially with children during dentition," would seem to point to *irritation* of the brain, whether idiopathic or reflex, we cannot decide, but would suggest an intestinal origin. Podophyllum has been much used against brain affections by electic physicians, but in such large doses as to act as a "revulsive" or "derivative" as they express it. I would not undertake to decide that it could not cause disease of the brain: it would need a pathological proving to elucidate that point. I will quote some eclectic testimony as to its value in their hands in brain affections, and the reader may judge of the nature of its action for himself. *Prof. Morrow* says: "In no class of cases has the medicine manifested a higher degree of value, so far as I have been able to observe its effects, than in those cases marked by strong determination of blood to the brain, producing either congestion or incipient inflammation of that organ. In several cases of this description, in the treatment of which I have witnessed its effects, I was agreeably surprised to find every trace of congestion eradicated by one or two thorough operations of this article. It seemed to exercise a more completely controlling influence on this pathological condition than any medicine I have ever used for this same purpose." It was given of course, in strong cathartic doses. Still a *mere* cathartic would not have such a "controlling influence," and it may after all have exercised some specific curative effect upon the condition of the brain; *i. e.*, the small amount of the drug which was absorbed by the stomach. *Dr. Coe*, strangely enough does not say much about its use in brain diseases, as he considers it specific for almost every other class of maladies. He says it does good, as a revulsive cathartic, in congestion of the brain and apoplexy. He mentions *one* case however, where it acted *mechanically* with good results, and if no better agent was at hand —castor oil, etc.,—the homœopathist might use it legitimately. "In a child eight months old" he says, "we removed by means of lobelia and podophyllin *one and a half pints of solid casein.* This matter so expelled was in a high state of putrefactive fermentation." This case he says was pronounced "congestion of the brain," but with the removal of the morbid material from the stomach, all the symptoms abated, and the child recovered. In a case of Jaundice, which had advanced so far as to cause comatose sleep, and partial insensibility, after every usual homœopathic remedy had been tried without much effect, the Podophyllin, one grain of the first trit., every half hour, removed all the dangerous symptoms. Improvement commenced about the time frequent *bilious* stools appeared. No bile had passed the bowels for nearly two weeks previously.

Eyes.—Smarting in the eyes; drawing sensation in the eyes, accompanying pain in the head; heaviness of the eyes, with occasional pains on the top of the head; pain in the eyeballs and in the temples, with heat and throbbing of the temporal arteries. Eyes sunken in their orbits.

Clinical Remarks.—In a conversation with the venerable Dr. Hering, relating to this remedy, he referred me to a remark of Dr. Barton (Allopath); namely, that he had noticed that frequently after administering the Podophyllum—no symptoms appeared on the same day, but the next morning the *eyes would appear inflamed.* This, according to Hering, would seem to imply that Podophyllum was indicated in ophthalmias which appeared, or were aggravated, *in the morning.* It has been used as a collyrium in chronic opthalmia or ulcers on the cornea, and is probably as useful as any escharotic, for all act upon the law of Similia.

Teeth.—*Grinding of the teeth at night; the teeth are covered with dried mucus in the morning.

Clinical Remarks.—The first symptom above recorded should perhaps be placed under the "Head" symptoms. However, children often grind the teeth (adults also) from a disordered state of the stomach, indigestion, acidity, and even hepatic disorder. I once noticed in a child to whom Mandrake had been administered by the parents, that each paroxysm of nausea and griping was preceeded by "grinding of the teeth." In this case there was a reflex symptom proceeding from the intestinal irritation. The teeth are said to become *loose* under the action of this medicine. (See mouth symptoms.)

Mouth.—Copious salivation; *offensive odor from the mouth; *offensiveness of the breath at night — perceptible to the patient; the taste of fried liver in his mouth at night; sourness of the mouth and tongue on waking in the morning. *white fur on the tongue with foul taste; putrid taste in the mouth.

Clinical Remarks.—Dr. Williamson contributes the curatin symptoms marked with a star. The effect of Mandrake upon the mouth is quite specific and note-worthy. All writers agree that it will cause symptoms like salivation. I have known it to cause severe ptyalism in numerous cases, when abused by electic physicians. Even in the 3d trit., this effect is quite noticeable in persons who are subject to stomatitis, or have been mercurialized. Dr. Coe says : "It has been said that Podophyllin is capable of producing ptyalism, but we have never seen any evidence of the fact in persons who had *never taken mercury*. The only symptoms of salivation we have ever observed have been in those cases where mercury has been taken at some previous time. Podophyllin is powerfully resolvent, and by its peculiar excitation of the glandular system will sometimes dislodge deposits of latent mercurial atoms, and so bring about a season of mercurialization. Lobelia, Irisin and Phytolaccin will frequently do the same." This is a species of special pleading, often resorted to by eclectic practitioners, but it is untenable. If these drugs will cause ptyalism when mercury is in the glands it will cause the same symptoms when mercury is not present. The only difference will be that the presence of mercury renders the glands more susceptible to the action of these agents. Podophyllin is homœopathic to ptyalism, even mercurial; to stomatitis and many inflammatary affections of the gums and buccal mucous membrane. It has been found curative in "nursing sore mouth," "canker in the mouth." I have cured with the dilutions, used as a wash, a case of chronic inflammation of the tongue, which was red, dry, cracked, and often bleeding, and somewhat swollen. It seemed idiopathic, as no greater derangement was noticeable.

Throat.—Sore throat, commencing on the right side and then going to the left; soreness of the left side of the throat, especially painful when swallowing liquids, and worse in the morning; *dryness of the throat;* soreness of the throat extending to the ears; *rattling of mucus in the throat; **goitre*; *sore throat, commencing on the right side and going to the left.

Clinical Remarks.—The three curative symptoms are from Dr. Williamson. The first is due to the excited secretory action of Mandrake upon the tonsils and mucous follicles of the throat. This medicine has made undoubted cures of Goitre in the hands of homœopathic as well as eclectic physicians. The testimony on this point appears conclusive, but I cannot say that I have ever seen much benefit from its use in my hands, at least no such decided effects as follow the use of Iodine, Bromine, and their salts, even in minute doses. Nor have I found it of much value in tonsillitis, in which it is inferior to Phytolacca or Iris versicolor.

Appetite.—Voracious appetite; regurgitation of food; loss of appetite; indifference to food; satiety from a small quantity of food, followed by nausea and vomiting; desire for something sour; thirst towards evening; putrid taste.

CLINICAL REMARKS.—The effects of Podophyllin in small doses (one-tenth of a grain) is, according to King and others, to cause increase of appetite, and healthy digestion; but, in large doses, it causes disgust for food, which if taken is regurgitated. Dr. Williamson cured many cases of dyspepsia in which the above symptoms were prominent. (See Gastric.)

Gastric Symptoms, and Stomach.—Regurgitation of food; food turns sour after eating; sourness of the stomach; acid eructations; belching of hot flatus which is very sour; acidity in the afternoon, with an unpleasant, sickly sensation in the stomach; nausea and vomiting, with fullness in the head; vomiting of food an hour after a meal, with a craving appetite immediately afterwards; extreme nausea, continuing for several hours; vomiting of food with putrid taste and odor; heart-burn; water-brash; heat in the stomach; sensation of hollowness in the epigastrium; throbbing in the epigastrium, followed by diarrhœa; gastric affection, attended by depression of spirits; heat in stomach; vomiting of hot frothy mucus; stitches in the epigastrium from coughing. (Williamson.) The nausea begins about two or three hours after the medicine, in material doses, is taken; it continues sometimes with great severity, and with vomiting of ingesta, mucus, and bile, for twenty-four or forty hours even. (Hale.) Great thirst, and the stomach contracting so hard and rapidly in the effort to vomit that the wrenching pain would cause them to utter sharp screams, one after another, for five minutes at a time; vomiting of bilious matter mixed with blood, the bile, dark green and very thick, the blood dark and coagulated; vomiting of thick bile and blood for eighteen hours." (Dr. Owen.)

CLINICAL REMARKS.—From its effects in the case of fatal poisoning, we should judge it indicated in acute Gastritis, when the pain and vomiting is unusually severe, and the matter ejected consisted of bile and blood as described above. The nausea which attends the action of Mandrake, is particularly distressing. It is "lingering and death-like, something like that caused by tobacco." It is attended generally with severe and painful vomiting of bilious matter, as well as copious bilious and watery discharges, and severe griping pain in small intestines from the bowels, when the dose is large. The critical physician will readily see by the pathogenetic and curative symptoms above, that Podophyllin is indicated in many conditions of gastric irritation, and even inflammation. Eclectic writers, particularly mention that it is contra indicated in gastritis, which observation implies to the homœopathist, that it will prove a valuable remedy in some forms of that disease. Some physicians value it highly as a homœopathic remedy for many forms of dyspepsia. (See curative symptoms above.) In its effects upon the gastric mucous membrane it is analagous to Iris versicolor, Mercurius, Arsenicum, Nux vomica, Pulsatilla, and others, and will rival them in the various affections of the stomach.

Abdomen.—Fulness in the right hypochondrium, with flatulence.

Colic with retraction of the abdominal muscles; pain in the transverse colon at three o'clock in the morning, followed by diarrhœa; rumbling of flatus in the ascending colon; pain in the ascending colon; pain in the bowels at daylight in the morning which is relieved by external warmth and by bending forwards whilst lying on the side, but is aggravated by lying on the back; the pain in the bowels is at first attended with coldness, which is followed by heat and warm perspiration; sensation of heat in the bowels, accompanying the inclination to go to stool; sensation of flatus in the left hypochondrium; faintness with sensation of emptiness in the abdomen after stool; cramp-like pain in the bowels, with retraction of the abdominal muscles occurring at 10 o'clock in the evening, and again at 5 o'clock in the morning, and continuing until 9; sharp pain above the right groin, preventing motion in the last months of pregnancy; distention of the abdomen; enormous swelling of the abdomen (in case of fatal poisoning).

Clinical Remarks.—The pains which are caused by Podophyllum are not confined to the intestines, but extend to the muscles of the abdomen. According to Inman irritation of the mucous coat of the intestines may, and does generally cause myalgic pains and *spasm*. There is some similarity in the pains caused by Plumbum and Podophyllum; but, the former drug acts directly upon the *nerves* which govern the contraction of muscles, while the latter causes pain and spasm in the same muscles by irritating a contiguous mucous membrane. Williamson recommends the Podophyllum in *Colica pictonum* (lead colic), and Eclectics claim to cure that disease with Mandrake. Perhaps the *similarity* of the two diseases may be sufficiently clear to empower the one to cure the other. I once attended a case of poisoning by Podophyllum, when the rectus and other muscles were drawn into lumps or knots; the pain was relieved by "doubling up" and very hot applications. Colocynth did but little good; Gelseminum, in drop doses, gave some relief; I did not try Plumbum, having none at hand. The colic caused by Podophyllum is generally attended with diarrhœa or dysentery, and often with *bilious* vomiting and diarrhœa. In *Peritonitis*, I do not consider it indicated, unless in exceptional cases. Certain intestinal and myalgic disorders simulate true peritonitis and may be mistaken for it; in such cases the Podophyllum may be useful. Eclectic physicians consider it almost specific for *Puerperal Peritonitis*, but it cannot be anything but injurious in that disease, given in the heavy doses in which they present it. The allopathic treatment of this disease shows some strange discrepancies. Some writers claim that blood-letting, Verat. v., Antimony, etc., are the only reliable remedies; others, rely wholly upon Opium, and narcotics; and still another portion of that school place their faith upon Turpentine. It is very probable that Podophyllin acts similarly to the latter drug. According to Inman (see Treatise on Myalgia), inflammation of serous membranes, as the pleura and peritoneum is *not necessarily accompanied with pain*, and, that myalgia or paralysis of the muscular parietes of the abdomen is *often* mistaken for Peritonitis. We have the same intense burning pain in certain localities, (the attachment of muscles) the same exquisite tenderness, and the same *distention*, noted as belonging to puerperal peritonitis. Any treatment, says Inman, which will give tone to the muscles, causing contraction of the muscles involved, will restore the patient. This statement accounts for the benefit which has accrued from the use of stimulants, tonics, Opium, and even Turpentine and Podophyllin. The two first give tone to the muscles—Opium gives them *rest*, which is so necessary to a cure; and the two latter by a certain specific influence which they seem to have over our muscular fibre; for turpentine cures tympanitis, in small doses, too small to irritate the bowel, (*it causes* tympanitis), and Podyphyllin causes all the symptoms of Peritonitis, as will be seen by reference to the cases of poisoning above. In the fatal case, Enteritis could not have been present, for the time was too short, and if the peritoneum was affected it was by the direct toxical action of the poison. No post mortem having been made of the fatal case, we do not know whether peritonitis was present, and the symptoms *may* have been due to some other lesion.

Liver and Spleen.—(1.) Fullness in the *right hypochondria;* hypochondrium with flatulence; stitches in the right hypochondrium, worse while eating; twisting pain in the right hypochondrium, with sensation of heat in the part; * fullness, with pain and soreness in the right hypochondrium; chronic hepatitis with costiveness; pains in the region of the liver. (2) Sensation of weight and dragging in the *left* hypochondrium, close under the ribs; sensation of flatus in the left hypochondrium; pains in spleen.

Clinical Remarks.—It is difficult to decide whether all the pains above mentioned are myalgic or really in the organs referred to in the headings. *Some* of the symptoms are undoubtedly myalgic. The curative symptoms of fullness, etc., has been so often verified by Dr. Williamson and others of our school, that we may safely say that it indicates *hepatitis*, or *congestion of the liver*. The "chronic hepatitis with costiveness," is also a valuable observation. It is not necessary, however, that constipation should be present; it is as useful when that disease is attended with diarrhœa, or the two states alternately. From many years, experience with, and observation of, the use of Podophyllin in diseases of the liver, I feel qualified to venture the following observation relative to its pathogenitive and curative action upon that organ. I believe the *Podophyllum* and its active principle to be a *direct stimulant of the liver*. I am aware that some of the most astute investigators of the allopathic school deny that *Mercury* has any direct or specific action on that organ. They would probably allege the same of the Mandrake, but there are certain reasons which I shall give further on, why I consider the arguments against Mercury not valid in the case of Podophyllum. The *primary* action of Podophyllum in large doses is generally to cause vomiting and diarrhœa of undoubted bilious matters. I have examined the evacuations caused by *Pn.* in case of jaundice, which before its administration were completely free from bile, and found that the green color was actually due to that secretion. The examination was made with the most approved chemical tests. The patient *felt* the action of the drug upon the liver, before it nauseated or caused any intestinal irritation. (The dose was one-fourth of a grain of the pure resinoid, triturated with ten of sugar of milk). In still smaller doses, third trituration, it wil cause bile to appear in the previously clay colored stools. I consider this medicince therefore *primarily* homœpathic to acute irritation, congestion and inflammation of the liver, bilious diarrhœa, and hepatic pains. A further proving is needed to give special indications. The powerfully irritating effect which this drug has upon the secretory functions of the liver, enables it to cause such excessive action as may pass over into *passive* congestion, chronic inflammation, suspension of function from exhaustion, suspension of biliary secretion, and even *retention* of that fluid. Podophyllum has been abused in the hands of eclectics as badly as Mercury in the allopathic school. I have known it to cause chronic hepatic diseases, as jaundice, enlargement, and even some organic affections. There is scarcely an acute or chronic disease of this important viscus, in which this medicine may not, in some of its stages, be found useful. A careful study of our proving, together with the observations of physicians of both schools, will give us much information as to its sphere of action. The *dose* in hepatic diseases, is a matter of great importance. I believe an adherence to the following rules will give the physician greater success with the medicine than he could attain without them. (1.) For the *primary* (acute) conditions, similar to those caused by large doses of Podophyllum, give the highest and middle attenuations. (The third or eighteenth of Podophyll*um*, and sixth or thirtieth of Podophyll*in.*) (2.) For Symptoms and conditions (chronic) simulating the secondary effects, give the lower actenuations, and in rare cases, even the one-tenth of the resinoids, (3.) In a few cases, as in *retention* of bile from obstruction of the gall duct., or in case of gall-stones, we must have the direct mechanical effects of Podophyllum. In such cases crude doses are required. This is best illustrated by the following case of "expulsion of gall stone," reported by me to the North American Journal, Vol. 12, p. 258:

"In Vol. 7, 304, of this Journal, my industrious colleague, Dr. Marcy, made mention of 'An Empirical Remedy for gall-stones,' and says: 'For the violent spasmodic pains which accompany their passage to the intestines, we have found the following treatment, derived from an empirical sourse, eminently efficacious: As soon as the pains have declared themselves, we give the patient six ounces of tepid Olive-oil, and then prescribe Nux and Aconite in alternation every half hour. We also apply hot water fomentations, and occasionally a warm bath, when the paroxysm is not speedily ameliorated.' The case which I will now report is a very interesting one. The patient, a young lady, residing at No. 53

Carpenter street, had been subject, for several years, to attacks of supposed gastralgia, which would pass off in a few days under the use of anodynes, leaving her slightly jaundiced. This attack had been much more severe, and she had been under the care of two professors in the allopathic colleges in this city for six weeks when I was called. They pronounced her disease "neuralgia of the stomach." The character of the pain had not changed, only to grow more severe since its onset. She had been drugged with *Blue-mass*, *Calomel*, *Opium*, *Dover's-powder* and *Chloroform*, and received only temporary benefit from their use. I found her emaciatied, jaundiced, (her skin of the hue of bronze), tongue coated white; no appetite; headache most of the time; pulse quick and hard, but small; urine very scanty, a yellowish brown color, and was found to contain *bile* when the usual tests were applied. The pains in the epigastrium extended to the right side, region of the gall-bladder, and were *remitting i. e.*, there were paroxysms of great intensity, but some pain all the time; excessive nausea, when the pain becomes severe; constipation and diarrhœa alternated, and in either condition the evacuations were now, and had been destitute of bile for several weeks. At my first visit I was undecided as to the pathological condition at the bottom of the difficulty, but gave Aconite and Nux-vomica. The next I decided that the malady originated from the presence of gall-stones in the gall-duct, obstructing completely the passage of bile into the intestines, and giving rise to the interior pain; no relief had been obtained from the remedies, and she had been obliged to resort to Chloroform all night. I now resolved to try Dr. Marcy's treatment. Six ounces of tepid Olive-oil were ordered, but she could only be induced to swallow three. This was at 3 P. M.; at 9 P. M., the other three ounces were administered. Nux and Aconite were continued as before. *Third day*—no improvement. She took Chloroform about half the time to get relief from the intense spasmodic pain; urine more scanty, and of a deeper color; slimy, white diarrhœa, not a trace of bile in the discharges; vomiting of mucus; no bile had been vomited for several weeks. I ordered a hot bath. In the attempt to take it, a very severe chill set in with fainting; this was followed by some fever. In the evening she became stupid, would not answer questions, and I feared she would go into coma. Dr. Coe, (Conc. Org. Med., page 247) gives the following treatment for gall-stones: He gives at bed-time a powder composed of Podophyllin, grs. ij., Euphorbin, grs. j., Caulophyllin, grs. ij. The next morning, 'as soon as the nausea attending the operation of the powder has subsided, administer eight ounces of pure Olive-oil.' 'We have known," he asserts, 'as many as two hundred of these concretions, varying in size from that of a small pea to that of a hazle-nut, to be passed after the administration of a single dose of Podophyllin and the Oil.' My patient was rapidly sinking, and I knew that if the obstruction was not soon removed, the blood would become irretrievably poisoned with bile. I did not deem it necessary to follow Coe's practice. Podophyllin is the *real* agent which dislodges the concretions from the gall-duct. This it does, I believe, by increasing the expulsion power or *peristaltic* action, so to speak, of the gall-bladder and its duct. The Olive-oil may aid in relaxing and dilating the duct, and carries the concretions off through the bowels, after they have been expelled. I accordingly gave *one grain* of Podophyllin in the evening; she was allowed Chloroform during the night. In the morning she swallowed *three ounces* of Olive-oil, at 6 o'clock. At 9 o'clock she vomited bile; at noon she had a free evacuation from the bowels, of a bilious appearance. At 3 P. M., another bilious stool, and with it a discharge of several gall-stones—they fell into the vessel with a metallic sound—as the nurse informed me. All pain ceased about the time she vomited, and did not return. The concretions were round, about the size of a cherry, rough externally, yellowish, and when broken in two, showed a radiating appearance from a common centre. No account was kept of the number passed, as the nurse was somewhat negligent, and failed to collect them. In a few days, under the use of Aconite and Nux, the jaundice had nearly disappeared; her appetite returned, and in two weeks she was able to ride into the country, and has since enjoyed good health. In the words of Dr. Marcy, I assert that 'this affords us example where the consistent homœopathist is justified in employing a chemical and purgative agent to rid the system of foreign substances which nature is struggling to throw off. It is not *disease* which we are to remove; not a *therapeutic* agent which we are to administer.' I recognize three methods of restoring health; viz: the *chemical*, the *mechanical*, and the *homœopathic*. By the first we can remove an irritating cause of disease, as by the use of Nitric-acid, in Oxalic-acid urine by the second, we can expel a biliary calculus with Podophyllin and Olive-oil; and by the last—the only law of cure—we can remove, with Aconite and Nux, the hepatic inflammation consequent upon the passage of the stones. I maintain that my treatment was as rational and cientific as that of the surgeon who removes the spiculæ of bones or the musket-ball, and *then* uses his specific remedies, and his surgical apliances."

It is amazing to witness the vast confidence which the eclectic physicians have in Podophyllin in nearly every disease of the liver. They use it almost indiscriminately in the most opposite states and conditions, and in functional organic affections of that organ. I have not space to quote their observations and praises, but would refer the reader to their works on Practice and Materia Medica. In *congestion of the portal circle*, this medicine appears to have an immense curative power, in which it is only equalled by Mercury and Leptandria. In *Diseases of the Spleen*, the Podophyllum has been found useful. It may be tried in acute inflammation, or chronic enlargement.

Enteric Symptoms.—Stool earlier in the morning than usual, but natural; frequent stools during the day, but of a natural consistence; six soft yellow stools a day, with some griping: (from grain doses of the third trit); profuse diarrhœa, worse in the morning; very frequent papescent, yellowish stools for forty-eight hours; diarrhœa early in the morning, which continues during the forenoon, followed by a natural stool in the evening; evacuations of green stools in the morning; diarrhœa immediately after eating or drinking; *extreme weakness and cutting pain in the intestines after stool; *painful diarrhœa, with screaming and grinding of the teeth, in children, during dentition; white slimy stools; *hot, watery evacuations; stools watery, frequent, profuse, and attended with prostration and cramps as in cholera; stools muco-gelatinous, small and infrequent, with flatulence, and pain in the *region of the sacrum*; after an evacuation of a large mass of gelatinous substance, like white of egg, the severe tormina ceased and did not return; *food passes the bowels in an undigested state; copious evacuations, with blueness under the eyes; *evacuations which consist of dark, yellow mucus, which smells like carrion; frequent chalk-like stools, which are very offensive; *with gagging and excessive thirst in children; *constant pain in the lumbar region, which is worse during evacuation, and particularly after stool; stools yellow, green or watery and brown; stools streaked with blood; evacuations in the morning, attended with strong urging in the bowels, with heat and pain in the anus; flashes of heat running up the back after a stool; sensation at stool as if the genital organs would fall out, (in a female); too much bearing down at stool, as if from inactivity of the rectum; severe and painful tenesmus after a watery stool; *chronic diarrhœa, worse in the morning; diarrhœa with prolapsus ani at every stool, (in children); *descent of the rectum from a little exertion, immediately followed by stool, or a discharge of thick, transparent mucus, sometimes of a yellow color, and mixed with blood; the prolapsus ani occurs most frequently in the morning; secretion of mucus from the anus; the anus feels very sore, sensitive and swollen; aggravation of existing hemorrhoids; several hard, painful hemorrhoidal tumors around the anus, one of which bleeds profusely, (primary symptoms): constipation for two days after the diarrhœa; constipation with headache and flatulence; the fæces are *hard* and *dry*, and voided with difficulty; constipation, with hemorrhoids and prolapsus ani; alternate constipation and diarrhœa, (secondary symptoms): hard stool, coated with yellow, tenacious mucus.

CLINICAL REMARKS.—It will be seen that I have arranged the above symptoms in a peculiar order, different from that adopted in the original proving. The plan of arranging the symptoms of a drug without reference to its primary and secondary action is much to be deprecated. The entire symptoms ("stool," etc.) of all our drugs begin with "constipation." Now, no one supposes that this is the first symptom of all drugs. On the contrary, frequent and loose evacuations are the rule. The first symptom from even small doses of Podophyllum is diarrhœa. It is not until the purgative action has subsided, or the irritability of the intestines exhausted, that we have constipation. In fact this medicine rarely causes constipation, and then only secondarily. To avoid repetition, I have designated those symptoms cured by Williamson and Jeanes with an asterisk, but all of the other symptoms are of *equal importance*, and have all been verified by clinical experience. I will briefly enumerate the disorders of the bowels in which this drug is indicated, without a useless repetition of the symptoms. *In acute or chronic mucous or follicular enteritis*, it is specifically and primarily indicated. No drug, not even Mercury, so surely causes these conditions. Whether the disease be present in children or adults, the Podophyllum will be found promptly curative. *Diarrhœa*, in nearly all its varied manifestations, finds a *similimum* in the pathogenesis of this potent drug. Drs. Hering, Jeanes, Pretchs, and many others lay much stress on the tendency to *morning aggravation* of the intestinal, and indeed all the symptoms of Podophyllum. There are only two forms of diarrhœa in which this medicine is secondarily indicated. I allude to that form which accompanies complete jaundice, and in which the evacuations are clay-colored and offensive; and the diarrhœa which *alternates* with constipation, in some chronic hepatic disorders. In these varieties it will be found necessary to use the lower dilutions and triturations, while in the former affections the middle and highest potencies will act curatively. Dr. Jeanes has cured many cases of relaxed bowels, when the stools were *too frequent but natural*, with the highest attenuations of this remedy. Acute and chronic *Colitis* is a disease which calls for the Podophyllum. The symptoms of the drug and disease bear a remarkable resemblance, as a comparison will show. *Dysentery* is one of the diseases in which this medicine has been found most useful. An abuse of this drug, and even its moderate and careful use, in some cases, is sure to bring on symptoms of acute dysentery. It is useful in chronic or acute dysentery, and in many cases will be found more beneficial in all the stages, than any other agent. One peculiar feature of the Podophyllum-dysentery, is the almost invariable presence of *prolapsus ani*, or a tendency thereto. I once attended two children, aged respectively three and six years, who had been dosed with Podophyllin by an Eclectic. Dysentery was present in both patients, and also prolapsus recti. The mucous membrane of the rectum was red, inflamed and exquisitely sensitive. Drs. Jeanes and Williamson noticed similar pathogenetic effects. I cured the children with Nux and Nitric acid. Many cases of prolapsus recti have been cured with Podophyllin, even when of *six years'* standing, and accompanied all that time with diarrhœa. Dr. Gatchell, gives the indications for this remedy in dysentery, "commencing with a watery diarrhœa, terminates in a muco-sanguineous dysentery, accompanied with sickness at the stomach. If the diarrhœa, which preceded the dysentery, especially manifested itself early in the morning, the case will be all the more appropriate." He advises six drops of the tincture in six ounces of water, a teaspoonful at a dose; which is to be repeated after each stool, until improvement commences. This prescription will cure many cases of dysentery. This remedy is chiefly indicated in the so-called bilious dysentery in which the stools look like pea-soup, and consist of a yellowish, greenish, or bloody mucus, having a disagreeable odor, and accompanied with violent pains in the region of the colon, rectum and anus; it causes and aggravates hemorrhoids, and severe tenesmus, with prolapsus ani, especially in children; sometimes nausea and vomiting go with the above symptoms. The active principle, or Podophyllin, at the third trituration, is often more effectual and prompt in its action, than the tincture. Altogether, it is one of the best remedies we possess for the cure of dysentery, enteritis, and many other inflammatory diseases of the intestinal track.—*H.*) Dr. G. also advises Leptandrin in typhoid dysentery, and mentions that Dr. Morrow was very successful with it, in that formidable form which appeared after the cholera of 1849. "In the practice of the writer, the second and third trituration, has often been used successfully in low conditions occurring in dysentery, chronic diarrhœa (especially the obstinate diarrhœa of soldiers), and in typhoid fever."—*Amer. Mag. Hom., vol.* 1, *p.* 370. In *Cholera morbus*, is sometimes treated very successfully by the use of Podophyllum. It causes, in large doses, similar watery, flocculent discharges, very profuse and exhausting, accompanied with cramps in the abdominal, and flexor muscles of the extremities. In this respect it is the analogue of Elaterium, Jatropha, Euphorbia cor., Arsenic, and Veratrum. *Asiatic Cholera*, in some of its phases, ought to find a specific remedy in this medicine. So abundant are the alvine evacuations of serum caused by Mandrake, that Eclectics use it as a *hydrogogue* cathartic in cases of dropsy. In *Cholera Infantum* it was found by Dr. Jeanes and Williamson to be eminently useful. I have used it in a good many cases of this disorder, as well as diarrhœa from teething, and nearly every intestinal disease to which children are subject, and have found it as useful as Mercury, Chamomilla, or Pulsatilla. In the bowel complaints of children the practical physician is cognizant of the colic with spasmodic retraction of the abdominal muscles, the spasmodic tenesmus, and tending to prolapsus ani; all strong indications for this medicine. *Hemorrhoidal affections* are admirably under the control of Podophyllum. The specific affinity which this drug has for the liver, portal system, and rectum, as shown in the pathogenesis, enables it to cause hemorrhoids from portal congestion, chronic hepatic affections, and primary irritation, congestion, and even inflammation of the veins and mucous membrane of the rectum. It will be found useful in internal or external piles—for those which bleed and those which do not. The *sensations* it causes in the rectum, anus, and hemorrhoidal tumors are similar to the effects of *aloes*, of which it is a congener.

Urinary Organs.—*Enuresis; *involuntary discharge of urine during sleep; *frequent nocturnal urination during pregnancy, (primary effects); pain in the region of the kidneys, followed by flow of urine with calculi sediment; *diminished secretion of urine; *suppression of urine; scanty urine, with frequent voidings, (secondary effects).

Clinical Remarks.—All the above symptoms are marked by Dr. Williamson as curative. They are also pathogenetic, as I propose to show by Eclectic authority. I quote such testimony because it may throw some light on the action of Podophyllum on the urinary apparatus. *King* says it has been found useful in "incontinence of urine, and some affections of the bladder;" a very ambiguous kind of testimony. *Jones* says it is almost specific in "incontinence of urine, and useful in some renal difficulties." Dr. Coe, writes, "in the suppression and retention of urine, we have found the Podophyllin of exceeding utility, as a radical remedy. We remember one case in which the catheter had been used, on an average, twelve times in twenty-four hours, for four weeks, and which was promptly and permanently relieved by a single dose of Podophyllin, rendering the further use of the catheter unnecessary. In all derangements of the urinary apparatus, Podophyllin will be found one of the best alterative diuretics that can possibly be employed. It operates not so much by increasing the flow of urine as by restoring the secreting power of the kidneys. It is very effectual in removing uric acid deposits, and corrects the diathesis. Frequently during its operation, *considerable pain will be felt in the region of the kidneys, followed by a flow of urine highly charged with calculous sediment.* It possesses also diuretic properties." If this last observation is reliable, it would seem to show that Podophyllin has some specific action upon the renal organs.

Organs of Generation of Men.—Sticking pain above the pubes, and in the course of the spermatic cords.

Clinical Remarks.—The Podophyllin has seemed to produce but few symptoms, nor has it been used in homœopathic practice in any of the affections of these organ. In the eclectic school, however, it is used quite extensively for *Syphilis, Gonorrhœa, Gleet, and diseases of the prostrate.* We are left in doubt, however, whether the medicine has any specific relation to those diseases, or was used in a spirit of blind empiricism, and the maladies got well in spite of the medication.

Organs of Generation of Women.—Retarded menstruation; suppression of the menses in young females, with bearing down in the hypogastric and sacral regions, with pain from motion, which is relieved by lying down; pain in the region of the ovaries, especially in the right; after-pains, with strong bearing down; leucorrhœa; discharge of thick, transparent mucus; leucorrhœa, attended with constipation and bearing down in the genital organs; *prolapsus uteri;* symptoms of prolapsus uteri, continuing for several weeks after parturition, with rumbling of flatus in the region of the ascending colon; symptoms of prolapsus uteri, with pain in the sacrum; flatulence unfrequent; muco-gelatinous stools.

Clinical Remarks.—Besides the symptoms marked as *curative* and pathogenetic, above, Dr. Williamson and Jeanes have cured the following: "Prolapsus uteri—many cases; numb, aching pain in the region of the left ovary, with heat running down the left thigh, in the third month of pregnancy; ability to lie comfortably only on the stomach in the earlier months of pregnancy; swelling of the labia during pregnancy; after-pains, attended with flatulency." Other homœopathic practitioners have found the

Podophyllum useful in many of the diseases of women, especially when involving the uterus and ovaries. It is still an unsolved question in what way the medicine affects the uterus; in some cases it would seem to do so by its action on the bowels and rectum, as is the case with aloes. It is well known that any drug which powerfully irritates the lower bowel will cause congestion and even inflammation of the womb, by extension of effect through contiguous tissues; thus, aloes may cause the above, as well as uterine cramps, menorrhagia, prolapsus, etc. It is thought by some that Podoph. has a similar action, but it would seem from our proving, as well as numerous clinical cases reported, that the medicine must have some direct action on the uterus and ovaries. *Prolapsus Uteri et Vagina.*—CASE 1.—A lady who had lately given birth to a still-born child, of large size, with a serious loss of blood, and had, undoubtedly, the symptoms of a severe prolapsus of the womb; Arnica was given a few days, followed by China and Carbo veg.; these greatly increased the strength of the patient, after which I gave Mercurius 3. four powders, and Podophyllin 3. four powders, on alternate days. In four or five days she was completely cured.—*Dr. Prowell, Amer. Mag. Hom.*, vol. i. p. 70. CASE 2.–A lady had been confined about four weeks previously, but had been suffering ever since, with violent bearing-down pains in the region of the womb; intolerable pain in the back; great degree of weakness; apthæ; and several scrofulous swellings about the neck. On examination, I found a moderate degree of prolapsus, swelling and induration of the os uteri, a profuse excoriating leucorrhœa, and great *ardor urinæ.* I gave, in this case, Mercurius sol., and Podophyllin, in alternation daily, which relieved in ten days the prolapsus, and reduced the os uteri to its normal size. The apthæ yielded at the same time, to a great extent, Belladonna, relieving this symptom; Sulphur, Sepia, and Merc. iod., removed the leucorrhœa, and swelling of the glands, in three weeks time. The 3d attenuation was used. (Ibid). CASE 3.–Prolapsus uteri, brought on by a violent strain, seven years ago; she was emaciated from violent suffering, loss of appetite, cold and debilitating night sweats, violent burning in hypochondriac region, extreme low spirits. Merc. viv. 3d removed the night sweats permanently; Podophyllin 3d removed the other symptoms, with the prolapsus, and she remains cured—more than one year.

Induration of Os Uteri.—Dr. Gatchell mentions, incidentally, that Dr. Brown, of Cincinnati, cured with a trituration of Podophyllin, an induration of the os. which had resisted the efforts of the distinguished Prof. Morrow, until he abandoned the case in despair. This remedy is used extensively by the eclectics in all diseases of the liver; uterus, and in dysentery; diarrhœa, acute and chronic; glandular enlargement; scrofulous and venereal diseases. (*Amer. Mag. Hom.*, vol. i. p. 63). According to some physicians, Podophyllin is useful in swelling and inflammation of the ovaries; its general specific action on the glandular system would lead us to suspect it of the power of causing disease of those organs. I once found it beneficial in a case of chronic ovaritis, with symptoms like those in the proving. It is also useful in many of the disorders of pregnant females, especially when caused by a *congested condition of the pelvic viscera;* the morning sickness, or excessive vomiting of pregnant women, will often be relieved by this medicine. Eclectic physicians praise it highly in simple, recent amenorrhœa, but they use it as the allopathist uses *aloes*, not homœopathically; in *congestive* amenorrhœa, however, it is homœopathic to the condition, and in minute doses will act curatively.

Larynx.—* Cough, accompanying remittent fever; * dry cough; * loose, hacking cough; * hooping cough, attended with costiveness and loss of appetite.

Clinical Remarks.—All the above symptoms seem to be curative. We are left in doubt as to the power of Podophyllin in causing laryngeal affections. Dr. Coe states that he seldom employs any other medicine in the *treatment of croup*, when called to treat the disease in its incipient stages; but, he applies cold water to the throat, and alcoholic baths, and then gives a "full dose" of Podophylin. This practice it is needless to say is needless torture, and the children who escape such practice are lucky indeed. It is too much like the allopathic treatment of croup with "full doses" of Calomel and Castor oil.

Chest.—Pains in the chest, increased by taking a deep inspiration; snapping in the right lung, like breaking a thread, when taking a deep inspiration; inclination to breathe deeply; sighing; shortness of breath; sensation in the chest as if the heart was ascending to the throat; sensation of suffocation when first lying down at night; *palpitation of the heart* from exertion or mental emotion; * palpitation of the heart with a clucking sensation rising up to the throat, which obstructs respiration; sticking pain in the region of the heart; * palpitation of the heart, from physical exertion, in persons subject to a rumbling in the ascending colon; heavy sleep, and a feeling of fatigue on waking in the morning, followed by drowsiness in the forenoon.

Clinical Remarks.—The first curative symptom above was a case reported by Dr. Ward. It is to be regretted that a physical examination of the heart was not made, that we might know the condition of that organ. Such omission is to be deprecated in all clinical reports. The last heart-symptom is not marked with an asterisk in the original pathogenesis. Dr. Hempel, however, placed it in the Symptomen Codex, probably upon good authority, in fact, the remark in parenthesis in the original, ("Jeanes' numerous cases") would seem to imply that he had cured that symptom in numerous cases, although it might imply only that it had been indicated as a pathogenetic symptom. The *condition* of the heart which gave rise to those symptoms, needs elucidation; taking the collateral symptoms into account, we should say it was a *sympathetic* derangement of that organ, from disease of the liver, occurring in a debilitated subject. I do not imagine that the Podophyllum is capable of curing or causing any organic disease of the heart. In pulmonary or pleuritic affections it does not seem to be often indicated.

Back.—Pains in the small of the back when walking or standing, with the sensation of the back bending inwards; pain in the lumbar region, with the sensation of coldness, worse at night and from motion; pain in the loins, increased by a false step and walking over uneven ground; pain between the shoulders, with soreness, worse at night and from motion; pain under right shoulder-blade; stiffness of the nape, with soreness of the muscles of the neck and shoulders; pain in the nape, with soreness increased by motion; pain between the shoulders in the morning.

Clinical Remarks.—Upon a careful analysis of the above symptoms, guided by Dr. Inman's treatise on Myalgia, I pronounce them of a myalgic character, *not* rheumatic. I do not consider Podophyllin capable of causing or curing rheumatism, like Bryonia, Colchicum, etc. It causes myalgia by its debilitating influence on muscular fibre. The pain under right shoulder-blade *may* have been from hepatic derangement.

Upper Extremities.—*Rheumatism in the left forearm and fingers; weakness of the wrists, with soreness to the touch.

Clinical Remarks.—My estimate of the sphere of action of Podophyllum would lead me to doubt if it cured a veritable *rheumatism* of the left forearm and fingers, inasmuch as Inman proves that myalgia of the muscles of the arm is often mistaken for that disease; the last symptom is purely myalgic.

Lower Extremities.—Pain and weakness in the left hip, like rheumatism, from cold, increased by going up stairs; pains in the thighs, legs, and knees, worse from standing; weakness of the joints, especially the knees; slight paralytic weakness of the left side, of one years duration; cracking in the knee joints from motion; heaviness and stiffness of the knees, as after along walk; stiffness on beginning to move; aching of the limbs, worse at night; pain in the left knee, leg, and foot; sharp pain in the outer and upper portion of the left foot; coldness of the feet; perspiration of the feet in the evening.

Clinical Remarks.—Here again, as above, I consider all the above pains as myalgic, arising from muscular debility. Dr. Jeanes, reports the cure, in a girl eighteeen years of age, of "slight paralytic weakness of the left side, of one years duration."

POLYGONUM HYDROPIPER.

(*Smart-weed.*)

This is a very common indigenous plant, known by the above vulgar name, and also as *Water pepper.* It is found in rich, moist ground, about barns, stables, and out-houses, and along small water courses, in most parts of the United States. It has but a slight odor, and a pungent, acrid taste. It yields its medicinal properties to water and alcohol.

GENERAL EFFECTS.

In allopathic works it is generally classed as an *Emmenagogue*, but is said to be "diaphoretic, diuretic, stimulant, antiseptic, rubefacient, and discutient." Probably no indigenous plant is in such general, almost universal use, in domestic practice in the country and city, and no remedy is so popular in a great variety of complaints. It *may* be one of the many popular delusions, but certain it is, that the remedy gives satisfaction to the patient in a majority of cases. In the country it is almost useless for the homœopathic physician to attempt to prohibit the *external* use of the Polygonum; and, as its use is no more objectionable than Arnica applications, and prevents officious friends from applying some worse article, it may as well be permitted, and even advised, as a fomentation in internal inflammations, spasms, pains, etc.

The green herb, bruised, and applied to the surface, acts promptly as a rubefacient. Anti-septic properties have been assigned to it, and from the testimony in its favor, we doubt not it may be advantageously employed as a local application for that purpose. "It constitutes an important fomentation in hysteritis, cystitis, nephritis, peritonitis, pneumonitis, pleuritis, articular rheumatism, local pains, sprains, bruises, indolent and painful tumors, etc., one of the best in use."—(*Eclectic Mat. Med.*)

Dr. B. L. Hill, when an eclectic, reported a "protracted case of epileptic fits entirely cured by the use of the extract, made into pills." "In combination with Sulphate of Iron and Gum Myrrh, it is said to have cured epilepsy—probably dependent on some uterine derangement."—(*King.*) *Which cured?* "The infusion, or a fomentation of the leaves, has been beneficially applied in chronic ulcers, hemorrhoidal tumors; also as a wash in chronic erysipelatous inflammations and as a fomentation in tympanitis and flatulent colic."—(*Ib.*) It has quite a reputation as an external application in poisoning by the different varieties of *Rhus.*

Dr. Small informs me that a proving of this remedy was once made by himself, aided by some of the students of the Philadelphia Homœopathic College, when he was Professor in that institution. The records of that proving, are, however, unfortunately lost. He states that its general sphere of action is quite similar to that of *Pulsatilla.* It acts upon the mucous membranes, skin, and sensory nerves. It has a great reputation in *acute catarrhal* affections, to which it appears to be homœopathic; also to some rheumatic disorders. We append to this notice of the Polygonum, Dr. Joslin's fragmentary provings. We shall not arrange the symptoms, nor attempt any clinical observations, except as relates to the

Sexual Organs of Women.—Drs. Tully, Eberle, Wood, and others, class it among the *emmenagogues.* Dr. Eberle states that it causes the following symptoms:—"Warmth, and a peculiar tingling sensation throughout the whole system; in most instances slight aching pains in the hips and loins; a sense of weight and tension within the pelvis." He states that he has used it in about twenty cases of amenorrhœa, and says:—"I can affirm that with no other remedy or mode of treatment have I been so successful as with this. I have seldom found it necessary to continue its use for more than six or seven days, before its emmenagogue powers were manifested." He says that those to whom he recommended it, found it effectual. He used it in the form of a saturated tincture, in doses of a teaspoonful three times a day. The warm infusion is used successfully in domestic practice—a wine glassfull every few hours. I have known this simple treatment to prove effectual after all the usual remedies failed.

FRAGMENTARY PROVINGS OF POLYGONUM HYDROPIPER, BY DR. B. F. JOSLIN, OF NEW YORK.

First Proving.—A specimen was collected September 12th, 1854.—A heavy rain a few days before had washed the leaves. The earth in the vicinity had not yet become dry, so that no dust had since fallen on the leaves. The weather and time of day were favorable, all dew having been removed by the sun shining in a clear sky. The flowering season of the plant had commenced. At noon, immediately after collecting the specimen, a leaf was thoroughly masticated and swallowed; the taste pungent, like that of black pepper.

Symptom 1.—At 12.30 p. m., momentary pain in the right frontal protuberance, and instantly afterwards in the right occipital protuberance, after half an hour. In the afternoon of the same day, two dozen of the leaves were thorougly bruised in a clean agate mortar, and not being sufficiently succulent to allow of the expression of juice, the mass was put into a vial with alcohol, reduced by water to about fifty per cent. At ten in the evening eat another leaf.

2.—September 13th.—Intolerable itching at the left shin, a little above the ankle, in the morning at six o'clock.

3.—Severe aching at the fore part of the left tibia, about four inches below the knee, from one till two o'clock, p. m.

4.—Aching in the left shoulder, when recumbent, about 11 p. m., soon after going to bed.

Second Proving.—On the 7th day of May, 1856, I decanted a second time a second sample of the tincture, from a specimen collected September 16th, 1854, and prepared in a similar manner. At 1.30 p. m. agitated one drop of this tincture with half an ounce of water, and took it at once.

1.—At 1.40 p. m., painful pressure on the palmar-radial side of the right fore-arm, an inch and a half above the wrist, at the spot where the radial artery is distinctly felt, lasting seven minutes, commencing ten minutes after the dose.

2.—Dry cough in the night, excited by titillation in the upper-anterior part of the chest, with a dry sensation in the larynx when coughing, after about twelve hours. May 8th.—At 1 p. m.. put one drop of the tincture, Polyg., in one gill of water, and after agitating it several times, occupied a minute in sipping it.

3.—Sensation of heat in the mouth and throat within the first quarter of an hour, commencing at the tip of the tongue and extending to much of the mouth, then to the throat at the right upper part.

4.—Cough excited by a pricking, tickling sensation, behind the upper part of the sternum, at 1.30 P. M.; *i. e.*, after forty minutes.

5.—May 9th and 10th.—Pain pressive and remittent, for two consecutive evenings, at the anterior-inner surface of the head of the left tibia.

6.—On the 9th, in the evening, the interior of the anus was studded with itching eminences, as from corrugation without contraction—a kind of hemorrhoidal tumor; they disappeared within two days.

The above is an exact copy of records made at the time of the provings. Short as they are, I call them two because the latter was made after such an interval as precludes the possibility of continuance of action.

NOTE.—It would seem homœopathic to hemorrhoids.

RUMEX CRISPUS.

(*Yellow Dock.*)

This plant is a native of Europe, though naturalized in this country. It follows closely the march of emigration, and even precedes it, so that it may almost be looked upon as belonging to the class of indigenous plants. It grows in fields, gardens, and waste places, and is so well known that it needs no accurate description. The *root* which is the officinal portion, is large, spindle-shaped and *yellow*; it has but little odor, and a bitter and astringent taste. It yields its medicinal properties to boiling water and alcohol. This is one of four species of dock used in this country in medicine, but of the others we have no provings or clinical experience. To the late lamented B. F. Joslin, M. D., of New York, the profession owe the valuable and accurate provings of this medicine. He first called the attention of the profession to it in the first and second volumes of the Philad. Jour., of Hom., afterwards in other Journals, and finally in the American Hom. Review, in which he published the "verified symptoms of Rumex Crispus." The original provings and clinical contributions, were made by some of the best men in our schools, namely Drs. Joslin Sr. and Jr., Bowers, Bayard, Kellogg, Houghton, Payne, Rhees, and others. We may implicitly rely upon the accuracy of their observations. I cannot omit in this place to render my tribute of respect and reverence for the genius, virtues, and sterling qualities of Dr. B. F. Joslin. He was one of those representative men of our profession and school, ranking with Hartmann, Hempel, Neidhard and a few others whose "mighty footsteps" will

"Echo down the Corridors of Time."

Among his many excellent qualities, the most to be admired were his *industry*, *honesty*, and consistency. In the domain of Materia Medica and Therapeutics, no man has done more in this country. He has given us some exact and reliable provings, and a volume on "Epidemic Cholera," which is one of the finest monographs ever published in our school. He was rigorously *honest* in that he allowed no prejudice to sway his judgment, but examined carefully the testimony relating to drugs, from any and all sources, selecting the reliable, no matter from what source it emanated, or how obtained. He also recorded his observations with that truthfulness and candor which commands our highest regard. Although a staunch champion for the "high potencies," he did not allow his enthusiasm to degenerate into bigotry, or his preference into prejudice. He was thoroughly *consistent*, always relying upon the higher dilutions, even in Cholera, and his success in their cure was something astonishing, but probably owing to his carefulness in selecting his remedies. We can admire such a man, as much as we can despise others, who, constantly harping upon the highest potencies, habitually resort to the lower, and even cruder drugs. For myself, who allow the largest lattitude, I can sincerely respect the consistency of a Joslin, even though I cannot adopt his practice altogether. According to Dr. Joslin's "verified symptoms," and clinical experience, the Rumex c., is closely analogous to *Sulphur Phosphorus*, Causticum, Calc., Mercurius, and Spongia. In fact it has many symptoms which are to be found in the pathogenesis of these remedies. This may partly be accounted for by a fact too little heeded by our school; namely, that the chemical analogue of a plant *is* some clue to its pathogenetic effects. *Rumex c.*, contains, besides starch, mucilage, lignin, etc., *Sulphur*, and various salts, among which are the *phosphate of lime*. Here we have *three* of our best remedies represented indirectly in the yellow-dock; namely, Calcarea, Phosphorus, and Sulphur. Its use in the old school, for diseases of the skin, and other obstinate affections, all of which are covered by the symptoms of the medicines above named, and its undoubted success, should have led us, without any proving, to decide nearly the sphere of action of this plant. The following provings, however, show its real properties, and proves the reliableness of the above assertion. The provings were made with the *mother tincture*, lower and higher dilutions; the thirtieth causing the same or similar symptoms, that were aroused by the crude tincture.

General Effects.—Allopathists have decreed the Rumex c., to be alterative, tonic, astringent and discutient. In the first volume of the Philad. Jour. of Homœopathy, Dr. Joslin comments on the Allopathic use and statements concerning this medicine. As it would be improper to copy his remarks entire I would refer the reader to that article (page 289). He remarks:—"Its only definite and well-ascertained property was its power of curing itch, when administered internally and applied externally. This was as well known to the laity as to the profession." He goes on to say that the Allopathist compounds the medical properties of the different varieties of Rumex, and would have us consider their effects nearly the same. Ignoring as they do the necessity of *proving* each drug, in order to ascertain its true action, they grope in the dark. They reverse the true order of investigation. "But these" he remarks "are not specially the faults of the professor (Wood); they are almost inseparable from the school." *Dr. Wood* remarks: "We have *placed together* the *three* officinal species of dock (i. e. R., aguaticus, R. brittanica and R. obtusifolius)," because their virtues are so nearly alike that a separate consideration would lead to unnecessary repetition. All the *other* species may be used indiscriminately with those which are considered officinal. The medical properties of dock root are those of an astringent and mild tonic. It is also supposed to possess an alterative property which renders it useful in scorbutic disorders, and cutaneous eruptions, particularly the itch. It is said to have been useful in scrofula and syphilis. The roots of some species unite a laxative, with the tonic and astringent property, resembling rhubarb, somewhat, in their operation." (Wood.) "Dr. Payne, in his judicious compend of the Allopathic Materia Medica, comes to the conclusion, that Rumex is similar but inferior to Rhubarb. Our school, after a comparison of the provings, would consider the difference to be more qualitative than quantitative." (*Iodine*).

The eclectic school estimate the docks more highly than their Allopathic brethren. Jones and Scudder in their Materia Medica say:—"The dock appears to exert its silent alteratve action upon the constitution in many chronic cutaneous eruptions, as scabies, the different forms of herpes, etc.; syphilis, when it has assumed a constitutional form, attended with an ulceration of the fauces, eruption or ulceration upon the surface, also in mercurio-syphilitic disorders, mercurial cachexy, cancerous tumors or ulcers, scrofula—whether manifested by a general depravation of the system, enlarged glands, or foul and indolent ulcers—or in any other form of ulcer, especially if dependent upon any constitutional taint. In caries, necrosis or other morbid conditions of the osseous system, in scurvy or scorbutic affections, and in numerous other abnormal states, its resolvent, depurative and detergent qualities, render it an excellent auxiliary and corroborant, all the agents desired under this class (alteratives) are either associated or alternated with other remedies and *not relied upon as individual curative agents.*"

This last sentence contains the elements of all the errors of Allopathic therapeutics. They mix a number of drugs together, and then affirm certain curative properties of *one* of these, because the *compound* seemed to cure. It is in this manner that the estimate of Rumex quoted above is made up. It is generally given in combination with Stillingia, Iodide of Potash, or some other drug. Nearly all the curative effects above named may be due to the latter medicines. It is also recommended for "dyspepsia, debilitated states of the intestinal canal, diarrhœa, and dysentery." Dr. J. Williams, says:—"Boiled in milk, and taken in hæmatemesis, it is an infallible remedy." It is said to be useful as a wash or gargle in spongy states of the gums, ulceration of the mouth, throat, etc. How much of value there may be in the above statements, will be shown by the proving.

GENERAL SYMPTOMS.—General languor; general pulsation or throbbing through the body; sensitiveness to the open air in cold weather, or to the cold.

CHARACTERISTICS.—*Locality and character.*—The *left* chest has more verified symptoms than any other region; they are generally sharp pains. The other regions which afford a considerable, and nearly equal number of symptoms, as compared with each other, are the head, stomach, abdomen, and inferior extremities. The symptoms of the head are, generally, dull pains in the frontal region. The symptoms generally appear to be either in a mucous membrane, or in a muscular locality, and to be about equally numerous in both. I leave it for others to decide whether the latter are neuralgic. They present about the same number as the former. (*Joslin.*) *Conditions.*—Headache, worse *on movement*; sensation of weight of a hard substance in the stomach, or pit of the stomach *after a meal;* liquid diarrhœa, evacuations *in the morning;* pain in the chest when *in bed at night;* unquiet sleep, with dreams of danger or trouble, *early in the morning;* itching of the skin, worse on uncovering, and exposing it to the air, especially on going to bed in the evening, or at night. (*Joslin.*)

The above careful remarks by the astute observer, Dr. Joslin, are very valuable, and quite practical.

Skin.—Itching in various parts of the body, either in this order: left portion of the back, left ear, left shoulder, and left loin, or else principally on the lower extremities. On various parts a stinging, itching, or pricking itching; itching on the shoulder in the evening, with itching in the lumbar or dorsal region; itching on the body, principally on the lower extremities; itching of the skin when uncovered and exposed to the air; eruption on the limbs, first perceived in the evening; itching of the vesicles on undressing in the evening to go to bed; an itching rash, in which numerous small red pimples are developed; the eruption itching in the evening, and worse on exposure to the air.

CLINICAL REMARKS.—For the allopathic use of Rumex, in skin diseases, see "General Effects." No clinical records of cures of skin diseases, treated with Rumex, have yet appeared in our school, but Dr. H. M. Payne, while experimenting with Rumex, got the following notable symptoms from the crude tincture: "While undressing and for some time after, considerable *itching of the surface of the lower extremities.*" This occurred several nights, when he says:—"There is no appearance of an *eruption* until after irritating the skin by scratching, and then rather a diffused redness, which soon disappears. Frequent scratching of the surface has produced a number of little sores, (which, however, readily heal,) on the calves of the legs, and about the knees, especially the posterior surfaces;

the rash is not usually troublesome until after the surface is exposed to the air while undressing at night, or on getting up in the morning; the warmth of the bed soon relieves the itching." (The contrary occurs in most cases of skin diseases, the itch especially; also in the provings of Mercurius, the opposite obtains.) Many persons are troubled with a peculiar irritability of the skin, like the condition above described. Exposure to air, working in water, scratching, wearing flannel or new cloth, will get up considerable irritation, and even cause erythematous and other eruptions. In such cases the Rumex will probably form an admirable remedy. I would also suggest its persevering use in those eruptions which seem constitutional, and which, when suppressed, or not appearing upon the surface, are replaced by cough, hoarseness, and other lung symptoms. May not the peculiar irritation which Rumex causes in the bronchial mucous membrane be analogous to the condition of the skin noted above? The remarks of Dr. C. Dunham are pertinent to this suggestion. They will be found under the head of "*chest.*"

Sleep.—Great propensity to sleep in the evening before the proper time; unquiet sleep at night; restless and uncomfortable in the bed at night; unquiet sleep, with dreams of danger and trouble early in the morning; dream of theft or burglary; an unpleasant dream in the morning between five and six o'clock, just before waking; unquiet dreamy sleep, followed by headache, and bitter taste on waking in the morning.

Fever.—Heat and other symptoms of fever in the morning, preceded by restlessness at night; increased frequency of pulse; sensation of heat, followed by that of cold without shivering.

Head.—Sensation of fulness in the head; headache after awaking in the morning, preceded by a disagreeable dream; headache worse by motion; dull pain in the head, between the time of waking and breakfast, preceded by a disagreeable dream in the morning; dull pain in the head in the forenoon, commencing at 10 o'clock; *dull pain in the forehead;* frontal headache on awaking in the morning; pain over the right eyebrow; pain on the right side of the forehead in the region of causality; pain in the left temple; darting pain, or sharp, piercing pain in the left side of the head, for half an hour or less; dull aching pain in the occiput.

Eyes.—Sore feeling in the eyes, without any external signs of inflammation.

Ears.—Ringing in the ears; itching in the ears; sensation as if the ears were obstructed; constant roaring in the ears, not relieved by pressing the fingers into the ears.

Nose.—Obstruction of the nose; fluent coryza, attended with painful irritation in nostril and sneezing; epistaxis; mucus discharge from posterior nares; violent and rapid sneezing; sensation of great dryness in the nose, day and night; feeling of dryness in the posterior nares.

Face.—Sensation of heat in the cheeks, within the first hour;

heat and redness of the face in the evening; heat and redness in the face with dull headache in the evening.

Teeth.—Toothache with aching in the head; grumbling, stinging toothache in right superior molars, while riding in cold wind, attended with dull aching in forehead.

Mouth.—Sensation as from a burn or scald on the tongue; sensation of excoriation, or slight stinging, at edge of tongue; flow of saliva within first hour; dryness of the mouth and tongne at night.

Throat.—Sensation of excoriation in the throat; sore feeling in the throat on swallowing in the forenoon; sensation as of a lump in the throat, not relieved by hawking and swallowing; raw feeling in throat, with secretion of phlegm; mucous secreted in upper part of throat; aching sensation in the throat, as if a lump were sticking fast in the œsophagus, aching in the pharynx, with collection of tough mucus in the fauces.

Gastric Symptoms.—Awoke with bitter taste in the mouth in morning; flatulency after meals; heaviness, or a sensation of hard substance in the stomach or epigastrium soon after a meal; after a meal has a sensation of weight in the stomach, like that produced by the presence of undigested food in it (the first symptoms in two provers, with the tincture*). Tasteless eructations; sensation of fullness or distension in the stomach or scrobiculous cordis, with eructations on going to bed or in evening; *nausea* in the morning and forenoon, also in the evening; nausea with eructations; nausea either with a sensation of fullness in the abdomen, as if diarrhœa were forming, or else with moving in the intestines as from a cathartic; *sharp pain* in the pit of the *stomach*, either worse on movement, or occurring while riding out in the open air; stitching, then cutting pain in stomach.

Clinical Remarks.—It has been used with alleged success in dyspepsia. Many of the above symptoms would seem to indicate its applicability in some forms of gastric derangement. Dr. Joslin reports the following cases in the "Review:"—"A young lady complained of shootings from the pit of the stomach into the chest in various directions; sharp pains in left chest; dull aching in the forehead and slight nausea; ordered her to take Rumex thirtieth, morning and evening. She called the next day; all her symptoms had been removed by a single dose, and her appetite, which had been defective, improved; having eaten an unusually full dinner, there is a partial return of the shootings; gave Rumex thirtieth, evening and morning; there was no further complaint." "A lady about fifty years of age, who had suffered about three weeks with pain in the pit of the stomach, aching in the left chest, flatulence, eructations, pressure and distention in the stomach after meals; was permanently cured of these dyspeptic symptoms in two or three hours by one dose of Rumex, two hundredth."—"A

* "Dr. Payne, who experienced this symptom several times, adds, that this sensation of weight in the stomach, was accompanied with a pressing sensation as far upward as the throat pit; it descends towards the stomach upon every empty deglutition, but immediately returned. have clinical confirmation of this, as well as the symptoms of the text."—(*Joslin.*)

young lady has a sensation of fulness and pressure in the pit of the stomach, extending up towards and to the throat, and afterwards carried down again towards the stomach when she swallows, and then rising again to the throat. This curious alternation has been observed in the proving of Rumex. She was cured by Rumex two hundredth." "A gentleman, not accustomed to the use of tea, took a cup of it, very weak, of the black kind; then followed aching in the pit of the stomach and aching and shooting above it in the chest, at, and especially on each side of the lower end of the sternum. These symptoms were removed in a few minutes by one dose of the Rumex, *thirtieth*."

Hypochondrium.—Pain in the hopochondrium in the afternoon, after dinner; worse on movement, or occurring while walking; hypochondrium pained by coughing, rapid walking, or deep inspiration.

Abdomen.—Dull pain in the abdomen in day time, continuing two hours; pain in the abdomen in the night; pain in the abomen in the morning; pain in the abdomen in the morning in bed; protuberance or hardness, or else sensation of fulness in the abdomen; rumbling in the bowels, or much flatus moving obout in them; pain in the abdomen, occurring or increasing during deep inspiration; moving in the intestines; flatulent colic near the umbilicus soon after a meal, mitigated by discharge of flatus; emissions of flatus in the morning; pain in the umbilical region, with eructation, soon followed by pain over eyebrow; pain in the abdomen, in the morning, followed by an evacuation of the bowels; griping pain in the bowels below the umbilicus, which is partially relieved by the discharge of very offensive flatus, after breakfast; sensation in the bowels as if diarrhœa would ensue. (See clinical remarks under "*stool.*")

Stool and Anus.—Dark-colored fæces; stool brown, or else black; constipation, or else scanty fæces; sensation in the bowels as if a diarrhœaic evacuation would ensue, the sensation passing off without subsequent evacuation; liquid diarhœaic stool in the morning; diarrhœaic stool in the morning, preceded by eructations; diarrhœaic stool in the morning preceded by pain in the abdomen; sensation as if from pressure of a stick in the rectum; itching in the anus; discharge of offensive flatus.

Clinical Remarks.—It is considered by allopathists, as similar in its action to Rhubarb, and has been used by that school in diarrhœa and dysentery. It is homœopathic to some forms of intestinal disorder. Dr. A. E. Small informs me that at one time he found it very useful in the bowel complaints of children. Dr. C. Dunham, writes (Am. Hom. Review, vol. ii, p. 533); "I have noticed in one case the cessation of a brown, watery diarrhœa after the administration of Rumex. A boy of five years, had brown, watery diarrhœa, chiefly in the morning, having five stools from 5 to 9 A. M., attended with moderate griping pain in the lower part of the abdomen; this continued several days, notwithstanding two prescriptions which I made for it. Observing that the boy had a cough, which presented the characteristic features of the rumex cough, I gave that remedy, and both diarrhœa and cough were speedily cured." A writer, ("I") in the Hom. Review, reports two cases. "A lady about the turn of life, had *diarrhœa in the morning*, four evacuations, between 6 and 10 A. M.; fæces very thin; evacutions painless; nausea on movement in the night, preceding the evacuations; mouth dry, tongue slightly coated yellow; the day previous had dull pain on the right side of the sternum; sharp pain on the left. Gave Rumex 30th., in solution, once in three hours. The next day all the symptoms were removed."—"*Diarrhœa in the morning with cough*—a lady about fifty years of age, has had diarrhœa every morning for four days; the evacuations, profuse, offensive, and thin, and have even become watery; she is also suffering from a cough, excited by a sensation of tickling in the throat-pit. It is usually dry, but when expectoration takes place, this is tasteless; the cough shocks the stomach, and is attended with a sensation of excoriation in the chest; it keeps her awake at night. Rumex 30th., every four hours, on 30th of March, in the evening the cough was immediately and decidedly improved, so that she slept all night. Next morning she awoke with the most severe headache she had ever suffered; it was a continuous aching in the temples, forehead and eyebrows, and lasted all the morning; the cough and diarrhœa were removed without any other medicines. All the above symptoms, except the fœtor of the fæces, have been observed as pathogenetic of Rumex."

Urinary Organs, etc.—Urine extremely pale, or colorless; very sudden and urgent desire to urinate; copious discharge of colorless urine in afternoon; complete loss of sexual desire for several days.

Larynx.—Pain in the larynx; in the second prover in a few minutes, and the first rumex symptom in six years; tenacious mucus in the throat or larynx, detached and removed by an expiratory effort, or attended with a constant desire to hawk and raise it; in the first prover it was the first symptom in the second proving, five years after the first; much mucus in the bronchi, or in the larynx; expectoration made by coughing and hawking, or attempted by hawking, worse at night; scraping and tenacious mucus in the throat, or else much tough mucus in the larynx, with a constant desire to hawk and raise it, but without relief; cough excited by tickling or irritation behind the sternum; cough excited by irritation in the chest; cough, attended with pain in the head. Sudden change of voice at the same hour on consecutive days; the first and second of the proving, it becomes suddenly hoarse at eleven at night, or else rose several notes in pitch at two in the afternoon.

Clinical Remarks.—The Rumex c. seems to have a specific affinity for the laryngeal and bronchial mucous membrane; the recorded clinical experience with this remedy is quite extensive. Dr. C. Dunham makes some valuable observations concerning its therapeutical properties. I copy a portion of his article (see Amer. Hom. Review, vol. ii., p. 530): "I have used the Rumex chiefly in acute catarrhal affections of the larynx, trachea, and bronchi. In these cases it seems to me to present a close analogy in its action to

Belladonna, Lachesis, Phosphorus and Causticum. Without assuming to present an exhaustive analysis of the action of Rumex on the respiratory organs, I proceed to state the indications for its use to which my studies of it, thus far have led me. Rumex diminishes the secretions, and at the same time exalts in a very marked manner, the sensibility of the mucous membrane of the larynx and trachea, exceeding in the extent of this exaltation, any remedy known to us. The cough, therefore, is frequent and continuous, to an extent quite out of proportion to the degree of organic affection of the mucous membrane. It is dry, occurs in long paroxysms, or, under certain circumstances, is almost uninterrupted. It is induced or greatly aggravated by any irregularity of respiration, such as an inspiration a little deeper or more rapid than usual; by an inspiration of air a little colder than that previously inhaled; by irregularity of respiration, and motion of the larynx and trachea, such as are involved in the act of speech; and by external pressure upon the trachea, in the region of the supra-sternal fossa." The subjective symptoms, are, rawness and soreness in the trachea, extending a short distance below the supra-sternal fossa, and laterally into the bronchi, chiefly the left; and tickling in the supra-sternal fossa, and behind the sternum, provoking the cough; this tickling is very annoying and very persistent, and is often but momentarily, and sometimes only partially, relieved by coughing. The cough occurs chiefly, or is much worse, in the evening after retiring, and at the time the membrane of the trachea is particularly sensitive to cold air, and to any irregularity in the flow of air over its surface; so that the patient often covers the head with the bed clothes to avoid the cold air of the apartment, and refuses to speak, or even listen to conversation, lest his attention should be withdrawn from the supervision of his respiratory acts, which he performs with the most careful uniformity and deliberation, and all in the hope of preventing the distressing tickling and the harrassing cough which would ensue from a neglect of these precautions. I have frequently witnessed this state of things during the last three years, and have invariably given prompt relief with Rumex. In the group of remedies in which I have placed Rumex (along with Bell., Lach., Phos., Caust.), it stands pre-eminent in respect to the extreme sensibility of the tracheal mucous membrane. All of these remedies produce symptoms identical in kind: the characteristic of each is to be found in the relative *degree* in which each symptom is pronounced in the different remedies, quite as much as in the possession by any one of them of symptoms not produced by the others. Thus, Belladonna, Lachesis, and Rumex produce each, a dry cough, induced by tickling in the larynx or trachea, and provoked by deep inspiration, by speaking, and by external pressure on the larynx or trachea. The cough of each is spasmodic and long continued, and is worse at night after retiring; but, apart from the fact that Belladonna and Lachesis act more upon the lower part of the trachea, we observe that, in the case of Lachesis, the slightest external pressure on the larynx or trachea produces violent and long-continued, spasmodic cough; the patient cannot endure the least constriction in that region, not even the ordinary contact of his clothing. There is, moreover, a sense of fulness in the trachea and a very painful aching in the whole extent of the os hyodes. In the case of Belladonna not only is cough produced to a moderate extent by pressing upon the larynx, but soreness and pain are experienced with a sense of internal fulness and soreness which at once suggests the presence of Acute Laryngitis sub-mucosa. In Rumex, on the other hand, there is no sensibility, strictly speaking, of the trachea, but simply such an instability of the mucous membrane that cough is produced by the change of position induced in that membrane by external pressure on the trachea. As regards the extent and intensity of this symptom, Rumex holds a lower rank than the other remedies named. But the irritability of mucous membrane by virtue of which cough is induced by hurried or deep inspiration, or by speaking, while it is common to Bell., Lach., Rumex, and Phosphorus is produced in the most exalted degree, as we have already seen, by Rumex, which, as regards this symptom, takes first rank. A sensation of rawness or roughness in the larynx, trachea and bronchia is produced by each of the four remedies above named, but the *locality* and the *degree* in which it is produced, vary in such a manner as to serve in some measure as a characteristic of each. It is most marked in Phosphorus and Belladonna, less prominent in Rumex, and least of all in Lachesis. In Belladonna and Lachesis it is most marked in the larynx; indeed it is almost confined to that region. Rumex produces it in the trachea and upper part of the bronchia, while Phosphorus induces it in the whole mucous tract, from the larynx to the smaller bronchia, and bronchi; and, moreover, in the Phosphorus proving this 'rawness' of the air passages is accompanied by a no less characteristic sense of weight and constriction across the upper part of the thorax, which indicates an affection of the finer air tubes, and of the air vesicles, of such a character as seriously to impede the function of respiration. In considering this last symptom we must mention Causticum also, which produces 'rawness,' extending the whole length of the sternum. All five remedies, again, produce *hoarseness:* Phosphorus, Causticum, and Belladonna most eminently, Rumex less decidedly, and Lachesis in a still less degree.—As regards complications, Belladonna and Lachesis apply especially to those which involve the fauces and pharynx, and are acute—the one of a sthenic, the other of an asthenic character:—Phosphorus, those of the pulmonary tissues of a definite inflammatory character; and, Rumex, to certain affections of the lungs and their envelopes of which their nature is not clearly defined in the proving. They are indicated by pairs, generally sub-acute, in the upper part of the lung, near the clavicle and axilla, and more frequent in the left than in the right lung. The following case from my clinical record will illustrate the character of the Rumex cough. M., aged twenty-two of feeble constitution, strumous, subject for several years to sub-acute rheumatism, has had a severe cold for several days, and is now confined to the bed. The pulse is quick, not hard, one hundred and ten, skin moderately hot and dry; face somewhat flushed; respiration embarrased, not so much by any constriction of the chest as by the violent and long-continued cough, which follows any attempt to make a full inspiration. A physical examination of the chest reveals no abnormal condition. The patient complains of roughness and soreness in the lower part of the trachea, and behind the upper third of the sternum, much more perceptible when she coughs. The cough is dry, slightly hoarse, very violent and fatiguing to the patient. It is provoked by a tickling in the supra-sternal fossa—is induced by pressure on the trachea in that region, and especially by talking, and by deep inspiration or by the inspiration of cool air. This irritability of the trachea increases very markably after 7 P. M., so that the patient suffers exceedingly from the constant tickling and violent cough. Can prevent them only by respiring with very great caution and deliberation, by avoid ing all distractions of speech and conversation, and finally, she draws the bed clothes over the head in order to avoid inhaling the cool air of the chamber. This patient states that she has frequently had such coughs as this, and they have proved very obstinate, although under skilful homœopathic treatment. I gave Rumex 12th in solution, a teaspoonful every two hours. After the second dose there was complete relief. The next evening a very slight disposition to cough. No further symptoms. I supplied the patient with Rumex 30th, and advised her to use it at once on the occurrence of such a cough, and I am informed that she always succeeded in subduing the cough within twelve hours. The following cases in the practice of Dr. P. P. Wells, of Brooklyn, were communicated in a letter to Dr. Joslin, some years since. We regret that these are the only cases of Dr. W.'s that we can at present report, but hope at some future time we shall be able to publish more, as the doctor's experience with this remedy has been very satisfactory. Mrs. ——, had been subject to eight miscarriages, all in the early stage of pregnancy, which in each case was early attended with dry, shaking, spasmodic cough, in paroxysms of great violence, which was regarded by herself and friends as instrumental in producing the abortions. At the beginning of the ninth pregnancy she came to Brooklyn to be under homœopathic treatment. She had her cough, which was very dry, harsh, loud, shaking, worse at night, preventing sleep, excited instantly by pressure on the trachea. The cough was relieved promptly by Rumex crispus, 30th. The following marked and rather important group of symptoms were relieved promptly, in the treatment of the case of our friend D., by Rumex 200th., Lehrman's preparation. Thinking a knowledge of the fact might interest you, to whom we are indebted for our knowledge of this interesting drug, I send it. The cough begins with tickling behind the top of the sternum, and sometimes in paroxyms of five to ten minutes duration. Trachea sore to outward pressure; feels excoriated through its whole extent, as do also the whole fauces; cough excited by pressure on throat pit; cough is violent, with scanty, difficult expectoration; shocks the head and chest, as if the head would fly in pieces, and he feels as if he might raise blood at any minute. He is greatly exhausted after the paroxysms of coughing; head aches during the cough. You have the group above in the order as written down for me by his brother, and upon which I prescribed the medicine, which was followed by the happiest results. Dr. J. M. Rhees, reports several cases of *Aphonia*: one of three months standing; with sore throat during deglutition; posterior surface of pharynx irritated and in places excoriated, edges of soft palate and uvula red and somewhat swollen, and covered with an eruption of minute red pimples; slight hacking cough produced by a tickling in larynx and upper part of trachea. Under Carbo veg., Caust., and Merc. she grew worse; her cough became almost constant; tickling at the root of the tongue; Hyos. and Rhus. were given, but gave no relief. *Rumex* 6th was then given, and she commenced to improve the day after. On the third day her cough was much better, and the pharynx looked almost natural. The eruption on the palate had almost disappeared, but there was still some redness on the edges, Rumex 6th as before, cured. Dr. B. F. Joslin, in the first Vol of Philad. Jou. of Hom., reported eleven cases of cough, cured with the 30th dilution of Rumex c. I give a brief abstract of the cases:—*Case* 1. Dry cough; tickling in the throat pit; excoriation in larynx and behind the upper portion of the sternum; cough worse on working; pain in chest. *Rumex* 30th cured the case; three doses only were given. The cough had lasted several weeks before the Rumex was prescribed. *Case* 2. Fluent coryza, with cough excited by tickling in the throat pit; sensation of excoriation behind the upper part of the sternum while coughing; Rumex 30th, morning and evening. Cured promptly. *Case* 3. A lady of highly nervous temperament, had confusion of the head; hoarseness in the evening; cough; excoriation behind the whole of the sternum on coughing, and inspiration, and coldness of the fingers; Rumex 30th, three times a day. Cured in a few days. *Case* 4. Severe, dry cough, excited by an irritated pressure in the throat pit; excoriation in the larynx, and chest; Rumex 30th morning and evening. Cured in a few days. *Case* 5. Cough excited by pressing on the throat, and attended with excoriation in the larynx and chest, and hoarseness. He took one dose of Rumex thirty drops, in the morning; in afternoon of same day was much better; no cough next day, nor did it return. *Case* 6. Violent cough in evening, worse about 11 o'clock at night; aggravated by lying down; excited by a tickling behind the sternum, and attended by a sprain-like aching near the sternum, and with accumulation of mucus in the fauces, near the posterior orifice of the nares. One dose of Rumex 30th, removed the paroxysm in a few minutes, and it did not return. *Case* 7. A young lady complained of shootings from the pit of the stomach into the chest, in various directions; sharp pains in the left chest; dull aching in the forehead, and slight nausea; Rumex 30th, morning and evening. Cured in two days. My own experience with Rumex, has been mainly with the third dilution I have cured many cases where Phos. Merc. and Caust., semed indicated, but failed. The remedy has not been used as much by the profession, as its merits seem to demand.

Chest.—Pain in the chest, right and left; either aching pain in the anterior portion of both lungs, which harrassed him day and night for five days, or else raw pain just under each clavicle while hawking mucus out of the throat; pain in chest when in bed at night; pain in outer-superior part of chest near the axillas; near the left axilla, pain undefined—near the right, sharp; both after the same dilution; first symptom in two provers; in one, in ten minutes, the first symptom ever produced in any proving of Rumex; in the other, two minutes, his first symptom—sharp pain in right chest; a burning pain in the left chest; dull pain in the left chest; sharp pain in left chest; shootings in the left chest; sticking pain in the left thoracic region; stitches in the left chest; sharp, cutting pain at or under the left breast; pain in the chest a little below and to the right of the left nipple; burning, sticking, or burning, stinging pain in the left chest; burning—smarting, or burning—stinging pain in the left chest; a very acute stitch, or burning—stinging pain in the left chest; shootings, or else dull pain in the left side near the back, a little above the seventh rib; pain in the left chest when recumbent; a sticking or stitch in the left chest while riding in the open air; painful sensation in the anterior part of the left chest, immediately after waking, about two o'clock at night, and between five and six hours after taking a low dilution; an acute stitch in the sternal region, or a severe stinging, which obstructs the respiration; itching at or near the sternum; dull pain in the region of the heart; burning pain in the region of, or near the heart; palpitation of the heart, or else a sensation in the left chest, as if the heart suddenly ceased beating, followed by a heavy throbbing through the chest.

Clinical Remarks.—Some of the provers, especially Dr. Rhees, experienced some peculiar, and severe cardiac symptoms, which we could hardly, at first thought, expect from this remedy. Yet we have no right to judge, before we prove a remedy thoroughly, of the probable effect of a drug. It does seem, however, if Rumex thus affects the heart, that of the thousands who have taken the Dock in large doses, some of them would have had dangerous heart-disease; but we hear of no such instances. Dr. M. J. Rhees, one of the original provers of this remedy, furnished the following interesting case: "Joseph H., aged thirteen years, subject to violent attacks of Inflammatory Rheumatism. In the spring of 1858 I attended him in a severe attack, in which the disease concentrated itself on the heart with so much violence that I almost despaired of his recovery. Pulsatilla cured the disease at that time. In December, 1858, he was again attacked, but the heart was the principal seat of the disease from the first. On the 24th of December, his symptoms were: violent palpitation of the heart, with throbbing of the carotid, and throughout the body, visible to the eye and shaking the bed; pulse 120; violent aching pain in the region of the heart; great dyspnœa, especially while lying, so that it was necessary to prop him up in a sitting posture in bed; face red and somewhat puffed up, especially about the eyes, which were red, heavy, and lustreless; tongue coated with white fur, with red tip and edges; excessive thirst; no appetite; bowels costive. I commenced the treatment by giving Acon. 3rd., and Puls. 3rd., alternately. Some relief followed the administration of these remedies, but the improvement was slow. From December 28th to January 9th, 1859, various other remedies were used, as they seemed to be indicated, but without decided improvement on the whole. On the latter date the patient complained of a stinging pain in the region of the heart, which was increased by lying down and by breathing deeply. In my arranged proving of Rumex crispus the following symptoms may be found:—"No. 41, burning, stinging pain in the whole of the left side of the chest; suddenly, when taking a deep inspiration while in the act of lying down in bed at night."—"No. 49, burning stinging pain in the left chest near the heart; came on soon after lying down in the bed at night. These symptoms were fresh in my memory, and I accordingly gave Rumex crispus 6th, in water, two tea-spoonfuls every three hours. January 10th, considerably relieved of the pain in the chest, and otherwise improved; continued Rumex. January 11th, the pain in the chest is almost removed. Rumex was continued several days after this, with the effect of entirely relieving the pain in the chest; but the improvement in other respects ceasing, Rumex was discontinued, and other remedies substituted. Bell. 30th, and Phos 30th; eventually cured the case, and there has been no return of the disease." This case is in many respects a marked one. But it will require further clinical experience to prove satisfactorily, that Rumex will cure serious heart-affections..

Spinal Region.—Sore or burning pain at or near the sacro-iliac symphysis; chilliness in the back; sensation of heat in the back; pressive or aching pain in back at the inferior angle of scapula; aching pain in the back, on the left side of the dorsal spine, either extending from the spine half way to the side, or else situated under and below the apex of the left scapula; stinging pain in the left dorsal region near the inferior angle of the scapula; pain in the back in the evening; itching in the evening.

Superior Extremities.—Pain in shoulder; either pain in the left shoulder, and from it along the upper arm to the elbow, including the joint, and leaving the arm with a sensation as if strained, commencing after four minutes, or else pain in the right shoulder on waking in the morning, ameliorated by rest, and passing off in two hours; itching on shoulder in the morning; pain in upper arm in the evening; numb sensation in the right hand about 10 P. M., or else in the left upper arm after lying down in bed; pain at the inner side of the right upper arm; dull, aching pain in the left upper arm; pain in the upper arm and elbow, undefined or dull; pain in wrist, the left aching, or ulnar half of the right, character undefined.

Inferior Extremities.—A sensation of weakness or fatigue in lower limbs; aching of the lower extremities; itching on lower extremities when the part is uncovered and exposed to cool air; stinging or prickling itching at an upper part of inferior extremity, either at the anterior part of the left thigh, or on the nates; pain in knee when in erect posture; stitch-like pain at the inner part when stepping, or rending aching in the flexure of the left while standing; the legs feel weak in the evening, or tired, then, though he had done but little walking; pain in an anterior part of both lower extremities, either rheumatic pain at the anterior part of the tibiæ, or rending in the anterior part of the ankle joints, running down the insteps; aching in the calves, or drawing pain in the right calf; itching on the calves of the legs; legs densely covered with a rash, composed partly of small red pimples; itching worse on exposure to the air in the evening when undressing to go to bed; aching or rending in the upper-anterior part of the tarsus, the instep: sensation of coldness of the feet during the forenoon.

SANGUINARIA CANADENSIS.

(*Blood-root.*)

This plant is indigenous, growing in open woods, in light, rich soils. It appears early in the spring, and flowers in April. The tincture for Homœopathic use should be prepared from the green root. The root is from an inch to two inches in length, and half an inch in diameter, terminating abruptly, as if bitten off. When the fresh root is broken, a light red fluid exudes, resembling blood; when dried the root becomes dark brown externally, contracted, wrinkled, breaking with a short waxy fracture, the broken extremities presenting an orange red color. Its odor is feebly narcotic and disagreeable, its taste acrid and bitter; the powder is a grayish red. The active principles of Blood-root are said to be Sanguinarina and Sanguinarin, the former a pure alkaloid, the latter an alka-resinoid. The Sanguinarin is supposed to represent the plant more nearly, and is the one generally used in practice. Homœopathists generally prefer the green root tincture and its dilutions, but triturations of the root or the Sanguinarin are not to be discarded.

General Effects.—"Blood-root is an acrid emetic, with narcotic and stimulant properties, it is also expectorant, sudorific, alterative, emmenagogue, tonic, anti-septic, detergent and escharotic, according to the mode in which it is employed. It is a very active agent, and is capable of exercising a powerful influence on the system. When given in small doses it stimulates the digestive organs, accelerates the circulation; in larger doses it occasions nausea and consequent depression of the pulse; in a full dose it produces active vomiting; in overdoses it causes violent emesis, a burning sensation in the stomach, tormenting thirst, faintness, vertigo, dimness of vision, alarming prostration and even death. (*King's Disp.*) "Sanguinaria is emetic, expectorant, diaphoretic, acro-narcotic, sedative, alterative, and in small doses, tonic and stimulant; in full doses it induces nausea and vomiting, with a sensation of warmth in the stomach, acceleration of pulse, and slight headache. It acts on the fauces, producing an acrid impression, and in some cases it proves cathartic. The leaves and seeds possess similar properties. The seeds however are said to exert a marked influence upon the brain and nervous system, occasioning torpor, languor, disordered vision and dilatation of the pupils; in large doses the emesis is violent, there is a burning sensation in the stomach, faintness vertigo, dimness of vision and alarming prostration. (*Jones and Scudder's Mat. Med.*) *Wood*, *Tully*, *Eberle* and other writers use about the same language in describing the general toxical effects of the Sanguinaria. It is undoubtedly one of the most powerful agents in the vegetable materia medica, and ranks as an analogue of such potent medicines as Arsenicum, Phosphorus, Tartar emetic and Veratrum viride.

SPECIAL EFFECTS.—**Nervous System.**—The toxical and pathogenetic effects of Sanguinaria indicates that it has a profound effect upon the nerves of sensation and motion, but the exact nature of this action has not been sufficiently investigated. Among the symptoms we find—"a quickly diffused and transient, but at the same time a very peculiar nervous thrill, which is often extended to the minutest extremity." In large doses it causes "torpor, languor and dilatation of the pupils."

Mucous Membranes.—There are a few drugs, like Pulsatilla, which seem to affect the mucous tissues of the whole system; others, like Squills, have a specific affinity for the pulmonary mucous membrane; Sanguinaria is an analogue of the latter to a certain degree, although it more nearly approaches the action of Tartar emetic. It was known as an expectorant, long before the allopathic profession brought it into use, and now, both that and the eclectic school value it highly for that purpose. (See Respiratory Organs.) Blood-root does not seem to notably increase the mucous secretions from the intestinal or other mucous tissues.

Serous Membranes.—Said to be useful in pleuritis, synovitis.

Muscular and Fibrous Tissues.—Sanguinaria seems to cause pains of a rheumatic or myalgic character. It is difficult to decide which of the two affections were cured by this medicine in the reported curative symptoms. I am inclined to the opinion, however, that Sanguinaria, although it may cure some neuralgias, will not, like Colchicum and Cimicifuga, act specifically in rheumatic affections. (For cases cured see "Extremities.")

Vascular System.—*Heart.*—Pressing pain in the regions of the heart; palpitation of the heart, with great weakness, (large doses;) extreme reduction in the force and frequency of the pulse, together with great *irregularity* of action, and palpitation of the heart.

Clinical Remarks.—We have no clinical record of any disorders of the heart treated with this medicine. The symptoms would seem to indicate that it was more adapted to *venous* hæmorrhages and congestions than arterial, (secondarily).

Fever, Pulse.—In the evening in bed, chill and shivering in the back; shaking chill with pain under the shoulder blade on motion; chill with headache; chill and nausea; heat flying from head to stomach; burning heat, rapidly alternating with chill and shivering; fever and delirium (from the seeds); pulsations through the whole body; a gradual increase in the force and frequency of the pulse, (from small doses); during the vomiting the pulse is frequent; slow pulse with the extreme nausea; strength and frequency of the pulse extremely reduced, with irregularity, and with insensibility, coldness, etc.; (from very large doses) suppressed pulse with fainting.

Clinical Remarks.—Sanguinaria has not been used in fevers, generally; but it has been administered successfully in Hectic fever. In the pathogenesis of no other medicine, except perhaps, Phosphorus and Lycopodium, do we find the hectic poroxysm as perfectly delineated; generally the hectic is associated with cough and other symptoms of lung affection, but there are exceptions. Dr. Bute, cured—(1.) In a lady, coldness of the feet in the afternoons, at the same time the tongue was painful and sore upon being touched, like a boil, and there was stiffness of the knee and finger joints." (2.) "Burning of the palms of the hands and soles of the feet, compelling him to throw the bedclothes off the feet for the purpose of cooling them. These paroxysms generally come on in the P. M., or evening." (3.) Paroxysm of fever in P. M., with circumscribed redness of the cheeks; cough and expectoration."

Hemorrhages.—Dr. Morrow relied on Sanguinaria as a remedy for hemorrhages in general, because of "its power of quieting excessive, or depressing the natural circulation," he advises it particularly in hœmoptysis; It has also been used in menorrhagia, epistaxis, etc.

General Symptoms.—Great weakness; great prostration of muscular strength, (by large doses); extreme weakness and debility in the limbs, whilst walking in the open air, during the evening of the first day; debility with vertigo and pain in the hypochondria; great weakness, with vomiting; great weakness, with suppression of the pulse—with irregular pulse; weakness and palpitation of the heart; a quickly diffused and transient, but at the same time a very peculiar nervous thrill, which is often extended to the minutest extremity; a slowly shooting pain, with long continued thrill, ending in a grumbling aching in a carious molar tooth of the upper jaw; fainting weakness; general sensitiveness and weakness; torpor and languor from the seeds. *Paralysis of the right side, of fourteen years duration, cured by the tincture, in the dose of a small tea-spoonful every three or four days; (verbally from Dr. B. Becker,) convulsive rigidity of the limb.

REMARKS.—We can sometimes comprehend the sphere of action of a drug, by comparing the *ensemble* of its symptoms with that of other drugs; a careful analysis of the symptoms and toxical effects of Sanguinaria show its marked resemblance to those of our most important medicines, namely: Arsenicum, Phosphorus and Tartar emetic; more remotely it resembles Belladonna, Verat. viride and Iris versicolor; Lycopodium, Sulphur, Kali carbonicum and Rumex c., have some symptoms in common with Sanguinaria.

Sleep.—Sleeplessness at night; he awakens at night with affright as if he would fall; dreams two nights in succession of sailing on the sea; dream of a frightful and disagreeable character; he awakens earlier than common.

Skin.—Heat and dryness; increased itching of an old tubercle-like eruption on the skin; itching and nettle rash before the nausea.

CLINICAL REMARKS.—The blood-root has been used successfully for *scaly* eruption; old indolent ulcers; ill-conditional ulcers with callous borders and ichorous discharge; the powdered root is escharotic, and when applied to fungous growths causes their rapid disappearance. I consider it the best application we have for this purpose; it has also cured warts, and polypi, when given internally and applied topically. Dr. Sholl uses it externally and internally for carbuncle with alleged success.

Mind and Disposition.—Extreme moroseness; anxiety before the vomiting; hopefulness; sanguine of recovery from illness.

CLINICAL REMARKS.—The last two symptoms were observed by me several times, from the blood root. Every physician is aware of the peculiarly *hopeful* condition of mind in phthisis. Sanguinaria is quite homœopathic to that mental state.

Sensorium.—Vertigo, with singing in the ears; flatulent eructation, and then tickling in the throat, which excites cough (immediately after taking it); frequent vertigo, and diminished vision before vomiting, after large doses; vertigo with nausea, long continuing, with debility and with headache; *vertigo on quickly turning the head, and looking upward.

CLINICAL REMARKS.—It has cured, "vertigo on quickly turning the head and looking upward."

Head.—Confused and dull feeling in the head, which became better after eructation; determination of the blood to the head, with whizzing in the ears, and a transitory feeling of heat; then a sensation as if vomiting was about to take place, but instead of this there succeeded slight cutting drawings in the abdomen, and then a stool; heaviness in the head; pressing drawing in the forehead; pain of a short duration in the right side of the forehead, like a pressing, only while standing still, better while walking; at the same time a pain deep in the ear; headache as if the forehead would split, with chill and with burning in the stomach; a pain occurs suddenly in the interior angle of the right eye, and thence to the forehead; about five o'clock in the evening a severe quick-darting pain in the forehead and temple on the right side, which continued for about five minutes; this pain re-appeared in the evening about seven o'clock; about eleven o'clock at night a sudden pain through the forehead, like an electric stroke, of short duration; a slowly-shooting pain in the forehead; periodic stitches in the left temple; pain in all the upper part of the head; in the abdomen, pain, like fulness; pain in the fore part of the head; pressing in the upper part of the head, in the region of the anterior fontanelle, disappears while walking; boring pain above, in the fore part of the head; severe pain above, on all the left side of the head, especially in the eye; at the same time similar pains in the left foot; nausea, disposition to vomit without being able to do so; then headache with rheumatic pains and stiffness in the limbs and neck; beating headache and bitter vomiting; headache in the evening, with tickling in the throat; headache, with chill; headache, with nausea and chill, then flying heat from the head to the stomach; headache, with vertigo and pain in the ear; the headache occurs paroxysmally; feeling as if the head is drawn forward; soreness of the scalp, on being touched; feeling of looseness of the scalp on the right side; sensation of looseness, and drawing in one side of the scalp, on raising the eyes.

CLINICAL REMARKS.—Dr. Bute found blood-root curative in headaches with "distention of the temporal veins which were painfully sensitive to the touch," also with "feeling of soreness on small spots on the head, especially in the temples." Other physicans have cured cephalalgias with "pains in the head, in rays drawing upward from the neck." Dr. Hering considers it homœopathic to the so-called North American sick headache. He has cured with the high dilutions the following symptoms: "Severe pains in the head, with nausea, and vomiting, frequently with bilious vomiting, in attacks, with hebdomadal or longer intervals, from very different inducements, commonly beginning in the morning, increasing in violence through the day, only diminished by lying quiet, and when possible, by sleep." (*Tran. Amer. Ins.* vol. 1.) Dr. Hering also gives (*New Archives*, vol. 2, part 2, p 132,) the following indications for Sanguinaria: "It is the best remedy in most cases of Migrana or sick headache. Still, it must prove most useful when the attacks occur paroxysmally, viz; every week, or at longer intervals; or when the pains begin in the morning, increase during the day, and last till evening; when the head seems to feel that it must burst, or as if the eyes would be pressed *out*, or when the pains are *digging*, attended with sudden *piercing*, throbbing lancinations through the brain, involving the forehead and top of the head in particular, and being most severe on the *right* side, followed by chills, nausea, vomiting of food, or bile, forcing the patient to lie down and preserve the greatest quiet, as every motion aggravates the sufferings, which are only relieved by sleep. *Case* 1. A man was attacked with frightfully severe headache; the only relief he could obtain was from pressing the back of his head against the head-board of the bed. An infusion of Rad. Sanguinaria removed the headache permanently. (*Hering.*) *Case* 2.—A lady suffered with frequent and severe attacks of headache, with such sensitiveness during the paroxysm, that no one dared to walk across the room. Sanguinaria 6th, was given, but the first dose produced such an aggravation that the patient became almost beside herself; after the second dose, she fell into a pleasant sleep, from which she awoke refreshed. Dr. Helfrig always gave Aconite and Belladonna during the paroxysm of sick headache, and used Sang. thirty, during the interval, unless some other remedy was more indicated. (*Ibid*). Many of the symptoms of Sanguinaria, are similar to those pains which Inman discribes as belonging to *Myalgic* headaches; particularly the superficial sensitiveness, and drawing pains. *Congestions of the head* are controlled by this medicine, when the *temporal veins are distended.* It is probable that it is also homœopathic to some of the varieties of Apoplexy. Its known carative influence over hæmorrhage from congestions, would suggest its use in *Sanguineous* apoplexy. The symptoms would seem to imply that *venous* congestions (if the term may be allowed) are most under the control of Sanguinaria.

Face.—Feeling of fulness in the face; distention of the veins of the face, with excessive redness, and a feeling of stiffness; severe burning, heat and redness of the face; paleness of the face, with disposition to vomit; twitching of the cheeks, towards the eyes.

Clinical Remarks.—It has caused the following symptoms when occurring during other affections: "A red cheek, with burning of the ears;" "redness of the cheeks, with cough," "cheeks and hands livid in typhoid pneumonia." These symptoms are also found in the provings of Phosphorus, Lycopod., Sulphur, and Lacnanthes tinctoria.

Nose.—Heat in the nose; smell in the nose like roasted onions; dislike to the smell of syrup; much sneezing; fluid coryza, with frequent sneezing; severe fluid coryza in the right nostril; watery, acrid coryza, which renders the nose sore; copious watering of the right eye; the eye painful, especially on being touched; and soon afterwards there occurred a copious watery discharge from the right nostril; in the evening two diarrhœic stools, and then all the symptoms disappeared; fluid coryza, alternating with stoppage of the nose.

Clinical Remarks.—No drug so surely produces intense irritation of the nasal mucous membrane, when inhaled, as the Sanguinaria. Even its internal administration causes coryza. It is not strange, therefore, that homœopathists have found it curative for acute and chronic coryzas, also for "loss of smell." It has cured "Influenza, with rawness in the throat, pain in the breast, cough, and finally, diarrhœa." This last is a characteristic peculiarity of the drug, and as many catarrhal affections tend to end in intestinal irritation, or diarrhœa, the Sanguinaria should be remembered in each instance. Dr. Barton (allopathic) says he has "heard of the application of the powdered root to a fungous tumor within the nostril, with the effect of producing detumescence, and bringing away frequently, small pieces of the fungous, which, in the first instance, impeded the progress of the air through the nostril, and was supposed to be a polypus." Dr. Smith (botanic) says: "Applied to fungous flesh it proves escharotic, and several *polypi* of the soft kind were cured by it." Dr. Becker (homœopathist) states that a polypus of the nose ceased to grow from the time the powder of the root was snuffed. Several physicians of my acquaintance claim to have cured nasal polypi by the internal administration of the tincture of blood-root. It was used in the lower dilutions, in some cases. The finely powdered root forms one of the ingredients, of many, of the "catarrh snuffs" sold in the shops. It is often used as a domestic remedy for chronic catarrhal affections of the nose. Dr. Powers, late of Coldwater, Mich., was very successful in the treatment of obstinate nasal catarrhs, and *ozœna.* He prescribed the 2d trit., of blood-root, as a "snuff," to be forcibly inspired up the nose, and gave at the same time Sanguinaria 3rd, or Nitric acid, internally. It has cured in my hands, many cases of ulcerative ozæna, also *epistaxis.*

Eyes.—Pain in the right eye; pressing pain in the left eye; stitch in the upper eyelid; watering and burning of the right eye, which is painful on being touched—then coryza; feeling as if the eyes were affected by sour smoke, afternoons about two o'clock; in the afternoons dimness of the eyes, and a feeling as if hairs were in them; very great glimmering before the eyes; diminished power of vision; dilation of the pupils (by the seeds).

Clinical Remarks.—It is homœopathic to catarrhal ophthalmia, granular lids, and even ulcers on the cornea. I once cured a case of the latter, very happily, by the use of Sanguinaria 3rd., internally and topically. The case had proved obstinate under ordinary treatment, and I bethought me of the beneficial effect of blood-root in indolent ulcers. A wash of about the strength of the third dilution was prepared in distilled water, and used as a collyrium. Under its use the ulcers healed in a week, leaving but a slight opacity.

Ears.—Beating under the ears at irregular intervals, frequently only a couple of strokes; * burning of the ears, with redness of the cheeks; pains in the ears, with headache; singing in the ears, with vertigo; humming in the ears, with determination of blood; slow stitches in the left ear during the pain in the forehead; beating-humming in the left ear; painful sensitiveness to sudden sounds; a crackling in the right ear when he draws his fingers lightly over his right cheek; on the left side this is not the case.

Jaws.—Stiffness of the jaws; pain in the upper teeth; pain in a hollow tooth, especially when touched by the food; toothache from picking the teeth; pain in one or more of the incisor teeth, and in a carious molar tooth; shooting and thrilling pain in a carious molar tooth of the upper jaw, which passes away gradually in that form of pain which is often termed a "grumbling toothache;" on awaking, toothache in an upper carious tooth on the right side, at the same time headache in the same side; the toothache is made worse by cold water, and better by drinking warm drink; pain in a carious molar after cold drinking, two mornings in succession; looseness of the teeth; salivation and looseness of the teeth; he supposes himself able to take them all out; spitting, with nausea; feeling of dryness of the lips.

Clinical Remarks.—Blood-root is useful in expulsive gingivitis, in cases where the gums become very spongy, bleeding, and fungous.

Throat.—Feeling of dryness in the throat, not diminished by drinking; heat in throat, alleviated by the inspiration of cool air; a long-continuing impression in the fauces; a transitory, but marked sensation in the fauces, as if he had swallowed something acrimonious; burning in the fauces after eating sweet things; burning in the œsophagus; a feeling in the throat as if it were swollen up, and would suffocate him, with pain in the throat when swallowing, and with aphonia; in the evening a pain with a feeling of swelling in the throat; worse on the right side, and most perceptible on swallowing; feeling of swelling in the throat when swallowing.

Clinical Remarks.—*Angina*, in several cases, particularly a species of pharyngitis. *Ulcerated sore throat.* I was once informed by intelligent persons, that they had been permanently cured of recurring quinsy with ulceration, by using a gargle of blood-root. Upon testing it in practice, I found it quite equal to Hepar sulphur in its power of preventing attacks of tonsillitis; also in actual ulcerations of the throat. The lower dilutions were used.

Mouth.—A prickling sensation on the tongue and roof of the mouth, as after chewing mezereum, but slighter; crawling on the point of the tongue, after which an acerb feeling extends itself over the whole tongue, in the morning on awaking; prickling on the point of the tongue; tongue feels as if burned; a feeling of dryness and rawness, as after acrid things; begins on the right side of the tongue, and spreads over the whole tongue, mornings on awaking; * tongue sore; pains like a boil; stitches on the left side of the tongue; white-coated tongue, with loss of appetite; loss of appetite, with uncertain cravings; * increase of appetite; loss of smell and taste; a piece of sugar-cake tastes bitter, followed by burning in the fauces; fatty taste in the mouth; slimy taste in the mouth; disinclination for butter, which leaves a disagreeable after-taste; dislike to the odor of syrup; craving for he knows not what, with loss of appetite; craving for piquant food.

Stomach.—Pressing in the stomach; soreness in the epigastrium, aggravated by eating; feeling of warmth and heat in the stomach; *burning* in the stomach from large doses; *burning* in the stomach, with headache; jerking in the stomach, as if from something alive; great weakness of digestion; loss of appetite; * strengthens the stomach; excites the appetite, and aids digestion; soon after eating a feeling of emptiness in the stomach; * inflammation of the stomach.

Clinical Remarks.—By reference to the "gastric symptoms," as well as the above, it will be seen how closely the symptoms similate those of Arsenicum, Phosphorus, and Tartar emetic. It will cure, according to Dr. Tully, "atonic, sub-acute, and chronic inflammations of the stomach." No remedy, however, is more decidedly homœopathic to *acute gastritis*. We have the terrible *burning*, the unquenchable *thirst*, the *pain*, *vomiting* and *prostration* which mark that disease. In acute gastritis, the sixth or thirtieth should be used. In chronic gastritis, the lower dilutions may be as useful. It ought to be useful in *ulceration* of the stomach.

Gastric Symptoms.—Severe nausea from large doses; nausea as if vomiting would succeed; nausea after eating; nausea which is not diminished by vomiting; loss of appetite and periodic nausea; nausea by stooping; nausea with much spitting; extreme nausea with great salivation; nausea, with flow of saliva, and constant spitting; long continued nausea, with chill; nausea without vomiting, then headache; nausea with headache, with chill and heat; nausea before the nettle rash; heartburn and nausea; regurgitation and disposition to vomit; flatulent eructation; spasmodic eructation of flatus; hiccough while smoking tobacco; frequent flatulent eructations of unpleasant odor, with disposition to vomit, and paleness of face; after the eructation of flatus, the dullness of the head becomes better. Vomiting with severe, painful *burning* in the stomach, and intense *thirst;* many unpleasant feelings previous to vomiting; before vomiting, great anxiety; before vomiting, slight pressure to stool; vomiting of bitter water; bitter vomiting, with headache; vomiting, with craving to eat in order to quiet the nausea; vomiting and diarrhœa; causes vomiting, without nausea or perceptible weakness.

Clinical Remarks.—Blood-root is fully indicated for *nausea* or *vomiting* from *irritation* of the coats of the stomach. Allopathists have cured *vomiting* of food and bilious vomiting with small doses of the tincture. It is doubtless homœopathic to many functional and organic diseases of the stomach, and I would suggest its use in gastric disorders not amenable to the ordinary remedies. Dr. F. W. Hunt in an article on "Dyspepsia, or Diseases of the Stomach," (U. S. Journal of Homœopathy, vol. i. p. 190,) thus speaks of the virtues of Sanguinaria canadensis: "This is one of the most important remedies for various diseases of the stomach, throat, liver, lungs, etc. In almost every form of indigestion, for many years, it has given me satisfactory results. It is especially useful in deficient gastric secretion, with loss of appetite and periodic nausea; heartburn, nausea, and irregular chills; torpid state of the liver; dyspeptic headache, terminating by regurgitation, and vomiting of bitter, greenish fluids; soreness in the abdomen, increased by eating; feeling of heat in the stomach; chronic gastritis; red tongue, which burns as if from contact with something hot; lips red and dry; throat hot and dry; tickling at the entrance of the larynx, which excites cough; cough peculiarly severe, not relieved by expectoration, with pain in the chest and redness of the cheeks. When digestion is imperfect from deficiency of the true gastric fluid; when the food undergoes chemical decomposition, and gas is evolved in large quantities, Sanguinaria will generally change the action of the stomach, and digestion becomes more complete. When the mucous membrane is congested, the flatus formed by fermentation is retained by a spasmodic constriction of the cardia. Its irritation is reflected through the pneumogastric nerve upon the lungs, exciting a feeling of 'tickling' in the entrance of the trachea, with *sympathetic cough.* This peculiar, dry cough does not yield to expectorants, but often persists for hours, and is only relieved by eructations. Aromatics and stimulants fail to expel the gas: they only increase the erethism of the coats of the stomach. The Sanguinaria affords a better resource. It not only relaxes the constricted cardia, permitting the flatus to escape, but excites a healthy, homœopathic reaction on the whole surface of the fauces, œsophagus, and stomach, superseding the morbid state by a healthy one. Dr. Coe and others (allopathists) caution against the use of blood-root when there exists "gastritis and enteritis, and whenever we have occasion to suspect ulceration or abrasion of the mucous surfaces of the bowels." This caution suggests to the homœopathist that the medicine will cure such conditions, if administered in dynamic doses.

Abdomen.—Severe and continual pain in the hypochondria; vertigo and debility; *pain in the left hypochondrium, worse by coughing, better by pressure and lying on the left side; diseases of the liver; torpor and atony of the liver; inflammation of the abdominal viscera; hot streamings from the breast towards the liver; beating in the abdomen; cramps in the abdomen, which passes from one place to another; sensation as if hot water poured itself from the breast into the abdomen, followed by diarrhœa; discharges of flatus upwards and downwards by raising himself up on account of the cough, which then ceases; bellyache; paroxysmal pain in the abdomen; slight cutting drawings in the abdomen; colic, with torpor of the liver; in the night digging pain in the sacrum; an hour after taking it severe cutting pain in the bowels, followed by a single watery stool; in the morning, colicky pain in the upper part of the abdomen, and then a diarrhœic stool.

Clinical Remarks.—Eclectic physicians claim that Sanguinaria has a specific action on the *liver.* The hepatic symptoms in this proving were collected from allopathic sources.—(*Barton McBride* and *Tully*). It is doubtful if they should have a place in the proving at all, as by reference to the original, (Trans. Amer. Ins.) it will be seen that they were mere assertions of the above named physicians, and *not* pathogenetic symptoms. It may not be amiss, however, to quote the statements of eclectics on this point. *King* says it has been used successfully in "jaundice, and other hepatic affections. In torpid conditions of the liver it is very valuable." *Jones* asserts that it "arouses the *liver* and glandular system in general." *Coe* admires it in "all cases of hepatic torpor, jaundice, biliary concretions, chronic hepatitis, etc." The first curative symptom above noted would seem to point to the spleen as the diseased organ, although it may have been the lung, or even a myalgic affection, accompanied with cough. It is said to have cured "*indurations of the abdomen,*" but no details are given, nor the name of the observer, and consequently we are at a loss to know their character.

Stool.—Pressure to stool without evacuation, with the sensation of a mass in the lower part of the rectum; this sensation recurred frequently during the day, without stool; inoperative pressure to stool, then vomiting; feeling to pressure to stool; in the afternoon frequent pressure to stool, but only discharges of flatus; frequent discharges of very offensive flatus; in the morning a hard stool; diarrhœic stools with great flatulence; purging; after cutting pains, stools; after severe pains, stool like water; diarrhœa in the evening, with disappearance of the coryza and catarrh; diarrhœa terminated the pain in the breast; dysentery; the food passes away undigested in the stool; five natural stools in the day; two small but not fluid stools the first day; the first days the stools more laxative and frequent, afterwards rather costive; hemorrhoids, a twisting pain on the left side above the groin, equi-distant from the symphysis pubis, and the crest of the ilium; worse whilst sitting, standing, or bending towards the right side, increased by pressure; better whilst walking erect; afterwards this pain passed towards the hip, around and upwards until it reached posteriorly on the short ribs and remained peculiarly sensible by bending to the right.

Clinical Remarks.—The blood-root does not generally purge unless given in large doses, hence it will not be found often indicated in *diarrhœa.* There is one variety of diarrhœa, however, in which it has been found curative, by Dr. Bute, namely: "With the diarrhœa, termination of the coryza and catarrh," also, "The affection of the breast always ended with the feeling as if hot water were poured from the chest into the abdomen, which was *followed by diarrhœic stool.*" The "*Dysentery,*" marked as curative in the original proving, is merely an observation of Rafinesque, (botanist). Some dysenteric symptoms, however, are found in the pathogenesis, which may be made use of. Dr. Bute asserts its curative power in *hemorrhoids*, but gives no special indications, nor do we find any in the proving. The last symptoms under "*Stool,*" would seem to be misplaced. It denotes either an affection of the left *ovary*, or was simply a myalgic pain. (Take it all in all, the so-called proving of Sanguinaria, as made up for the "Transactions of the American Institute," cannot be considered a commendable production. Some of the most notable of the symptoms marked * (curative) were the mere assertions, or theoretic deductions of allopathic observers, *not* verified by homœopathic physicians. I would advise the student or physician, before he attempts to use this drug upon the information obtained in that proving, to study the original, and judge of its merits for himself.)

Urine.—*Frequent urination, also at night; large and frequent discharges of urine, as clear as water; frequent and copious nocturnal urination; seminal emissions during sleep, two nights in succession, after which he feels very well; *gonorrhœa.

Clinical Remarks.—The first curative symptoms belonged originally to the following group reported cured by Dr. Bute, namely: "In a lady, pain in the left hypochondria, which was rendered worse by coughing, but was better from being pressed, and by lying on the left side; very *copious irritation* at night." The whole group of symptoms may have been of *renal* origin. According to Dr. Coe, Sanguinaria is very useful in many functional disorder of the *kidneys.* Our provings are, however, too meagre to give us any clue to its action on those organs. I cannot ascertain who reported the curative observation "*Gonorrhœa.*" Dr. Coe advises it for chancres, buboes, secondary and tertiary syphilis, but says nothing of its use in gonorrhœa, nor does any other writer. I can readily imagine it might be useful in phagadenic chancre, used internally and as a topical application.

Generative Organs of Women.—Abdominal pains, as if the menses would appear; abdominal pain the whole night, like the menstrual; at times it increases menstruation; the menses appear a week too early, with a discharge of black blood; abortion on account of too strong operation on the uterus; causes uterine hemorrhage; amenorrhœa; the menses appear at the proper time, but still much more freely than at other times, with less pain and weakness in the sacrum, but with pain in the right side of the head and forehead, and a feeling as if the eyes would be pressed out of the head, worse on the right side.

Clinical Remarks.—*Rafinesque* used it successfully in *Amenorrhœa. Dr. O'Connor*, (allopathist), writes:—"For the last twelve years I have used the tincture of Sanguinaria exclusively, in the treatment of *amenorrhœa*, and have recommended it to others, who speak favorable of its effects. In that time I have treated as many cases of this disease, as usually falls to the lot of a village practitioner, and, as yet, have no cause to find fault with the efficiency of the remedy. I consider it superior to Eberle's great remedy, the tincture Polygonum hydropiper. I commence a fortnight before the expected return of the menses, and give teaspoonful doses of the tincture three times a day, and a teaspoonful on going to bed (preceded by a warm foot-bath). If the secretion is not restored at the time, I remit the use of the remedy for a fortnight, and proceed as before. When the full effect of the remedy is produced, it is characterized by slight nausea, *pains in the loins*, extending through the *hypogastric and iliac regions, as well as down the thighs.* These symptoms sometimes manifest themselves once or twice before the discharge is completely established."—(*Cin. Lancet and Observer.*) The symptoms which I have placed in *italics* are worthy of being noticed, as purely pathogenetic. I esteem the blood-root a good remedy in *suppressed menses*, but chiefly indicated when the suppression has been *followed, or preceded by pulmonary disease.* Its use in such cases has generally been attended with good results. Dr. Miller, (eclectic), advises it in *dysmenorrhœa*, when occurring in torpid subjects, but says it is "contra-indicated in patients of plethoric habit." This would indicate to us that it would be useful in dynamic doses in dysmenorrhœa, when menses too frequent in such patients, when there is a tendency to congestion of the brain or lungs. It is homœopathic to threatened *abortion*, when the symptoms mentioned by Dr. O'Connor are present, accompanied with some hemorrhage. It is used for this criminal purpose in domestic practice, and by unprincipled physicians. Dr. Bute reports the following case cured with the blood-root, "a female who had distention of the abdomen in the evening, and flatulent discharges per vaginum, from the os uteri, which was constantly open, at the same time a pain passing in rays from the nape of the neck to the head." This was probably an instance of that rare disease in which the lining membrane of the uterus secretes a gas. Dr. Bute also reports cases of affections of women at the climacteric period, characterized by "burning of the palm of the hands and soles of the feet, compelling her to throw the bed clothes off the feet for the purpose of cooling them." Used internally and topically, (by injection), it has cured ulcerations of the os uteri, corrosive and fœtid leucorrhœa, and polypi of the uterus.

Catarrhal Symptoms.—Much sneezing; fluid coryza, with frequent sneezing; severe fluid coryza in the right nostril; watery, acrid coryza, which renders the nose sore; copious watering of the right eye; the eye painful, especially on being touched; and soon afterwards there occurred a copious watery discharge from the right nostril; in the evening two diarrhœic stools, and then all the symptoms disappeared, (five hours after taking it); fluid coryza alternating with stoppage of the nose; aphonia, with swelling in the throat; tickling irritation to cough; influenza; coryza; rawness in the throat; pain in the breast; cough, and finally diarrhœa.

Respiratory Organs.—Slight cough, especially whilst eating; tickling in the throat in the evening, with slight cough and headache; a slight cough from tickling in the throat, many evenings after lying down; a dry cough, awakening him from sleep, which will not cease until he sat upright in bed, and flatus was discharged both upwards and downwards; *chronic dryness in the throat, and sensation of swelling in the larynx, and expectoration of thick mucus.—(*Dr, Neidhard.*) *Continued severe cough, without expectoration, with pain in the breast, and circumscribed redness of the cheeks.—(*Dr. Burt.*) *Feels stronger and freer in the breast in the mornings, and in the afternoon, and in the evening the customary dyspnœa does not appear.—(*Dr. Husman.*) A hot, burning, streaming in the right breast, begins under the right arm and clavicle, and draws itself downwards towards the region of the liver, (afternoon of the third day,) acute stitches in the right breast in the region of the nipple.

Clinical Remarks.—Sanguinaria has always had an extensive regutation in the cure of coughs. The aborigines of the Eastern States often astonished the early settlers by the cures they effected with this remedy. It is said that the most obstinate coughs disappeared during the use of the blood-root. The physicians of an early day seem to have used blood-root more frequently than their successors. Rafinesque, Barton, Tully and others, all assert its great curative power in many varieties of cough. They even assert its power to cure pulmonary consumption. Besides the above curative symptoms the following are reported: "Cough, with coryza; then diarrhœa;" "tormenting cough, with expectoration and circumscribed redness of the cheeks." Several instances have come under my observation, where the blood root really appeared to cure phthisis.

Breast.—Whooping cough; hydro-thorax, (a); asthma, (a); pneumonia, (a); typhoid pneumonia, with very difficult respiration, cheeks and hands livid, pulse full, soft, vibrating and easily compressed, (a); diseases of the lungs, (a); pain in the breast, with periodic cough, (h); pain in the breast, with cough and expectoration, (h); pain in the breast with dry cough, (h); burning and pressing in the breast, then heat through the abdomen, with diarrhœa, (h); slowly shooting pain in the right side of the chest about the seventh rib; acute stitch in the right breast; slowly shooting pain in the left side of the chest near the axilla; stitches from the lower part of the left breast to the shoulder; pressing pain in the region of the heart; stitches in the left side in the region of the short ribs, by moving and turning the body; continued pressure and heaviness in the whole of the upper part of the chest, with difficulty of breathing; slowly shooting pain under sternum numb pain the whole length of the scapula, along the inner edges, which is also increased by breathing; pressing pain in the breast and back; palpitation of the heart, from immoderate doses, with great weakness; stitches in both breasts; severe soreness under the right nipple, aggravated by being touched; the nipples are sore and painful.

Clinical Remarks.—The "curative" symptoms above, which are designated (a) are from allopathic sources; (h) from homœopathic sources. Eclectic physicians use it in thoracic diseases where the allopath censiders Tartar emetic indicated. In this they are not far from the truth. Sanguinaria, in affections of the lungs, occupies a place midway between Phosphorus and Tartar emetic. It has many symptoms in common with both, and others possessed by neither. I have used the blood-root for many years in *bronchitis*, *pneumonia*, and other diseases of the respiratory organs, and have obtained from it some very satisfactory results. In the massive doses of the old school given to nausea and emesis, it was productive of great injury, but in dynamic doses its use is never attended with any aggravations; a few drops of the mother tincture may be used in some chronic affections of the pulmonary organs, while in acute diseases, with a high grade of irritation, the 30th is the safest and best attenuation. In the majority of cases of pneumonia, there occurs a group of symptoms for which we have generally used phosphorus or sulphur, with good results, although the convalescence under those remedies is apt to be lingering. But when those symptoms and conditions are met with, under Sanguinaria, 2nd dil. (decimal), or Sanguinarin, 4th trit., a rapid subsidence of the diseased action occurs. At the second, and during the existence of the third stage of the inflammation, we have as physical signs: dullness on percussion, bronchial respiration, etc., denoting the presence of red, or even gray hepatization, and purulent infiltration of the pulmonary parenchyma. Watson considers it doubtful whether recoveries take place from the third stage of pneumonia; but under homœopathic treatment, I do not believe such recoveries impossible. The general symptoms indicating Sanguinaria are extreme dyspnœa, short, accelerated, constrained breathing, the speech ceases to be free, the sputa becomes tenacious, rust-colored, and is expectorated with much difficulty. The position of the patient is upon the back; there is not much pain in the chest, unless the pleura are involved, and then it is of a burning, stitching character. The pulse is quick and small—the face and extremities inclined to be cold, or the hands and feet burning hot, with circumscribed redness and burning heat of the cheeks, especially in the afternoon. Under the use of this remedy, the dyspnœa subsides, the bronchial breathing disappears, we hear afresh the small crepitation, and first, alone, then mixed with the natural respiratory murmur, which in its turn becomes alone audible. The sputa becomes again less tenacious, less red and yellow, and more like the expectoration of catarrh, and is expectorated in large, heavy masses; the febrile symptoms gradually abate, and a favorable convalescence is established. I give the medicine every two hours, generally alone, but occasionally in alternation with Phosphorus or Tartar emetic. In its power over chronic, bronchial or laryngeal coughs, it rivals Lycopodium and Sulphur. It relieves, and often cures, "coughs with chronic dryness in the throat, and sensation of swelling in the larynx; continual severe cough without expectoration, with pain in the breast, and circumscribed redness of the cheeks;" "cough, with coryza, then diarrhœa." This last symptom is an important indication for the use of Sanguinaria. After a severe cold, or undue exposure, some persons are attacked with coryza, catarrhal headache, severe pains in the chest, with tightness of breathing, and dry harrassing cough, all of which subsides upon the recurrence of diarrhœa. In such cases Sanguinaria is eminently indicated, as it causes a similar group of symptoms. Dr. Morrow praises it very highly in *hæmoptysis*. In one case which came under my observation it seemed to correct the bleeding, promptly. Cases have been reported to me, where the tincture of blood-root, cured spitting of blood, which had resisted other means. It will undoubtedly be found useful in some cases of Asthma, Croup, Larygnitis, and perhaps *Pleurisy*, but we have no homœopathic testimony of its effects in those diseases.

Back.—Pain in the nape of the neck; soreness of the nape of the neck on being touched; pain in the left side of the nape of the neck; pain in the right side of the neck, as if sprained; stiffness of the nape of the neck; pain in the back; pain in the sacrum and bowels—(Dr. Bute); *pain in the sacrum from lifting; pain in the sacrum, which is alleviated by bending forward; rheumatic pains in the nape of the neck, shoulders and arms; pain in both shoulders; severe pains in the left shoulder, in the evenings; pain under the sholder-blade, with chill; pain from the left breast to the shoulder; rheumatic pain in the right shoulder, worse in the forenoon when she has retained the arm for a long time in the same position, drawing itself downwards to the elbow; pain on the top of the right shoulder; sudden rheumatic pains in the shoulder joints; in the upper part of the shoulder joint, severe pain on every motion; *rheumatic pain in the right arm and shoulder, worse at night, in bed; cannot raise the arm,—(Dr. Bute); *pain in the right shoulder, and in the upper part of the right arm, worse at night on turning in bed.—(Dr. Jeanes).

Clinical Remarks.—Nearly all the symptoms of the back, etc., are purely *myalgic*, and are easily mistaken for rheumatism; in prescribing this medicine, this distinction should be made. The curative symptoms appear to have been rheumatic, all but the "pain in the sacrum from lifting."

Superior Extremities.—Rheumatic pains in the arms and hands; rheumatic pains in the right forearm, in the evening; severe pain in the hand, with aching in the arm when lying quiet and warm in bed; it is also often felt in the left foot, now above, then in the instep, and then in the toes; in the right palm near the index finger, a severe pain as from a boil; *burning of the palms redness of the hands, and severe burning; *lividity of the hands in pneumonia; numb pain in the ball of the right thumb; cutting pain on the left joint of the left middle finger; sticking in the point of the right small finger; stiffness of the finger joints; pain, as from a boil, at the root of the right thumb nail, then in the left, from this to all the fingers, one after another, from the thumb to the small finger, alike on both hands; *ulceration of the roots of the nails on all the fingers of both hands.

Inferior Extremities.—Rheumatic pain in the left hip; pain as from a bruise in the left hip joint, whilst walking, but worse on rising from a seat; *a rheumatic pain on the inside of the right thigh; *a bruise-like pain in the thigh, alternating, with burning and pressure in the breast; *stiffness of the knees; stiffness and tightness in the bend and sides of the knees; cramp and pain in the calf of the left leg; drawing in the calves and into the instep, worse right than left; sticking pain in the right ankle; continual stitches under the right exterior ankle bone, as from the sting of a bee; pain in the left foot, with headache, and during the pain in the right arm; sticking as from a needle in the instep, in the morning in bed, and in the afternoon; coldness of the feet; *burning in the soles of the feet, worse at night; burning of the hands and feet in the night; pain in the corns; great weakness of the limbs, with pains in the sacrum whilst walking; *acute swelling of the joints of extremities.

Limbs.—Rheumatic pains in the limbs; acute, inflammatory, and arthritic rheumatism; acute swelling of the joints of the extremities; stiffness of the limbs and rheumatic pains, with headache; pain in those places where the bones are least covered with flesh, but not in the joints; on touching the painful part, the pain immediately vanished and appeared in some other part.

Clinical Remarks.—The clinical symptoms above, are mostly from homœopathic sources. The physician can draw his own deductions from them.

SARRACENIA PURPUREA.

(*Huntsman's Cup.*)

A perennial plant, indigenous to the United States, with leaves of a singular character. The curious pitcher-shaped leaves, "are usually half filled with water and drowned insects; the inner face of the hood is clothed with stiff bristles pointing downward." Dr. C. H. Cleaveland, of Cincinnati (*Journal of Rational Medicine*), says: "Of the Sarracenia, there are several varieties. As long since as the writer's earliest recollection, an aged female living near his father's residence, was famous for the *syrup* which she made for the cure of chlorosis and other derangements of the uterine organs, and for the relief of dyspepsia and other gastric difficulties. Not all the ingredients of the syrup were made known to those who purchased of her; but, after a time, it was discovered that it owed all its active properties to the Sarracenia, with perhaps the mucilage of the *Osmundia regalis*. Within the last five years, I have again had my attention called to the side-saddle plant, from learning that it was used by a Canadian French doctor as a regulator of uterine derangement; and, for several years, I have, with satisfactory success, prescribed it in many cases of gastric disease, in the form of an infusion, or in that of a syrup, made from the leaf or the root. During the year 1847, Dr. F. P. Porcher, of South Carolina, experimented with the *root*, or that portion of the stem which is below the surface of the ground. He thinks the *bitter* and *astringent* principles of the plant are imperfectly extracted by water, and that the *decoction* is even more destitute of these properties than the cold infusion. He made trial of the root, in a recent state, as well as of the dried root, on his own person, and gives the following, as the result of one of his experiments: 'Dec. 4th.—We again commenced experimenting with it. It had become dry, having been rolled into pills of three grains each. Of these we took sixty (180 grs.) between ten and twelve o'clock P. M., upon a comparatively empty stomach, swallowing them at intervals, six or eight at a time. Its diuretic action in this instance was frequently repeated, the secretion being increased in quantity—pure, limpid, and colorless, with scarcely any sediment after several hours' standing. Its action on the stomach resembled that following its first employment, being attended with the same phenomena. A feeling of emptiness was produced in the course of an hour. After retiring to bed, the whole abdominal region was in a state of commotion, extending along the track of the ascending and descending colon, all of which appeared to participate in a kind of rolling motion produced by it. To these were added involuntary rumbling sounds, as if the entire alimentary tube was stimulated, and apparently forewarning a cathartic effect. We are led to believe that its astringent property prevented this result. There was, also, tenderness on pressure of the epigastrium. The feeling of congestion about the head, with irregularity of the heart's action, which *lasted several days*, was again observed. Before morning, the pulse rose to 100 by the watch, resuming its usual frequency after a time. We were prevented by sleep, which was much disturbed, from ascertaining positively the co-existence of strange impressions on the sensorial functions. The general vigor of the digestive apparatus was increased. The appetite following, the next day, was unusually active, seeming to demand much more to satisfy its requirements; but there was a sense of pain about the stomach like that following inflammation, or that felt in the muscular tissue after a limb has been overtasked.' In the first experiment, in which Dr. Porcher took 140 grains of the *fresh* root, the symptoms produced were very similar to those detailed in the above quotation, pointing distinctly to the parts of the system influenced by the drug; namely, *the gastric filaments of the ganglionic or organic system of nerves.* This produced an increased action of the circulatory system, and drove the blood to the head. It also increased the peristaltic motion of the entire alimentary canal, and promoted the renal and other glandular secretions, without any apparent effect upon the nerves of animal life. As the experiments of Dr. Porcher are directly corroborative of those made by the writer, and confirmatory of the utility of the plant in all cases where there is a sluggish or torpid condition of the stomach, the intestines, the liver, the kidneys, or the uterus—producing co-tiveness, dyspepsia, amenorrhœa, dysmenorrhœa, and the various functional derangements which are so commonly to be met with—it must be evident that this plant possesses valuable properties, which render it well worthy the attention of the enlightened practitioner. Within the past year, several articles have been published in regard to it, of such a nature as to attract considerable attention; and, although some of the statements made in regard to it are certainly erroneous, and others may prove to be too strong and positive, it seems entirely proper to place them on record, and in the way of repeated and thorough tests."

The Am. Medical Times has the following letter by Fred. W. Morris, M. D., Resident Physician of the Halifax Visiting Dispensary: "*Sir*—You have by this time, in all probability, heard something of an extraordinary discovery for the cure of small-pox, by the use of 'Sarracenia purpurea,' or Indian cup, a native plant of Nova Scotia. I would beg of you, however, to give full publicity to the astonishing fact, that this same humble bog-plant of Nova Scotia is the remedy for small-pox, in all its forms, in twelve hours after the patient has taken the medicine. It is also as curious as it is wonderful that, however alarming and numerous the eruptions, or confluent and frightful they may be, the peculiar action of the medicine is such that very seldom is a scar left to tell the story of the disease. I will not enter upon a physiological analysis now; it will be sufficient for my purpose to state, that it cures the disease as no other medicine does—not by stimulating functional re-agency, but by actual contact with the virus in the blood, rendering it inert and harmless; and this I gather from the fact that if either the vaccine or variolous matter be washed with the infusion of the Sarracenia, they are deprived of their contagious properties.

The medicine, at the same time, is so mild to the taste, that it may be mixed largely with tea or coffee, as I have done, and given to connoisseurs in these beverages to drink, without their being aware of the admixture. Strange, however, to say, it is scarcely two years since science and the medical world were utterly ignorant of this great boon of Providence; and it would be dishonorable in me not to acknowledge that had it not been for the discretion of Mr. John Thomas Lane, of Lanespark, County Tipperary, Ireland, late of Her Majesty's Imperial Customs of Nova Scotia, to whom the Mec-Mac Indians had given the plant, the world would not now be in possession of the secret. No medical man before me had ever put this medicine upon trial, but in 1861, when the whole Province of Nova Scotia was in a panic, and patients were dying at the rate of twelve and a half per cent., from May to August, Mr. Lane, in the month of May, placed the 'Sarracenia' in my hands to decide upon its merits; and, after my trials then and since, I have been convinced of its astonishing efficacy. The only functional influence it seems to have, is in promoting the flow of urine, which soon becomes limpid and abundant, and this is owing perhaps to the defecated poison or changed virus of the disease exclusively escaping through that channel. The 'Sarracenia,' I have reason to believe a powerful antidote for all contagious diseases, lepra, measles, varicella, plague, contagious typhus, and even syphilis, also a remedy in jaundice. I am strongly inclined to think it will one day play an important part in all these."

Report by Dr. Herbert Miles, of the British army:—"Early in the last winter a small coasting vessel landed a portion of her crew at an obscure seaboard village a few miles from Halifax, N. S. These persons were sick with small-pox, and the disease soon spread, first among the cottagers, with whom the fishermen mixed, and subsequently among those from the capital, who resorted to the village for purposes of trade. Through the early weeks of spring, rumor constantly asserted that vast numbers of the seafaring population were attacked with the complaint; but it was not until early in March that the large Civil Hospital of Halifax, by the number of its weekly admissions for variola, began to corroborate rumor, and to authenticate the justice of public anxiety. The disease, in process of time, extended to the troops in the garrison, but the proportion of attacks to those among the civil population, was singularly small. While certain portions of the inhabitants of Halifax were suffering from the epidemic, alarming accounts reached that place, relative to the terrible ravages of the scourge among the Indians, and colored people generally. Variola is the special plague of the Indians; and when they are invaded by this pestilence, it sweeps them off by scores. Like the fire of the prairies, it passes over their encamping grounds, destroying all of human kind in its path. On this occasion the most painful details were given of whole families being carried off by this loathsome disease. After some time, however, it was said that the pestilence had been stayed. One of the Indian race, it was asserted, had come into the disease-stricken camp, possessed of a preparation which had the extraordinary power of curing the kind of cases that had hitherto proved so fatal. This remedy was believed by the Indians to be so efficacious, that if given to them when attacked with small-pox, they looked forward with confidence to a speedy and effectual cure. An old weird Indian woman was the fortunate possessor of the remedy in question. She had always been known as the Doctress of her tribe, and had enjoyed celebrity for many years in consequence of her reputed knowledge of Medicine, and wonderful acquaintance with the herbs and roots of the woods. So well established was her fame among the Indians, that when sick they resorted to her in preference to the white doctors, whom they considered to be 'No good.' Captain Hardy, of the Royal Artillery, an accomplished and intelligent officer, who has been for years among the Indians, says that 'the old squaw's remedy had long been known to them as an infallible cure for small-pox,' and that 'the Indians believe it to be successful in every case.' From the information gathered from the Indians, the following observations have been carefully sifted: 1. In the case of an individual suspected to be under the influence of small-pox, but with no distinct eruption upon him, a wine-glassful of an infusion of the plant, 'Sarracenia purpurea,' or pitcher-plant is to be taken. The effect of this dose is to bring out the eruption. After a second and third dose, given at intervals of from four to six hours, the pustules subside, apparently losing their vitality. The patient feels better at the end of each dose, and in the graphic expression of the 'Mec-Mac,' 'knows there is a change within him at once.' 2. In a subject already covered with the eruption of small-pox in the early stage, a dose or two will dissipate the pustules, and subdue the febrile symptoms. The urine from being scanty and high-colored becomes pale and abundant, whilst from the first dose the feelings of the patient assure him that 'the medicine is killing the disease.' Under the influence of the remedy, in three or four days the prominent symptoms of the constitutional disturbance subside, although as a precautionary measure, the sick person is kept in the camp until the ninth day. No marks of the eruption (as regards pitting, etc.,) have been left in cases examined, if treated by the remedy. 3. With regard to the medicine acting (as is believed by the Indians) in the way of a preventive, in those exposed to infection, it is curious to note, that in the camps where the remedy has been used, the people keep a weak infusion of the plant prepared, and take a dose occasionally during the day, so as to 'keep the antidote in the blood.'"

We find also that the following result of a trial of the Sarracenia has been communicated to the London Times by Mr. Cosmo G. Logie, Surgeon-Major Royal Horse Guards (Blue). Eleven men of Mr. Logie's regiment, which is stationed at Windsor, contracted the disease. After expressing his disbelief in the perfect protecting power of vaccination, he writes: "Some time ago, seeing a paper written by Assistant Surgeon Miles, of the Royal Artillery, on the efficacy of the North American plant, called the Sarracenia purpurea, or pitcher-plant, in the treatment of small-pox among the Indians, my colleague (Mr. Agnis) and myself have given this remedy. Four of the cases in my hospital have been severe confluent cases; they have, throughout the disease, all been perfectly sensible, have had excellent appetites, been free from pain, and have never felt weak. The effects of this medicine which I have carefully watched, seemed to arrest the development of the pustules, killing, as it were, the virus from within, thereby changing the character of the disease and doing away with the cause of pitting, and thus avoiding the necessity of gutta percha and India rubber applications, or opening the pustules. In my opinion, all anticipations of disfigurement from pitting may now be calmed, if this medicine is given from the commencement of the disease."

A proximite analysis of the Sarracenia by Theobald Frohwein, of New York, gave: "Organic elements—traces of volatile oil, gum, starch, vegetable albumen, tannin, resin, bitter principle, with acid reaction and extractive matter. Inorganic elements—sulph. lime, carb. acid, sulph. acid, phosph. acid, traces of lime, magnes., potass. and soda, iron and silicic acid." A committee of the New York Med. Society (Allopathic) made a report on Sarracenia, which will be found in full, pages 7 and 19, American Med. Times, Jan., 1864. They thus close their report: "Your committee has endeavored to lay before the Society the history and recorded experience thus far in the use of the Sarracenia purpurea, for the treatment of small-pox; and, in conclusion, would respectfully submit the following as their deductions from the testimony here accumulated:—1st. That the analyses already made of the plant do not give any active principle or elements which would indicate any great medicinal potency. 2d. That the discoverers and advocates of the specific remedial power of the Sarracenia purpurea over variola have given, apparently, too great credit to the 'post hoc' circumstances, as being 'propter hoc' influences, (one reason for this latter inference being suggested by the loose, unscientific, and eulogistic style of the communications). And, 3rd, that the reliable experience thus far, appears to preponderate against the remedial efficacy of this plant in those forms of disease which do not generally recover under the administration of ordinary remedies." From these allopathic deductions we dissent. 1. The analysis showing the presence of sulph. lime, carb. acid, sulph. acid, phosph. acid, and traces of lime, magnes., potass. and soda, and silicic acid, also tannin, bitter principle, etc., would evince that it is a remedy of considerable power, rather than an inert substance. 2. Although the reports have been exaggerated in many instances, the recommendations, homœopathic and allopathic, are too numerous to be discarded.

The testimony relates to the empirical use of the plant. Until we obtain a thorough proving, we shall not have any reliable data for its homœopathic application.

SCUTELLARIA LATERIFOLIA.

(*Scull Cap.*)

This is an indigenous plant, growing in most parts of the United States, in woods, meadows, and near small streams and ponds. There are several varieties of this plant, and they should not be confounded with each other by our pharmaceutists. The *whole plant* is officinal; it should be gathered while in flower. The tincture is best when made from the green herb. For my estimate of the general therapeutic and pathogenetic effects of this plant, I would refer the reader to my notice of the Cypripedium pubescens; not that I consider these two remedies as possessing *identical* properties, but they are such close analogues, and affect the system in such a *similar* manner, generally, that many of my remarks applied to Cypripedium, will be applicable to Scutellaria. I have used the latter in *diseases of children, and affections of the nervous system*, similar to those in which I recommended the former, and with like good results. That a careful proving would elicit *different* symptoms, I do not doubt. If I were to attempt a differential estimate of the two remedies, I should say that the *Scutellaria affected the spinal cord more, and the brain less, than the Cypripedium.* I believe this statement will be verified by experience and observation. As substantiation, in part, of this opinion, I quote the following from Jones and Scudder's Materia Medica: "It has been found remarkably efficacious in Chorea, or St. Vitus' dance. Dr. Beach states that he has cured a great number of cases with it. We have used it in several instances with apparent benefit. In cases of great nervous excitement, with severe tremors, also in attacks of delirium tremens, it has in several cases afforded prompt relief." It has been highly extolled in many of the nervous and spasmodic affections so very common among women. It has attracted much attention in *Hydrophobia*, and at one time it enjoyed a high reputation in the treatment of that formidable disease, although the same reliance is not now placed on it that was some years ago; still, it is resorted to, both as a prophylactic and curative agent, in cases of canine madness. Testimony is not wanting to establish the fact that many persons have been bitten by rabid animals, and avoided the development of the disease by the free use of Scutellaria; while others, bitten at the same time, by the same animal, became hydrophobic. So many circumstances may concur to prevent the inception of the canine virus at the time of the bite—as the interference of clothes, or the speedy removal of it from the parts bitten and thus preventing it from being absorbed—that we must view many of the cases said to have been cured by the exhibition of this article, as highly equivocal. "A physician, bitten by a mad dog, has assured me," says Rafinesque, "that himself, alone, had avoided the disease by using it, while others bitten by the same dog, died." Dr. Vandesveer, who is said to have introduced it to the notice of the profession in 1772, or, rather, to have discovered its prophylactive powers against hydrophobia, is said to have prevented 400 persons, and 1000 cattle from becoming hydrophobic; and his son is said to have relieved or cured forty persons who had been bitten, by the use of the same agent. These favorable reports of its efficacy are strongly questioned, and even denied by eminent physicians, while many of the reformed school report very favorably of its efficacy in that disease. It would seem that there *ought* to be *some* grains of truth among so much testimony. My observations have not fallen upon any such cases; but in one patient to whom I gave the Scutellaria, first dec., for a nervous affection, its administration was always followed by the symptom—"spasmodic or constrictive closing of the jaws, and a *tightness* of the muscles of the face." A proving might elicit symptoms which would account for its efficacy in hydrophobic conditions. I have used it successfully in several cases of *tremors*, and *twitchings* of the limbs, in typhoid fever; also in mild form of hysteric spasms, nervous irritation in pregnant females, etc.; doses same as recommended for Cypripedium.

SENECIO GRACILIS.

(*Life Root. Unkum. Female Regulator.*)

This plant is indigenous, growing in rocky, poor ground, in many parts of the United States. The S. aureus and some other species possess similar properties, though not near as active. The whole herb is medicinal. The root grows just below the surface of the ground, and runs along horizontally. It is from half an inch to six or eight inches in length, and about two lines in diameter; reddish or purplish externally, purplish-white internally, with an aromatic taste, and having scattered fibers. It is found in the shops, mixed with the leaves, etc. It yields its best properties to alcohol. The *Senecin* is the concentrated, active principle of the Senecio gracilis. It is a greenish brown powder, of a peculiarly pungent smell and taste. We can use the dilutions from the *tincture*, prepared from the green plant, and triturations from the Senecin.

General Effects.—This medicine belongs peculiarly to the eclectic practice, or *did*, until I introduced it to the notice of the homœopathic school a few years since. It has been decreed to be emmenagogue, diaphoretic, diuretic, expectorant, alterative, tonic, and is said to have a peculiarly specific, *regulating* influence on the functions of the female generative organs. We have not been able to obtain any reliable proving, but present the following clinical suggestions and experience.

Nervous System.—Although its influence on the nervous system is not mentioned by any writer, yet my observations have convinced me that it ranks with Coffea, Chomomilla, Valerian, and Ambergris, and is in many respects a "nervine." It has been suggested by those familiar with its use, that it acts as a nervine, by subduing the irritation of the uterine organs, and thus prevents the nervous irritation, which might have been of a reflex character. This may be the true explanation of its action. It has a great reputation among the country people, who, under the name of "Unkum" (a name borrowed from the Aborigines) and "Wild Valerian," use it extensively for nervousness, hysteria, lowness of spirits, and sleeplesness, especially when these conditions occur in females. Under the head of "Organs of Generation," will be found a case which illustrates its action in this regard.

Mucous Membranes.—I am strongly impressed with the idea that this remedy acts upon the mucous tissues similarly to *Pulsatilla.* It causes increased secretion from the bronchial, intestinal, and vaginal mucous membranes, and has been found curative in abnormal conditions characterized by mucous discharges. It seems to me to be indicated when a catarrhal affection has appeared in *one organ, and caused, or is consequent, upon the suppression of a natural discharge in another;* thus, profuse leucorrhœa, or a bronchial, and even a nasal catarrh will set in upon the suppression of the menses, or appear in place of the menses. A catarrhal diarrhœa often appears at such times. It is in these conditions that Pulsatilla and Senecio prove so successful as curative agents, by curing the catarrhal discharge, and permitting the natural functions to go on. The Senecio has also proved useful in *hæmorrhages* from mucous surfaces, appearing upon the suppression of habitual discharges.

Skin.—It causes, in large doses, free perspiration.

Sleep.—Has proved curative in obstinate sleeplesness, or restless, uneasy sleep.

Fever.—Is considered by some as a "febrifuge," but probably is not indicated in any but *catarrhal* fever, in which condition it seems indicated.

Head, etc.—From some experience with this remedy I would suggest its use in catarrhal headache; also in catarrhal affections of the eyes, nose, and ears, particularly if these occur after suppressed perspiration, or menstrual discharge.

Gastric and Intestinal.—It may prove useful in certain *nervous* affections; also *catarrhal* conditions of the bowels. It is said to have been used successfuly in *dysentery* and *diarrhœa* (catarrhal).

Urinary Organs.—Increased flow of urine; clear, limpid urine; frequent and profuse urination.

Clinical Remarks.—This medicine has long had an extensive reputation in domestic practice as a diuretic, and used as such in cases of dropsy, suppression of urine, and irritable bladder; "As a diuretic it has been employed with advantage in calculous affections to subdue the irritation." (H. S.) "It is said to be diuretic and specific in strangury." (K.) In those anasarcous states which attend chlorosis, or attacks of women at the climacteric age, and seem to be caused remotely by some disorder of the generative organs, the Senecio gracilis may prove a very efficient remedy; also in ovarian dropsy, or dropsy occurring after suppression of the menses. The *Senecio aureus* is said to possess more specific action on the renal organs than the S. gracilis. Dr. Small has used it with benefit in some affections of the kidneys and bladder; also in diabetes.

Generative Organs of Men.—It is recommended by some physicians for the cure of gonorrhœa, in which it is asserted to have been used with benefit.

Generative Organs of Women.—It is upon these organs that the *Senecio* is reputed to exert its peculiar and specific curative influence. In accordance with the plan I proposed in the preface to this work, I shall proceed to give the suggestions, clinical experience, etc., of the eclectic and allopathic schools, and then that of our own school, together with my own. From the testimony thus adduced, the reader can come to some conclusion as to the value of the remedy. "It exerts an especial influence upon the female reproductive organs. In Amenorrhœa, not connected with some structural lesion, it has proved very efficacious. In dysmenorrhœa it has also proved valuable. It is serviceable in menorrhagia, administered both at the time of the discharge and during the interval."—(*King*). "It appears to exert a specific influence upon the uterine organs, and may with propriety be termed a *uterine tonic.* We have employed it in many cases of *Amenorrhœa*, both in retention and suppression, and almost invariably with the most gratifying results; indeed, so certain is it to restore the uterine secretion, when suppression does not depend upon organic disease, that we almost view it as a specific. Its action is peculiar; it seems to possess the power of restoring the secretion when suppressed; of promoting it when deficient; of alleviating pain in dysmenorrhœa, and of controlling or lessening the secretion when redundant; hence one of its common names, "*female regulator.*" "We have employed it to check free and too long continued lochial discharges, after other remedies had failed, and with the most gratifying results. It has proved a valuable remedy in leucorrhœa, and in displacements of the uterus, attended with dragging pains in the lower part of the abdomen and pelvic region, and with leucorrhœal discharges, when combined with Trillium." (*Jones & Scudder's, Mat. Med.*) "Senecin has proved eminently successful in the treatment of *Amenorrhœa.* When the obstruction has arisen from cold, this remedy in connection with warm alkaline pediluvia is generally sufficient. When the affection is uncomplicated, we know of no remedy so generally reliable. It operates kindly and without excitement, and the catamenial flow is restored in a manner so natural that the patient is scarcely aware of being under the influence of medicine." "We have derived equally happy effects from the employment of Senecin in the treatment of *Dysmenorrhœa.* The most beneficial results are obtained by exhibiting it during the intermenstrual period. It acts as a special tonic upon the uterine system, invigorating the menstrual function, and restoring equilibrium of action. If the menstrual secretion be *profuse* use Trillin in combination. If *scanty*, Macrotin or Baptisin may be employed." (alternated). "We have been equally successful with the Senecin in the treatment of *Menorrhagia.* It may seem somewhat paradoxical to the reader that we should prescribe the same remedy in what are generally conceived to be opposite states of the system. (Here Dr. Coe, launches out into a verbose explanation of the reason why this remedy is thus indicated, but his logic is lame, and based upon incorrect physiological doctrines.) "No matter in which direction the scale may be turned if we can but restore and equalize the functional activity of the parts, we shall effect a cure. For this purpose we employ the Senecin simply because it possesses the power of recalling or restoring lost or healthful action. This then explains the seeming paradox of giving the same remedy in dissimilar derangement of the same organ." *Chlorosis* is another of those incidental female affections in which the Senecin will be found an excellent remedy. It is particularly servicable when the chlorosis occurs in a strumous diathesis." (*Coe's concent org. med*). The following case treated with Senecio gra., is reported to me by Dr. A. R. Smart: A lady, aged forty-eight, presented the following symptoms: inability to sleep, nervous irritability, loss of appetite, coated tongue, bowels constipated, constant feeling of lassitiude, disinclined to move about, wandering pains in the back and shoulders; had been in this condition six months, during which time the catamenia, which, previous to this, had been regular in *appearance*, have not appeared; has been treated allopathically for the last three months, with no permanent benefit. I gave *Macrotin*, *Sepia*, *Secale cornutum*, *Zincum val.*, *Pulsatilla*, *Cypripedium* etc., with but little or no success. At last the *Senecio* was given in doses of twenty drops, three times per day; this was followed by a marked improvement, and after the lapse of one week she reported herself able to sleep well all night. Under the continued use of the remedy all the symptoms disappeared in the space of two weeks longer. A relapse presenting the same phenomena, which occured about six months later, was in like manner cured by the *Senecio.* The following case was reported by me to the Amer. Hom. Observer (Vol. 1, No 3). A lady, the mother of one child, had had an abortion three years ago, and another—at the second month of pregnancy—four months since. Since the date of the last abortion she had suffered much from painful menstruation, which had not been the case previously. The menses came on too soon—every three weeks; were very profuse, lasting eight or nine days; and were accompanied with a great deal of pain, of a cutting, grinding character, referred to the region of the sacrum, hypogastrium and groins. She was pale, weak, and "nervous," and had a slight cough, generally at night. Thinking this a good case in which to test the vaunted virtues of the *Senecio gracilis*, I prescribed five drops of the mother tincture three times a day, and continued its use until the next menstrual period. To the patient's gratification and my own, the menses appeared at their proper time (in 29 days), and were normal in quantity, and unaccompanied with pain or suffering of any kind. Since reporting the above case I have treated several cases of a similar nature, and with success. In one case the first dec. dilution was used; in another the first of Senecin, and in still another the second decimal. I have used it in but one case of Amenorrhœa; Pulsatilla failed to restore the discharge, but Senecin second, apparently had the desired effect.

Respiratory Organs.—Increased secretion from the bronchial mucous membrane; loose cough; rattling in the chest.

Clinical Remarks.—It affects the respiratory organs in a manner somewhat similar to Asclepias tub., Dulcamara and Pulsatilla. "In coughs, colds, and other complaints of the chest, Senecin in one of the most valuable remedies we possess. *It is especially serviceable in mucus coughs.*" (Dr. Coe.) "It has acquired considerable reputation in chronic coughs, catarrhal affections, hæmoptysis, incipient phthisis, attended with troublesome cough, *the result of obstructed menstruation*, with unequivocal advantage. (J. & S. Mat. Med.) I have used it in a few cases of cough occurring in females, according to the indication given above. It seemed to act admirably. These suggestions may seem bare and valueless, unless backed up by more pathogenetic symptoms. But it must be recollected that many of our best remedies started from just such small beginnings.

The following case reported by Dr. Thomas Irish, to the American Homœopathic Observer, seems to prove that it ranks high as a remedy in pulmonary affections. "In the year 1822, in the State of New York, I was taken suddenly with *profuse hæmorrhage from the left lung.* Physicians were sent for; consultation took place; they manifested much wisdom in endeavoring to stay the red current of life by tapping my arm. The blood refused to flow in that direction, but the lung continued to perform its office in opposition to these endeavors to change its current, by cutting the cephalic vein. All to no purpose; the life current continued to flow until it would hardly stain a white cloth. They gave me up as lost without hope, and then gave rules and ordered medicine taken. I refused to take medicine. I became a living skeleton; the dry, hacking cough, the hectic flush and sleepless nights were my companions for day and night for about five months, and still living in opposition to the wisdom of the prophets, I was in the daily habit of wandering about the fields on my father's farm, and pulling and testing of roots and herbs. The *Senecio* was before me, near a small stream. I tasted and was impressed to try its virtues. I had it gathered, roots and tops—a pailful, and prepared a strong decoction, of which I took half a table-spoonful four times a day. Improvement set in soon after commencing the use of the Senecio. In six weeks the cure seemed complete. This was in the fall. I continued well through the winter; in the spring went to work; in a month was prostrated by hæmorrhage from the lung again; continued to work until fall. Again the life root was taken, chewing the root and drinking a tea of the same. Again, contrary to the expectation of all, health was mine in the spring of 1824. I came to Michigan; worked hard all summer; in fall was taken sick; continued feeble until spring. At every attack of the disease the lungs would sympathize, so as to have it terminate in a lung fever with bloody expectoration. I employed no physician, but always used the Cure-All, as I often called it. In the too free use of the *green root* it proved a laxative, which was not favorable to the healing process. At every attack, for eleven years or more, of lung fever, which were many, I always used the same remedy with the same success. I have never known it used in such attacks without some benefit, and the number would be hundreds. I saw the blood spirt the size of a common straw from a cut in the leg. The Senecio, roots and tops bruised and applied, immediately stopped the blood; it was the only dressing. The person was not kept from his work an hour in all. It was a bad cut, and healed in a few days. It is the best dressing for cuts, bruises and sores, known to me. It has more power over diseases of the *Uterine Organs* than any other medicinal plant, in my opinion. In Erysipelas it has with me proved a useful remedy, internally and externally."

It would seem by the last paragraph to have a general curative influence over hæmorrhage, making it analogous upon some points with Erigeron, Trillium, and Lycopus. With this I leave the consideration of the plant, and hope my colleagues will prove it, and at the same time collect clinical data, illustrating the sphere of the remedy.

SILPHIUM LACINIATUM.

(*Compass Weed.*)

This is an indigenous, perennial plant, found on the prairies of the United States, from Michigan southward to Texas. The lower leaves present their edges north and south, hence the name "*compass-plant.*"

Dr. King, speaking of the S. gummiferum and S. laciniatum, says: "They are emetic in decoction. They have effected cures in intermittent fever, and are beneficial in dry, obstinate coughs. Said to have cured heaves in horses."

Dr. A. E. Small, uses and advises it in asthma and moist coughs with dyspnœa. Its present use in our school is quite limited, and until we have a thorough proving of the plant, we do not expect it will be much favored. The testimony, however, of homœopathic physicians, in regard to its curative power in *gleet*, is unequivocal. In the acute stage of gonorrhœa it does not appear to be of much service, but in the chronic stage, as well as in blennorrhœa, leucorrhœa, and vesical catarrh, it is of great value.

We hear of its use in allopathic practice in nasal catarrh, asthma, and other diseases of the respiratory organs.

It is doubtless an analogue of Copaiva, Thuya, etc., and possesses similar properties. The *peculiar* range of action of the Silphium remains to be developed by future provings.

STICTA PULMONARIA.

(*Lungwort.*)

*Nov. 9th, 1859, I commenced proving this plant, having previously prepared a strong tincture. At 7 o'clock, A. M., I took ten drops of tincture. About one hour after I had sharp, darting pains in the arms, legs, and shoulders, commencing first in the muscles of the arms, then in the finger-joints and shoulders; next in the thighs, knee-joints, and toes; also dull sensation in the head, with sharp, darting pains through the vertex, side of the face, and lower jaw. There was a feeling of fulness at the root of the nose and in the left hypochondriac region. These symptoms were well marked; they continued for two or three hours, and were followed by a general feeling of dullness of two or three hours duration.

Nov. 10th, 7 o'clock, A. M., took ten drops. The symptoms which followed were similar to those produced by the first dose. There was also, a dull, oppressive pain in the cardiac region; slight oppression of the lungs; dull pain in the right hypochondrium. Duration from three to four hours.

Nov. 11th, took at 7 o'clock, A. M., twenty drops of the tincture. About one hour after, I experienced the previous dull sensation in the head, with dull, heavy pressure in the forehead and roots of the nose; darting pains in the temporal region; burning in the eyelids, with soreness of the ball on closing the lids, or turning the eyes. There were burning, biting, sticking pains all over the body; lancinating pain in the second joint of the middle finger; inability to concentrate the mind upon any one subject; a general confusion of ideas. The above symptoms continued to increase in intensity during the entire day, and most of them continued until the 13th, without repeating the drug.

---

* Partial proving and clinical observations by S. P. Burdick, M. D., from the North American Journal of Homœopathy. (*Sticta Sylvatica.*)

CLINICAL OBSERVATIONS.—1. A few weeks previous to the above experiments, I was attacked with catarrh of the head, to which I was subject, and had been for five years; at times it was very severe, obliging me to keep my room for a week at a time. The above attack was one of the severest I had ever experienced. I discharged quantities of bloody pus from the nose and throat, and it left me with a distressing cough, and oppression of the lungs, causing the feeling of a hard mass collected in them. The cough was at first dry and hacking, from tickling in the larynx, which finally extended to the lungs. During the day I was comparatively free from cough, but it returned every evening about 6 o'clock, and would continue the entire night, being almost incessant. I could not sleep nor lie down. All treatment failed to afford the slightest relief, and I had become completely worn out from the cough and want of sleep. I now prepared a tincture from Sticta, and put a few drops in a tumbler of water. At 1 o'clock, P. M., I took a teaspoonful, and continued to repeat it every hour during the afternoon. At 10 o'clock, P. M., my cough had not returned, as I had coughed but once or twice during the evening, but on retiring that night there was a slight return, lasting perhaps for a half hour, after which I slept quietly all night. The next day I took of the medicine several times, and had no return of cough.

2.—Some two weeks after, I took a slight cold, which brought on catarrh in the head again. There came with it a slight cough, which increased, and in the evening it was quite troublesome. I took of Sticta two or three times during the evening; and, to my great surprise, I awoke the next morning perfectly free from catarrh and cough. These results of trials of Sticta on myself in disease, induced me to attempt the proving above reported. The following notes of cases treated by this remedy may show its ordinary operations in the forms of disease in which its powers have been most frequently tested.

3.—Dec. 12th, Mrs. S——— had taken a severe cold, had a hard, racking cough, aggravated by every inspiration, and there was considerable oppression of the chest. At 6 o'clock, P. M., I gave her Sticta tincture, a few drops in a tumbler of water, a tea-spoonful to be taken every half hour. The next morning she coughed but very little, said she was well, and the medicine was discontinued. A few days after she was caught out in the rain, got her feet wet, took a severe cold, and coughed worse than before. In the evening I gave her Sticta as before; the cough ceased after she had taken a few doses; and the next morning she was feeling quite well.

4.—January, 1860, Mr. B———, aged fifty-six years, was suffering from soreness of the throat of long standing, I gave Mercurius third, with favorable results. A few days after, I found him suffering from coryza, I gave him Sticta tincture, a few drops in a tumbler of water, a teaspoonful to be taken every hour. But a few doses had been taken when great relief was experienced. He had been subject to frequent attacks of a similar character for ten or fifteen years. I continued the remedy, night and morning, for a week or more, as it appeared to affect his throat favorably. While taking the remedy, he was exposed a good deal, and took a severe cold; but he was entirely free from those distressing symptoms of coryza, which had for many years accompanied the slightest cold. He had been treated by several homœopathic physicians, besides taking quantities of allopathic medicines; but he had never experienced any decided benefit from any of them. In February following, he had a slight attack, and I gave him Sticta tincture as before. He said the first dose gave him great relief. This was in the evening. The next morning he was entirely free from all traces of the troubles of the previous evening. I met him almost daily for two years after, during which time he had no return of the disease.

5.—The next case was that of a young lady who was subject to coryza. During one of these attacks, which came on in the morning, I was requested to see her. In the afternoon I found her sneezing almost incessantly, with a feeling of fulness in the right side of the forehead, extending down to the root of the nose, with tingling in the right side of the nose. Sticta tincture was given as in previous cases. Two doses effected the cure, and the next day she was feeling perfectly well. Previous attacks lasted from three days to a week.

6.—August 21st, 1862. Mr. F———, aged fifty years, came to me, saying he had rheumatism all over him, and could get no relief, he said he had tried everything, had been to two or three allopathic physicians, but was getting worse every day. His troubles commenced about six months ago, with sharp, darting, lancinating pain, first in the knee-joints, then in the elbow and shoulder. The finger-joints were next involved, and it gradually extended to every joint in the body; the pain in the neck and head were intense. At the present time the joints are all swollen and stiff. He cannot sleep for the pain, and can scarcely walk. By comparing the above with the provings of *Sticta pulmonaria*, I found a perfect type of the disease before me in this drug, and I at once determined to test its curative power; the following are the results:—I gave Sticta 1st, five drops to a tumbler of water, a table-spoonful to be taken every hour. August 23.—Mr. F—— reports himself greatly improved; pains not so severe—has *slept* better. Sticta 1st, as before. Aug. 26th.—Reports a great deal better; can walk better than at any time during the past five months; pain in the head and neck gone; all the pains are less severe, and the joints are not so much swollen. Continued Sticta, 1st, as before. Aug. 28th.—Reports himself entirely well; has no pain; swelling all gone; says he feels better than at any time during the past nine months; stiffness of the joints all gone; he is getting young again, and walks as sprightly as a young man.

7.—At the time the above was under treatment, I was also treating a Mrs. G———, aged about forty, for rheumatism of the wrist-joints. She had been under treatment for nearly three months, with very little, if any, improvement. The wrists and hands, with little if any redness; very painful on moving them. I had given her nearly all the remedies that are usually given in rheumatic troubles; none of them had afforded relief to any extent. After the results produced in the last case by Sticta, I determined to try it in the case of Mrs. G———. I accordingly gave her five drops, first, in a tumbler of water, a tablespoonful every two hours. On the second day after, I called, and on entering the room, she exclaimed, "Doctor, you have done it this time!" To my great surprise, I found her sewing. The pain and swelling were nearly gone. Sticta, first, was continued for a few days, and the cure was permanent. (This last case is reported from memory.)

8.—Aug. 20th. Mrs. M——— came to me, complaining of headache with severe pain in the eyes, which felt very sore on closing the lids or turning the eye-ball. The pains and soreness as she described them, were very similar to those I experienced while making the above provings, and I prescribed Sticta, first, five drops to a tumbler of water, a tablespoonful to be taken every two hours. Aug. 27th.—Reports greatly relieved soon after taking the medicine. Sticta continued as before. Aug. 28th—Reports perfectly well.

9.—In the month of February, 1862, while treating a patient very susceptible to the influence of medicine, I had administered Sticta one-tenth. Very soon after taking it she said, "Doctor, I feel that medicine all over me." In a few months after, she said her leg felt as though it was floating in the air, feeling light and airy, without any sensation of resting upon the bed; this continued for some time, and gradually passed off.

10.—Mrs. F———, age about forty years, had hemorrhage of the bowels. She had lost large quantities of blood during the previous weeks, looked pale and ghastly, and could scarcely walk, she had become so reduced. I gave Hamamelis, which arrested the hemorrhage; but she could not sleep, and had not for over a week; saying that as soon as it came night, her feet and legs would dance and jump around in spite of her; so that she was compelled to either hold them down on the floor with her own hands, or have some one hold them for her; and as soon as she would lie down, her limbs felt as though they were floating in the air as light as feathers. This brought to mind what had happened to the last patient, and I administered Sticta, first, a few drops in a tumbler of water. To commence taking a tablespoonful as soon as the above symptoms should re-appear, and repeat every hour. The next morning at about six o'clock, the dancing commenced. The medicine was repeated every hour until eleven o'clock, when she slept for the first time in over a week, did not awaken until seven next morning. Medicine discontinued during the day. Next evening symtoms returned, but not so severe. Medicine repeated every hour. Fell asleep at 10, P. M. Slept quietly until awakened next morning. Next evening slight recurrence. Two or three doses of Sticta were given, and she slept quietly all night. Next evening no recurrence; Sticta one or two doses; slept at 7 P. M., did not awaken until the next morning. Medicine discontinued. Recovery rapid without any further medication.

11.—A lady about fifty yeaıs of age, complaining of attacks of great anxiety about the heart. Very nervous. Had had a good deal of mental trouble. Ignatia and Digitalis afforded great relief; but after two or three months she called, saying that she was troubled at night by awaking with a strange sensation about the heart, and for a few moments after she would feel as though she was floating in the air. A few doses of Sticta first, effected a complete cure. In coughs and colds, it has proved very efficient. And I have never used a remedy which has been so efficacious in procuring quiet, refreshing sleep as *Sticta.* I have given it when all other remedies have failed, and have never, save in one or two cases, had it disappointed me; and now if I have a patient who cannot sleep, it is my first resort. I have reported two cases of rhematism which it has cured almost by magic. I have also given it in several cases in which it produced not the slightest effect; but in these cases there was not a perfect representation of the drug in the disease. The following cases are from the Case Book of the *Northern Homœopathic Dispensary*, New York, where this remedy has acquired some reputation:

1.—Ellen Murphy, aged nineteen, scrofulous; had hæmoptysis three years ago. Every cold, damp spell brings on cough with expectoration of dark blood. Suffers now with loose cough in the morning, expectoration less free during the day; pain in left side below the scapula, foul taste in the mouth, tickling in the larynx and bronchia; costiveness; courses regular. Bry. 3rd. Aug. 5—Pain in the left side less, other state the same. Sticta first. Aug. 8—Great relief. Aug. 12—Nervous headache which she complained of in the temples improved. Cough steadily improving. Sticta. Aug. 20—Cured.

2.—Anna Ernst, aged fifty-one, oppression in the pit of the stomach; great thirst, no appetite, tongue clean, disgust for food; soft cough with expectoration. Vertigo, restless at night. Bry. third. Aug. 5.—Some relief. Bry. twelfth. Aug. 9—Cough the same. Morning cough. Symptoms of change of life. Sticta first. Aug. 19—Cough improving. Raises more easily, especially mornings. Sticta first. Aug. 29—Cough well. Only some vertigo yet. Puls. sixth. Aug. 31—Cough all right. Vertigo the same. Cyclamen third.

3.—Joseph Weidner, aged forty. Dyspepsia. Cannot bear anything tight on the stomach. Vomits phlegm. Hemorrhoids. Nux. Aug. 8—Cough raw and sore. Better otherwise. Sticta. Aug. 11—Cough only after meals. Bry. Aug. 16—Cough easier, but very hoarse. Puls. Aug. 20—Cough worse, expectoration tighter. Bry. Aug. 24—Morning cough continues. Well every other way. Bryonia.

4.—Ellen Minaman, aged twenty-five. Cough for six weeks. Hoarseness; nightly expectoration of whitish phlegm. Sticta. Aug. 12—Greatly improved. Does not cough near so much. Sticta.

5.—Ida Hatfield, eighteen months old. Tussis morbillosa. Had measles two weeks ago. Sticta. Aug. 8—Greatly improved.

Sticta. Aug. 17—Has whooping cough. Sticta. Aug. 19—State the same. Worse at night. Corallia thirtieth. Aug. 24—State the same. Bell., Ipec. Aug. 29—Improving. Bell., Ipec.

6.—Kate Winkler, aged fourteen. Nasal catarrh. Nose always dry and stuffed up; swollen with tickling in it. Constant dripping down throat, which feels and looks raw. Tongue clean. Sticta. Aug. 9—Improving. Sticta. Aug. 12—Discharges a great deal of phlegm, with great improvement. Sticta. Aug. 19—Is getting well. Sticta.

7.—Martin Wyman, aged two years, febris catarrhalis. Acon. Aug. 15—Less fever. Rattling in the chest, coryza. Sticta. Aug. 18—Improving. Sticta. Aug. 21—Cured. We cured a great many such cases with Sticta.

8.—Magd. Hauser, aged forty-two. Influenza. Sticta. Sept. 29—Cough gone; pressure in the chest and abdomen, more in the left side. Caught cold when her courses were on. Sticta. Oct. 1—Cured.

9.—Emma Russ, aged sixteen years, Otalgia, noise and beating in the back part of the head. Pimples on the face. Sticta. Sept. 11—Well, except the pimples. Sepia thirtieth.

10.—Louis Walker, aged thirty-six. Influenza with bilions diarrhœa. Sticta. Sept. 7—Improving. Sticta. 9th, cured.

11.—Anne Wiebold, thirty-five years old. Loose cough with free expectoration. Worse from midnight to morning. Sticta. Sept. 9—Cured.

12.—William Coleman, aged sixty-six. Coryza, the result of sunstroke, comes back every middle of August, when not exposed; if exposed to the sun in July, it comes on then. Itching in the nose. When careless, it goes to the chest. Suffers now severely with it in the chest and head. Sticta. Aug. 31—No better. Acon. 3rd. Greatly improved. Acon. Sept. 5—Cured; never cured in so short a time before.

13.—Stephen McCue, aged four years, had measles five weeks ago, which never came out well. Cough worse night and morning; some emaciation; restless sleep on account of the cough. Sticta. Sept. 15-19—Steady improvement and cure. Sticta first.

14.—John Holt, aged seven years. Barking cough like whooping cough, from catching cold. Cured by Sticta in a few days.

15.—Rose Caen, aged thirteen years. Sept. 23—Had small-pox a few weeks ago, and has ophthalmia varilosa yet. Conjunctiva inflamed. Says she cannot see plainly. Pains worse when shutting the eyes. Sticta. Sept. 26—Great improvement. Ball clearer; vessels in the lower part of the eye full yet. Sticta. Sept. 29—Improvement continues. Sticta. Oct. 3—Caught fresh cold. Keratitis and conjunctivitis with great photophobia. Acon. followed by Apis. Oct. 4—Improving. Apis. Nov. 6. Was nearly well, till she caught cold again; has now conjunctivitis, burning pains, photophobia, hepatic eruption on the face. Apis during the day, Tr. Sulph. at night. Oct. 12—Improvement. Sulph. Nov. 4—Cured.

16.—Peter Weidman, aged forty-three. Oct. 1—Influenza,

when cough comes on he can hardly breathe; choking sensation in the throat, free expectoration; slime coated tongue with indigestion. Sticta. Oct. 2—State the same. Sticta. Oct. 4—No improvement. Bry., Merc. Oct. 6—Cured.

17.—Philip West, aged seven months. Oct. 3—Diarrhœa mucosa, and loose cough. Sticta. Oct. 5-6—Some rattling in the throat yet. Cough and diarrhœa improving. Sticta. Oct. 7—Only restless at night now. Oct. 9—Cured.

18.—Julie Eitler, aged nine months. Oct. 22—Diarrhœa, dentition, cough, and rattling in the chest. Passages green, like chopped eggs. Oct. 24—Diarrhœa improving, but cough the same still. Sulph. Nov. 4—Slimy diarrhœa again. Cough abating. Sulph. Nov. 12—Cured.

19.—Charles Bennet, aged twelve years. Oct. 26—Catarrh of the head for four years. Sneezing mornings with greenish discharges; frontal headache and epistaxis. Sticta. Oct. 25—Less bleeding from the nose. Left foot and right arm often benumbed and cold. Sticta. Nov. 4—Free from catarrh, but full of boils. Sticta. Nov. 20—Entirely well.

The following brief references to the Sticta are found in the *American Homœopathic Observer*, for July, 1864:

Dr. F. W. Bathrick cured a case of Catarrh with Sticta, after failure with the ordinary remedies. He proposes trying it in the form of inhalation.

Dr. B. M. Pettitt, finding that an epidemic Influenza prevailing in Cayuga county, New York, would not yield to the usual remedies, resorted to Sticta, and had the most gratifying success.

Timothy Baker, Esq., says, "that Mrs. Baker has been very much benefitted by Sticta, used for her cough, (character of cough not reported.)

Dr. Jno. C. Fall, says, "I have used the Sticta pulmonaria with very happy effect. I wish I had time to write of the remedy *in extenso*, but may in future."

Dr. C. W. Boyce writes, July 16th, 1864:—"Dr. Lodge,—*Dear Sir:*—In the July number of your 'Observer,' I notice a reference to Sticta, in Catarrh. This remedy has been of the greatest value in this vicinity, in that troublesome disease. During the past spring, there was an epidemic influenza which affected nearly every one, and which produced symptoms quite unusual here. These consisted of an extensive dryness of the nasal mucous membrane, which became painful. The secretions were so quickly dried, that they were discharged after great effort, in form as hard as scabs; the soft palate felt like dried leather; deglutition became painful from the same cause. Often, the catarrh extended to the chest, leaving an irritation lasting for weeks. There was, usually, a distinct exacerbation in the latter part of the day, and fore part of the night; the morning hours were nearly free from distress. *Sticta was the only remedy that relieved.*"

TRILLIUM PENDULUM.

(*Birth Root*).

This is but one of eight species of Trillium, growing in the Northern States. Few of our indigenous plants surpass them in elegance and beauty, and they are all endowed with active medicinal properties. The root of the *T. atro-purpureum*, or purple species, is generally believed to be the most active. "The Trillium has somewhat tuberous roots, having a faint, slightly terebinthinate odor, like cedar, and a peculiar, aromatic taste. Tannin, and a bitter extractive, however, form two of its active ingredients, to which its medicinal effects are doubtless owing." (Lee.) Nothing seems more ridiculous and puerile to the rational physician, particularly the homœopathist, than the senseless reiteration, that "certain drugs owe their medicinal power to the *tannin*, or other chemical principle, which they happen to contain." Thus, they (the allopaths) decree that Trillium arrests flooding, etc., because it is an *astringent*, and the *tannin* is the curative principle; they blindly deny the *specific* (*dynamic*) action of drugs, and, therefore, are obliged to take up with all such absurd subterfuges. Geranium mac. contains more tannin than any other plant, yet possesses no specific control over hemorrhages, which the Trillium undoubtedly does. (H.) Prof. Lee says:—"From all I have observed, and can gather from others, I am led to believe that the Trillium is one of our most valuable tonics, astringents, alteratives, and especially beneficial in most cases of passive, atonic hemorrhages, as menorrhagia, etc. Less astringent than many other plants, it is far more alterative and tonic, yet it has decided efficacy, as an astringent, when this indication is present." The late Dr. Williams used the powdered root in all kinds of active hemorrhages, in doses of one drachm to an adult, repeated according to the urgency of the symptoms. Dr. Stone, of Mass., has made very extensive use of it, in all forms of bleeding, especially from the womb and lungs, and, as he thinks, with great and decided benefit. In the various forms of scrofula and cutaneous diseases, he has also seen great advantage from its use. In popular practice, the *Birth-root* is used in parturition, and is believed to facilitate the birth of the child, hence its name. *Dr. Lee* found it employed extensively for this purpose, among the Chippewa Indians, on Lake Superior. They also believed it to be a certain specific for the bite of the rattlesnake. It seemed to be their favorite remedy in all female complaints, especially *those attended with discharges*; indeed the evidence in its favor, in cases of vaginal and uterine leucorrhœa, is very strong and satisfactory; also in passive bronchorrhœa and hæmoptysis." *Dr. Coe* (Concentrated Organic Med.) says: "Its dynamic influences are chiefly directed towards the mucous surfaces, over which it seems to exercise a special control. Though mostly employed in affections of the uterine system, it is nevertheless, of great utility in the treatment of all diseases involving the mucous membranes. It is decidedly antiseptic, and is useful in correcting a tendency to putrescency of the fluids, and the fœtor of the critical discharges. Slight hemorrhages occurring from wounds, cancerous ulcerations, etc., may be corrected by its local application."

Skin.—Applied to erysipelatous and other ulcers, it is said to restrain the profuse discharges; slight hemorrhages, occurring from wounds, cancerous ulcerations, etc., may be arrested by the same means.

Nose.—"A solution of the Trillin, or the dry powder, snuffed up the nostrils, will immediately check an epistaxis." (*Coe.*) This use of Trillium is quite common in domestic practice. It is asserted, on good authority, that epistaxis may be arrested by smelling of the recent root. I found it to act promptly in a case of obstinate *passive* epistaxis, after other remedies had failed; it was given in five drop doses of the first dilution and a solution of the same strength, was snuffed up the nostrils.

Teeth.—A small quantity of the powder, or cotton saturated with the tincture, introduced into the cavity from which a tooth has been extracted, will effectually arrest the hemorrhage.

Mouth.—"It is useful in cancrum oris; putrid sore throat, etc., and as a wash or gargle." (*Coe.*)

Stomach, etc.—Heat in the stomach; burning in the stomach; thirst; increase of appetite; heat rising up from the stomach into the œsophagus.

Clinical Remarks.—The above symptoms were noticed in several cases from the 1st dec. trit. It is recommended in dyspepsia by eclectic physicians. Theoretically, I would suggest it in "gastric catarrh;" erosion of the mucous coat, with hæmatemesis.

Abdomen, Stool, etc.—Constipation; hard, dry stool.

Clinical Remarks.—It is undoubtedly useful in chronic diarrhœa, where the discharges are mainly of mucus, or of bloody mucus; in dysentery, when the amount of blood is considerable, and the discharges are fœtid, after the acute stage, and when the disease threatens to become chronic. It is evident that a remedy which exercises such specific power over passive discharges from nearly all mucous membranes, should be useful in chronic intestinal discharges of that character.

Urinary Organs.—It is highly recommended in hæmaturia. Its action on the urinary organs is similar to that of Uva ursi, Chimaphila, and Copaiva. *Dr. King* says: "An infusion of equal parts of Trillium and Lycopus v. has been highly recommended for the cure of diabetes." Dr. Jones (Mat. Med.) asserts: "I have used it freely in diabetes, and from the advantages derived from its use in those diseases, we think it merits a conspicuous place among the list of our therapeutical agents, and one upon which much reliance can be placed in that formidable disease." Judging from its curative action in other diseases, it should prove useful in chronic catarrh of the bladder, chronic urethritis, gleet, and even in some conditions found in chronic nephritis. Dr. E. G. Wheeler reports the following cases illustrative of its effects in flooding, menorrhagia, and leucorrhœa. (*Jour. of Mat. Med.*, vol. ii., p. 448.) CASE 1.—Mrs. G., at the third month of pregnancy, was taken at 6 o'clock, A. M., with a bloody discharge from the uterus, with pain in the back, considerable sickness at the stomach, and occasional chills. I was called in at 9 o'clock; the flooding had greatly increased during the last hour, and the patient fainted as I entered the room. The pains had ceased—os uteri dilated to the size of a twenty-five cent piece, but rather tense; loss of blood very great. I made a strong infusion of the Trillium root, and gave her two table-spoonfuls every ten minutes; in half an hour the bleeding had greatly diminished; the infusion was continued, but given at rather longer intervals, and in two hours from the time I was called in, the hemorrhage had ceased altogether; pains returned during the following night, and the fœtus was expelled with but very trifling loss of blood." CASE 2.—"Was called in at 4 o'clock, P. M., to see Mrs. S., at the full term of pregnancy; os uteri dilated to the size of a half dollar; no pains; flooding excessive. Administered the Trillium as in the preceeding case; it acted promptly, so that in an hour from the time of giving the first dose, the bleeding had entirely ceased. In about four hours more, labor pains came on, and she was shortly delivered of two healthy children, with no more than the usual amount of hemorrhage." CASE 3.—"Mrs. M., at about the third month of pregnancy, had had slight uterine hemorrhage, for two or three days previous. At 8 o'clock in the evening of the third day, she became alarmed by sudden and excessive flooding. I was immediately called in, but her fainting turns were so frequent and so protracted, that I could not give the remedy as fast as I desired; and notwithstanding I brought all the means to my aid, that I could command, I greatly feared I should lose my patient; in about three hours, however, she had taken an infusion, made with about three drachms of the bruised root as nearly as I could judge, and the hemorrhage was perfectly controlled. Thirty-six hours after this, pains came on, and the fœtus was expelled without further trouble. It may not be amiss to state, that I think I have found this remedy of decided utility in facilitating labor. I have treated cases of leucorrhœa, satisfactorily. The plant I made use of is the *Trillium atro-purpureum*." This is allopathic testimony, and better than the average; it is surprising that the medicine was given alone. According to their general usage, the physician should have given it in combination with Kino, Plumbum aceticum, or some powerful drug, and then claimed it as a cure with the Trillium. The medicine was given in large doses, yet not inordinately so—not more than two or three drachms of the mother tincture in each case. The specific curative action was promptly manifested, apparently without inducing any pathogenetic effects, showing that no injury was done by the material doses. In the cases which follow, it will be seen that more minute doses act just as well. It is decreed by some writers, that the Trillium is most useful in *passive* hemorrhages, but the cases above reported were of an opposite character. We have no proving of this remedy, showing its pathogenetic action upon the generative organs of women, nor can we decide with any certainty, as to the pathological states which it would induce in the uterine tissue. To say it acts by giving *tone* to the uterus would not convey any *exact* idea, although it actually has that effect; it stimulates the uterine nerves to healthy action, and as a consequence, we have muscular tonicity, and a healthy condition of the mucous membranes. Hemorrhages from the uterus, either arise from relaxation, or laceration of the blood-vessels of that organ, or from abrasion or relaxation of its mucous coats. Any drug, therefore, whose symptoms correspond, will possess the power of causing just such pathological changes, and will, therefore, cure similar lesions. The analogues of Trillium are Terebinthina, Sabina, Pulsatilla, and Erigeron canadensis. The following clinical cases occurred in my own practice:—CASE 1.—*Menorrhagia*—Mrs. M., aged twenty-eight, had been subject for several years, to frequent and profuse menstruation. The menses came on every fourteen days, and lasted seven or eight. In the intervening periods, there was profuse leucorrhœa, of a yellowish color, and creamy consistence. The blood was once bright red, and but lately, owing to her anæmic condition, has been pale and mixed with a leucorrhœal discharge. She took Crocus, Platina and Sabina, but with no apparent benefit. Trillium second dec. was then given, in doses of one grain, four times a day. The first effect noticed was a diminution of the leucorrhœa, then the menses delayed one week. The medicine was continued, and the next menstrual period came on at the end of four weeks, and was not followed by leucorrhœa. She was then put upon the use of Ferrum met. 1st dec. and Helonin 1st dec., one grain of the former after meals and a similar dose of the latter, before eating; and in a few weeks the strength and color returned. Several other similar cases were treated with the same medicine, and all recovered. CASE 2.—*Metrorrhagia*—Mrs. S., aged forty-six, passing through her climacteric, had occasional attacks of profuse flooding, at irregular times, so profuse as to bring her down very low; the blood was thick, dark, and clotted, and would continue several days. The attacks had been partially controlled by the use of Sabina, and Crocus, but being called during the first day of a seizure, I determined to test the Trillium. Ten drops of the 1st dec. dilution was given every half hour; in a few hours the flooding had decidedly diminished, and subsided completely in two days. This was continued, in alternation with Sanguinaria 3d., and she had no more attacks, but menstruation ceased normally. CASE 3.—Mrs. T., aged fifty, had been subject to attacks, similar to the above, but anæmic, dropsical, and much debilitated. Apis. 2, relieved the dropsy promptly; Helonin gave her more strength, and better digestion than she had had for months; and when an attack of "flooding" came on, Trillin 2nd decimal arrested it in two days. These attacks were of a peculiar character; the discharge was pale, watery, only slightly tinged with blood, but very profuse, accompanied with prostration, vertigo, dimness of sight, palpitation of the heart, and a painful sense of "sinking at the pit of the stomach."

All these symptoms, which usually lasted eight or ten days under allopathic treatment, with Sulphuric acid, and Mur. tinc. Iron, subsided in two days, under the action of minute doses of Trillin. In this case the discharge was *really* blood as much as though it had been red; but such was her anæmia, that the red globules were very deficient. She had become jaundiced, but under the use of Leptandria 2nd decimal, the liver resumed its normal functions, and her increased appetite and digestion, soon brought some color to her hitherto pallid cheeks. CASE 4.—*Hemorrhage after abortion*—The fœtus and placenta came away properly, but imprudence kept up the hemorrhage, which was dark, sanious, and accompanied with pain in the back, dragging in the loins, and soreness in the hypogastric region. All these symptoms subsided after using Trillin 2nd decimal for a few days. "In the treatment of vaginal and uterine leucorrhœa, particularly when of an atonic character, the Trillin will be found one of the most reliable remedies." In fœtid discharges from the vagina and uterus, it may be employed in the form of injection, one drachm of the powdered root to one quart of hot water—used when cool. "But among the most valuable of its hæmostatic properties, is its power of restraining profuse lochial discharges. * * * We have found the Trillin exceedingly valuable in the treatment of prolapsus uteri, particularly when of an asthenic character, and dependant upon an atonic condition of the uterine supports. In engorgements of cervix uteri, chronic vaginitis, passive hemorrhages of the uterus, it is an efficient remedy." The above is extracted from Dr. Coe's article "Trillin," and is in the main correct, for it has been used in similar conditions, in minute doses, and with success. I have found the 1st dec. or even the 3d trit. as successful as he claims massive doses are. Dr. Chamberlain (N. A. Jour. of Hom., p. 438) recommends the "Trillium, in cases of uterine hemorrhage, and profuse flooding after confinement." He prescribes half a tea-spoonful of the powdered root, in molasses, repeated every ten or fifteen minutes. Dr. Freeland has used it for thirty years, with success.

Catarrhal Affections.—It is recommended generally for *chronic* catarrhal affections, especially for cough when dependent upon chronic bronchitis, or larygnitis. In such cases it would seem to have an effect similar to Copaiva, Stannum, or Pulsatilla.

Respiratory Organs.—Dr. Coe says: "In chronic cough, accompanied with spitting of blood, the Trillin is useful, and may be combined with Lycopin." It has quite a reputation in hæmoptysis, in the eclectic school. "Trillium has been found by us, a valuable agent in hæmoptysis, also in the incipient stages of phthisis, with bloody expectoration; even in the more advanced stages, with copious, purulent expectoration, hectic fever, troublesome cough, etc., we have found it useful." (Jones & Scudder, Mat. Med.) It has even been recommended in asthma (humid) and whooping cough, but upon rather unsatisfactory data.

REMARKS.—I would recommend my colleagues to test this remedy in their practice, carefully noting its pathogenetic symp toms, and curative results. The above is mainly suggestive and clinical, but may serve as the basis upon which to build a proving. *Mode of administration.*—It may be used in the dilutions from the mother tincture, triturations of the root, or the *Trillin.* I have usually used the 2nd decimal trituration of Trillin.

VERATRUM VIRIDE.

(*American Hellebore*).

This plant, known also by the names of Swamp Hellebore Indian Poke, and Itch Weed, is indigenous to many parts of the United States, usually growing in swamps, wet meadows, and on the banks of mountain streamlets, flowering from May to July. For homœopathic use a tincture is made of the green root. The root is said to contain a principle nearly identical with *Veratria*, but Dr. King thinks it is like *Colchicia*, a distinct, though analagous principle. From *old school* and *eclectic* sources, we glean the following estimate of the properties and uses of this medicine. We have no regular and exhaustive proving, only fragmentary ones, but enough to guide us pretty correctly. Dr. W. C. Norwood, who has done much to bring this plant into notice, states that actual experiments made by himself, have proved. 1.—"It is slightly acrid, and confining this action mostly to the mouth and fauces. 2.—Expectorant, and unsurpassed by any other remedy for which this property is claimed. 3.—Diaphoretic, being one of the most curative belonging to the materia medica; often exciting great coolness or coldness of the surface; sometimes rendering the skin merely soft and moist, and at others, producing free and abundant perspiration, without reducing or exhausting the system. 4.—Adenagic, deobstruent or alterative, far surpassing Iodine, and from which much advantage may be expected in the treatment of Cancer and Consumption. 5.—Nervine, and never narcotic. This property renders it of great value in the treatment of painful diseases, and such as are accompanied with spasmodic action, convulsions, morbid irritability, and irritative mobility, as in chorea especially, epilepsy, pneumonia, puerperal fever, neuralgia, etc. And it produces its effect in this respect, without stupefying and torpifying the system, as opium is known to do. 6.—*Emetic*; it is slow but certain in its operation, efficient, rousing the liver to action during its operation, and vomits without occasioning the prostration or exhaustion which follow the action of most other emetics. It is also superior to most other emetics in not being cathartic. It is peculiarly adapted as an metic in hooping cough, croup, asthma, scarlet fever, and in all cases when there is much febrile or inflammatory action. 7.—*Arterial sedative.* This he considers its most valuable and interesting property, and for which it stands unparalleled and unequalled as a therapeutic agent. 8.—In small doses it creates and promotes appetite beyond any agent with which we are acquainted." Dr. Norwood was doubtless too enthusiastic in his praises of this medicine, just as the ancients too highly estimated the value of the Veratrum *alb.*, its nearest analogue. He has reduced the pulse by use of the tincture to thirty-five beats per minute, without exciting the least nausea or vomiting. The antidotes to its excessive action, are morphine, ginger, brandy, and laudanum. *Dr. Osgood* says it is an emetic, and its action violent and long continued. He denies its cathartic action. It increases most of the secretions, and when freely taken, exercises a powerful influence on the nervous system, indicated by faintnes, somnolency, vertigo, headache, dizziness of vision, and dilated pupils. Prof. Tully regarded it as an excellent substitute for Colchicum, in gouty, neuralgic and rheumatic affections, to which diseases it seems best adapted. Prof. Wood classes it among the "nervous sedatives" along with Digitalis, Aconite, Verat. alb, etc., and records many symptoms resulting from its use, which will be found recorded in the pathogenesis. We present the bold and heroic proving of this powerful drug, by Dr. Burt. It is a faithful record of the symptoms caused by large doses. In a note to the proving, Dr. B., writes. "I am confident that had I not assumed the horizontal posture when on the point of fainting, the syncope would have proved fatal," he intimates that a "heart-clot" would have formed, but it is doubtful if that effect would have happened: paralysis of the heart would have been the most probable result.

PHYSIOLOGICAL EXPERIMENT WITH VERATRUM VIRIDE.

By Wm. H. Burt, M. D., of Lyons, Iowa.

Dec. 21st.—In perfect health; bowels regular, once a day; pulse seventy-four; respiration twenty; took thirty drops of the 3d dec. dilution of fluid extract of Veratrum viride, prepared in water. At 10 A. M., ten minutes after, sharp drawing pain over the left eye, with a contracted feeling of the skin of the forehead; one-half after ten, constant, dull, frontal headache, with neuralgic pains in the right temple, close to the eye; eleven A. M., dull pains over the eye with quite severe drawing pains in the umbilical region—pulse sixty-seven, took fifty drops; 12 M., slight frontal headache with prickling pains in the region of the heart, frequent drawing pains in the umbilical region; pulse seventy, took sixty drops; 2 P. M., dull drawing pains in the forehead, natural stool, took one hundred drops; 3 P. M., dull, heavy, frontal headache, with prickling pains in the præcordial region; took 150 drops; 5 P. M., slight frontal headache, neuralgic pains in the region of the heart and cardiac portion of the stomach; took 200 drops; 7 P. M., very frequent neuralgic pains in the cardiac portion of the stomach; took 175 drops; slight, dull, frontal headache, neuralgic pains in the right side of the umbilicus, passing down to the groin; slight drawing pains in the right elbow and calves of the legs; sharp flying pains in the epigastric and umbilical regions, pulse sixty-six.

Dec., 22d.—Slept well, but had frightful dreams of being on the water, feeling well, pulse 79; 9 A. M., took three drops of fld. ext. one-half after nine, pulse seventy-six; slight, dull, frontal headache, with a contractive feeling of the skin of the forehead; 10 A. M., respiration twenty; took four drops; 11 A. M., dull frontal headache with neuralgic pains in the temples; sharp pains in the epigastric and umbilical regions, passing down to the pubes; pulse seventy-one; 12 M., took five drops; 2 P. M., very severe frontal headache, with dull aching pains in the umbilical region; pulse seventy-four; took six drops; 4 P. M., constant dull headache, pulse seventy; took six drops; 9 P. M., dull frontal headache, with neuralgic pains in the right temple; tongue feeling as if it had been scalded; dull aching pains in the epigastrium; very sleepy, took eight drops.

Dec. 23rd.—Had a restless night, frightful dreams of people drowning; flat taste in the mouth; tongue coated yellow along the centre; soft papescent stool, at 9 A. M., took ten drops; pulse seventy; 10 A. M., there has been constant and severe cutting, aching pains in the umbilical region with rumbling in the bowels, with a soft stool; took twelve drops; dull heavy aching pains in the region of the gall-bladder, with dull pains in the umbilical region; arms ache; 12 M., took twelve drops; 1 P. M., very severe aching in the back of the neck; very difficult to hold my head up; constant burning distress in the region of the heart; am very weak and tremble all over; pulse forty-six, soft and very weak; can hardly be felt; mushy stool without pain; 2 P. M., dull frontal headache; face is very pale; nose looks pinched and blue; constant hiccough with violent and constant spasms of the upper part of the œsophagus; cannot swallow; profuse vomiting of thick glairy mucus and water; profuse secretion of tears, and mucus from the nose, also saliva; neck aching severely, pulse forty-four, soft and very weak; twenty minutes after 2, violent vomiting; with severe frontal headache and hiccough; cannot walk; if I attempt it, I am very faint and completely blind; obliged to keep in the horizontal position; 4 P. M., pupils dilated; neck and arms ache severely; dull aching pains in the umbilical region with rumbling; cannot walk across the room without becoming blind; pulse forty-four, soft and very weak; 5 P. M., constant dull aching pains in the umbilicus, with sharp neuralgic pains in the left groin; can walk about ten rods, when I become blind, and am compelled to sit down; pulse forty-six; 8 P. M., feeling much better, pulse sixty-one, soft and weak, constant dull pain in the umbilicus, and pain in the region of the gall-bladder, took eight drops and retired.

Dec. 24th.—Slept sound, frightful dreams of the water as usual; flat, bitter taste in the mouth; tongue coated yellow along the centre; slight dull pains in the bowels; pulse sixty-four, soft and full; took ten drops; at 8 A. M., dull aching pains in the umbilicus; by spells they are very sharp and shooting, dull pains in the region of the gall-bladder, tongue feeling as if it had been scalded; took ten drops at 10 A. M.; 12 M., dull frontal headache; dull pains in the umbilicus; natural stool, followed by aching in the rectum; pulse fifty-five, soft and very weak; took ten drops; 1 P. M., very severe frontal headache; hiccough with constant and severe spasms of the upper part of the œsophagus; violent vomiting of my dinner, and then a thick glairy mucus; the secretion of saliva, mucus from the nostrils, and tears is profuse; dull aching pains and distress in the umbilical region; back of the neck and arms ache severely; almost impossible to hold my head up; pulse forty-four, soft and very weak; can just be felt; can walk about four rods, then I become blind and faint, but can sit up without any trouble; 2 P. M., hiccough lasted two hours, also the spasm of the œsophagus; dull frontal headache; severe aching in the neck very much worse by moving; dull pain in the bowels; pulse forty-six sitting or lying down; constant dull aching, burning pain in the region of the heart under the sternum; ringing in the ear; moving quickly makes me very deaf; 3 P. M., dull, hot aching pain in the region of the heart, dull pain in the umbilical region, pulse forty-six, soft and very weak; 5 P. M., pulse fifty-seven, soft and weak, burning distress in the region of the heart; dull pains in the umbilicus; 6 P. M., pulse sixty, burning distress in the region of the heart; dull pains in the bowels; 10 P. M., pulse sixty-six; dull pain in the umbilicus, with desire for stool, mushy stool, followed by an aching sensation in the rectum. Morning, feeling well; pulse sixty-six, small, quick and hard.

Nervous System.—Wood places the Verat v., among the "nervous sedatives," and nearly all writers contend that its sedative action on the heart is through the nervous system.

Nerves of Sensation.—Its action on these nerves is quite similar to that of Aconite and Verat alb.; yet, there are points of difference worthy of being noticed. It does not actually produce anæsthesia, but allays pain and hyper-catharsis. When given in rheumatism and neuralgia the pain abates as soon as the system is under the influence of the medicine. An external application of the tincture to painful swellings, eruptions, etc., is said to mitigate the painful sensations.

Nerves of Motion.—"We have observed as a result of the administration of Veratrin very singular contortions of the muscular system, particularly of the muscles of the face, neck, fingers and toes; the head would be drawn to one side, the mouth drawn down at one corner, and the facial muscles affected with convulsive twitchings; at times these contortions would take the form of tonic spasms, while at other times the action would simulate a series of galvanic shocks, frequently of such violence as to precipitate the patient out of bed; during all this time the intellect of the patient remained undisturbed, and he was conscious of all that was going on."—(*Coe* Con. Org. Med.) It would certainly seem that the Veratrum was homœopathic to chorea in some of its forms. The Veratrum viride seems to exert a *sedative* influence over the nerves, as specifically as Nux vomica and its analogues *irritate* them. Its primary action is the opposite of the primary action of Strychnine. It is secondarily homœopathic to convulsive affections. As a prompt and reliable remedy I prefer it to Aconite in hysterical, epileptiform, or puerperal convulsions; also in the convulsions of children. I have succeeded with the first decimal dilution, rarely having to resort to the mother tincture, and then only giving it in one and two-drop doses. The following allopathic experience with the Verat. v. in nervous and spasmodic affections, is worthy of place here: It is stated that animals poisoned with the Veratria from Verat. viride "*lost the power over the locomotive muscles*, and after death the galvanic current did not exercise the same convulsive movements as in cases of death from other causes."—(*Amer. Med. Times.*) Experimenters all notice a peculiar "weakness and inability to move the muscles;" also, stiffness of the voluntary musles. Dr. Baker, in the Southern Medical and Surgical Journal, gives an account of the value of the drug in the treatment of certain neuroses. *Case* 1:—"The patient was a stout, healthy man of sober habits. I found him sitting on the side of the bed, seemingly well and perfectly intelligent, unaware, however, that he had had convulsions. All that I could ascertain of his previous history was, that he had been similarly affected in childhood. While conversing with him he was suddenly, and without apparent premonition, seized with a frightful convulsion, occasioning frothing at the mouth, and the most violent jactitations of all the voluntary muscles. I immediately opened a vein and bled him profusely, but without the desired result; for, after the lapse of a certain period, with as perfect a return of consciousness as before, there occurred another convulsion of equal severity. In this emergency, the excessive muscular relaxation capable of being produced by the Veratrum viride occurred to my mind, and I reflected that such an effect could only be produced by an influence primarily exerted upon the cerebro-spinal system of voluntary nerves. I administered the Veratrum in full and repeated doses, desiring, and confidently expecting to produce the same train of distressing symptoms that so alarmed me some years previously; these were nausea, vomiting, purging, (rarely observed) *muscular relaxation*, and coldness of the surface. In this I was disappointed; for, though the *convulsions were arrested*, there occurred no other symptom than a relaxed skin, with profuse perspiration. Since then I have administered the Veratrum in numerous cases of eclamsia of children, with such satisfactory results as to establish beyond all doubt, the power of this agent to arrest convulsions." Dr. Baker, in June, 1858, undertook the cure of a case of chorea in a young lady. It had been gradually coming on for two months. When first visited, her symptoms were distressing to the last degree, the entire muscular system being in continuous and tumultuous motion. The case passed on from bad to worse, notwithstanding the most assiduous attention and energetic treatment. Tonics, anti-spasmodics, and anodynes were exhausted without avail; the spine and nucha were cupped and blistered, without benefit; chloroform was administered internally and by inhalation; opium and its preparations seemed to make her worse; so, after all the family had given up all expectation of recovery, upon the suggestion of a medical friend, who had twice used the Verat. viride, in three cases of chorea, with the most satisfactory results, "I at once commenced its administration. And as she was gradually brought under its influence, the turmoil began to cease; the face, which had been worked by its muscles into the most ludicrous and horrible distortion, became placid and intelligent; the head ceased its everlasting jerking, the extremities lay still, the body left off writhing, and the patient quietly passed into a peaceful and profound slumber. This sleep was deep and long, as it was the first, with few and slight exceptions, that she had had in nearly two weeks; and the quiet that the muscles now received was all that had occurred, save during those few and short slumbers. At a subsequent visit, I found the family cheerful and hopeful, and the patient quiet and sleeping, the pulse but little depressed; there had occurred no vomiting—I roused her, and to my great satisfaction, when awake, there was no jactitation of the extremities, and but very little twitchings of the muscles of the face. The Veratrum was continued, and for the first few days, if withheld, the commotion began to return; under the quiet induced, the sleep was so continuous at the outset, that the family called the preparation 'the laudanum mixture.' After a time the convulsions ceased altogether, and the patient was restored to health under a course of tonics." Dr. Terry reports three cases of chorea, in which the Verat. v. was employed. The first was a child, *æt.* twelve. "It had been confined to bed for three weeks, and was reported to have been under treatment for about six weeks; first, for worms, with spigelia, worm-seed, etc., and subsequently, for chorea, with cimicifuga rac., iron, quinine, and the usual routine treatment, until the child was apparently dying. It is not in the power of language to convey a proper conception of the truly pitiable state in which I found this child. It had slept none, neither taken any nourishment for days. It was evidently dying from exhaustion and inanition. The muscular commotion was violent, universal, and unaffected by sleep; the lips embossed with foam, worked up by a continued champing of the teeth. Three drops of the tincture of Verat. viride were administered every three hours, the vehicle being gum water. In twenty-four hours, I had the gratification to see the symptoms greatly improved; the muscles were much quieter, and the child could swallow without difficulty. The trouble in this respect had constituted the greatest embarrassment in the treatment. At the end of the fourth day, all convulsive action had ceased. *Case* 2, was an ordinary one, in a girl of fifteen. After purging, four drops of the Verat. v. were given every three hours. Prompt convalescence ensued. *Case* 3.—A woman *æt.* thirty-six, childless, and subject to menorrhagia, immediately after an attack of which, she had a continual nodding of the head, and violent convulsive action in one arm, together with jactitation of one leg. In this case six drops of the tincture of Verat. v. were given every three hours. The fourth dose occasioned slight nausea, and after the fifth dose, the convulsive action ceased, when the Veratrum was withheld. In eight or ten hours the symptoms returned. Upon resuming the medicine, they again disappeared—the doses were then reduced. The case recovered. Dr. Baker also mentions a case of *puerperal convulsions* in which Chloroform by inhalation, copious bleeding and forceps were employed; child dead; weighed eleven and a half pounds. Patient was left quiet and comfortable. Seen after four or five hours had elapsed; she was found in a most violent convulsion, which was said to be the seventh since delivery. Fifteen drops of the tincture of Verat. viride were given, and ten more were directed to be given in two hours, after which the intervals should be prolonged to three or four hours. *There occurred no more convulsions*, and the woman recovered perfectly. She was not even nauseated, though the medicine was given at regular intervals during the whole night. *Dr. Woodward*, of Galesburg, Illinois (Philadelphia M. and S. Reporter), writes:—"In a late case of puerperal convulsions, I did not resort to the Veratrum, but used the lancet twice, taking away forty-five ounces of blood before the convulsions ceased; but in about four hours after the last convulsion, the lady became furiously delirious, requiring to be held on the bed. Two doses, of ten drops each, of tincture Verat., v., quieted her so completely that she slept for hours, and had no return of the delirium."

Skin.—Coldness of the skin, which is usually perspiring; the sweat is often warm, but sometimes cold and clammy; it causes vesication of the skin, when applied externally; tingling and prickling of he skin.

Clinical Remarks.—We have no proof in our proving, or in the cases of poisoning on record, that it causes any eruptions when taken internally; externally it causes erythema and vesications. Prof. Lee says it is an "epispastic;" it causes perspiration, not like Opium, which stimulates the skin, but like Tartar Emetic. In other words, the sweating is *passive* from depression of function. In Tilden's Journal we read that the Verat. v. has been used externally in local inflammations. The tincture should be combined with Glycerine two parts to six. Apply by saturating lint, and putting it on the inflamed spot. It is reported to have cured a case of shingles, applied externally in the form of diluted tincture. In chronic skin diseases, it has been used according to Prof. Lee, with much benefit. A popular ointment for the cure of scabies, tinea capitis, etc., is made from this plant, but its external use in such cases is not devoid of danger.

Sleep.—Sound sleep every night, but has frightful dreams of being on the water; restless night, with frightful dreams of being drowned.

Clinical Remarks.—The above symptoms, are quite commonly experienced in cerebral congestions. In the incipient stages of meningitis, or hydrocephalus, dreams of being on the water are not unusual. Dr. Coe says it is a "soporific," but decrees that it is *not* a narcotic. Drs. Tully and Ives proved to their own satisfaction, that it was possessed of narcotic properties.

Fever.—Chilliness with nausea; coldness of the whole body with cold perspiration, especially upon the hands, feet and face; coldness, with pale skin, flabby muscles, and quick weak pulse; excites great coolness or coldness of the surface, sometimes renders the skin merely soft and moist, at other times causes profuse, cold perspiration; cool skin, pulse reduced from 100 to 60 in fever; coldness of the whole body, with cold sweat; pulse 35 slow and soft, with nausea and vomiting. When given in fever it does not always cause *slowness* of the pulse, but will render a pulse of 140, softer and weak without diminishing its frequency; weak, scarcely perceptible pulse, and reduced from 68 to 52; feeble, *irregular*, scarcely perceptible pulse, with cold clammy perspiration.

Clinical Remarks.—The Veratrum viride belongs to the group of remedies of which Aconite, Veratrum alb. Gelseminum semp., etc., are members. The primary action of all these remedies when given in medicinal doses, is to *depress* the circulation, through the agency of the nervous system. With this depression, there is always present coldness or coolness of the skin, warm or cold perspiration, chilliness or coldness, and, in short all the symptoms which generally characterize the *cold* stage of fevers. I have not been able to find, in any of the cases of poisoning by Verat. v., any general reaction following this cold stage. The same may be said of the other members of this group. It is only in careful and exhaustive provings, with small and repeated doses, that we get continuous febrile symptoms. But we may properly accept this statement, namely:—that it is with medicinal, as with natural diseases, a fact that a febrile reaction always follows the cold stage, if the vital powers do not prevent. Any *cause* capable of depressing the nervous and vascular system (primarily) will cause excitation and irritation of the same systems (secondarily). The secondary (reactive) symptoms will vary in nature, symptoms, and intensity, with the cause. Thus, the secondary febrile symptoms following the primary febrile symptoms of Aconite are very different from those of Gelseminum or Veratrum. In *fevers* in general, Veratrum viride enjoys the confidence of a great portion of the allopathic and eclectic schools of medicine. But like, all other powerful medicines, it has its enthusiastic adherents, and its bitter opposers. Some very high authorities are extravagant in their laudations of its safety, efficiency, and curative power over many other diseases besides fevers; at the same time, other authorities equally high, denounce it as a dangerous drug. Prof. Lee says:—"The same objections will apply to it, as has been brought against Aconite, namely: the difficulty of regulating its effects, and its dangerously depressing effects, *even in small doses.* From what we have seen and know of its use, we have little doubt *that it has caused more deaths in one year than chloroform has since its discovery.*" I am sorry for the sake of humanity, that I can agree with Prof. Lee in his estimate of its danger, *but only when used in the recklessly* large doses of his school. Aconite, Tartar emetic, and Mercury, are equally dangerous and fatal when used by the dominant school; yet, in the hand of the homœopathist, these poisonous agents become potent instruments for the removal of disease. He regulates the dose to suit the over-sensitive, diseased organism, and the result is that Veratrum viride, as well as Verat. alb., Aconite, Tartar emetic, Gelseminum, and others, become invaluable to suffering humanity. In simple *Ephemeral fever*, without local inflammation, but accompanied by vertigo, headache, dimness of sight, nausea, weakness, and restlessness, this remedy is as useful as any. (Drop doses of the first decimal dilution.) In *Irritative fever* it may sometimes be of great utility. In this disease the pulse often runs as high as 140, or even 160. It differs not less in strength and fulness than in frequency. Sometimes it is strong, full, and moderately accelerated, and sometimes small and feeble; and the latter is most apt to be the case when the frequency is the greatest. When the fever is accompanied with a tendency to drowsiness, throbbing of the temporal arteries, a full, frequent, hard pulse, vomiting of mucus and bile, constipation, tendency to spasms, (as is frequently the case in the *Infantile remittent* of children), the Veratrum viride in suitable doses will soon effect a favorable change. To a person over ten years, may be given five or ten drops of the first decimal dilution, every hour or two; to children from *one* drop to five drops will suffice, although in cases of cerebral congestion large doses may be used. When this fever is caused by teething, the irritation of worms, or any cause acting through the nervous system, this remedy is the best we can use. As stated above, the pulse is often quick, febrile, and very feeble. This may arise from an affection of the nervous centres, and the pulse may be the pulse of oppression and of weakness. In the former case the Verat. viride in the doses above recommended will often cause the pulse to become less frequent, fuller, and softer. When debility is the cause of the small pulse, Phos. ac. and China are indicated. *Intermittent fever* is not controlled by any remedy of the Aconite group. They do not seem to possess the anti-periodic power, which is essential. I cannot subscribe to the doctrine taught in our school, that "*any* medicine will cure ague if indicated by the symptoms." I practiced in a malarious district over twelve years, and my experience in the treatment of miasmatic fevers led me to adopt this conclusion, namely, that there is a certain class of remedies which possess *antidotal* virtues, or are capable, when introduced into the system, of antidoting the malarious poison. I believe this poison to be a specific miasm, and not a mere "correlated force," as some teach. Not all intermittents are due to the action of this poison, and some such fevers may be cured by others than members of the *China*-group, namely:—Quinine, Nux vomica, Arsenicum, Salicine, Cornus florida, etc. Veratrum viride, although not indicated for the disease itself, is often of great use in the hot stage, when the reaction is intense, and the vascular system is excited strongly. In such cases, in adults, we may have congestion of the brain, delirium, powerful action of the heart, and a hard, rapid pulse; and in children severe spasms and convulsions. In these cases this remedy is superior to Aconite or Belladonna. Under its use the intensity of the paroxysm will soon subside, and the threatened convulsions be arrested. I have sometimes given one or two drops of the mother tincture every half hour to an adult, and half as much to a child, with the happiest results. *Remittent or bilious fever*, when not dependent on miasmatic influences, will often be amenable to the therapeutic influence of Veratrum viride; but will have to be alternated with other remedies like Bryonia, Mercurius, Podophyllum or Leptandria, as the symptoms and conditions demand. When the gastric symptoms are predominant, this remedy will have to be used in smaller doses (2nd or 3rd dil.) than when the stomach or bowels are irritated. When this form of fever assumes the character of a *pernicious* remittent, the Verat. v. is to be used with extreme caution. It is still indicated, but *primarily*, for the primary action of the drug is to cause conditions very similar to a pernicious fever; namely, prostration of the vital forces, with typhus symptoms, etc. My experience in such fevers has taught me that the best and safest treatment is to use Baptisia, Verat. viride, Aconite, or Verat. alb., 3rd, in alternation with a remedy secondarily indicated; namely, China, Quinine, Nitric acid, etc., in material doses. Indeed, it is often necessary in those low conditions which occur during pernicious fevers, to give Quinine in five or ten grain doses, repeated in brandy, every hour. Those who have had to combat with these terrible malarious diseases will know and appreciate the necessity of resorting in some cases to such doses; and those who know the least, practically, of these diseases, are they who are loudest in denouncing what they term "gross medication." In *Yellow Fever*, the Veratrum has been used by the dominant school, with alleged success. Drs. White and Ford of Charleston, S. C., treated many cases with Verat. v. In the Charleston Medical Journal and Review they give the results of their treatment. They gave from eight to ten drops to adults, and from one to six drops to children, repeated every hour or two. "By the administration of the Veratrum in this manner, the pulse was sooner or later subdued, and as it sank, became somewhat irregular. The first doses were often vomited, in severe cases, but the succeeding ones were commonly retained, and the patient did not vomit again until the pulse was reduced, when the effect of the remedy was occasionally marked by emesis. This vomiting was rarely severe, ceasing of itself upon a temporary discontinuance of the medicine, or yielding readily to common restoratives. The reduction of the pulse was accompanied by a notable cooling of the body, by a well-marked diminution of the headaches, pain in the back and limbs, of the restlessness and anxiety, of the frequency of the respiration, of the congestion of the skin, flushing of the face, tumefaction of the tongue, and injection of the conjunctiva. The patient felt much relieved, and slept tranquilly as soon as the vomiting had ceased; nor would the symptoms tend to recur for some hours, as they would always do, however, if the drug were not again prescribed."

The pulse was kept by the Veratrum fifteen beats below the normal range. If the pulse was small and frequent, it was given in small doses; if black vomit supervened, and the pulse was slow, the Veratrum plainly was not required; if, however, the pulse was rapid, the Veratrum was continued in doses proportioned to its frequency, which were usually small, and repeated every two or three hours. Without regard, therefore, to the ordinary accidents of the disease, whenever it was required, and only then, the Veratrum was uniformly, or specially administered, until convalescence was declared." Together with the Veratrum, however, Mercury was given, pushed to salivation and catharsis; also, saline, diuretic and refrigerent mixtures; so that the results are anything but satisfactory to the investigator, who would ascertain the pure effects of drugs in disease. Of the whole number treated with Veratrum; namely, 117, there recovered 102; died 15. Adults, 80, recovered 66; died 14. Children 37, recovered 36; died 1. The subjoined table shows the mean range of the pulse under the Veratrum viride, as compared with its mean range before the Verat was given:

Mean Frequency.	Adult Males.	Adult Females.	Children.
When Veratrum v. was first given	102.5	114.2	137.5
Seven hours after	61.3	65.2	71.0
Remainder of disease	52.8	64.7	74.8

This table shows the power which the medicine exercises over the pulse and the heart's action *in disease*, and by it we can judge pretty correctly of its action on the healthy organism.

In Typhoid fever, the Veratrum viride has not been used much in homœopathic practice; not as much, as in our opinion, it is entitled to. Many of its symptoms strongly resemble the symptoms of typhoid, particularly the abdominal and cerebral varieties. The only cure on record in our literature, illustrating the action of this remedy in typhoid fever, is reported in the Philadelphia Jour. of Hom., by Dr. Henry. He says: "It is the best remedy I have ever used in the treatment of those diseases which have a tendency to assume a typhoid form of fever. As far as I have been able to test this remedy, in fever of all descriptions, I must say I am better pleased with it than with Aconite." *Case* 1.—A little girl, aged thirteen, had been suffering with continued fever for ten days. She complained of violent pain in the back; inclined to sleep most of the day; very sick at the stomach, but not so as to produce vomiting; black diarrhœa; pulse varying from ninety-eight to one hundred and ten during the day; pain and weakness in the lower limbs. I took the case to be a mild form of typhus. I immediately put five drops of the mother tincture in a tumbler half full of water, and ordered a tea-spoonful to be taken every half hour, until perspiration was produced. I called in two hours, found the pulse down to eighty-four; the patient was in a general perspiration; she recovered without any other remedy, in two days. *Case* 2.—Mr. H., a young man, aged eighteen, sick two weeks. Found him with a very high fever; pulse 120; face very much flushed; fulness, with slight pain, and great buzzing in the head; gnats and bugs fly before the eyes; inclined to jump out of bed; talking at random; slight bearing down pains in the bowels, attended with black diarrhœa; great weakness of the lower extremities, with general prostration. Six drops of the mother tincture of Verat. v. was mixed with twelve tea-spoonfuls of water, a tea-spoonful to be taken every half hour. In three hours found the pulse down to ninety-five; before the day was out he was in a fine perspiration; no fever for three days; has now a slight fever, which lasts two or three hours a day; every other symptom right." There is no question in my mind, but that a continuance of the pathogenetic action of Verat. v. would result in such lesions of the intestinal canal, as result in the typhus process. Rubbed on the skin, or held in the mouth, it causes erosions and vesicular eruptions, and it will probably affect, similarly, the whole intestinal tract. I regard it as secondarily indicated in all fevers of the synochal or inflammatory type, and even in some typhoids. The above cases have many symptoms which resemble those caused by Verat. v.; but Baptisia, Belladonna, Phosphoric acid, and Muriatic acid, are more generally indicated. A large amount of testimony could be produced from allopathic sources, in regard to the value of Verat. v. in typhoid fevers, and many grains of truth gleaned from the chaff, but we cannot give the space. In *Small Pox, or Variola*, when the fever is intense, with excessive pain and restlessness, the Verat. viride will prove as reliable as Aconite, and in some cases, even more satisfactory. I have used it in but one case of variola—four drops of the 1st dec. were given every hour, with the effect of mitigating the severity of the fever, and hastening the occurrence of the eruption. The recent use of the *Saracenia pur.*, in this dreaded disease, now attracts much attention, and bids fair to supersede all other remedies. In *Measles*, during the febrile stage, and especially if pulmonary congestion is feared, the Verat. v. is a most useful remedy. Under its use the dyspnœa, cough, and pain, rapidly subside. In children, convulsions often precede the outbreak of the eruption. If Verat. v. is given at the outset, this accident will generally be prevented. The next most useful remedies in this disease are, Gels., Puls., Euphr., and Merc. iod. In *Scarlatina*, it is infinitely superior to Aconite, Gelseminum, or any other remedy, except Belladonna. I allude to the Scarlatina simplex, and S. Anginosa, during the first, or febrile stage. It controls the pulse, even when given in the low dilutions, better than any other remedy, and hastens the normal appearance of the eruption. The testimony of some of the most prominent physicians of the homœopathic school sustain this assertion. Dr. Small prefers it to any other remedy, when the arterial excitement is intense, and there is danger of cerebral congestion, or irritation of the spinal centres. It is well known that in this disease the arterial excitement is more severe, the pulse more frequent, and the heat of the skin greater than in any other; the Verat. v. will sooner modify this condition than Aconite or Gelseminum. It should be given in alternation with Belladonna; the doses must be varied to suit the severity of the case. For children, the dilutions from the 1st to the 3d (dec); for adults, drop doses of the mother tincture may be required. The best is, to *give enough to control the arterial excitement.* It is useful in certain *Sequelæ* of scarlatina, acute rheumatism, dropsy, etc., when febrile symptoms are manifested. In *Erysipelas*, it is often useful. Besides its specific action in controlling the arterial excitement, it appears to be homœopathic to the *vesicular* variety; for the application of Verat. v. to the skin often causes an eruption closely resembling that form of the disease, and even its internal administration is said to have caused a similar eruption all over the body. When cerebral symptoms occur from a supposed metastasis of the inflammation to the brain, and we find the pulse hard and *full*, or hard and *small*, we may expect much benefit from this remedy, in alternation with Belladonna, Apis, or Arnica. If the febrile symptoms assume a low, or asthenic type, Rhus tox., Arnica, Muriatic acid, or Baptisia, will be more applicable. The Verat. v. has been used as an external application, with alleged benefit in cases of erysipelas—a weak solution—one drachm to one pint of water, may be applied with soft cloths.

Head.—Headache, with vertigo; dimness of vision, and dilated pupils; headache, proceeding from the nape of the neck; heaviness of the head; sharp, drawing pain over the left eye, with a contracted feeling of the skin of the forehead; dull, frontal headache, with neuralgic pains in the right temple, close to the eye; dull, drawing pains in the forehead, with drawing, dull pains in the umbilical region; very severe, frontal headache, with vomiting; constant, dull, heavy headache.

Clinical Remarks.—The Veratrum v. acts upon the brain, similarly to Aconite, and Gelseminum; yet, its effects are far from identical. The therapeutic range of Veratrum over affections of the brain is far greater than that of the latter. I know of no drug, not even Belladonna, so useful in affections of the head, when they are of a *congestive* character. In *Cerebral Congestions*, it is immensely superior to any known drug. This assertion is made understandingly, and based upon an experience of six years with the medicine. It is most useful when the congestion arises from *plethora*, *vascular irritation*, *coup de soliel*, *alcoholic stimulants*, *teething in children*, and especially when it occurs from *suppressed discharges*. When the congestion occurs from rheumatic irritation, Cimicifuga, or Aconite are better indicated. The symptoms calling for Verat. v. are, a sense of fulness; heaviness; weight, or distention of the head; giddiness; intense headache, with fulness and throbbing of the arteries, sometimes with stupefaction; increased sensitiveness to sound, with buzzing, roaring, etc.; double, partial, luminous, painful, dim, or otherwise disorered vision; nausea and vomiting; tingling, numbness, etc., in the limbs; mental confusion; loss of memory; convulsions, or paralysis of motion. For these congestions of the head in young children, from teething, I have for several years given this medicine the preference over Belladonna, or Aconite; also in cerebral oppression, occurring during the progress of a pneumonia. I consider it as perfectly homœopathic to these before-mentioned congestive conditions, as any other drug in our materia medica, for it has caused all the symptoms of such morbid states. It does not cure by "depressing the action of the heart," as bleeding does. Those who denounce the use of Verat. v. in vascular irritation, fever, etc., might as well denounce Aconite and Gelseminum, for they all act in a similar manner. The increased action of the vascular system is a secondary effect of these medicines. In *Meningitis*, the Verat. v. should be used promptly, and in the lowest dilutions, alternated with Belladonna, when the latter remedy seems indicated. I believe it to be more useful in this disease, as well as *Cerebritis*, than Aconite. In Tubercular meningitis, or Hydrocephalus, it can do no good, except in the stage of active inflammation, if that stage exists; but it may be palliative in preventing or arresting spasms in the later stages.

Face and Nose.—Pale, cold face; face cold, bluish, and covered with cold perspiration; convulsive twitching of the facial muscles; mouth drawn down at one corner; paleness of the lips, and around the alæ of the nostrils; nose looks pinched, cold, and blue; profuse secretion of mucus from the nostrils; singular contortions of the muscles of the face. (See spasmodic symptoms.)

Clinical Remarks.—We have in the above facial symptoms these conditions indicated, namely: collapse of the general system, spasmodic or chorectic states, and a congested or apoplectic condition of the brain. It has cured several cases of chorea, and is of great value in cerebral congestion. The "drawing down of a corner of the mouth" would point to a sanguineous effusion into the brain substance.

Ears.—Ringing in the ears; moving quickly produces complete deafness; dull roaring in the ears; the ears are cold and pale.

Clinical Remarks.—Most of the effects of Veratrum upon the ears and eye arise from a depressed state of the circulation. The same condition is present, as after excessive bleedings, or loss of any of the vital fluids. In high potencies it may prove useful in similar affections. But Veratrum v. causes, secondarily, congestion of the brain, with ringing of the ears. In low dilutions, it is one of the best remedies for the latter condition. It is well known that anæmia and plethora will produce nearly the same array of brain *symptoms*, although opposite pathological states are really present. Thus, *acute* hydrocephalus is often simulated by the *hydrocephaloid* disease, which arises from sheer debility.

Eyes.—Profuse secretion of tears; dimness of sight; walking brings on blindness with faintness; dimness of vision with dilated pupils; immense circles of a green color appeared around the candle, which, as vertigo came on, and I closed my eyes, turned to red; double vision.

Clinical Remarks.—It is primarily homœopathic to Amaurosis from anæmia, or from loss of fluids, or from debility during convalescence (should be alternated with China, Phos. acid 1st), and given in the 6th dilution). It is also indicated in amaurosis from imitation or congestion of the optic nerves, when the symptoms correspond with its pathogenesis.

Mouth, Fauces, and Œsophagus.—Tongue feels as if it had been scalded (constant symptom); tongue coated yellow along the centre; flat, bitter taste on the tongue; copious secretion of saliva; intense burning in the fauces, with constant inclination to swallow; burning in the œsophagus; spasms of the œsophagus; burning and spasm of the œsophagus, with rising of frothy, bloody mucus into the mouth (this symptom was intensely disagreeable, lasted several days, and was relieved by Phosphorus 3d, after several remedies had been tried in vain); sensation as of a ball rising in the œsophagus.

Clinical Remarks.—The yellow coating on the tongue, and the bitter taste, were both noticed in the *morning*, and point to irritation of the liver. The Veratrum v. produces undoubted inflammation of the mucous membrane of the œsophagus, with superficial erosion, spasm, etc. We have here a truly homœopathic remedy for œsophagitis. It is also homœopathic to spasmodic stricture of that tube.

Stomach.—Uneasy constriction of the stomach, with tendency to sickness; excruciating pain in the lower part of the stomach, the pain extending to about the size of the hand; the constrictive pain is increased by warm drinks, which seem to go *under* the pain; violent nausea and vomiting; vomiting of glairy mucus with blood, with running from the nose and eyes; excruciating pain in the pit of the stomach, with heat and constriction of the throat; vomiting of, first food, then mucus, finally a small quantity of blood; painful, empty retching; sensation of dryness and heat in throat, extending to the stomach, with disposition to hiccough; severe hiccough of fifteen or twenty times per minute; violent vomiting, coming on in about ten or fifteen minutes; great irritability of the stomach, the smallest quantity of food or drink is immediately rejected—this irritation continued for three weeks (from thirty drops); great uneasiness, followed by intense pain in the stomach; the pain was drawing, twisting, and pressing; the stomach felt as if drawn tightly against the spinal column, causing pain in the back, in the dorsal region; the stomach seemed to press against the spine when lying upon the back; the pain in the stomach would culminate every five or ten minutes, with powerful and expulsive vomiting; the pain was aggravated by the least noise; vomiting, not preceded by nausea.—(Various sources.) Vomiting of bile and blood; hiccough before and after vomiting; very frequent neuralgic (?) pains in the cardiac portion of the stomach; sharp, flying pains in the epigastrium and umbilical region, passing down to the pubes. —(Dr. Burt's proving.) Dr. Osgood—an allopathic observer—noticed in his own case, that the vomiting was effected by a spasmodic contraction of the stomach itself without participation of the diaphragm, and abdominal muscles; and in another individual was preceded by a sensation as of a ball rising in the œsophagus—the result no doubt of spasmodic contraction of the tube. Dr. Norwood says: "We have seen it produce emesis in very susceptible persons, and the contractions of the stomach were so rapid as to be almost continuous, and uninterrupted" He also remarks that: "there need be no danger apprehended of causing inflammation of the stomach; we have given especial attention to that particular. It is peculiar, and at the same time interesting in its effects, from the fact of its acting as a sedative on almost every other portion of the system, diminishing the vascular and muscular action and motion of every other part, and *increasing* that of the stomach." Dr. N. asserts that it *increases the appetite and desire for food.*

CLINICAL REMARKS.—We have in the above a notable array of symptoms, pointing to excessive gastric irritability. Its action on the stomach is quite similar to that of Verat. alb., Tartar emetic, or Arsenicum. It is evidently homœopathic to cardialgia, gastralgia, and neuralgic or spasmodic affections of the stomach, when accompanied by vomiting, retching and excessive irritation. Dr. Burt considers it the best remedy in such cases—better than the V. alb. He uses it at the 3rd or 6th. It should not be given lower. It should prove curative in gastritis, erosion of the stomach, and ought to palliate the pain and vomiting in cancer of the stomach. It causes all the symptoms of pyrosis, water-brash, and many of the symptoms of "dyspepsia."

Bowels, Stool, etc.—Frequent drawing pains in the umbilical region; neuralgic (?) pains at the right side of the umbilicus, passing down to the groin; sharp, flying pains in the epigastrium and umbilical regions, passing down to the pubes; dull, heavy, aching pains in the umbilical region (constant symptom); cutting, aching pains in the umbilical region, with rumbling in the bowels, and desire for stool; soft, mushy stool *preceded* by cutting pains in the bowels, and *followed* by cutting pains in the rectum and anus. "At three different times, on the second day of the proving, I had severe neuralgic and long-lasting pains in the rectum; neuralgic pains in the left groin; I never had such pains before."—*Dr. Burt.* "The first day after I left off proving the Verat. v. I had neuralgic pains in the anus and rectum. They came on twenty or thirty times a day for three weeks, when there appeared a large tumor which pained me constantly. One-half the tumor was very red, the other half dark blue. I never had piles before in my life. My alvine evacuations were natural all the time."—*Burt.*

CLINICAL REMARKS.—It is agreed by all allopathic medical writers who speak of this plant, that it irritates the bowels much less than the Veratrum alb. Some, however, claim that it should not be used in diseases where any intestinal irritation exists. *Wood*, however, does not mention it as a purgative. Dr. Coe remarks: "The employment of Veratrum v. in the treatment of diarrhœa and dysentery affords occasion for some remarks in regard to the action of this remedy upon the bowels. We have seen it stated by some writers, that Veratrum is objectionable on account of its irritating influence upon this organ. Such has not been our experience. We have employed it much in the treatment of bowel complaints, and with the most happy results." Yet he admits that it has an "emeto-cathartic" action, and says it is contra-indicated in "intestinal ulcerations." He says it is useful in all cases of "torpor and debility of the abdominal organs," and is of utility in mania, epilepsy, hysteria, convulsions, melancholy, etc., when arising from "functional obstructions" of the abdominal viscera, and disturbed and discordant action of the abdominal nervous plexus." All this, however, is quite conjectural, although it is apparently indicated in abdominal congestions. Dr. Norwood says, "it is not cathartic," but he speaks of "avoiding its drastic effect," and mentions that "the only cases in which we have seen it purge, were when given in combination with Tartar emetic. In most of these cases it excited a violent *cholera morbus*. Concerning its therapeutic effects, he states: "We have found it of great value in the treatment of typhoid dysentery, and would feel unable to combat that disease without it, or some other remedy of equal power." It seems homœopathic to about the same condition of the bowels as Verat. alb.; also to hæmorrhoids.

Kidneys, Urine, etc.—Profuse urine; increased secretion of pale urine.

CLINICAL REMARKS.—Its action on the kidneys has been pretty well investigated by allopathic observers. Prof. Lee says: "its diuretic action has been established by numerous experiments. It is worthy of particular note that it does not act as a mere renal hydragogue, but like colchicum it increases the solid constituents of the urine. While it increases the amount of organic and inorganic solids, it is not positively established that it augments the quantity of uric acid. Like colchicum it increased the amount of urine, as well as the total amount of solids eliminated, but it is pretty certain that this is mainly dependent on an increase of organic matter. Its curative influence in gout and rheumatism may thus be explained. It is said to eliminate lithic acid through the kidneys." Dr. Abbott made some experiments which proved that it causes a considerable increase in the amount, and a corresponding decrease in the specific gravity, of the urine. It would seem to be homœopathic primarily to certain forms of diuresis, enuresis, and perhaps diabetis. It is curative in acute inflammation of the kidneys and bladder.

Male Generative Organs.

CLINICAL REMARKS.—It is used successfully in severe inflammatory diseases of these organs. Dr. Osgood considered it almost specific for *Orchitis*. It will probably prove as useful as Aconite in affections of these tissues.

Generative Organs of Women.—We have yet no symptomatic proving of Veratrum viride upon the female organism. It is said to have caused *abortion* in numerous instances, yet Drs. Ford and White, who used it so freely in yellow fever, thought it *prevented* that accident. It may not cause abortion directly, as Sabina or Cimicifuga, but indirectly, by the great prostration of the general symptoms, the severe efforts to vomit, etc. In the same way it would cause hemorrhage from the uterus. It is probably homœopathic *primarily* to *passive* congestions of that organ. My experience with the Veratrum viride in this class of diseases, is confined principally to acute inflammation of the uterus, or *puerperal metritis*, in which I place a high estimate upon its value. I think I have arrested the inflammation, or materially modified it, by the use of the lower dilutions. There are certain conditions attending uterine disorders, in which the Verat. v. has proved very successful in my hands. I allude to those congestions of the head or lungs which occur during uterine disorders, such as *menstrual* congestions of the head (menstrual headache), also congestion of the head or lungs from suppressed menses, suppressed lochia, etc. In these accidents a few drops of the lowest dilutions has never failed to prove promptly curative in my practice. It is highly recommended by Dr. Miller (eclectic), in *Dysmenorrhœa*, occurring in plethoric subjects (*i. e.* congestive dysmenorrhœa). In anæmic subjects he pronounces it decidedly injurious. It is probably indicated in this affection, for similar symptoms to Aconite and Belladonna. It has been found useful in palliating violent attacks of *hysterical convulsions.* Many allopathic writers, among them Dr. Simpson, of Edinburg, extols it highly in *puerperal fever.* It may prove useful in the *vomiting*, *pyrosis*, and other symptoms occurring during *pregnancy.* Many of the symptoms occurring during the *change of life*, are simulated by this medicine. In *acute mastitis*, with high febrile action, and great tumefaction of the breasts I have used it alternately with Belladonna with very satisfactory results. It has been used boldly —recklessly—by the allopathic school, in puerperal convulsions (eclamsia) as a substitute for blood-letting, but in such doses as to be nearly as injuriously pernicious as the abstraction of blood. I have never used it in that affection, but I have administered it in cases where I thought convulsions *would* ensue if not warded off, and with the apparent result of preventing that terrible array of symptoms. In *puerperal mania* it has proved curative. (See a case reported by Dr. Woodward.) Dr. Atlee reports a case as follows: "The labor had been preternatural, child delivered dead, by podalic version. She did well until ten days after confinement, when she became silent, suspicious, and distrustful of those about her, without any obvious cause. In the hope that the change was temporary, opium and perfect rest, with careful watching was enjoined. Two days after, symptoms of puerperal mania were still more developed; it was impossible for the doctor to come near her; his presence seemed to terrify her, and her husband told him that since the previous visit, she expressed strong apprehensions that the doctor had poisoned her and meditated her destruction. She had slept little or none, and it was difficult to keep her confined to her bed and her room. In the hope that some benefit might result by controlling the general circulation and diminishing the nervous excitement, five drops of the tincture were given every three hours, as long as it did not produce nausea, vomiting, or prostration. On the following morning, on entering the room, he found his patient lying quietly and calmly on the bed, with a total absence of the sinister expression of the day before. She answered him slowly but in a whisper, put out her tongue, and let him feel her pulse without resistance. Upon inquiry he found that soon after the administration of the third dose of Veratrum on the previous evening, she had become calm, had rested quietly, and had remained so. Pulse fifty-six. She was cheerful and obedient, conversed rationally and freely, and without allusion to her previously unhappy condition. She recovered perfectly in a few days. Dr. Coe (Art. Veratrin, Conc. Org. Med.) states that a majority of the cases of mental aberration arise from and are dependent upon a morbidly increased activity of the nervous structure of the abdomen." "This," he says, "would seem to explain why Veratrin is of utility in the treatment of mania, melancholy, and mental weakness." (Very doubtful, H.) "In cases of mental aberration, accompanied with torpor and debility of the abdominal organs, Veratrum will be found serviceable." (Mere theory, H.)

Chest.—Oppression of the chest; sensation as of a heavy load on the chest; anxious oppression of the chest; constant, dull, burning pain in the region of the heart, under the sternum; burning pain in the region of the heart; oppression of the chest with nausea. The respiration decreases from 30 and 40 to 16 and 12 (in pneumonia;) respirations 12 to 14 (in healthy persons under the influence of the drug).

Remarks.—The symptoms of *oppression* enumerated above are due principally to the debility caused by the drug; the oppression comes on just before the vomiting, and *with* nausea. Dr. Burt's experiments with the Veratrum v. on cats, seem to show that it causes intense engorgement of the lungs. We would refer the reader to his paper, published herewith. In Dr. Burt's proving, made on himself, he makes no mention of any pains which may be termed pneumonic, or pleuritic; the pain in the heart, only, was noticed. It is a notable fact, however, that in the proving of Tartar emetic, we have the same absence of acute thoracic pain; yet the latter drug has a high reputation, even in the homœopathic school, in the treatment of pneumonia. It is well known by all practical physicians that severe cases of pneumonia may run their course with little or no *pain* at any time being present. The Veratrum v. has not been extensively used by homœopathists in the treatment of thoracic diseases. Satisfied with that time-honored remedy, Aconite, they prefer to adhere to that drug. But many of my colleagues, both East and West, agree with me in considering the Verat. v. as superior to Aconite, in *pneumonia* in particular. My own experience with it has, so far, been satisfactory. In the incipient stage of that affection, when simple engorgement only exists, I believe it has the power of arresting the disease, and in the later stages it proves a valuable auxiliary to such remedies as Bryonia, Phosphorus, Tartar emetic, and Sanguinaria. I usually give the lowest dilution, ten or fifteen drops of the 1st dec. every thirty or sixty minutes to adults, and half the quantity to children. In a few cases only have I been obliged to resort to the mother tincture. In one case, that of a strong, robust man, five drops were given every two hours; after ten hours, profuse vomiting with sweating set in; the previously intense fever subsided, and *did not return*, and a rapid convalescence followed. It was given on the third day of the fever, when there was bloody sputa, severe oppression and pain in the chest (left side), and all the physical signs of the first stage of pneumonia. I deem it my duty, in this place, to give some of the large amount of allopathic testimony, for and against, the use of this remedy; for, as with their experience with Tartar emetic, we may gain valuable hints from their observations. Dr. Davidson (Nashville Journal of Medicine), says: "I have followed no other particular treatment for the last two years in pneumonia and pleurisy, than this medicine, and I am happy to say I have never seen a case terminate unfavorably under the treatment. I look upon the Veratrum as being worth all the other treatments combined, for pleurisy, pneumonia, and all other diseases of an inflammatory character." Dr. Wood, in his Therapeutics, does not give you his personal experience, but says: "The testimony in its favor is so strong, and from so many sources, that it is impossible to refuse it credence." Dr. A. F. Patton (Tilden's Journal of Mat. Med., vol. i., p. 369,) writes: "Pneumonia is the disease in which Veratrum viride is particularly indicated. It seems to have more controlling power in this than any other disease, reducing the inflammation, and favoring the expectoration in a very few hours; in some instances, vomiting is induced, which is generally of tough, viscid mucus; the pulse now rapidly declines, if not affected before; the breathing becomes very easy, and the patient falls into an easy sleep, with, perhaps, a gentle perspiration—the dose, now, is to be managed so as to sustain the depressed circulation. I find that, in pneumonia, it is better to reduce the pulse as soon as possible. The inflammation being in a degree arrested, the lung is saved from the more severe consequences of the *second stage*, or that of *red hepatization*, for the concrete fibrinous exudation being caused by a peculiar inflammatory action—thus, the cause being in part removed—this exudation is, in a great degree, arrested, and the patient, in a majority of cases, enters into a favorable convalescence." I have quoted the first authorities that came to hand, but I have looked on the immense amount of material, which is to be found scattered through the various periodicals, etc., and the opinions expressed above coincide with a majority of physicians who have written concerning the use of this medicine in pneumonia. There are, however, many of the most enlightened minds in the allopathic profession, who sturdily and rationally oppose its indiscriminate use. Among the most prominent of these, is Prof. Charles A. Lee. His objection can also be aptly applied to the use of Tartar emetic, an article so much abused by his school in the (mal) treatment of pneumonia. That drug, and the Verat. v., act in a similar manner. In poisonous or pathogenetic doses, both cause engorgement and passive congestion of the lungs (primarily), and *inflammation* of those organs (secondarily). The allopath who uses Veratrum viride for pneumonia, in the doses usually prescribed by his school, brings about the very conditions which *caused* the disease, namely, congestion. The homœopath who administers this remedy, in the first stage of pneumonia, in minute doses,—a drop of 1st or 2d dec. —gives it upon the law of *Similia*, and arrests the disease, or notably modifies it. In the *second* stage, when the inflammation is fairly established, it should be given in alternation with Phosphorus, or Sanguinaria; but, the moment the pulse ceases to be the pulse of *sthenic* action, that moment the Verat. must be omitted. The same may be said concerning the use of Aconite or Gelseminum; or, if these remedies are administered at all, in such conditions, only the highest potencies should be selected. No greater error can be made, than to give Aconite, Bryonia, Gelseminum, or Veratrum, in the *low* potencies, because the pulse is *quick*. A quick pulse must have many other qualities, to be the pulse of active inflammation, and to indicate these medicines. In *Pleuritis*, the Veratrum, will probably never be a very useful remedy. Like Tartar emetic, it does not seem to affect the serous tissues, as does Aconite or Bryonia.

Cardiac Symptoms.—Prickling pains in the region of the heart; dull, aching pains in the region of the heart; *constant, burning distress* in the cardiac region; faintness after rising from the recumbent position; syncope when walking, only relieved by lying down. (Burt.) The heart's pulsations reduced from sixty-eight to twenty-four (in health); and from one hundred and forty to thirty-three, in fevers; beats of the heart, low and feeble, scarcely perceptible (primary symptoms); palpitation of the heart; fluttering sensation in the region of the heart; palpitation on taking the least exercise; strong, loud beating of the heart, with quick pulse; palpitation with dyspnœa (secondary effects).

Clinical Remarks.—It is generally believed that the Veratrum viride acts upon the heart, through the nervous system, paralysing the nerves of motion. It is supposed that Aconite and Verat. alb. act in a similar manner. (Gelseminum, I believe, to act more directly upon the muscular structure of the heart.) The *Verat. viride* is primarily indicated in cardiac oppression, with passive congestion; cardiac debility, with fainting and collapse therefrom. In those heart affections, occurring during prostrating diseases, after hemorrhages, etc., it may be used, but *always in the minutest doses.* No remedy exercises a more depressing action on the heart, than the Verat. v. in large doses. It is *secondarily* indicated in increased activity of the heart, after previous depression. In *carditis*, and *pericarditis*, it has been used with alleged success by allopathic practitioners. In *rheumatic* affections of the heart, it is especially lauded, but may do as much injury as bleeding, if used in large doses. Having a similar action to Aconite, it will, perhaps, be found as useful as that medicine in heart affections. It does not, however, cause that intense cardiac anxiety, with fear of death, which Aconite does. It will be found palliative in many organic diseases of the heart, but should be used with great caution. It is not a "*cardiac tonic,*" in material doses, as the Digitalis is said to be. It will alleviate, according to my experience, those palpitations, attended with faintness, or dyspnœa, which occur in many diseased conditions of the heart, or attend the "change of life" in women. Some of the symptoms felt by Dr. Burt, resemble those found in the pathogenesis of Spigelia. It may be a matter of doubt, whether the "burning sensation," experienced by Dr. Burt, was really in the heart; the *œsophagus* may have been the seat of the sensation.

Back.—Very severe, and constant, aching pains in the back of neck and shoulders, so that it was almost impossible to hold the head up.

Clinical Remarks.—By some practitioners it is valued very highly, as a remedy for Lumbago, also for neuralgic pains in the back. It may prove valuable for some forms of spinal irritation, and even myelitis. We do not know what pathological changes it effects in the spinal cord.

Extremities.—Drawing pains in the right elbow, and calves of the legs; cramp of the legs (Burt); the fingers and toes cramped as in cholera; galvanic shocks in the limbs, frequently of such violence as to precipitate the patient out of bed (Coe); coldness, blueness, and dampness of the hands, feet, and limbs, with cramps of the extremities; weakness and loss of power in the extremities; paralysis of the lower limbs; prickling, and partial loss of sensation in the extremities.

XANTHOXYLUM FRAXINEUM.

(*Prickly Ash.*)

* Nat. Ord. Xanthoxylaceæ.—This shrub is known by the various names of Yellow-wood, Toothache-bush, Northern Prickly Ash, etc. It is an indigenous shrub, ten or twelve feet in height, with alternate branches, which are armed with conical, brown prickles, at the insertion of the young branches. The leaves are alternate and pinnate; the leaflets about five pairs with an odd one, nearly sessile, ovate, acute, with slight vesicular serratures, somewhat downy underneath. The common petiole is round, usually prickly on the back. The flowers are in small, dense, sessile umbels and have a somewhat aromatic odor. The Prickly Ash is a native of North America, growing from Canada to Virginia, and west to the Mississippi, in woods, thickets, and the river banks, flowering in April and May before the appearance of the leaves. The entire plant contains medicinal properties. The fragrance is due to a volatile oil which may be extracted by ether or alcohol. Both the bark and berries are officinal. The bark from which the tincture was prepared for proving, comes in fragments

* A Report of the Committee on Materia Medica of the Massachusetts Medical Society. By Charles Cullis, M. D., Boston, and contributed to this work by him.

of various sizes, quilled, light or ash-colored externally, internally white and glossy; it is faintly odorous, and has a slightly aromatic taste. The bark of the Prickly Ash has been found to contain a fixed oil of a greenish color, volatile oil, resin, coloring matter, gum, and a crystallizable matter, which has been named Xanthoxylin. Dr. King, in his Dispensatory, speaks of Prickly Ash as "a stimulant, tonic, alterative and sialagogue. Taken into the stomach, it causes a feeling of warmth, slightly accelerates the pulse, and determines to the skin, causing a gentle moisture. It is used as a stimulant in languid states of the system, and as a sialogogue in paralysis of the tongue and mouth. It has proved highly beneficial in chronic rheumatism, colic, syphilis, hepatic derangements, and wherever a stimulating alterative treatment is required."

First Proving.—Mr. S., aged twenty-nine, light hair, nervous temperament, July 9th, 1862, took at 10 P. M., four drops of Xanthoxylum tinct.. Immediately a smart peppery taste in mouth and fauces; slept hard all night; on the morning of the 10th, took ten drops followed by the same smarting or prickly sensation in the mouth and throat, which soon extended to the stomach, followed by an increased pulse and a degree of heat all over the body. In five minutes a dull headache in space not larger than half a dollar over the nose; in fifteen minutes, sharp, shooting pains in right side (like pleurisy pains) occasionally extending through to the shoulder blade; these pains increased in severity and lasted half an hour, during this time there was a continual desire to take a long breath; in one hour a dull pain in the right ear, seeming to affect the jaw socket, the kind of pain which one has when he doen't know whether it is his tooth or ear that aches; this pain lasted two hours and then gradually wore away. Two days after, took twelve drops at 8 o'clock in the evening, followed by dryness of both nostrils, constant desire to take a long breath; flatulence; gaping; one half hour after, throbbing headache over right eye with nausea; sharp pains in right side, of a neuralgic character; severe pain in the right arm, commencing just above the bend of the elbow; severe pain in the wrist and extending to the thumb; in three quarters of an hour, ringing in ears, more particularly in right ear; throbbing headache, pulse 100; slept hard all night; awoke in the morning, languid and depressed; no appetite. July 14th, 3 P. M., same prover took twenty drops; in five minutes severe frontal headache, with dizziness; continual desire to take long and deep respirations; terrible, nervous frightened feeling; head feels full; pain over right eye; pain in right side; sharp, shooting pain; decided catarrhal symptoms; watering of the eyes and nose; tightness of the head, with the pain increasing over the eyes; in fifteen minutes increased desire for long respiration; flatulence; pain in right arm; pain in right knee; drowsiness all the evening; urine at night, and the next morning, scanty and high colored. September 3d, 8 P. M., took twenty-five drops, almost immediately experienced the same desire for deep and long respirations; in five minutes, pulse 100; frontal headache; nausea; twenty minutes after, pulse still at 100, but more feeble; one hour after, pulse 82, feeble and irregular.

SECOND PROVING.—Mr. A., twenty-seven years of age, dark brown hair, fair complexion, phlegmatic temperament. July 9th, took three drops at bed-time; slept hard and heavy; dreamed of flying about over tops of houses; in the morning, felt pain in right leg; bowels constipated; took three drops, felt sleepy all the morning; great depression; after dinner felt a bunch in the left side of the throat when swallowing; after supper, discharge from bowels; on going to bed bunch in throat shifted to right side. July 11th, at 6.30 A. M., took five drops; in fifteen minutes discharge from bowels; also another after breakfast; sleepy feeling all the morning with headache. At 6 P. M., another discharge from bowels; flatulence; slight hacking cough. July 11th, took twelve drops, strong, peppery sensation in mouth and throat; five minutes after, had a darting pain under and back of the right ear; right nostril seems filled up; sensation of soreness in right side of throat; fifteen minutes after, had a darting pain in the left temple, recurring again and again; drowsy symptoms appear prominent; also, about the upper part of the cranium an achy feeling accompanied by flashes of throb-like pain, as if the top of the head were about being taken off; flatulency; slight pain inside right arm, just above elbow; one hour after felt a good deal of tightening about the chest, which continued with much inclination to gape. At 10.30 P. M., or two hours after, some pain in right side below ribs; continued gaping; head dull, and aching; a flash of pain in right thumb, extending to hand; another in calf of right leg; legs and feet feel tired. July 12th, had a discharge from bowels before breakfast, and one after; soreness of throat with expectoration of tough mucus.

THIRD PROVING.—Prover, light complexion, sanguine-nervous temperament, active habit, uniform health, age thirty-three. Took two drops of tincture followed by these symptoms: burning and dry feeling in the mouth and tongue; diffused pain in the upper part of the forehead; worse in the right side; pain extends to the base of the brain, with soreness; shaking the head produces a feeling of looseness or quivering of the brain followed by dizziness; rumbling of the abdomen, with soreness on pressure; discharge of mucus from the nose with congested feeling, as if it were about to bleed; dull, heavy, grinding pain in the left eye; feeling of fulness or pressure at the epigastrium; empty eructations with slight taste of ingesta; slept soundly without dreaming, but soon after waking at 7 o'clock next morning, had severe griping abdominal pains with thin brown, diarrhœic discharge, mixed with some mucus; anorexia, could eat but a few mouthfuls at breakfast, and could only drink a half cup of coffee, which was vomited soon afterwards; griping pain continued at intervals, with a general feeling of indifference and malaise; discharge of dry and bloody scales of mucus from the nose; hoarseness with some husky feeling in the throat; obliged to clear the throat frequently. This hoarseness and obstruction of the throat continued some days after the other symptoms had subsided.

PROVINGS BY WOMEN.—1st. Miss D., aged twenty-six; black hair; active habit; good health. Took twelve drops of the tincture. In five minutes felt pressure in the head, with fulness of the veins. In ten minutes, dull pain in right knee. In fifteen minutes, pain in both elbows, and back of the head, also a bewildered sensation; pain in the lid of the right eye. Half an hour after sense of heat all over the veins, with a desire to be bled; flash of heat from head to foot. One hour after taking the medicine, pain in ankle; flash of heat; pain in left heel; a feeling of enlargement of the throat; pain in right side of the throat; dull pain in left elbow, passing to the palm of the hand, then to the shoulder; pain in left side; heavy feeling in the top of the head; pain in the left leg between the hip and knee; pain in left elbow and left side of the head; dull pain in left knee, also in left elbow, extending to the hand, then in left side and top of the left foot; a feeling of numbness through the whole of the left side of the body from head to foot, the division made perceptible in the head, affecting half of the nose—this feeling lasted two or three minutes; pain in left knee. Two hours after, pain in left knee, very severe; slight pain in left side, and under the left shoulder-blade, also the left hip; the pain in the left knee has lasted, without cessation, a little more than half an hour; pain in lower jaw and left side; the whole left arm and shoulder numb; pain in both feet, shooting up to the knees.

2nd. Mrs. H., aged 30. Took ten drops of the tincture at 9:20 P. M.; pulse, 80. Soon after taking it began to experience a feeling of depression and weakness; weakness of the lower limbs, with pain in the knees. At 9:30 P. M., pulse 74 soft; slight nausea, with sense of oppression at the stomach; nausea increased as did the pains of the extremities, accompanied with frequent chills. Next evening same prover took twenty drops of the tincture; did not experience the feeling of depression in so great degree as the night before; the weakness of the limbs and pain in the knees about the same; some pain in the left side; *menses appeared next morning, being one week* before the usual time; *was attended with a good deal of pain.*

3rd. Mrs. J., aged twenty-eight; light complexion; sanguine temperament; good health. Took twenty drops of the tincture at 8 o'clock P. M. In about twenty minutes noticed a tightening of the scalp, and heavy pains in temples, with a twitching in left knee, and trembling in right. On the following day took at 11 o'clock A. M., twenty drops; felt same feelings in head; did not notice lower limbs. 2 o'clock P. M., took twenty-two drops; felt the same headache, or severe pain and tightening. 3 o'clock P. M., took twenty-five drops; increase of head difficulties, with a great heat and a quiet flowing (menstrual), being two days in advance of proper time. 8 o'clock P. M., took twenty drops; some headache; all the system quiet, with an unnatural forcing of nature; went to sleep as usual, and in *dreadful distress* and *pain*, baffling description; profuse flowing; the pain (or agony) continued until noon of next day, when it gradually subsided.

Classification of Symptoms.—**Head.**—Headache over both eyes; throbbing headache; pressure over nose; grinding pain in head with nausea; head feels heavy, particularly the right side; pressure in the forehead; pressure and pain over the eyes; severe pain in the top of the head; pain directly over the root of the nose; feeling of fulness in the head; head seems as if divided—the division seeming to extend to the nose; pain in the top of the head as if the top would come off.

Sleep.—Hard; *unrefreshed in the morning;* drowsiness; sleeps heavy, and dreams of flying about over tops of houses; annoying dreams.

Skin.—Skin feels hot and sore.

Fever.—Fever, followed by *great depression;* flashes of heat from head to foot; nausea followed by chills; pulse quick; face flushed and hot.

Moral Symptoms.—Great despondency; irritability; anguish about the chest; fearfulness.

Sensorium.—Heaviness of the head; head feels full; vertigo; bewildered feeling; insensibility.

Eyes.—Lachrymation; pain in the lid of the right eye; dull, heavy pain in the left eye.

Ears.—Dull pain in the left ear; ringing in the right ear.

Nose.—Pressure in the nose; fluent coryza; discharge of bloody mucus from the nose, particularly from the right nostril.

Jaw.—Pain in the right jaw socket; dull pain in the left side of the lower jaw.

Mouth.—Ptyalism; tongue coated yellow; foul taste in the mouth; tongue and mouth feel hot.

Throat.—Throbbing in the throat; right side of throat feels sore; sensation of swelling; hoarseness; soreness of throat, with expectoration of tough mucus.

Stomach.—Fluttering in the stomach; a feeling of heaviness in the stomach; eructations with nausea.

Abdomen.—Colic pain in right iliac region; fulness and pressure at the epigastrium; griping in the bowels; rumbling, with soreness on pressure.

Stool.—Inodorous discharges, with tenesmus; thin, brown discharges, with mucus.

Urine.—Profuse and light-colored.

Chest.—Oppression of the chest, with desire to take deep inspirations; shortness of breath; tightness of the chest; difficulty to inflate the chest; pain in the left side under fourth rib.

Arms.—Pain in the right shoulder and arm; pain inside the arm just above the elbow; pain in right elbow; pain and pricking feeling in right arm, extending to the third finger; pain in little finger of right hand; numbness of the left arm; pricking and throbbing sensation in left arm and fingers.

Legs.—Excessive weakness of the lower limbs; pain in the calf of right leg; pain in left leg between hip and knee; pain in the top of the left foot; pain in the third toe of the left foot.

55

Generative Organs of Women.—Appearance of the menses too soon. *Profuse menses* with *violent pains.* Leucorrhœa.

Clinical Remarks.—Clinically, I have used this remedy in *Dysmenorrhœa* and *Amenorrhœa* with marked success. One or two cases will serve for illustration: Miss A., aged twenty-five; brunette; has suffered from menstrual irregularities since their first appearance; the catamenia appearing in three, four, or five months, and at that time her sufferings were excruciating. Her general health otherwise was good. At the time of consulting me, she had not had her catamenia for two months. I gave her Xanthoxylum 1st dilution, five drops three times a day. In three days her menses appeared, and much to her joy, with little pain. Miss B., light complexioned, nervous temperament, aged twenty-five, consulted me for suppression of menses received by getting her feet wet, she being then about one week past her time. I gave her Xanthoxylum 1st dec., five drops every three hours. Her menses appeared the next day. Mrs. C., aged thirty-two, mother of ten children, a large, fleshy woman, had not menstruated for five months, and previous to that time had not for three or four months. Gave Xanthoxylum 1st, to be taken three times a day. Menses appeared in four days.

In Dysmenorrhœa, I have used this drug with very satisfactory results. I will quote one marked case: Mrs. D., aged twenty-six; spare habit; scrofulous diathesis; had suffered for years from dysmenorrhœa. Her sufferings were so great that she would be confined to her bed for two or three days. She had tried all sorts of treatment, but without any relief. She came under my care, saying the only way she could live through her menstrual period was to drink whisky or gin until she was intoxicated. For several months I treated her with the usual remedies, but without any beneficial result. I then gave her Xanthoxylum 3rd dec.; this completely cured her. She was extravagant in the praise of this remedy. It has never failed to relieve her.

I think Xanthoxylum more especially indicated in females of spare habit, nervous temperament, and delicate organization. In some cases of plethoric habit it has failed me. In *Leucorrhœa* with Amenorrhœa, it has proved very successful. In *after-pains* in obstetric practice, I have found it of inestimable value; also, in profuse flowing and threatened abortion. I have used it in *Opthalmia*, both locally and internally, with excellent results.

APPENDIX.

DIOSCOREA VILLOSA.

[This was received too late for insertion in its proper place.]

DR. W. H. BURT'S PROVING.

May 5th, 1864, 10 A. M.—Took 30 drops of the fluid extract of Dioscorea. Half an hour after taking the medicine, commenced to have pain in the whole epigastrium, and region of the gall-bladder, quite severe, of a cutting, tearing character, at times spasmodic. 3 P. M.—Slight distress in the stomach; took forty drops. 5 P. M.—Slight, dull, frontal headache; frequent empty eructations, constant dull pain in the epigastric and umbilical regions, with frequent colicky pains of a cutting, tearing nature; great depression of spirits. 8 P. M.—Slight frontal headache; frequent, sharp pains in the stomach and region of the gall-bladder; frequent, sharp, cutting pains in the umbilical region, aggravated by walking; frequent drawing pains in the left shoulder and neck; drawing pains in the knees and ankles, the knees are very weak when walking; constant dull pain in the lumbar region, aggravated by stooping or walking; took fifty drops.

May 6th.—Awoke three times in the night with severe cutting pains in the umbilicus. There is constant dull aching pains in the umbilicus, with occasional colicky pains; severe frontal headache; thick yellowish-white coating on the tongue; rough, flat taste in the mouth; black, dry lumpy stool; dull heavy pain in the lumbar-sacral region, very much worse by stooping; fingers ache and are quite stiff; drawing pains in the ankles and feet. Took sixty drops, 9 P. M.—Slight, dull headache; rough feeling in the fauces, with constant inclination to swallow; constant aching distress in the umbilicus; dull aching pains in the back; drawing pains in the calves of the legs and ankles. Took 100 drops, 11 A. M.—Dull, frontal headache; dry, rough feeling in the fauces, with frequent inclination to swallow; constant, dull, aching pains in the whole umbilical region, with frequent, sharp, cutting pains all through the small intestines; dull drawing pains in the fore-arms and wrists; drawing pain between the shoulders; constant, severe drawing pains in the calves of the legs and ankles; knees are feeling very weak; disposition to yawn and stretch. 3 P. M.—The pains are all the same, only more mild, took 200 drops. 5 P. M.—Slight frontal headache; rough feeling in the fauces, with frequent inclination to swallow; constant distress in the umbilical and hypogastric regions, with severe cutting, colicky pains every few minutes in the stomach and small intestines; bearing down prolapsed feeling of the anus; feeling very weak, hands and legs tremble constantly, can hear my heart beating after walking a little. Pulse 80; sharp pulsating pain just at the top of the sternum, lasting an hour; severe drawing pains in my elbows, wrists and fingers, at times the pain in the fingers is very sharp; constant dull aching pain in the lumbar sacral region, very much worse by bending the spine; dull drawing pains in the knees and ankles, very sharp cutting pains in the bottom of the feet and toes; the right ankle and foot has the most pain in it. 9 P. M.—Slight frontal headache, with occasional sharp pains in the right temple; dryness of the fauces; constant aching distress in the whole of the bowels, with frequent sharp cutting pains in the stomach and small intestines. Three hemorrhoidal tumors have made their appearance, and are partially prolapsed; there is constant dull pain and distress in the anus; the pulsating pain at the upper part of the sternum is still there, it is very distressing; flying pains all through the chest and back (cervical portion); constant dull pain in the small of the back, and hips, cannot bear to stoop down, it is so painful; constant, dull, drawing pains in the elbows, wrists, hands and fingers; the pain in the fingers is very severe, of a cutting, tearing nature; constant, dull, aching pain in the ankles, feet and toes; the pain the toes is of a tearing, cutting character; took 150 drops.

May 7th, A. M.—Slept soundly, but perspired a good deal, awoke at 2 A. M., with great burning distress in the stomach; dull frontal headache, tongue coated white; flat pappy taste; tonsils slightly congested; constant aching distress in the stomach and bowels; stomach is quite painful when pressed upon; stool, first part black, very dry and hard, last part mushy and white. The stool was followed by the protrusion of four hemorrhoidal tumors, the size of large red cherries, with great pain and distress in the anus; constant dull backache; hands and fingers ache and are very stiff; closing the hands is very painful; ankles, feet, and toes are also very stiff, and ache constantly. After exercising two hours my hands and feet felt quite free from pain. Took 100 drops, at 10 A. M.—Slight headache; constant distress in the umbilicus. The hæmorrhoidal tumours are constantly prolapsed, which is very distressing and painful; dull aching pains in the wrists, hands, and fingers, ankles, feet and toes; they are feeling quite stiff. Took 200 drops. 12 M.—Slight frontal headache; constant aching, burning distress in the epigastric and umbilical regions; dull, heavy aching distress in the right lobe of the liver; constant, dull, aching pain in the whole lumbar region; bending the spine produces sharp, cutting pains all along the lumbar region; dull pains in the hands and feet; three of the hæmorrhoidal tumors are of the color of the mucous membrane of the anus, and are the size of very large red cherries; the other one is not so large, and is of a very dark, livid, blue color. 4 P. M.—Very severe frontal headache; feeling very faint and weak; hands and legs tremble constantly; vertigo with great faintness; have to lie down to keep from fainting; seems to all centre at the stomach; great distress in the stomach, with frequent, sharp, prickly pains in it; sharp, cutting pains every few minutes in the umbilical region; dull, aching distress in my wrists, hands, fingers, ankles, feet and toes. Fearing that I would have spasms, I took three doses of camphor with no relief. I then inhaled chloroform every few minutes until 7 P. M. The chloroform gave great relief, but would last only a short time, when the great faintness would come on again; at 7 P. M., the faintness left me. 9 P. M.—severe frontal headache; constant and very severe burning distress in the whole of the epigastrium; distress in the umbilicus, and desire for stool; very hard, dry, lumpy stool, followed by prolapsus of the anus, with great pain and distress in the hæmorrhoids; feeling very weak in the knees; constant, aching distress in the hands and feet; very weak in the knees, can just walk; constant trembling of the arms and legs; very severe backache.

May 8th.—Slept well until midnight, after that, was very restless until morning; skin dry and hot; pulse 62, while lying down; dull, frontal headache; great distress in the stomach, but not so much of the burning; tongue coated yellowish white; flat, rough taste; stomach is very tender, cannot bear to have it pressed upon; very severe pain in the upper portion of the lumbar region, when bending the spine; soft mushy stool, very yellow, at 8 A. M., followed by a very weak, faint feeling; hands and fingers ache all the time; fingers are very stiff; dull pain in the ankles and feet, 8 P. M.; felt quite well until 2 P. M., when the great burning distress came on again in my stomach; dull headache; very lame back; the hemorrhoids are very troublesome; my hands and feet have been feeling quite easy all day after the first hour; exercise relieves all of the rheumatic symptoms.

May 9th.—Slept well; awoke at 5 A. M., with severe pain in the umbilical and hypogastric regions, and great distress for stool; very profuse thin, yellow stool, that did not relieve the pain in the bowels; feeling very faint at the stomach, and weak; 7 A. M., another very thin deep yellow stool, which relieved the pain a good deal, followed by the great faintness at the stomach; eating would not relieve it; 9 P. M., have been feeling quite well all day, but since 6 P. M., the great burning distress in the stomach has been constant; severe neuralgic pain in the left groin all the evening.

May 10th.—Slept well; this morning have the great burning in my stomach; slight distress in the bowels, with a deep yellow diarrhœic stool; hands and feet are quite stiff; dull back-ache; the hemorrhoidal tumors are free from pain and are getting smaller. The backache lasted one week after taking the remedy.

Characteristic Peculiarities.—The rheumatic symptoms are worse at night and early in the morning; first hour the pains are very much aggravated by motion, after that, motion relieves them;

diarrhœa early in the morning; all the pains are worse while sitting still; relieved by motion.

Mind.—Great depression of spirits; no desire to move; very sad.

Nervous System.—Great weariness and loss of strength; constant trembling of the hands and legs; pain and spasms of the bowels; slowness of the heart's action; vertigo with great faintness at the stomach; disposition to faint; disposition to yawn and stretch.

Head.—Constant, dull, frontal headache, more in the top of the forehead; very severe frontal headache; sharp cutting pains in the right temple.

Mouth and Tongue.—Tongue coated white and yellowish-white; flat pappy taste in the mouth; dryness of the fauces with frequent inclination to swallow; rough feeling of the fauces; tonsils slightly congested.

Stomach.—Frequent empty eructations; constant distress in the stomach, more in the afternoon and evening; severe cutting, tearing pains in the stomach and region of the gall-bladder; at times the pains are of a spasmodic character; constant dull pain in the stomach; great burning distress in the stomach, with sharp prickling pains in it and faintness; great faintness at the stomach; stomach very painful on pressure.

Liver.—The appearance of the alvine evacuations shows that it has a marked effect upon the liver; sharp, cutting pains in the region of the gall-bladder; dull, heavy, aching pains in the right lobe of the liver; the stools are very black, dry and hard; large, deep, yellow, papescent stools, showing an increased secretion of bile, then light-colored stools.

Urinary and Genital Organs.—No special effects observed.

Abdomen.—Constant, dull pain in the epigastric and umbilical regions, with frequent colicky pains of a cutting, tearing character; frequent sharp, cutting pains in the umbilicus, aggravated by walking; awoke three times in the night with severe colicky pains in the umbilicus; constant, dull pains in the umbilicus, with frequent sharp, cutting pains all through the intestines.

Stool and Anus.—Black, dry, hard, lumpy stool, last part of it soft, white and mushy; dry, black stool, followed by prolapsus of the anus; the anus has four hemorrhoidal tumours on it as large as red cherries; three are the color of the mucous membrane of the intestine; the other is of a livid, dark, blue color, the prover never had hæmorrhoidal tumors in his life, excepting one tumor after proving the Veratum v. and strong symptoms of it while proving Aesulus. He considers these hemorrhoidal tumors truly a pathogenetic symptom of the Dioscorea; obstinate constipation followed by bilious diarrhœa; severe pain in the umbilical and hypogastric regions, with great desire for stool; very profuse, deep yellow, thin stool, followed by a very weak, faint feeling. and without relieving the pain in the bowels. This continued two days, in the morning, then was followed by constipation. The hemorrhoidal tumors were prolapsed all the time, with great pain and distress in them.

Chest.—Sharp pulsating pain in the top of the sternum; sharp stitches all through the chest and cervical portion of the back; drawing pain between the shoulders.

Back.—Constant dull pain in the lumbar region; dull aching pain in the lumbar-sacral region very much aggravated by bending the spine; dull pain in the small of the back; bending the spine produces sharp cutting pains in all of the lumbar vertebra; back is quite stiff, especially in the morning.

Arms.—Frequent drawing pains in the elbows, wrists, hands and fingers; severe, cutting pains in the elbows, wrists and fingers; constant dull pains in the wrists, hands and fingers, with frequent sharp pains in the fingers; fingers are very stiff, can hardly close them, they are so painful.

Lower Extremities.—Dull drawing pains in the knees and ankles; very sharp pain in the bottom of the feet and toes; constant dull pains in the ankles, feet and toes, with sharp pain in the toes; the toes are very stiff, especially in the morning.

ÆSCULUS HIPPOCASTANUM.

PROVING BY C. H. LEE, M. D.

(Received too late for insertion with the other Provings of same Medicine.)

Prover healthy; temperament nervous—sanguine.

December 26, 1863. Took one drop of the third attenuation.

December 27. Felt drowsy; tongue coated white.

December 28. Very dull and stupid; disposition to sleep all the time; felt weak; very severe lancinating headache at the base of the brain as if too full; white coating on the tongue; borborygmus and flatus which was fœtid; abdomen swollen and tympanitic; took two drachms.

December 29. Same symptoms as yesterday, with sore throat, which was inflamed; throat felt hot; worse on left side; left tonsil very much swollen and painful on deglutition; stools, of a light brown color and very soft—frequent, but not to extent of a diarrhœa; no appetite; no more of the drug taken.

December 30. Same symptoms as above, but worse; about 4 o'clock, P. M., severe chill which lasted three hours; heat of the fire relieved me; from 7 to 12 at night, very high fever; pulse about 130; no thirst during the chill or fever, but rather an increase of saliva; head aches all over as if it would burst; photophobia; profuse hot perspiration with the fever; dyspnœa with rapid breathing; lungs feel heavy and as if they were engorged;

heart's action very rapid and heavy—would jar me while lying down, and could feel the pulsation all over the body; my stomach felt as if it would fall down into the intestines; urine scanty and of a mahogany color, and as it passed through the urethra it burned like hot water; a sore spot on the right parietal bone, which upon pressure, felt as if a knife was piercing through; took no medicine to-day.

December 31. Fever gone; pulse about ninety; neck very stiff and swollen; both tonsils swollen and of a fiery red color; difficult deglutition; head not aching so much, but is worse on stooping or getting up from a chair; breathing more natural; spitting of blood on getting up in the morning; no cough; stools hard and dark brown; urine not so high colored, with a brown sediment; took none of the drug.

January 1, 1864. I have severe shooting pains in the left temple; eyes of a pinkish hue; dull pain in the region of the spleen; stools hard; no other symptoms.

January 2. Stools soft; urine yellow, with a thick, white mucus sediment; took four drops of the tincture.

January 3 and 4. Appearance of hæmorrhoids like ground nuts, of a purple color; very painful, and with sensation of burning—(the prover never had hæmorroids before).

January 6. Felt a dryness in the soft palate; a fulness in the head; stools natural; urine dark, some little sediment; took eight drops.

January 8. Throat dry as if it was scraped, and swollen; borborygmus; flatus fœtid; took one drachm.

January 10. Dryness of the back part of throat; severe headache as if the head would split; desire to pass water often, but little at a time.

January 11. Symptoms same as above; a dry, burning sensation of the fauces and palate; a quantity of thick, yellow phlegm in the mouth; tongue coated yellow; bowels loose; stools brown; urine scanty, and dark brown, no sediment; pulse hard and frequent; dull, aching pain in elbow joint of left arm; took no more of the drug.

January 12. Symptoms begin to diminish.

January 14. No symptoms.

CLINICAL INDEX.

www.ingramcontent.com/pod-product-compliance
Lightning Source LLC
LaVergne TN
LVHW021131110826
845150LV00005B/993

* 9 7 8 1 4 2 5 5 5 0 1 4 1 *